Pearson Nursing Reviews & Rationales

Pharmacology

Fourth Edition

SERIES EDITOR

MaryAnn Hogan, PhD(c), MSN, RN, CNE

Clinical Assistant Professor

College of Nursing

University of Massachusetts–Amherst

Amherst, Massachusetts

CONSULTING EDITORS

Sharon Burke, EdD, RN, CCRN, CEN

Assistant Professor

Thomas Jefferson University

Philadelphia, Pennsylvania

Margaret M. Gingrich, MSN, RN

Professor

Harrisburg Area Community College

Harrisburg, Pennsylvania

Nancy C. Dentlinger, EdD, MS, RN

Associate Professor

University of Central Oklahoma

Edmond, Oklahoma

Pearson

Vice President, Health Science and TED: Julie Levin Alexander
Portfolio Manager: Hilarie Surrena
Development Editor: Rachel Bedard
Portfolio Management Assistant: Taylor Scuglik
Vice President, Content Production and Digital Studio: Paul DeLuca
Managing Producer Health Science: Melissa Bashe
Content Producer: Michael Giacobbe
Vice President, Product Marketing: David Gesell

Executive Field Marketing Manager: Christopher Barry
Field Marketing Manager: Brittany Hammond
Managing Producer, Digital Studio, Health Science: Amy Peltier
Digital Producer: Jeff Henn
Full-Service Vendor: SPi Global
Full-Service Project Management: Michelle Gardner, SPi Global
Cover Image: Hybrid Images/Cultura/Getty Images

Library of Congress Cataloging-in-Publication Data

Names: Hogan, Mary Ann (Nurse), author, editor. | Burke, Sharon Ogden, editor. | Gingrich, Margaret M., editor. | Dentlinger, Nancy C., editor.
Title: Pharmacology / series editor, MaryAnn Hogan; consulting editors, Sharon Burke, Margaret M. Gingrich, Nancy C. Dentlinger.
Other titles: Pearson nursing reviews & rationales series.
Description: Fourth edition. | Boston : Pearson Education, Inc., [2018] | Series: Pearson nursing reviews & rationales | Preceded by Pharmacology / MaryAnn Hogan; consulting editors, Sharon Burke, Margaret M. Gingrich, Traci Taylor. 3rd ed. c2013. | Includes bibliographical references and index.
Identifiers: LCCN 2017053258 | ISBN 9780134517155 | ISBN 0134517156
Subjects: | MESH: Pharmaceutical Preparations | Test Taking Skills | Examination Questions | Nurses' Instruction | Outlines
Classification: LCC RM301.13 | NLM QV 18.2 | DDC 615.1/9—dc23
LC record available at https://lccn.loc.gov/2017053258

1 17

ISBN 10:   0-13-451715-6
ISBN 13: 978-0-13-451715-5

Contents

Welcome to the Pearson Nursing Reviews & Rationales Series!

This series has been specifically designed to provide a clear and concentrated review of important nursing knowledge and concepts in the following content areas:

- Nursing Fundamentals
- Fluids, Electrolytes, & Acid–Base Balance
- Medical-Surgical Nursing
- Pathophysiology
- Pharmacology
- Maternal–Newborn Nursing
- Child Health Nursing
- Mental Health Nursing

The books in this series are designed for use either by current nursing students as a study aid for nursing coursework and NCLEX-RN® exam preparation, or by practicing nurses seeking a comprehensive yet concise review of a nursing specialty or subject area.

This series is truly unique. One key feature is that it has been developed and reviewed by a large team of nurse educators from the United States and Canada to ensure that each chapter is edited by a nurse expert in the content area under study. The series editor, MaryAnn Hogan, designed the overall series in collaboration with a core Pearson Education team to take full advantage of Pearson Education's cutting-edge technology. The consulting editors for each book, also experts in that specialty area, then reviewed all chapters and test questions submitted for comprehensiveness and accuracy. Finally, MaryAnn Hogan reviewed the chapters in each book and their corresponding questions for consistency, accuracy, and applicability to the latest NCLEX-RN® Test Plan.

All books in the series are identical in their overall design for your convenience. As an added value, each book comes with a comprehensive support package, including access to additional questions online and an appendix of valuable information for clinical reference and quick review.

What's New in this Edition

- Completely updated review material reflecting the 2016 NCLEX-RN® Test Plan.
- Online access to Nursing Reviews and Rationales. com where students can complete quizzes on a computer or other device to practice for the NCLEX® experience.
- Hundreds of updated or brand-new NCLEX®-style practice test questions.
- Dozens of new alternate-item format questions.
- The latest test prep advice from MaryAnn Hogan, trusted expert in what nursing students need to know.

Study Tips

Use of this book should help simplify your review. To make the most of your valuable study time, also follow these simple but important suggestions:

1. Use a weekly calendar to schedule study sessions.
   - Outline the timeframes for all of your activities (home, school, appointments, etc.) on a weekly calendar.
   - Find the "holes" in your calendar, which are the times in which you can plan to study. Add study sessions to the calendar at times when you can expect to be mentally alert and follow your plan!
2. Create the optimal study environment.
   - Eliminate external sources of distraction, such as online social media, smartphones, television, etc.
   - Eliminate internal sources of distraction, such as hunger, thirst, or dwelling on problems that you cannot work on at this time.
   - Take a break for 10 minutes or so after each hour of concentrated study both as a reward and as a physical and mental break to reenergize you.
3. Use prereading strategies to increase comprehension of chapter material.
   - Skim read the chapter headings (because they identify chapter content).

- Read the definitions of key terms to learn new words that will help you comprehend chapter information.
- Review all graphic aids (figures, tables, boxes) because they are often used to explain important points in the chapter.

4. Read the chapter thoroughly but at a reasonable speed.
   - Comprehension and retention are actually enhanced by not reading too slowly.
   - Do take the time to reread any section that is unclear to you.

5. Summarize what you have learned.
   - Use the accompanying online resource, NursingReviewsandRationales.com, to test yourself with hundreds of NCLEX-RN®-style practice questions.
   - Review again any sections that correspond to questions you answered incorrectly or incompletely.

Test-Taking Strategies

Test-taking strategies accompany the rationales for every question in the series. These strategies will assist you to select the correct answer by breaking down the question, even if you don't know the correct response. Use the following strategies to increase your success on nursing tests or examinations:

- Get sufficient sleep and have something to eat before taking a test. Eat carbohydrates that have a low glycemic index and a low-fat protein source to help maintain energy and focus. Avoid eating concentrated sweets (which have a high glycemic index) to prevent a rapid upward and then downward surge in your blood glucose. Also avoid high-fat foods that will make you sleepy.
- Take deep breaths periodically during the test. Remember, the brain requires oxygen to function well, not just calories.
- Read each question carefully, identifying the stem, the four options, and any key words or phrases in either the stem or options.
- Key words in the stem such as *most important* indicate the need to set priorities, since more than one option is likely to contain a statement that is technically correct.
- Remember that the presence of absolute words such as *never* or *only* in an answer option is more likely to make that option incorrect.

- Determine who is the client in the question. Often this is the person with the health problem, but it may also be a significant other, relative, friend, or another nurse.
- Decide whether the stem is a true response stem or a false response stem. With a true response stem, the correct answer will be a true statement, and vice versa.
- Determine what the question is really asking, sometimes known as the core issue of the question. Evaluate all answer options in relation to this issue, and not strictly to the "correctness" of the statement in each individual option.
- Use these strategies to answer questions in which only one option can be selected, such as standard multiple-choice, exhibit, or graphic options questions:
  - Eliminate options that are obviously incorrect, then go back and reread the stem and any associated information. Evaluate those remaining options against the stem once more to make a final selection.
  - If two answers seem similar and correct, try to decide whether one is more global or comprehensive. If the global option includes the alternative option within it, it is likely that the more global response is correct.
- When answering multiple response questions, which commonly contain the instruction "select all that apply," read each option and evaluate it as a true–false statement. If the wording of the question indicates the answers would be true/correct statements, select all of those that would represent appropriate nursing practice. If the question is worded negatively (with words such as *contraindicated*, *unsafe*, etc.), select those that would not represent appropriate nursing practice. Remember that nurses need to practice safely but also must be able to identify threats to safe client care.

The NCLEX-RN® Licensing Examination

Upon graduation from a nursing program, you will need to pass the NCLEX-RN® licensing examination to begin professional nursing practice. The NCLEX-RN® licensing examination is a Computer Adaptive Test (CAT) that ranges in length from 75 to 265 individual (stand-alone) test items, depending on your performance during the examination. The blueprint for the exam is reviewed and revised every 3 years by the National Council of State Boards of Nursing using the results of a job analysis study of new graduate nurses practicing within the first 6 months after graduation. Each question on the exam is coded to a *Client Need* and an *Integrated Process* category.

Client Needs Categories

There are eight *Client Needs* categories being tested on the licensing examination. Each exam will contain a minimum and maximum percent of questions from each of these categories. The percentages of questions from the *Client Needs* categories for the NCLEX-RN® Test Plan effective April 2016 are:

- Safe, Effective Care Environment
  - Management of Care (17–23%)
  - Safety and Infection Control (9–15%)
- Health Promotion and Maintenance (6–12%)
- Psychosocial Integrity (6–12%)
- Physiological Integrity
  - Basic Care and Comfort (6–12%)
  - Pharmacological and Parenteral Therapies (12–18%)
  - Reduction of Risk Potential (9–15%)
  - Physiological Adaptation (11–17%)

Integrated Processes

The integrated processes identified on the NCLEX-RN® Test Plan effective April 2016, with condensed definitions, are:

- Nursing Process: a scientific and clinical reasoning approach to nursing practice that consists of assessment, analysis, planning, implementation, and evaluation.
- Caring: client–nurse interaction(s) characterized by mutual respect and trust and that are collaboratively directed toward achieving desired client outcomes.
- Communication and Documentation: verbal and/or nonverbal interactions between nurse and others (client, family, health care team); a written or electronic recording of activities or events during client care to demonstrate accountability and adherence to standards of care.
- Teaching/Learning: facilitating client's acquisition of knowledge, skills, and attitudes that lead to behavior change.
- Culture and Spirituality: interaction of nurse and client (individual, family, or identified group) that recognizes and considers the client-identified preferences for care as well as applicable standards and legal instructions.

More detailed information about this examination may be obtained by visiting the National Council of State Boards of Nursing website at www.ncsbn.org and viewing the *2016 NCLEX-RN® Detailed Test Plan*.[1]

---

[1] Reference: National Council of State Boards of Nursing, Inc. *2016 NCLEX-RN® Test Plan*. Effective April 1, 2016. Retrieved from https://www.ncsbn.org/testplans.htm.

HOW TO GET THE MOST OUT OF THIS BOOK

Each chapter has the following elements to guide you during review and study:

Chapter Objectives describe what you will be able to know or do after learning the material covered in the chapter.

Objectives

- ➤ Describe general goals of therapy when administering gastrointestinal system medications.
- ➤ Describe the use and side effects of antacids.
- ➤ Identify the actions of various forms of laxatives.
- ➤ Discuss the effects of H_2-receptor antagonists, proton pump inhibitors, and mucosal protectants on the gastrointestinal tract.
- ➤ Describe client-centered nursing care related to administration of antiemetics.

NCLEX-RN® Test Prep

Access the NEW Web-based app that provides students with additional practice questions in preparation for the NCLEX experience.

Review at a Glance contains a glossary of key terms used in the chapter, with definitions provided up-front and available at your fingertips, to help you stay focused and make the best use of your study time.

Review at a Glance

antacid agent that reduces or neutralizes acidity

anticholinergic antagonist to parasympathetic action or other cholinergic receptors

antispasmodic agent that prevents or relieves spasms

cathartic agent with purgative action

H₂ antagonist antagonist agent against histamine that decreases gastrin secretion

Helicobacter pylori bacteria found in gastric mucosa that produces urease

and is associated commonly with gastric and duodenal ulcers

laxative agent used to cause a bowel movement or loosening of the bowels

surfactant a surface-active agent also known as a wetting agent, tension depressant, detergent, and emulsifier

Pretest provides a 10-question quiz as a sample overview of the material covered in the chapter and helps you decide in what areas you need the most—or the least—review.

PRETEST

1 A constipated client is given a prescription to use psyllium mucilloid. What information should the nurse provide during client education about the medication?

1. Refrain from physical activity for 2 hours.
2. Follow the initial dose with an additional 240 mL (8 oz) of water.
3. Take an antiemetic.
4. Sprinkle the powder formulation on food.

Practice to Pass questions are open ended, stimulate critical thinking, and reinforce mastery of the chapter information.

Practice to Pass

A proton pump inhibitor has been prescribed for a client who recently had a stroke (cerebrovascular accident or CVA). What nursing assessment should be performed?

NCLEX Alert identifies concepts that are likely to be tested on the NCLEX-RN® examination. Be sure to learn the information highlighted wherever you see this icon.

Case Study, found at the end of the chapter, provides an opportunity for you to use your critical thinking and clinical reasoning skills to "put it all together." It describes a true-to-life client case situation and asks you open-ended questions about how you would provide care for that client and/or family.

Case Study

A 45-year-old male client comes to the nurse practitioner stating he wakes often at night with coughing and burning he describes as heartburn. He drinks one or two alcoholic beverages per evening, usually with distilled liquor, and then wine with dinner. He eats heavy dinners with dessert. He prefers mint ice cream and coffee for dessert. The nurse practitioner prescribes a regimen with omeprazole (Prilosec) every morning and Maalox 30 mL qid.

1. How should you instruct the client about gastroesophageal reflux disease and its relationship to symptoms?

2. What information will you provide to the client about his diet, particularly the evening meal?

3. What type of medications are likely to be prescribed if the client is diagnosed with *H. pylori*?

4. What information and instructions should you provide to the client about his medications?

Posttest provides an additional 10-question quiz at the end of the chapter. It provides you with feedback about mastery of the chapter material after review and study. All pretest and posttest questions contain comprehensive rationales for the correct and incorrect answers, are coded according to cognitive level of difficulty, and the NCLEX-RN® Test Plan category of Client Need and Integrated Process. Each question also contains one or more suggested strategies for selecting answer(s).

POSTTEST

2 The nurse should consult with the prescriber if oral mineral oil is prescribed for which of the following clients? Select all that apply.

1. Client with dysphagia following a cerebral vascular accident (CVA)
2. Client who has suspected appendicitis
3. Client who has a fecal impaction
4. Client who has infrequent heartburn
5. Client who has steatorrhea

NCLEX-RN® Test Prep: NursingReviewsandRationales.com

For those who want to prepare for the NCLEX-RN®, practicing online will help you become more familiar with the computer-based testing experience, especially for alternate item format questions. With this new edition, use the code printed inside the front cover of the book to access Nursing Reviews & Rationales, which offers hundreds of practice questions using a variety of NCLEX®-style formats. This includes the practice questions found in all chapters of the book as well as 30 additional questions per chapter. Nursing Reviews & Rationales allows you to choose the two ways to prepare for the NCLEX-RN®. Both approaches personalize your practice experience according to where you are in your NCLEX® preparation.

Pearson Nursing Notes Appendix

This appendix provides a reference for frequently used facts and information. These are designed to provide quick and easy access to information that is useful in the clinical setting and that is important for the NCLEX® licensing examination.

About Pharmacology

Chapters in this book cover "need-to-know" information about medications that belong to a wide variety of drug classes and associated nursing management. The first chapter reviews general principles of pharmacology with an emphasis on safety. Chapter 2 explores the use of herbal agents as supplements and phytomedicines. Chapters 3 through 16 explore drug classes used to treat health problems that affect specific body systems. Each chapter provides information about specific drug classes and reviews their action and use, administration considerations, contraindications, significant drug or food interactions, significant laboratory studies, side and adverse effects and toxicity, client-centered nursing care, and client education.

Pharmacology is an ever-evolving field because drug therapy changes over time as new research evidence becomes available. Care has been taken to ensure that drug information in this book is accurate and current; however, this is a condensed review book, not a full pharmacology textbook or official drug reference. Before administering any medication, check the manufacturer's product literature to verify recommended dose, route, duration of therapy, and any contraindications. Neither the publisher nor the author assumes liability for any injury or damage arising from information contained in this condensed review book.

Acknowledgments

This book is a monumental effort of collaboration. Without the contributions of many individuals, this edition of *Pharmacology: Reviews and Rationales* would not have been possible. Thank you to all the contributors and reviewers who devoted their time and talents to the fourth edition. The contributors for this edition are Sharon Burke, EdD, RN, CCRN, CEN, Thomas Jefferson University, Philadelphia, PA; Nancy C. Dentlinger, EdD, MS, RN, University of Central Oklahoma, Edmond, OK; and Margaret M. Gingrich, MSN, RN, Harrisburg Area Community College, Harrisburg, PA. The reviewers for this edition are Sophia Beydoun, AA, ADN, BSN, MSN, Henry Ford Community College, Dearborn, MI; Sharon Burke, EdD, MSN, BA, CEN, Penn State University Ogontz Abington, Abington, PA; Lynette DeBellis, RN, MA, Westchester Community College, Valhalla, NY; Rachel Choudhury, MSN, RN, CNE, Brandman University, Irvine, CA; Nancy Ebersole, PhD, RN, Salem State University, Salem, MA; Brandon Johnson, MSN, RN, CHSE, Texas Tech University, Lubbock, TX; Sara Kaylor, EdD, RN, CNE, University of Alabama Tuscaloosa, Tuscaloosa, AL; Alice Kindschuh, DNP, APRN-CNS, GCNS-BC, CNE, Nebraska Methodist College, Omaha, NE; Cristina Perez, PhD, RN, Ramapo College of New Jersey, Mahwah, NJ; Katherine Poser, RN, BScN, MNEd, PhD, St. Lawrence College, Ontario, Canada; Diana Rangaves, PharmD, Santa Rosa Junior College, Santa Rosa, CA; Stacy Veach, MSN, Ed, Brandman University, Irvine, CA; Benson Yeung, RN, California State University Los Angeles, Los Angeles, CA.

Thanks also to the contributors and reviewers who assisted with the previous editions of this book: Julie A. Adkins, RN, MSN, FNP, Private Practice, West Frankfort, IL; Carolyn M. Burger, MSN, RN, C, OCN, Miami University, Middletown, OH; Janet Courtney, RN, MSN, Holyoke Community College, Holyoke, MA; Geralyn M. Frandsen, EdD, MSN, RN, Maryville University, St. Louis, MO; Joseann Helmes DeWitt, MSN, RN, C, CLNC, Alcorn State University, Natchez, MS; Suzanne Kay Marnocha, PhD, RN, MSN, CCRN, University of Wisconsin, Oshkosh, WI; Caron Martin, MSN, RN, Northern Kentucky University, Highland Heights, KY; Lee Murray, MSN, RN, CS, CADAC, Holyoke Community College, Holyoke, MA; Lynn Wemett Nicholls, PhD, RN, St. John Fisher College, Rochester, NY; Donna Polverini, RN, MS, America International College, Springfield, MA; Roni Ruhlandt, MSN, RN, CCRN, CNRN, University of Phoenix, Grand Rapids, MI; Susan K. Steele, MN, RN, AOCN, Southeastern Louisiana University College of Nursing, Hammond, LA; Bethany Hawes Sykes, EdD, RN, CEN, Salve Regina University, Newport, RI; Traci Taylor, RN, MSN, Nursing Instructor, West Texas A&M University, Canyon, TX; Daryle Wane, MS, APRN, BC, Pasco-Hernando Community College, New Port Richey, FL; Nathaniel M. Apatoy, MHS, MSN, PhD, CRNA, University of Miami, Coral Gables, FL; Ilene Borze, MS, RN, Gateway Community College, Phoenix, AZ; Pattie Garrett Clark, RN, MSN, Abraham Baldwin College, Tifton, GA; Skip Davis, PhD, MSN, BSN, San Francisco State University, San Francisco, CA; Janice Hausauer, MSN, BSN, ANCC-FNP, Montana State University, Bozeman, MT; Mercy Popoola, RN, CND, PhD, Georgia Southern University, Statesboro, GA; Anita K. Reed, BSN, MSN, St. Joseph College, Rensselaer, IN. Their work will surely assist both students and licensed nurses to extend and/or freshen their knowledge of pharmacology.

I owe a special debt of gratitude to the wonderful team at Pearson for their expertise and encouragement during development of this fourth edition. Hilarie Surrena, Nursing Portfolio Manager, oversaw this revision and fostered a culture of collaboration and teamwork. Rachel Bedard, Developmental Editor, shared her immense expertise with warmth and enthusiasm while coordinating different facets of this project. Her high standards and attention to detail contributed greatly to the final "look" of this book. Portfolio Management Assistant, Taylor Scuglik, helped to keep the project moving forward on a day-to-day basis, and I am grateful for her efforts as well. A very special thank you goes to the designers of the book and the production team, led by Michael Giacobbe, Managing Editor, who brought the ideas and manuscript into final form.

Thank you to the publishing team at SPi Global, led by Michelle Gardner and Karen Berry, Project Managers, for the detail-oriented work of creating this book. I greatly appreciate their diligence, attention to detail, and spirit of collaboration.

Finally, I would like to acknowledge and gratefully thank my children—Michael Jr., Kathryn, Kristen, and William—whose love and unending support enrich my life beyond words. I would also like to thank my nursing students, past and present, for continuing to inspire me daily with their quest for knowledge and passion for nursing. You are indeed the future of nursing!

–MaryAnn Hogan

Basic Principles and Safety in Pharmacology

1

Chapter Outline

Pharmacology and the Nursing Process

Legal Regulation

Prescription and Nonprescription Medications

Medication Classification Systems

Terminology Related to Pharmacology

Issues Related to Medication Administration

Objectives

➤ Describe legal regulatory issues related to medication administration.

➤ Identify the difference between generic and trade names.

➤ Identify differences between prescription and over-the-counter medications.

➤ Define terms commonly used in pharmacology.

➤ Describe differences between a side effect and an adverse or toxic effect of a medication.

➤ Describe factors that affect medication absorption and response.

➤ List the rights of safe medication administration.

➤ Calculate medication dosages accurately.

➤ Explain nurses' roles and responsibilities related to client education regarding medication therapy.

➤ Describe cultural considerations related to medication therapy and associated client education.

NCLEX-RN® Test Prep

Access the NEW Web-based app that provides students with additional practice questions in preparation for the NCLEX experience.

Review at a Glance

absorption what happens to a drug from time of introduction into body until it reaches circulating fluids and tissues

biotransformation enzymatic alteration of drug structure; most biotransformation takes place in liver; also called *drug metabolism*

critical concentration amount of a drug needed to cause a therapeutic effect

distribution movement of a drug to body tissues following absorption

drug chemical that is introduced into body to cause some sort of change; used interchangeably with the term *medication*

drug abuse use of a drug in a fashion inconsistent with medical or social norms

excretion removal of a drug from body, such as via skin, saliva, lungs, bile, kidneys, or feces

first-pass effect a phenomenon that occurs following ingestion of an oral drug in which a large percentage of drug is destroyed in gastrointestinal system and never reaches tissues

half-life time it takes for an amount of drug in the body to decrease to one-half of a peak level previously achieved

negligence failure to provide care that a reasonable person would provide in a similar circumstance

pharmacodynamics process of how a drug affects body

pharmacogenetics area of pharmacology that examines how heredity affects one's response to drug therapy

pharmacokinetics process of how body acts on a drug

pharmacology study of drugs and their interactions with living systems

pharmacotherapeutics branch of pharmacology that involves use of drugs to treat, prevent, or diagnose disease; also known as clinical pharmacology

selective toxicity ability of a drug, such as penicillin, to attack only those systems found in foreign cells

PRETEST

1 When administering medication to a hospitalized client, what would be the most consistently accurate way for the nurse to check a client's identity?

1. Ask the client to state name and date of birth.
2. Scan the client's identification bracelet and compare it with the medication record.
3. Check the client's room number and bed assignment.
4. Match the medication with the client's diagnosis.

2 The mother of a pediatric client asks the nurse, "What is the difference between Advil and ibuprofen? I can buy ibuprofen at a cheaper price, but the instructions from the clinic say to use Children's Advil Liquid." What would be the nurse's best response?

1. "Similarities do exist, but the liquid medication is a different formulation designed for children."
2. "There is no difference between Advil and ibuprofen."
3. "Advil and ibuprofen are two different drugs with similar effects."
4. "You need to talk to the healthcare provider who prescribed the drug."

3 A pregnant client tells the clinic nurse at the first prenatal visit that she heard it is good to take an over-the-counter (OTC) iron preparation during pregnancy. Which statement by the nurse would be the best response?

1. "You should not take any OTC products during pregnancy."
2. "Most prenatal vitamins contain iron, so there is no need to take additional iron supplements."
3. "It is safe to take iron during pregnancy, but tell your healthcare provider you are using it; many prenatal vitamins also contain iron."
4. "There may be staining of your baby's first teeth if you take this medication during pregnancy, so you should avoid taking any iron supplements."

4 A client taking an antihypertensive medication by mouth four times per day is experiencing symptoms of toxicity. Which intervention by the nurse should take highest priority?

1. Assess for elevation of body temperature.
2. Evaluate rate, depth, and regularity of respirations.
3. Assess for weight loss by obtaining a daily weight.
4. Evaluate client's intake of foods and other medications.

5 The nurse is caring for a 78-year-old client who has multiple medications prescribed to treat various health problems. The nurse should consider that which common age-related physical changes are most likely to require a reduction in medication dosage for this client? Select all that apply.

1. Increased rate of drug retention
2. Decreased total body fluid proportionate to body mass
3. Decreased efficiency in drug distribution
4. Decreased rate of drug metabolism by the liver
5. Significant weight gain

6 A 3-year-old client weighing 15 kg (33 lb) is to receive liquid ibuprofen 150 mg PO q6h prn for a temperature above 38°C (101°F). The nurse should administer how many mL to the client from a bottle labeled 100 mg/5 mL? Provide a numeric answer.

_____ mL

7 A client receiving nadolol for hypertension tells the nurse, "I get dizzy when I stand up." What is the most appropriate response by the nurse?

1. "This is an expected side effect of the drug, and you should use caution and move slowly when standing up."
2. "You may be experiencing a toxic effect of the drug, and I will notify the healthcare provider."
3. "Dizziness is not related to the drug, but I will need to ask you a few more questions."
4. "Episodes of dizziness when moving are common symptoms of elevated blood pressure."

8 An older adult client is given a prescription for an analgesic/anti-inflammatory medication to treat pain and stiffness from osteoarthritis of the hips and back. The nurse should take which action first?

1. Complete a thorough medication assessment to see what other drugs the client is taking.
2. Provide client with a printed pamphlet describing the drug and its uses.
3. Inform client where a medication organizer can be purchased.
4. Give a short, simple, verbal explanation about drug and its side effects.

9 The medication administration record shows that a client is to receive lisinopril 10 mg PO at 9:00 a.m. The pharmacy has sent tablets labeled fosinopril 20 mg. What action should the nurse take next?

1. Give one 20-mg tablet sent by the pharmacy.
2. Give one-half tablet of medication from the drug supply.
3. Ask the client if the 20-mg tablet looks familiar.
4. Read the original provider prescription to verify the drug and dose.

10 The nurse plans to administer an oral medication to a client. To safely administer the medications, in which order should the nurse complete the following interventions?

1. Review client's medication history and drug allergies.
2. Record drug administration in medication administration record.
3. Identify the client and explain the intended action of the medications.
4. Administer medication after verifying proper drug, route, time, and dose.
5. Obtain medication and compare the drug label against the healthcare provider's prescription.

➤ *See pages 19–21 for Answers and Rationales.*

I. PHARMACOLOGY AND THE NURSING PROCESS

A. Assessment of client

1. Client's current condition, health history, and presence of factors that are relative or absolute contraindications for some drugs (i.e., pregnancy, lactation, liver or renal disease)
2. Determine client's history of allergies and types of reaction
3. Drug history, including prescription and over-the-counter (OTC) medications, herbal therapies, home remedies, and recreational drugs
4. Lifestyle factors that could affect medications, including caffeine intake and nicotine use, alcohol consumption, and dietary patterns (number of meals per day and food restrictions)
5. Client's ability to swallow oral medications
6. Client's understanding of purpose of medication(s), how to self-administer, adverse effects to report, and routine follow-up care, including how to slow or reduce effects of illness
7. Presence of access devices (i.e., IV PICC or central lines, gastric or jejunostomy tubes)

    B. Assessment of drug
1. Medication prescription
2. Need for conversion when preparing drug dose
3. Review medication prescription for completeness and accuracy
4. Determine client history of allergies and type/level of reaction to drug
5. Review client's condition for which medication is prescribed

    C. Analysis/priority nursing concerns
1. Potential injury
   a. Can occur if client takes a medication to which he or she is hypersensitive (allergic)
   b. Can occur if medication is taken incorrectly
      1) An insufficient dose will lead to development of signs and symptoms of original disorder
      2) An excessive dose can lead to signs and symptoms of toxicity or other adverse effects
2. Insufficient knowledge
   a. Often pertinent when a client is given a prescription for a new medication
   b. Should also be assessed with each client encounter to ensure ongoing knowledge
   c. Insufficient knowledge of medication therapy may lead to suboptimal results of therapy or other complications

    D. Planning/goal setting
1. Client will remain free of injury
2. Client will verbalize purpose of medication, how to take it, expected effects, side effects and adverse effects, and proper storage of medication
3. Client will respond appropriately to medication

    E. Client-centered nursing care
1. Measure client's vital signs if indicated
2. Determine need for conversion when calculating correct dose of medication
3. Prepare and administer medication dose correctly
4. Determine client's understanding of the prescribed medication
5. Teach client about medication, including name, dose, route, frequency, purpose, any follow-up labwork, side/adverse effects including when to notify prescriber, and how to store medication properly
6. Document medication administration
7. Assess and document client's response to medication

    F. Evaluation
1. Client receives correct medication and dosage
2. Client's vital signs remain within normal limits
3. Client responds appropriately to medication
4. Client does not experience adverse effects of medication

II. LEGAL REGULATION

    A. Food and Drug Administration (FDA)
1. An agency of the United States Department of Health and Human Services (USDHHS) that regulates development and sale of **drugs** (chemicals that exert an effect on body) to ensure safety and efficacy
2. Drug legislation in Canada includes the Canadian Food and Drugs Act and the Canadian Controlled Drugs and Substances Act
3. Controls the process of scientific testing to evaluate therapeutic and toxic effects of a chemical that may potentially become a drug/medication

Box 1-1	*Investigational Drug Studies:* New drugs must be tested *in vitro* in animal studies prior to testing in humans; allows for determination of presumed effects on living tissue and also adverse effects.
Phases of Drug Development	*Phase 1 Clinical Trials:* A tightly controlled study is conducted that involves the use of healthy human volunteers to test the drug.
	Phase 2 Clinical Trials: The drug is administered to clients who have the disease that the drug was intended to treat.
	Phase 3 Clinical Trials: The drug is used in the clinical setting to determine any unanticipated effects or lack of effectiveness.
	Food and Drug Administration (FDA) Approval: Drugs that complete Phase 3 are evaluated by the FDA after submission of a New Drug Application (NDA), and if FDA approval is received, the drug may be marketed.
	Phase 4 Post-Marketing Surveillance: A phase that involves continual evaluation of the drug following approval for marketing.

4. Phases of drug development
   a. A drug must pass through several stages of development before receiving final FDA approval to be marketed to public
   b. Stages of development include preclinical research, Phase 1 clinical trials, Phase 2 clinical trials, Phase 3 clinical trials, FDA approval, and post-marketing surveillance (Phase 4) (Box 1-1)
5. Generic formulations of currently marketed drugs may be approved using an expedited process known as an Abbreviated New Drug Application
6. In 2002, the USDHHS reauthorized the Prescription Drug User Fee Act of 1992 and provided resources to review drug applications in an expedited fashion

B. **Controlled substances**
1. Substances that are considered to have potential for **drug abuse**, use of the substance in a manner inconsistent with medical or social norms
2. The Comprehensive Drug Abuse Prevention and Control Act (also known as the Controlled Substance Act) of 1970 regulates the manufacturing, distribution, and dispensing of drugs that are known to have abuse potential
3. The FDA studies a drug and determines its abuse potential
4. The Drug Enforcement Agency (DEA), a part of the Department of Justice, enforces the control of a drug
5. The DEA monitors the prescription, distribution, storage, and use of a controlled substance in an attempt to decrease substance abuse of prescribed medications
6. Controlled substances are assigned to one of five DEA schedules based on their potential for abuse and physical and psychologic dependence (Table 1-1)

Table 1-1 Drug Enforcement Agency Schedules of Controlled Substances

Schedule Number	Description	Examples
Schedule I	High abuse potential and no accepted medical use	Heroine, cocaine
Schedule II	High abuse potential with severe dependence liability	Opioids, amphetamines, barbiturates
Schedule III	Less abuse potential than Schedule II drugs and moderate dependence liability	Nonbarbiturate sedatives, nonamphetamine stimulants, limited amounts of certain opioids
Schedule IV	Less abuse potential than Schedule III drugs and limited dependence liability	Some sedatives, nonopioid analgesics, anti-anxiety agents
Schedule V	Limited abuse potential	Drugs that may contain small amounts of opioids such as codeine, used as antitussives or antidiarrheals

C. Pregnancy categories (Box 1-2)
1. Guidelines for use of a particular drug during pregnancy
2. Indicate a drug's potential or actual teratogenic or adverse effects on fetus
3. FDA requires that each new drug be assigned a pregnancy category
4. FDA recommends that no drug be administered during pregnancy regardless of pregnancy category, unless drug's benefit clearly outweighs risks of use

D. Investigational medications and informed consent
1. *Informed consent*: an autonomous decision made by a specific individual based on nature of health problem, treatment options, and risks involved
2. Client must be competent to give consent for procedures and treatment
3. Informed consent should be in writing; it should include explanation of procedure, medication, or treatment; description of benefits and harmful results; and an opportunity for client to ask questions
4. Information should be written in language understandable to client
5. Consent must be obtained by healthcare provider prescribing the medication, treatment, or procedure
6. A nurse administering a medication explains drug's purpose and answers client's questions
7. Client has a right to decline information and waive informed consent and undergo treatment; this decision must be documented in medical record
8. Informed consent can be waived during urgent medical or surgical intervention, such as severe bleeding, fractured skull, or gunshot or stab wounds
9. When client is a minor, unconscious, or incompetent, consent must be obtained from a responsible family member or legal guardian
10. When a nurse is involved in informed consent process, in most states the nurse is only responsible for witnessing client's signature on informed consent form
11. Most common concern regarding use of investigational drugs is that all adverse effects have not been identified; because client is not able to be fully informed about these, the decision-making process is not ideal
12. A placebo-controlled study implements use of placebos on certain clients; neither research staff nor clients know whether they are receiving a placebo or an actual drug

Practice to Pass

A pregnant client experiences occasional headaches and backaches. She asks you what over-the-counter (OTC) medication she can take to relieve these discomforts. How should you respond?

Box 1-2

Pregnancy Categories

Category A: Controlled human studies in pregnant women fail to demonstrate a risk to the fetus in the first trimester of pregnancy, and there is no evidence of risk in later trimesters.

Category B: Animal studies have not demonstrated a risk to the fetus but there are no adequate studies in pregnant women. Or, animal studies have shown an adverse effect, but adequate studies in pregnant women have not demonstrated a risk to the fetus during the first trimester of pregnancy, and there is no evidence of risk in later trimesters.

Category C: Animal studies have shown an adverse effect on the fetus but there are no adequate studies in humans; the benefit from the use of the drug in pregnancy may be acceptable despite its potential risks. Or, there are no animal reproduction studies and no adequate studies in humans.

Category D: There is evidence of human fetal risk, but the potential benefits from the use of the drug in pregnant women may be acceptable despite its potential risks.

Category X: Studies in animals or humans demonstrate fetal abnormalities or adverse reactions and reports indicate evidence of fetal risk. The risk of use in a pregnant woman clearly outweighs any possible benefits.

E. **Regulation of nursing practice related to medication therapy**
1. Nurse Practice Act
   a. A series of statutes enacted by each state legislature to regulate practice of nurses in that state
   b. The Nurse Practice Act describes role of nurse in relation to medication administration
   c. Advanced practice nurses may have prescriptive privileges; check statute for individual state or jurisdiction to determine laws governing prescriptive authority in that jurisdiction
2. Standards of care
   a. Some standards of care are global guidelines by which nurse should practice, without a specific focus on medication therapy
   b. Other standards of care may be based on research of specific health problems and include recommendations for care including medication therapy
   c. An example is the "stepped-care" approach to treating hypertension; medication therapy is recommended in specific sequences based on client response
3. *Professional misconduct*: a violation of Nurse Practice Act that can result in disciplinary action against a nurse; examples of professional misconduct are failing to wear an identification badge or sharing client's personal information with others without client's consent; medication therapy as part of client's plan of care can be construed to be personal information
4. *Disciplinary action*: denying or suspending any license to practice by boards of nursing because of unprofessional conduct; nurses who are involved in drug diversion are subject to disciplinary action
5. *Malpractice*: a form of **negligence** or professional misconduct; includes actions that are poor, wrong, or injudicious in the professional care of a client that result in injury, unnecessary suffering, or death to client (such as a serious medication error); this may also occur through omission of a necessary act, such as failure to give a prescribed medication

F. **Legal liability**
1. Administration of medications by nurse includes several aspects of legal liability
2. A legal prescription from a healthcare provider with prescription-writing authority, such as a healthcare provider or nurse practitioner, begins the process of medication delivery to a client; see Box 1-3 for a list of elements of a complete drug prescription
3. Nurses are responsible for their actions even when there is a written medication prescription
   a. If a drug prescription is incorrect (inaccurate dose or prescribed drug is not indicated for client's health condition), nurse who administers drug is liable for error along with prescriber
   b. Nurse must question any prescription that appears inappropriate and can refuse to administer drug until prescription is clarified
4. Nurses, healthcare providers, and pharmacists participate in systems used in a healthcare agency to maintain medication safety
   a. One important feature of such a system is documentation of client-reported allergy to medications
   b. Nurse is "last stop" in the system and has a crucial role in ensuring accuracy in medication administration
   c. System for use, storage, dispensing, and documentation of controlled substance drugs is a highly regulated part of a healthcare agency's medication administration system

Box 1-3	The following items must be included in a complete drug prescription:
Elements of a Drug Prescription	• Full name of the client • Date and time the drug prescription is written • Name of the drug to be given to the client • Dosage of the drug • Frequency of drug administration • Route of drug administration • Signature of person writing the prescription

   d. Nurse participates in a process of system analysis that addresses entire medication administration system, which includes the prescription and method of dispensing, as well as preparation, administration, and documentation
5. The nurse ensures that *right client* receives *right medication* in *right dose* via *right route* at *right time*; the nurse then completes *right documentation* (time of medication administration and client responses to medication)
   a. Included in this process is ensuring that dosage is appropriate for client's size and age
   b. It is critical to verify client's identity prior to medication administration by using two unique identifiers, such as checking identification band (or bar code scanning, when facilities have this technology) and asking client to state his or her name and date of birth
6. Nurse is responsible for assessing client's condition as it relates to prescribed medication, and client's response to medication (including expected or unexpected responses)
7. Nurse must have knowledge of effects and potential effects of every drug administered to a client
8. Nurse also takes measures to protect client from any safety hazards that may be expected from a medication's effects; an example is taking measures to protect client from falling if a medication has a sedative effect or can cause dizziness
9. Professional liability insurance: nurses need their own liability insurance for protection against malpractice lawsuits, including those involving medication errors

III. PRESCRIPTION AND NONPRESCRIPTION MEDICATIONS

A. **Generic, chemical, and trade names**
   1. *Generic name*: original designation that is given to a drug when drug company makes an application to begin approval process; each drug has only one generic name such as acetaminophen
   2. *Chemical name*: name that reflects chemical structure of a drug; often long and complex; of use to pharmacists and researchers
   3. *Trade name*: also known as brand name; a name given to an approved drug by pharmaceutical company that developed it; there can be multiple trade names; for instance, acetaminophen has several trade names, including Tylenol
B. **Nonprescription or over-the-counter (OTC) medications**
   1. Products that are available without a prescription for self-treatment of a variety of minor problems
   2. The regulation and evaluation of OTC drugs is under FDA supervision
   3. OTC medications may have been previously approved as prescription medications, usually at a higher strength

4. Advantages of using OTC medications include reduced healthcare costs, less time lost from work, less travel, and fewer side effects
5. Potential problems with OTC drug use include improper use, lack of counseling, labeling concerns, and possible delay in obtaining needed treatment

IV. MEDICATION CLASSIFICATION SYSTEMS

A. Two possible approaches
   1. Medications with similar characteristics might be classified together based on clinical indication; an example is analgesic medications, which relieve pain
   2. Medications can also be grouped together by body system upon which they act; an example is central nervous system medications

B. Benefits of a classification system
   1. Knowledge of a drug's classification helps the nurse to understand intended effects and common side effects of a drug being administered
   2. It also assists the nurse to organize knowledge of thousands of drugs that are used for a wide variety of therapeutic indications

V. TERMINOLOGY RELATED TO PHARMACOLOGY

A. Critical concentration: also called therapeutic level; amount of a drug needed to cause a therapeutic effect

B. Distribution: transport of a drug in body fluids from bloodstream to various tissues of body and then to its site of action

C. Drug: any substance used in diagnosis, treatment, or prevention of a disease or condition; this term is used interchangeably with *medication*

D. Drug–enzyme interactions: drugs can cause interference with enzyme systems

E. First-pass effect: a phenomenon that occurs following ingestion of an oral drug, in which a large percentage of drug is inactivated in liver after being absorbed from gastrointestinal (GI) tract as drug is carried from GI circulation through hepatic portal circulation; this explains why oral medication doses need to be larger than parenteral doses (e.g., an oral dose of morphine sulfate is 10 mg, but an intravenous dose is 1–2 mg)

F. Half-life: time required to reduce to one-half the amount of unchanged drug in the body at the time equilibrium is established (e.g., with a drug containing 500 mg with a half-life of 6 hours that was given at 0800, 250 mg will have been excreted by 1400, leaving 50% or 250 mg in the body; in another 6 hours, that 250 mg will again be reduced by half, so at 2000, 125 mg will remain)

G. Orphan drugs: drugs that are not profitable financially, but may be useful in treating rare diseases

H. Pharmacodynamics: what drugs do to the body and how drugs interact with body tissues

I. Pharmacokinetics: what the body does to a drug or how a drug is altered as it travels through body; involves four processes of absorption, distribution, biotransformation (metabolism), and excretion (discussed later in chapter)

J. Pharmacology: study of drugs and their interactions with living systems

K. Pharmacotherapeutics: also known as clinical pharmacology; branch of pharmacology that involves using drugs to treat, prevent, or diagnose disease

L. Selective toxicity: ability of a drug, such as penicillin, to attack only those systems found in foreign cells

VI. ISSUES RELATED TO MEDICATION ADMINISTRATION

A. "Rights" of safe medication administration: right medication, right dose, right client, right route, right time, and right documentation; additional "rights" may include right assessment, right to refuse, right response, and right education

    B. Factors affecting absorption and response
1. **Absorption:** movement of a drug from its site of administration into blood
2. Physiological factors affecting drug absorption
   a. Weight: the recommended dosage of a drug is based on drug evaluation studies and is targeted at a 70-kg (150-lb) person
   b. Volume of distribution (Vd): may be used along with client weight to calculate a loading dose of a drug needed by a client
   c. Age: a factor to be considered primarily in children and older adults
   d. Gender: because males have more vascular muscles than females, an effect of an intramuscular (IM) injection is noted sooner in a male than in a female; females have more fat cells than males; therefore, drugs that deposit in fat may be slowly released in a female and cause effects for a longer period of time than in a male
3. Chemical and physical factors affecting drug absorption
   a. Lipid solubility: highly soluble drugs are absorbed more rapidly than drugs whose lipid solubility is low
   b. pH partitioning: difference between pH of plasma and pH at site of administration is such that drug molecules will have a greater tendency to be ionized in plasma
   c. Range of dissolution: the faster the dissolution of medication, the more rapid the onset of drug absorption will be
   d. Blood flow: medications are absorbed most rapidly from sites where blood flow is high
   e. Routes of administration: barriers to absorption associated with each route are different, so patterns of absorption differ among routes

C. Unintended responses to drugs
1. Side effect: unavoidable secondary drug effect produced at therapeutic doses (e.g., gastric irritation caused by aspirin)
2. Adverse drug reaction: undesired response to a drug; may range from mild to life-threatening
   a. Toxicity: an adverse drug reaction caused by excessive dosing (e.g., coma from morphine overdose); some drugs have a narrow therapeutic index, that is, the dose required to produce a therapeutic effect is close to the toxic dose
   b. Allergic reaction: an adverse physiological reaction of immunologic origin; in order for an allergic reaction to occur, there should be prior sensitization of immune system; drug dosage has no effect on intensity of allergic reactions
   c. Idiosyncratic effect: an adverse drug reaction based on a client's genetic predisposition
3. Iatrogenic disease: a drug- or healthcare provider–induced disease
4. Teratogenic effect: a drug-induced birth defect
5. Carcinogenic effect: ability of a drug to cause cancer

D. Medications and children
1. Children metabolize drugs differently than adults in that they metabolize medications faster
2. Children have immature body systems for handling drugs
   a. Drug responses may be unusually intense and prolonged
   b. Absorption of intramuscular (IM) medications in neonates is slower than in adults; Figure 1-1 shows the vastus lateralis site for IM injection for a newborn and children up to 3 years of age
   c. Absorption of IM medications in infants is more rapid than in adults
   d. Neonates are more sensitive to medications that affect central nervous system (CNS) because blood–brain barrier is not fully developed

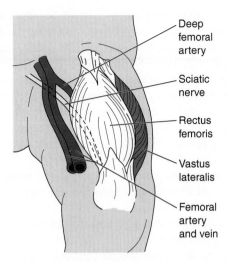

Figure 1-1

The vastus lateralis muscle is used for IM injections in newborns, infants, and children up to 3 years of age

Deep femoral artery

Sciatic nerve

Rectus femoris

Vastus lateralis

Femoral artery and vein

    e. Medication-metabolizing capacity of neonates is low

    f. Renal **excretion** (a process whereby drugs and pharmacologically active or inactive metabolites are eliminated from body) of medications is low in neonates

    g. Most pharmacokinetic parameters in children 1 year and older are similar to those in adults

E. Medications and older adults

    1. Older adults undergo physical changes as part of aging process that affect response to an administered drug

    2. Altered response may be due to less effective absorption, less efficient **distribution** (transport of a drug in body fluids from bloodstream to various body tissues and then to its site of action), less efficient perfusion, altered metabolism, and less efficient excretion

    3. Rate of drug absorption may be slowed in older adults or altered by a lowered gastric acidity

    4. Concentrations of water-soluble drugs may be high and concentrations of lipid-soluble drugs may be low in older adults

    5. Reduced liver and/or renal function may prolong medication effects; with reduced metabolism and/or excretion of a drug, it may continue to work for a prolonged amount of time or toxic effects may become apparent

    6. Adverse drug reactions are more common in older adults than in younger adults

    7. Nonadherence is more common among older adults; factors contributing to nonadherence include low income, forgetfulness, complex regimens, side effects, failure to follow instructions, and inability to obtain medications

    8. Polypharmacy: older adults often take multiple medications and may have multiple healthcare providers

F. Calculating medication dosages

    1. Calculation of medication dosage by body weight

       a. 1 kg = 2.2 lb

       b. To convert from pounds to kilograms, divide by 2.2

          1) Example: a client weighs 154 pounds: $154 \div 2.2 =$ the client weighs 70 kg

       c. To convert from kilograms to pounds, multiply by 2.2

          1) Example: a client weighs 20 kg: $20 \times 2.2 =$ the client weighs 44 lb

    2. Calculating daily dosages

       a. Dosages are expressed in terms of mg/kg/day or mg/lb/day

!

Practice to Pass

A client with chronic renal failure is taking medications to control hypertension and other health problems. What are the priority nursing considerations for this client in relation to the drug regimen?

        1) Example: the drug vancomycin can be given to a pediatric client with pseudo-membranous colitis in doses up to 40 mg/kg/day

        2) The pediatric client above, who weighs 20 kg (44 lb), can receive 40 mg × 20 kg/day; 40 mg × 20 kg = 800 mg/day in three to four divided doses

    b. Total daily dosage is usually administered in divided doses per day

        1) Example: from above drug prescription for vancomycin, 800 mg ÷ 4 = 200 mg each dose; this dose is within recommended range for this client

    c. Nurse is responsible for verifying that a drug prescription is within recommended dosage range; if not, prescription should be questioned and clarified

3. Intravenous fluid calculations

    a. First step: determine how many milliliters (mL) per hour (volume) needs to be given; this may be part of original prescription or may need to be calculated when total volume and hours are given

        1) Example: provider prescribes 1,000 mL IV solution to be given over 8 hours

        2) 1,000 ÷ 8 = 125 mL per hour (mL/hr)

    b. Second step: calculate drops per minute (gtts/min); when the mL/hr is given, calculate the gtts/min

        1) Example: client's IV set delivers 10 gtt/mL

        2) 125 mL/60 min × 10 gtts/mL = 1250 gtts ÷ 60 minutes = 20.83 gtts/min

        3) Since a fractional drop cannot be counted, nurse will set IV drip rate at 21 gtts/min after rounding decimal appropriately

    c. The drop factor is the number of drops in 1 mL; drop factors of 10, 15, and 60 are most common (drop factor is determined by manufacturer and is found on IV tubing box)

G. Routes of medication administration

1. See Table 1-2 for a detailed description of very commonly used routes for administering medications

2. Enteral (via GI tract): including oral administration as well as administration via a GI feeding tube; classic routes include:

    a. PO: typical oral administration

    b. SL: sublingual, under the tongue

    c. Buccal: between cheek and gum

    d. Via feeding tube

3. Parenteral

    a. Intravenous (IV): through an IV catheter into a vein; is fastest-acting route; effects should be experienced beginning in as little as a few minutes

    b. Subcutaneous (subQ): Figure 1-2 illustrates angle of insertion for subQ injections; typical volume is 0.5–1 mL per injection but should not exceed 1.5 mL; needle gauge is 25–29 and a 3/8- to 5/8-inch needle should be used

    c. Intramuscular (IM): Figure 1-3 illustrates angle of insertion for IM injections using Z-track method; total volume varies by age and injection site, commonly 1–2 mL in adults and 0.5–1 mL in children; needle size varies by age, commonly 21- to 23-gauge and 1–1.5 inches long

    d. Intradermal (ID): used for diagnostic testing, such as allergens or tuberculosis screening; uses a tuberculin syringe, usual dose is 0.01–0.1 mL using 25- to 27-gauge, ¼- to ½-inch needle

4. Topical

    a. Transcutaneous: some medications may be applied to skin as a paste (e.g., nitroglycerin) or a patch (e.g., nitroglycerin or scopolamine), so medication is absorbed continually over time

---

Practice to Pass

The healthcare provider prescribes morphine sulfate 15 mg subcutaneously for a client with pain. The medication is supplied as morphine sulfate 25 mg/mL. What volume of the drug will the nurse prepare to administer the right dose?

Practice to Pass

A client with a history of angina has an prescription for a topical nitroglycerin patch that is to be placed daily in the morning and taken off at hour of sleep (hs). Why is this route of administration desirable for this client? Explain your response.

Table 1-2	Commonly Used Routes of Administration			
Routes	**Barriers to Absorption**	**Absorption Pattern**	**Advantages**	**Disadvantages**
Intravenous	No barriers	Instantaneous and complete	Rapid onset Control over levels of drug in the blood Use of large fluid volumes Use of chemically irritant drugs such as anticancer	High cost Difficulty and inconvenience Irreversibility Fluid overload Infection Embolism
Intramuscular and subQ	Capillary wall	Rapidly or slowly; depends on the water solubility of the drug and blood flow to the site of the injection Intramuscular absorption faster than subQ because of better blood flow to muscle tissue	Poorly soluble drugs in water Depot preparations (preparations from which medication is absorbed gradually over an extended time)	Discomfort and inconvenience Possible nerve damage
Oral	a. The layer of epithelial cells b. The capillary wall	Varies according to: a. Solubility and stability of the drug b. Gastric and intestinal pH c. Gastric emptying time d. Food in the gut e. Co-administration of other drugs f. Special coatings on the preparation	Easy and convenient Inactivation Inexpensive Safer than parenteral injection	Variability of absorption Client requirements (i.e., cooperation, local irritation)

Figure 1-2

Inserting a needle for subcutaneous injection

Figure 1-3

Inserting a needle using the Z-track method for IM injections

        b. Instillations or irrigations: medications may be administered to various body orifices or cavities, such as ophthalmic (eye), otic (ear), intranasal (nose), vaginal, rectal, or into joints or urinary bladder

        c. Inhalations: some medications may be inhaled into respiratory tract using an inhaler, nebulizer, or positive pressure breathing machine

   5. Intrathecal (less common): some drugs, such as chemotherapy, are administered into spinal fluid in the subarachnoid space, using a device such as an Ommaya reservoir

H. Medication interactions

   1. *Drug–food interaction* is important because it can result in toxicity or therapeutic failure

        a. Impact of food on drug absorption: food may increase or decrease a drug's absorption rate and consequently affect extent of absorption; for example, if tetracyclines are administered with milk products or calcium supplements, absorption is reduced and antibacterial effects may be lost

        b. Impact of food on **biotransformation**: food may alter metabolism of certain medications; grapefruit juice produces a 406% increase in blood levels of some calcium channel blockers used to treat hypertension

        c. Impact of food on drug toxicity: interaction between monoamine oxidase (MAO) inhibitors and foods rich in tyramine (including yeasts, extracts, aged cheese) can raise blood pressure to a life-threatening level and cause other symptoms such as headache, nausea and vomiting, tachycardia, sweating, and rarely brain hemorrhage

        d. Impact of food on drug action: food may have direct impact on drug action, such as foods rich in vitamin K (e.g., broccoli, cabbage), which can reduce therapeutic effect of anticoagulant sodium warfarin

        e. Timing of drug administration with respect to meals: may result in significant increase or decrease in drug absorption

   2. *Drug–drug interaction* can occur whenever a client takes two or more medications; some interactions are intended and desired, but others are unintended

        a. Mechanisms of drug–drug interaction

           1) *Direct chemical or physical interaction*: when drugs are combined in IV solutions and cause formation of a precipitate; nurse must carefully inspect any solution that has been mixed with a drug to detect crystals or cloudiness

           2) *Pharmacokinetic interaction*: may alter absorption, distribution, biotransformation (metabolism), and excretion; for example, heparin cannot cross GI tract membrane, so absorption via oral route is not possible; drug must be given via parenteral route

           3) *Pharmacodynamic interaction*: includes interactions at same receptors or interactions at separate sites; for example, naloxone is a drug that blocks access of opiate drugs to receptor sites, so it is used to reverse action of opiates following opiate overdose

        b. Consequences of drug–drug interactions

           1) Increased/decreased therapeutic effects

           2) Increased/decreased adverse effects

           3) Creation of a unique response

   3. Incompatibility: occurs when the mixture of one medication with another results in an undesirable reaction

        a. Reactions could include chemical alteration, destruction, or pharmacological effect

        b. An example is diluting phenytoin in 5% dextrose in water will result in precipitation of solution, which can be fatal if administered to a client

I. Client education

1. Process of client education
   a. Assessment of need to learn
   b. Assessment of motivation
   c. Formulation of a nursing diagnosis or problem statement and setting objective goals with client
   d. Teaching–learning activities aimed at client's preferred learning style and general ability and educational level
   e. Evaluation and reteaching if necessary, depending on achievement of learning objectives

2. Nursing roles and responsibilities
   a. Applying nursing process to client teaching
      1) Assessment: assess for client's readiness for education; organize, analyze, and summarize collected data
      2) Diagnosis: formulate nursing problem statements to address learning needs
      3) Planning and goals: assign priority to nursing problems; identify teaching strategies appropriate for goal; establish expected outcome
      4) Client-centered nursing care: put teaching plan into action; encourage client participation in learning
      5) Evaluation: evaluate collected objective data; identify alterations that need to be made in teaching plan; make referrals to appropriate sources
   b. Establish a good teacher–learner rapport
   c. Plan best time for teaching and reduce noise and distractions in teaching environment
   d. Match teaching methods to client's primary learning style, such as visual, auditory, and/or tactile, for optimum effectiveness
   e. Use teaching tools appropriate to client's primary learning style, such as lecture or verbal teaching, demonstration, written materials, videotapes, or visual materials or physical models
   f. Identify barriers to learning, such as cognitive or psychomotor impediments, cultural or socioeconomic factors, communication, and excessive volume of learning materials

3. Client adherence
   a. A goal of client education is that clients adhere to therapeutic regimen; direct teaching program toward stimulating client motivation to adhere to therapy
   b. Perform ongoing assessment of variables that affect client's ability to accept specific behaviors; examples are age, gender identity, socioeconomic status, education, severity of illness, complexity of regimen, religious or cultural beliefs, and costs associated with a prescribed regimen
   c. Identify potential nonadherence to therapeutic regimens and plan counteractive strategies
   d. Establish comprehensive adherence-enhancing interventions (see Box 1-4)

4. Cultural considerations: cultural competence refers to a complex integration of attitudes, knowledge, and skills that direct the nurse to provide care in a culturally sensitive manner (Table 1-3)
   a. Recognize special dietary needs for clients from selected cultural groups; sometimes foods that clients prefer may be those that interact with prescribed medications
   b. Review drug information to be aware of variations in individual response to medications based on **pharmacogenetics**; some clients may require lower doses and some may have faster clearance rates of selected drugs based on genetics

---

Practice to Pass

A client who does not speak English is being discharged with three prescriptions for medications. What strategies should the nurse use to meet responsibilities for client teaching in this situation?

Box 1-4	Consider using these interventions to promote client adherence to treatment plan:
Enhancing Adherence to Treatment Plan	1. Provide verbal instruction in small amounts, specific to activity.
	2. Dispense optimal amounts of printed instructions.
	3. Use material at client's comprehension level.
	4. Dispense materials over time.
	5. Assess level of client's understanding.
	6. Encourage questions.
	7. Augment verbal instructions with demonstrations.
	8. Refer to community resources for additional skill development.
	9. Goal setting: make goals attainable and very specific.
	10. Reinforce learning by providing feedback and praise for attempts.
	11. Do problem solving; identify problems and potential solutions for adherence.
	12. Encourage habit building, such as placing bedtime medication on bedside table.
	13. Provide cueing; set up system of reminders to take medications, such as calendars or medication box.
	14. Establish social support by involving others in behavior change plan.

Table 1-3 **Comparative Characteristics of Culturally Diverse Clients**

Cultures	Communication	Social Roles	Health Risks	Implementation
African Americans	Nonverbal communication is very important	Large extended family networks are important	Hypertension, coronary heart disease, sickle-cell anemia, cancer	Be flexible and avoid rigidity in scheduling care Encourage involvement with family An herbalist may be consulted before an individual seeks medical care
Asian Americans	Silence is valued, eye contact considered rude, the word "no" considered disrespectful	Large extended family networks, devoted to tradition, education is highly valued	Hypertension, cancer, lactose intolerance, thalassemia	Limit eye contact Avoid gesturing with hands A healer may be consulted prior to medical treatment
European Americans	Eye contact indicates trustworthiness	The nuclear family is the basic unit; the man is the dominant figure	Breast cancer, thalassemia, diabetes	Eye contact is acceptable
Hispanic Americans	Eye contact indicates disrespect	The nuclear family is the basic unit; men are the decision makers; extended family is highly valued	Diabetes, parasites, lactose intolerance	Protect privacy Offer to call priest or other clergy
Native Americans	Silence is valued, eye contact is avoided	Family oriented; elders are honored	Diabetes, tuberculosis, alcohol abuse, heart disease, gallbladder disease, accidents	Be attentive Clarify communication Obtain input from members of extended family May consult a medicine man
Arab Americans	Direct eye contact often avoided	Family is the key social unit; patriarchal and hierarchal; men and women may have separate living areas	Cardiovascular disease, tobacco use, diabetes mellitus	Protect privacy and modesty May consult a "bone setter" for broken bones Same-sex interpreter preferred

Box 1-5	Consider using these interventions to assist in overcoming a language barrier:
Enhancing Communication to Overcome Language Barriers	1. Greet client using the last or complete name.
	2. Smile.
	3. Pay attention to any effort by the client to communicate.
	4. Avoid talking loudly.
	5. Use short and simple sentences.
	6. Summarize and repeat frequently.
	7. Use a qualified interpreter to ensure appropriate communication about plan of care and prescribed medications; family members may not be the best choices for this task, depending on a number of variables, including age and sensitivity of information.
	8. Identify cues that may signal a lack of effective communication, including absence of questions, efforts to change the subject, inappropriate laughter, and nonverbal cues.

  c. Create an environment in which client's traditional healing practices are respected; recognize that some clients may not value drug therapy as a primary mode of treatment for a health problem

  d. Establish effective communication by overcoming language barriers (see Box 1-5)

  e. Establish flexible regulations pertaining to visitors, such as length of visits

  f. View each client as an individual and avoid stereotyping

  g. Be aware of client's cultural preferences regarding space and distance, eye contact, time, touch, observance of holidays, and diet

  h. Maintain a broad and open attitude; expect the unexpected

  i. Try to understand reasons for any behavior that you do not understand; ask for clarification

  j. Use any words you know in client's primary language

 5. Healthcare beliefs

  a. Values are beliefs and attitudes that may influence a client's decision making process and behavior; they evolve from personal experiences

  b. Decisions about whether or not to use drugs as therapy for health problems are often influenced by a client's overall healthcare beliefs

  c. Ethical principles are codes that direct a person's actions

   1) Include an ability to make choices without external constraints, a need to maintain a balance between benefits and harms, and an obligation to tell the truth

   2) These are some areas in which ethical concerns arise for nurses and for clients related to treatment with drugs

  d. Ethical codes: provide broad principles for determining and evaluating client care

  e. American Nurses Association (ANA) Code of Ethics: an ideal framework for nurses to use in ethical decision making

  f. Ethical dilemma: occurs when there is a conflict between two or more ethical principles, including confidentiality, use of restraint, trust issues (not lying to client, communicating to family and healthcare provider), refusing treatment or care, and end-of-life issues; drug therapy may play a role sometimes when such issues arise; nurse's role is to maintain ethical behavior when administering drug therapy

Case Study

A 78-year-old male is admitted to the hospital following a motor vehicle accident in which he incurred a head trauma and began having seizures. He has a history of heart failure and atrial fibrillation and is currently on metoprolol succinate 25 mg bid, furosemide 20 mg bid, warfarin 5 mg daily, and ibuprofen 200 mg as needed for arthritis pain. He has been started on phenytoin 100 mg PO for seizure control.

1. Should the nurse be concerned for any drug interactions with the addition of phenytoin?

2. What role does protein-binding play with these interactions?

3. What adverse effects of medications should the nurse monitor in the client?

4. What laboratory values would the nurse want to monitor and why?

5. What are some important nursing implications to consider related to administration of the phenytoin?

For suggested responses, see page 537.

POSTTEST

1 When administering a pain medication via the intravenous route, the nurse should anticipate that the client will begin to have pain relief within which time frame?

1. Within the first minute
2. Within a few to several minutes
3. Within 30 minutes
4. Within 60 minutes

2 When administering a medication to a frail 89-year-old client with a body mass index (BMI) of 18, the nurse places priority on assessing for which adverse drug reaction?

1. Allergic reaction
2. Toxic effects
3. An idiosyncratic reaction
4. A teratogenic effect

3 A client who is taking several prescribed oral medications to treat chronic heart failure tells the nurse, "I usually take all of my medications with my breakfast." The nurse's best response should include which statements? Select all that apply.

1. "It might be a good idea to review each drug to determine the best times and conditions for taking it."
2. "That depends on what you eat at breakfast."
3. "Has the swelling in your lower legs decreased?"
4. "What time do you usually have breakfast?"
5. "That's a great idea."

4 The client received isophane (NPH) insulin 30 units subcutaneously at 7:30 a.m. What time is the nurse most likely to observe signs and symptoms of hypoglycemia?

1. 9:30 to 10:30 a.m.
2. 11:30 a.m. to 2:30 p.m.
3. 11:30 a.m. to 7:30 p.m.
4. 3:30 to 7:30 p.m.

5 The client taking theophylline 16 mg/kg PO for asthma has a serum theophylline level of 22 mcg/mL. Because the client is experiencing nausea and vomiting and headache, which action should the nurse take?

1. Seek a prescription for an antiemetic from the prescriber.
2. Withhold the next scheduled dose and notify the prescriber.
3. Ask if client expectorated any mucus after the last respiratory therapy treatment.
4. Stop prescribed doses of theophylline for 24 hours.

POSTTEST

6 Morphine sulfate 10 mg PO is prescribed for a first-day postoperative client with a large abdominal wound. The nurse should consider which action most appropriate?

1. Request a prescription that changes the route from oral to parenteral.
2. Administer drug with food.
3. Dissolve tablet in a small amount of warm liquid.
4. Encourage coughing and deep breathing 2 hours after ingestion.

7 A pregnant client who visits the clinic for a routine evaluation asks the nurse about continuing to take her routine medications. The nurse should provide a response based on which principles established by the Food and Drug Administration (FDA)? Select all that apply.

1. No drug should be administered during pregnancy unless the benefits outweigh the risks.
2. The Pregnancy Categories were established in order to indicate the potential for a drug to cause birth defects.
3. A Pregnancy Category A designation indicates that studies demonstrate abnormalities or adverse reactions in the fetus and that the risk of use outweighs any benefit.
4. The Pregnancy Category guidelines were developed in order to rank the abuse potential of various drugs in pregnancy.
5. Schedule V medications have limited abuse potential and are generally safe for pregnancy.

8 A healthcare provider prescribed 12.5 mg of an antiemetic suppository for a client with severe nausea. The nurse has on hand a 25-mg suppository. What is the next step that the nurse should take?

1. Cut suppository in half and insert the rounded edge.
2. Administer drug orally.
3. Contact pharmacist if unable to locate the correct dosage.
4. Clear rectal vault of the contents before administering half of the suppository.

9 A healthcare provider prescribes 1,000 mL 5% dextrose in 0.9% sodium chloride over 6 hours. The nurse calculates the flow rate for this infusion to be how many mL per hour? Provide a numerical response rounded to a whole number.

_____ mL

10 The home health nurse plans to provide additional education after hearing an older adult client taking glyburide 1.25 mg PO daily make which statement?

1. "I take the tablet with breakfast every day."
2. "If I forget the dose on one day, I will take two tablets the next day."
3. "I will avoid drinking alcohol while taking this drug."
4. "I will keep appointments to have my HBA_{1c} checked every 4 months."

➤ *See pages 21–23 for Answers and Rationales.*

POSTTEST

ANSWERS & RATIONALES

ANSWERS & RATIONALES

Pretest

1 **Answer: 2 Rationale:** The most accurate way is to scan the client's own identification bracelet, provided the facility has this mechanism in place. The alert client could also be asked to state name and date of birth. Two forms of identification are recommended. Asking the client to state his or her name is an accurate way to identify a client, but would not be a good method when the client is confused, disoriented, or comatose. Hospitalized or ill clients are often anxious, medicated, or confused and might respond incorrectly to this question. Because clients' bed assignments are sometimes changed to meet unit needs, simply checking the client's room number and bed assignment poses a risk for incorrect client identification. Because the same diagnosis with the same medication may be appropriate for more than one client, matching the medication to the diagnosis or need will place the client at risk. **Cognitive Level:** Applying **Client Need:** Pharmacological and Parenteral Therapies **Integrated Process:** Communication and Documentation **Content Area:** Pharmacology **Strategy:** Analyze each option and select the option that minimizes the risk for obtaining incorrect information. Recall that having the client provide information directly is a preferred option when there is no bar code system in place. **Reference:** Adams, M. P., Holland, N., & Urban, C. (2017). *Pharmacology for nurses: A pathophysiologic approach* (5th ed.). New York, NY: Pearson, p. 19.

2 **Answer: 1 Rationale:** Stating that similarities exist but that instructions were specific to the child answers the question and reaffirms the healthcare provider's instructions. Changing from brand-name drugs to generic drugs should be done by the healthcare provider. Advil, an enteric-coated tablet, is a brand name of ibuprofen. Not all ibuprofen is enteric-coated, although the active ingredient is the same—ibuprofen (which is also the generic name). Answering that Advil and ibuprofen are two different drugs with similar effects is inaccurate. It is inappropriate to make a referral when the nurse is capable of meeting the need of the client. **Cognitive Level:** Applying **Client Need:** Pharmacological and Parenteral Therapies **Integrated Process:** Communication and Documentation **Content Area:** Pharmacology **Strategy:** Select the option that is most accurate and that places the client at the least amount of risk. **Reference:** Wilson, B. A., Shannon, M., & Shields, K. (2016). *Pearson nurse's drug guide 2016.* New York, NY: Pearson, pp. 768–770.

3 **Answer: 3 Rationale:** Iron is a Pregnancy Category A drug, and this category is assigned to drugs that have not been shown to have adverse effects on fetal development. Therefore, it is safe to ingest the drug during pregnancy. The statement that no OTC products should be taken during pregnancy is inaccurate because of the word *any*. An example of a safe product to use during pregnancy is a multivitamin. Answering that "most prenatal vitamins contain iron" is accurate; however, it does not answer the client's question directly. Staining of the teeth is a side effect of tetracyclines. **Cognitive Level:** Analyzing **Client Need:** Pharmacological and Parenteral Therapies **Integrated Process:** Teaching and Learning **Content Area:** Pharmacology **Strategy:** To answer this question correctly, recall the Pregnancy Category of iron and use knowledge of the safety of Pregnancy Category A drugs to select the option that most closely correlates with that category. **Reference:** Wilson, B. A., Shannon, M., & Shields, K. (2016). *Pearson nurse's drug guide 2016.* Upper Saddle River, NJ: Pearson, pp. 639–641.

4 **Answer: 4 Rationale:** Interactions with foods or other medication can change the metabolism of the drugs and lead to increases in serum drug levels. This can lead to toxicity manifested by dysrhythmias (heart block, bradycardia), angina, heart failure, and hypotension. The highest priority is assisting the client to ingest this drug safely. Identification of the cause of the toxicity takes the highest priority. There is no direct relationship between elevated body temperature and toxic levels of antihypertensive drugs. Assessment of respiratory pattern may be important because of the toxicity, but does not address the primary problem directly; assessment should focus on the cause. Weight gain (not loss) is not an adverse effect of antihypertensive drugs. **Cognitive Level:** Analyzing **Client Need:** Pharmacological and Parenteral Therapies **Integrated Process:** Nursing Process: Assessment **Content Area:** Pharmacology **Strategy:** The core issue of the question is knowledge of factors that could increase the risk of toxicity. Recall that drugs can interact with other drugs and many foods. **Reference:** Adams, M. P., Holland, N., & Urban, C. (2017). *Pharmacology for nurses: A pathophysiologic approach* (5th ed.). New York, NY: Pearson, p. 308.

5 **Answer: 1, 2, 4 Rationale:** Since older adult clients experience a decreased rate of drug excretion, a reduction in dosage would be appropriate. The decreased total body fluid proportion that accompanies physical aging increases the concentration of water-soluble drugs and requires lower dosing in older adults. Older adult clients experience a decreased rate of drug biotransformation. Decreased efficiency in drug distribution would not correlate with a need to lower the dosage. Many older adults tend to lose weight, not gain weight, because of lean muscle mass loss. **Cognitive Level:** Analyzing **Client Need:** Pharmacological and Parenteral Therapies **Integrated Process:** Nursing Process: Diagnosis **Content Area:** Pharmacology **Strategy:** The core issue is the effect of age-related changes on drug biotransformation. Select the options that would place the client at greatest risk and that correlate closest to the information in the stem. **Reference:** Adams, M. P., Holland, N., & Urban, C. (2017). *Pharmacology for nurses: A pathophysiologic approach* (5th ed.). New York, NY: Pearson, pp. 73–74.

6 **Answer: 7.5 Rationale:** Use the following formula as one way to calculate the dose: 100 mg/5 mL = 150 mg/x mL 100x = 750; x = 7.5 mL. **Cognitive Level:** Analyzing **Client Need:** Pharmacological and Parenteral Therapies **Integrated Process:** Nursing Process: Implementation **Content Area:** Pharmacology **Strategy:** Use the "solving for x" equation or any other pharmacological dosage calculation formula to determine the correct amount. **Reference:** Olsen, J., Giangrasso, A., & Shrimpton, D. (2016). *Medical dosage calculations: A dimensional analysis approach* (11th ed.). New York, NY: Pearson, pp. 142–148.

7 Answer: 1 Rationale: Feeling dizzy when moving from lying or sitting to standing position is referred to as orthostatic hypotension and is a common side effect of beta-blocker drugs such as nadolol. The client should be instructed to change positions slowly. Signs and symptoms should diminish after a few weeks of treatment. Dizziness is not a sign of toxicity, but is related to the body's adjustment to reduced decreased cardiac output and reduced central circulating volume. Dizziness can be a sign or symptom of hypertension, but since the client is ingesting an antihypertensive drug, postural hypotension related to decreased central circulating volume should be suspected. Cognitive Level: Analyzing Client Need: Pharmacological and Parenteral Therapies Integrated Process: Teaching and Learning Content Area: Pharmacology Strategy: The core issue of the question is the ability to recognize a drug side effect and provide appropriate teaching to protect the client from falls and possible harm. With this in mind, select the option that provides the greatest safety to the client, which is to ask the client to use caution and move slowly when standing up. Reference: Wilson, B. A., Shannon, M., & Shields, K. (2016). *Pearson nurse's drug guide 2016.* New York, NY: Pearson, pp. 1049–1050.

8 Answer: 1 Rationale: Older clients often take other pre-scribed drugs, herbs, or other alternative remedies, and client may be ingesting an over-the-counter (OTC) remedy for arthritis. Because there is a potentially high risk for drug–drug or drug–herb interaction, getting a thorough picture of the client's current drug regimen is the first step in planning for client education when a new drug is prescribed. Providing written materials is appropriate as a supplement after the nurse has taught the client about the medication. Because of cognitive changes, the client may need a strategy to help in main-taining the drug schedule (like a meds organizer), but it should not be the first action. The first action is based on the potential risk to the client. Teaching about the drug is very relevant to the management of the client's health needs, but assessing the risk to the client should occur before implementation. Cognitive Level: Analyzing Client Need: Pharmacological and Parenteral Therapies Integrated Process: Nursing Process: Assessment Content Area: Pharmacology Strategy: The critical term in the question is *older adult*. Correlate knowledge associated with older adult clients and drug therapy. Assessment is the first step in managing client needs. Reference: Adams, M. P., Holland, N., & Urban, C. (2017). *Pharmacol-ogy for nurses: A pathophysiologic approach* (5th ed.). New York, NY: Pearson, pp. 467–470.

9 Answer: 4 Rationale: The nurse should check the original healthcare provider prescription. Giving medications that are different from what was prescribed is danger-ous. The nurse should recheck the original healthcare provider prescription in the medication administra-tion record (MAR). Asking the client if the pill looks familiar is not an appropriate means of validating the accuracy of a prescription. Cognitive Level: Analyzing Client Need: Pharmacological and Parenteral Therapies Integrated Process: Nursing Process: Planning Content Area: Pharmacology Strategy: The core issue of the question involves application of the principles of the *rights* of medication administration. Use the process of elimina-tion and select the option that best ensures delivery of the *right drug*. Reference: Adams, M. P., Holland, N., & Urban, C. (2017). *Pharmacology for nurses: A pathophysiologic approach* (5th ed.). New York, NY: Pearson, p. 19.

10 Answer: 1, 5, 3, 4, 2 Rationale: First, review the client's medication history and drug allergies as part of the assessment phase of medication administration. The client's medical history can influence a drug's effect; knowledge of client history and allergies can prevent inadvertent administration of a medication that could cause harm to the client. Second, obtain the medication, compare the drug label against the healthcare pro-vider's prescription, and prepare the medication. Third, identify the client and explain the intended action of the medication before administration, to prevent errors. Fourth, verify proper drug route, time, and dose, and then administer the medication. Fifth, record the drug administration at bedside in the medication admin-istration record. Cognitive Level: Applying Client Need: Pharmacological and Parenteral Therapies Integrated Process: Nursing Process: Implementation Content Area: Pharmacology Strategy: Visualize the correct and safe sequence of events; apply knowledge of appropriate drug administration techniques. Reference: Adams, M., & Urban, C. (2016). *Pharmacology: Connections to nursing practice* (3rd ed.). New York, NY: Pearson, p. 72.

Posttest

1 Answer: 2 Rationale: A drug given via the intravenous route enters the bloodstream immediately and has a very rapid onset of action. It should begin to act within a few minutes to several minutes depending on the actual drug. One minute is too soon. It should not take as long as 30–60 minutes to provide relief. Cognitive Level: Applying Client Need: Pharmacological and Parenteral Therapies Integrated Process: Nursing Process: Planning Content Area: Pharmacology Strategy: Remember that parentally administered medications have a rapid onset of action. Reference: Adams, M., & Urban, C. (2016). *Pharmacology: Connections to nursing practice* (3rd ed.). New York, NY: Pearson, p. 30.

2 Answer: 2 Rationale: The client is elderly with a BMI of 18, which reflects being underweight or malnourished; this will affect drug absorption and metabolism of drugs. Since there are fewer binding sites available, this places a risk for elevated drug levels and toxicity. Allergic responses can occur in anyone. Idiosyncratic reactions

ANSWERS & RATIONALES

are related to genetic predisposition, and teratogenic effects affect a developing fetus. **Cognitive Level:** Analysis **Client Need:** Pharmacological and Parenteral Therapies **Integrated Process:** Nursing Process: Assessment **Content Area:** Pharmacology **Strategy:** The core issue of the question involves analyzing the age of the client and BMI, recognizing the changes in drug absorption and metabolism that occur in the elderly and may be affected by malnutrition. **Reference:** Adams, M. P., Holland, N., & Urban, C. (2017). *Pharmacology for nurses: A pathophysiologic approach* (5th ed.). New York, NY: Pearson, pp. 39–43, 56.

3 **Answer: 1, 3 Rationale:** The nurse needs to be sure there are no significant risks to the timing of the drugs rather than just affirming the client's plan. Drug interactions, drug side effects, drug actions, and drug absorption should be examined before ingesting multiple prescriptions. Reaching the goals of the drug therapy such as a decrease in peripheral edema would indicate that this approach is appropriate. Stating "that depends on what you eat at breakfast" contains a correct statement, but is not comprehensive. Time is only one of the elements of concern. Stating "That's a great idea" is not a therapeutic response. **Cognitive Level:** Analyzing **Client Need:** Pharmacological and Parenteral Therapies **Integrated Process:** Nursing Process: Planning **Content Area:** Pharmacology **Strategy:** Select the option providing the most effective approach to the drug therapy. **Reference:** Adams, M. P., Holland, N., & Urban, C. (2017). *Pharmacology for nurses: A pathophysiologic approach* (5th ed.). New York, NY: Pearson, pp. 324–330.

4 **Answer: 3 Rationale:** Four to 12 hours is the peak time period for NPH. Two to 3 hours is the peak time period for regular insulin. Four to 7 hours is the peak time period for Semilente. Eight to 12 hours is the peak time period for Lente. **Cognitive Level:** Applying **Client Need:** Pharmacological and Parenteral Therapies **Integrated Process:** Nursing Process: Planning **Content Area:** Pharmacology **Strategy:** Associate this drug with an intermediate range and then select a time frame that is not the shortest range available but also not the longest. **Reference:** Wilson, B. A., Shannon, M., & Shields, K. (2016). *Pearson nurse's drug guide 2016.* New York, NY: Pearson, pp. 805–806.

5 **Answer: 2 Rationale:** Since the drug has a narrow therapeutic range, toxicity can develop quickly. The normal therapeutic dose level is 10–20 mcg/mL. Hence, the signs and symptoms indicate toxicity. The nurse should suspend the prescription until the prescriber is contacted. Procuring and administering an antiemetic would reduce the signs and symptoms but would not resolve the problem. The lab test validates that toxicity exists. The nurse should suspend the prescription until the dosage can be changed. The drug's duration is 4–8 hours. Asking whether client expectorated mucus does not address lab imbalance. Holding it for 24 hours could

create the opposite problem. **Cognitive Level:** Analyzing **Client Need:** Pharmacological and Parenteral Therapies **Integrated Process:** Nursing Process: Planning **Content Area:** Pharmacology **Strategy:** Recall that this drug has profound effects on GI tract and cardiac function. Then consider that toxicity is likely to have an effect on the two systems. **Reference:** Wilson, B. A., Shannon, M., & Shields, K. (2016). *Pearson nurse's drug guide 2016.* New York, NY: Pearson, pp. 1492–1495.

6 **Answer: 1 Rationale:** Because a parenteral route (IM or IV) is a more efficient route, the drug is likely to be effective more rapidly. Food will delay absorption. Dissolving the tablet would not address the issue of GI absorption soon after surgery; drug characteristics might also be altered when dissolved. Encouraging coughing and deep breathing does not address concerns related to absorption. **Cognitive Level:** Applying **Client Need:** Pharmacological and Parenteral Therapies **Integrated Process:** Nursing Process: Implementation **Content Area:** Pharmacology **Strategy:** Associate the route with the magnitude of the client's needs. **Reference:** Wilson, B. A., Shannon, M., & Shields, K. (2016). *Pearson nurse's drug guide 2016.* New York, NY: Pearson, pp. 1037–1040.

7 **Answer: 1, 2 Rationale:** Regardless of the FDA's designated Pregnancy Category, the recommendations include to not administer any drug during pregnancy unless necessary. Differentiation between the categories depends on adequate and reliable documentation and the risk–benefit ratio. The categories are intended to indicate birth defect potential. The FDA developed the Schedules of Controlled Substances to regulate drugs known to have abuse potential; these are not specific for pregnancy. Client education about medications would be based on the FDA's Pregnancy Categories, not the controlled substance schedules. The Schedules of Controlled Substances do not address pregnancy specifically, and routine medication that the pregnant woman receives should be based on the Pregnancy Categories. **Cognitive Level:** Analyzing **Client Need:** Pharmacological and Parenteral Therapies **Integrated Process:** Teaching and Learning **Content Area:** Pharmacology **Strategy:** Base knowledge of safe medication administration considerations and FDA recommendations to the education of a maternal client **Reference:** Adams, M., & Urban, C. (2016). *Pharmacology: Connections to nursing practice* (3rd ed.). New York, NY: Pearson, p. 18.

8 **Answer: 3 Rationale:** The nurse should consult with the pharmacist before contacting the prescriber. Drug companies do not guarantee that the medication is equally distributed throughout the medium, so cutting is not an option. The dosage is not stable across routes. Nurses may not change prescriptions. After the dosage problem is resolved, the rectal vault should be cleared adequately to guarantee maximum absorption; this is not the first step. **Cognitive Level:** Analyzing **Client Need:** Pharmacological and Parenteral Therapies **Integrated Process:** Nursing Process:

Planning **Content Area:** Pharmacology **Strategy:** Recall that the active drug in a suppository may not be evenly distributed and use the process of elimination to make a selection. **Reference:** Wilson, B. A., Shannon, M., & Shields, K. (2016). *Pearson nurse's drug guide 2016*. New York, NY: Pearson, pp. 277–287.

9 **Answer: 167 Rationale:** The rate for administration is calculated by dividing 1,000 mL by 6 hours: $1,000/6 = 166.66$ mL/hr, which rounds to 167 mL/hr. **Cognitive Level:** Applying **Client Need:** Pharmacological and Parenteral Therapies **Integrated Process:** Nursing Process: Planning **Content Area:** Pharmacology **Strategy:** Note that this is a simple calculation. Divide the total volume in mL by the number of hours and calculate the number of mL/hr. **Reference:** Olsen, J., Giangrasso, A., Shrimpton, D., & Dillon, P. (2016). *Medical dosage calculations* (11th ed.). New York, NY: Pearson, pp. 277–287.

10 **Answer: 2 Rationale:** Because of the drug's action (hypoglycemic), duration (24 hours), and the half-life (10 hours), the client could be at significant risk if the dose is doubled. The common dosage is once daily before or with breakfast. Ingestion of alcohol with the drug can result in a disulfiram reaction or excessive sympathomimetic reaction. HbA_{1c} provides information regarding the glucose level over a 4-month period. **Cognitive Level:** Applying **Client Need:** Pharmacological and Parenteral Therapies **Integrated Process:** Teaching and Learning **Content Area:** Pharmacology **Strategy:** Determine the client's health maintenance ability based on the content of the statement. The incorrect statement is the correct answer based on the wording of the question. **Reference:** Wilson, B. A., Shannon, M., & Shields, K. (2016). *Pearson nurse's drug guide 2016*. New York, NY: Pearson, pp. 713–715.

References

Adams, M. P., Holland, N., & Urban, C. (2017). *Pharmacology for nurses: A pathophysiologic approach* (5th ed.). New York, NY: Pearson.

Adams, M., & Urban, C. (2016). *Pharmacology: Connections to nursing practice* (3rd ed.). New York, NY: Pearson.

Agency for Healthcare Policy and Research, www.ahcpr.gov.

Berman, A., Snyder, S., & Frandsen, G. (2016). *Kozier & Erb's fundamentals of nursing: Concepts, process, and practice* (10th ed.). New York, NY: Pearson.

Burchum, J. (2016). *Lehne's pharmacology for nursing care* (9th ed.). St. Louis, MO: Elsevier.

Food and Drug Administration, www.fda.gov.

Ignatavicius, D. D., & Workman, M. L. (2016). *Medical-surgical nursing: Patient-centered collaborative care* (8th ed.). Philadelphia, PA: Elsevier.

Kee, J. L. (2017). *Pearson's handbook of laboratory and diagnostic tests* (8th ed.). New York, NY: Pearson.

National Institutes of Safety and Health, www.cdc.gov/niosh.

Olsen, J., Giangrasso, A., Shrimpton, D., & Dillon, P. (2016). *Medical dosage calculations: A dimensional analysis approach* (11th ed.). New York, NY: Pearson.

Smith, S. F., Duell, D. J., Martin, B. C., Gonzalez, L., & Aebersold, M. (2017). *Clinical nursing skills: Basic to advanced skills* (9th ed.). New York, NY: Pearson.

Wilson, B. A., Shannon, M., & Shields, K. (2016). *Pearson nurse's drug guide 2016*. New York, NY: Pearson.

ANSWERS & RATIONALES

2 Herbal Agents

Chapter Outline

Overview of Phytomedicines   Specific Phytomedicines   Nursing Management

NCLEX-RN® Test Prep

Access the NEW Web-based app that provides students with additional practice questions in preparation for the NCLEX experience.

Objectives

➤ Define the terms commonly associated with the use of herbs as supplements.
➤ Describe the general goals of therapy when administering specific herbal supplements.
➤ Describe the uses and dosages of various herbs used as supplements.
➤ Identify the cautions associated with the use of specific herbal supplements, including adverse effects, contraindications, and drug interactions.
➤ List the key client teaching points related to the use of herbs as supplements.

Review at a Glance

bulk unpackaged, loose body of plant used for tea or decoction

decoction liquid form of herb brewed from seeds, bark, and root; herb is covered with boiling water and covered, boiled, simmered, and then strained with water added for consumption

extract a solution or preparation containing active ingredient of herb made by pressing herb and then soaking it in alcohol or water, which is allowed to

evaporate; usually, it is put in a small amount of water for use

phytomedicine therapeutic agents or preparations made or derived from plants or plant parts

phytotherapy science of using plant-based medicines to treat illness

standardization act of conforming to a basis of comparison in size, weight, quality, strength, or the like

tea a liquid preparation using fresh or dried herb; boiling water is poured over the herb and allowed to steep for a period of time

tincture liquid extracts of herb most often alcohol-based, used internally or externally, taken in drops in small amount of juice or water; glycerin-based extracts are available when alcohol should be avoided

PRETEST

1 When a client asks the nurse about a magazine advertisement related to the therapeutic use of ginger, on which item should the nurse focus?

1. Client's ability to accurately assess reliability of information sources
2. Title and author of the article
3. Type of magazine in which the advertisement was found
4. Client's level of education

2 When a female client taking feverfew to prevent migraine headaches suspects she may be pregnant, the nurse should take which most appropriate action?

1. Instruct client to discontinue use of the feverfew.
2. Encourage client to have a pregnancy test performed.
3. Arrange for client to see her healthcare provider.
4. Suggest that client reduce the dosage of the feverfew.

3 The nurse interprets that a client is able to self-administer valerian root safely as a sleep aid after hearing the client state which information about valerian?

1. It is best to take the drug on an empty stomach.
2. It should not be taken with benzodiazepine derivatives.
3. It may be used safely in children over the age of 5.
4. It is not effective in capsule form.

4 A client weighing 150 lb wants to verify she is taking a safe dose of bilberry. Since doses of greater than 1.5 grams/kg/day could be fatal, the nurse informs the client to avoid exceeding which dose per day? Record your answer rounding to two decimal places.

_____ grams

5 After it is determined that a 50-year-old client's hot flashes and night sweats are not related to any underlying disease process, the nurse could support the client's use of which herbal phytomedicine?

1. Echinacea
2. Black cohosh
3. Bilberry
4. Valerian

6 The nurse should interpret that which client statement best indicates that a client has sufficient knowledge of the potential therapeutic effectiveness of garlic?

1. "The effectiveness of garlic is based on scientific research."
2. "Garlic may be used safely with ginger."
3. "There are no remedies for bad breath caused by garlic."
4. "I can take garlic safely with over-the-counter medications."

7 The nurse is conducting a seminar for clients interested in the use of herbal remedies. Which statement by the nurse about hawthorn would be most accurate?

1. "You may use hawthorn for acute episodes of chest pain or angina."
2. "Hawthorn may increase your heart rate."
3. "You should not take hawthorn while taking captopril."
4. "Hawthorn is known to produce the same effects as verapamil."

8 To increase mental concentration and physical stamina, a client has been ingesting nutritional bars containing ginseng for the past 2 weeks. The nurse should provide which instruction to the client?

1. Avoid operating machinery or driving a car while taking the nutrition bar.
2. Refuse to take this form of the herb, since it is known to increase adverse effects.
3. Avoid use of the nutrition bar with coffee, tea, or cola.
4. Continue use of the nutrition bar daily as desired.

9 Because a client is taking St. John's wort capsules to treat mild depression, which statements should the nurse make to provide the client with appropriate information? Select all that apply.

1. "You may need to switch to another form of the herb."
2. "One dose of the drug may remain in the body for up to 24 hours."
3. "It may take several weeks for the therapy to become effective."
4. "You may find that the drug helps your arthritis as well."
5. "St. John's wort may not be effective for your type of depression."

10 Prior to supporting a client's decision to select evening primrose to manage a long history of insomnia, the nurse should make which assessment?

1. Ability to swallow
2. History of a seizure disorder
3. Where client learned about this function of the drug
4. Most recent red blood cell (RBC) count result

➤ *See pages 43–45 for Answers and Rationales.*

I. OVERVIEW OF PHYTOMEDICINES

A. General information

1. The Food and Drug Administration (FDA) classification of herbs is as dietary supplements
2. Other than **phytomedicine** (therapeutic agents or preparations made or derived from plants or plant parts), names for herbal therapies also include botanicals, nutraceuticals, and dietary supplements
3. Herbal supplements are not substitutes for conventional medicine
4. The science of using plant-based medicines to treat illness is called **phytotherapy**
5. Doses of herbs are not yet standardized in many countries other than Germany; dosage of herbs is according to product literature, although in most cases a research-based safe dose is yet to be determined
6. Most herbs, except ginger, are contraindicated during pregnancy and lactation
7. The pharmacologically active chemicals in herbal products may come from one specific plant part or all parts, including leaves, stems, flowers, rhizomes, or roots

B. Frequency of use

1. More than 28 million Americans report taking one or more herbal supplements
2. Primary users tend to be college-educated women between the ages of 35 and 49
3. Many people use herbal products in addition to a conventional treatment, rather than a replacement

C. USP Verification Program

1. Manufacturer submits products for examination of ingredients
2. If product meets stringent standards of USP it may carry USP label, which verifies that product has been manufactured under acceptable standards of purity, has been tested for active ingredients stated on label, and is free of harmful contaminants
3. USP label is not a guarantee that product is either safe or effective

II. SPECIFIC PHYTOMEDICINES

    A. Bilberry (*Vaccinium myrtillus*, European blueberry, huckleberry, whortleberry)

        1. Description

            a. Relative of blueberry and cranberry

            b. Shrub with small, sweet black berries

            c. Active ingredients: anthocyanoside (antioxidant bioflavonoid), pectin (soluble fiber)

            d. Stabilizes collagen activity

            e. Prevents production and release of compounds that promote inflammation, such as histamine and prostaglandins

            f. Relaxes smooth muscle in vasculature

            g. Inhibits platelet aggregation

            h. Strengthens capillary wall membrane and reduces membrane permeability

        2. Uses

            a. Most commonly used for treatment of simple diarrhea

            b. Prevention and treatment of eye disorders: diabetic retinopathy, night blindness, macular degeneration, glaucoma, cataracts

            c. Diabetes mellitus

            d. Antioxidant

            e. Possible treatment of varicose veins, hemorrhoids

            f. Lowers cholesterol

            g. Cardiovascular problems

        3. Dosage

            a. Dosage varies considerably

            b. **Standardization** (act of conforming to a basis of comparison in size, weight, quality, strength, or the like) should contain 25% anthocyanoside

            c. 240–480 mg bid or tid of standardized **extract** (a solution or preparation containing active ingredient of herb made by pressing herb and then soaking it in alcohol or water, which is allowed to evaporate; usually, it is put in a small amount of water for use)

            d. 20–60 grams of dried fruit daily

        4. Cautions

            a. May increase coagulation time

            b. May interfere with iron absorption when taken internally

            c. Use cautiously with acetylsalicylic acid (aspirin), anticoagulants, vitamin E, fish oils, feverfew, garlic, ginger, ginkgo

            d. Contraindicated in pregnancy and lactation

            e. Avoid long-term large doses, doses over 1.5 grams/kg/day may be fatal, doses over 480 mg/day may be dangerous

    B. Black cohosh (*Cimicifuga racemosa*, black snakeroot, bugroot, rattleweed, rattleroot, squawroot, cimifuga)

        1. Description

            a. Active ingredients: triperpenoid glycosides, isoflavonones, aglycones

            b. Binds to estrogen receptors

            c. Inhibits luteinizing hormone

            d. Apparent estrogen-like activity

         2. Uses

            a. Primarily used to treat premenstrual syndrome (PMS) and postmenopausal symptoms

            b. Promotes labor of pregnancy

            c. Decreases blood pressure

            d. Treatment of snake bites

            e. Rheumatoid arthritis

            f. Recommended uses by herbalists: dysmenorrhea, antispasmodic, astringent, diuretic, expectorant, sedative

        3. Dosage

            a. Research-based safe dosage yet to be determined

            b. 40 mg daily

            c. Possible stimulation of estrogen synthesis with 8 mg/day for 8 weeks

        4. Cautions

            a. Contraindicated use with antihypertensives or hormone replacements

            b. May cause bradycardia, hypotension, joint pain

            c. Contraindicated in lactation

            d. Use in pregnancy only when birth is imminent to promote labor

C. Chamomile (*chamomilla recutita*)

    1. Description

        a. Derived from dried heads of German/Hungarian chamomile flower

        b. Flower heads and essential oil used

    2. Uses

        a. Commonly used as a mild sedative to aid in sleeping

        b. Antiflatulent and antispasmodic; often used to quiet GI spasms and upset

        c. Antimicrobial; may be useful for wound healing

        d. Anti-inflammatory

    3. Dosage

        a. Usually consumed in amounts of 1–4 cups daily as a **tea** (a liquid preparation using fresh or dried herb); boiling water is poured over the herb and allowed to steep for a period of time

        b. If taken by tablet, 400–1,600 mg daily

    4. Cautions

        a. Vomiting may occur with highly concentrated tea

        b. May increase bleeding if taken with antiplatelet agents, anticoagulants, NSAIDs

        c. **Tincture** (liquid extracts of herb most often alcohol-based, used internally or externally, taken in drops in small amount of juice or water) often contains alcohol; glycerin-based extracts are available when alcohol should be avoided

        d. Contraindicated in children, pregnancy, and lactation

        e. Do not use if allergic to asters, ragweed, or chrysanthemums; may cause severe allergic response

D. Cranberry (trailing swamp cranberry, marsh apple, bog cranberry)

    1. Description

        a. Active ingredients: anthocyanins, proanthocyanins, catechin, triterpenoids, and organic acids (citric, malic, quinic, benzoic, and glucoronic)

        b. Prevents *Escherichia coli* from adhering to bladder wall, teeth, and gums

        c. Acidifies the urine

    2. Uses

        a. Primarily used to prevent urinary tract infections

        b. Decreases incidence of urinary calculi

        c. Decreases blood pressure

        d. Reduces urine odor in incontinent clients

        e. Decreases symptoms of chronic pyelonephritis

        f. As unsweetened juice, may prevent accumulation of gum bacteria and reduce plaque formation

        g. May be used in drug overdoses to help with urinary excretion of phencyclidine

   3. Dosage
      a. Capsules: 300–500 mg twice daily; may use up to 9/day
      b. Juice: 3–10 oz unsweetened juice daily
   4. Cautions
      a. Avoid use in presence of urinary obstruction
      b. Excessive use may cause diarrhea
      c. Instruct clients with diabetes mellitus to use sugar-free solution if using cranberry mixes
      d. Notify healthcare provider if signs of UTI persist
      e. May reduce oral clearance of nifedipine, leading to increased serum concentrations
      f. May increase INR when taken in combination with warfarin

E. Echinacea (*Echinacea purpurea*, snake root, purple or American cone flower, sampson root, black sampson, hedgehog, survey root)
   1. Description
      a. Member of daisy family with nine species
      b. Active ingredients: polysaccharides, alkylamides, flavonoids, caffeic acid derivatives (echinacosides), essential oils, and others
      c. Available in capsule, tablet, candle, glycerite, hydroalcoholic extract, fresh-pressed juice, lollipop, lozenge, tea, and tincture forms
      d. Activates T lymphocytes and intensifies phagocytosis of macrophages
      e. Stimulates tumor necrosis factor, interferon, and interleukin
      f. Nonspecific stimulation of immune system
      g. Stabilizes hyaluronic acid (a component of connective tissue) to protect cells and connective tissue from microorganism invasion and attack from free radicals
      h. Inhibits lipoxygenase to reduce inflammation
   2. Uses
      a. Most common: prevention or reduction of symptoms of cold or influenza
      b. Boost immune system and increase body's resistance to infection, particularly upper respiratory and urinary infection
      c. Treatment of herpes simplex and *Candida* infection
      d. Topically: improve wound healing, antioxidant protection from ultraviolet A and B light rays
   3. Dosage
      a. Standardized preparation should contain 3.5% echinacoside
      b. Available in capsule of powdered herb, expressed juice, tincture, water- or alcohol-based formula, fluid extract, solid extract, lozenge forms
      c. Dosage dependent on formula potency; varies according to source consulted
      d. Typically supplied in 380-mg capsules: 1–3 capsules tid at mealtime with water
      e. Regime should consist of 8 weeks on and 1 week off to reduce decreased effects with continued use
   4. Cautions
      a. Not to be used in presence of autoimmune disease (e.g., HIV/AIDS, collagen disease, multiple sclerosis [MS], tuberculosis), severe illness or allergy to sunflower or daisy family
      b. Not to be used with immunosuppressants (e.g., corticosteroids or cyclosporine)
      c. Prolonged use (longer than 8-week cycle) may cause hepatotoxicity and suppression of immune system
      d. Not to be used with other hepatotoxicants (e.g., anabolic steroids, amiodarone, methotrexate, antifungals such as ketoconazole)
      e. May influence fertility by spermatozoa enzyme interference

  f. Many tinctures contain large amounts of alcohol

  g. Contraindicated in alcoholism, children, pregnancy, and lactation

  h. Adverse effects: allergic reaction and anaphylaxis

 5. Herb-to-drug interactions

  a. Amiodarone

  b. Anabolic steroids

  c. Ketoconazole

  d. Methotrexate

F. Feverfew (*Tanacetum parthenium*, bachelor's button, febrifuge plant, feather few, feather foil)

 1. Description

  a. Short, bushy perennial; member of daisy family with yellow flowers and yellow-green leaves resembling chamomile

  b. Active ingredients: sesquiterpene lactones, especially parthenolide, essential oils

  c. Suppresses secretion of granules in platelets and neutrophils to inhibit platelet aggregation

  d. May suppress production of prostaglandins (thromboxane, leukotriene)

  e. Inhibits release of serotonin

 2. Uses

  a. Principle use: prevent recurrent migraine headaches, treat arthritis

  b. Relief of menstrual pain

  c. Asthma

  d. Dermatitis, psoriasis

  e. Antipyretic (promotes diaphoresis)

 3. Dosage

  a. Dosage varies according to source consulted

  b. Standardized preparation should contain 0.2% parthenolide

  c. Available in freeze-dried leaf, dried plant part, capsules, infusion

  d. Supplied in 380-mg capsules containing pure leaf and 250-mg capsules of leaf extract

  e. Most sources recommend anywhere from 50 to 125 mg of dried herb taken with or after meals to reduce GI colic

  f. Migraine: 250–500 mg to prevent attack; 1–2 grams to control attack

  g. May chew one fresh or frozen leaf/day to obtain dose, but may cause mouth sores or gastric distress

  h. Infusion: ½ to 1 tsp of herb in 1 cup boiling water, steep for 5–10 minutes, 2 cups daily

 4. Cautions

  a. Long-term studies not done

  b. Contraindicated in pregnancy, lactation, and under age 2 years

  c. Cross allergy to ragweed

  d. Adverse effects: allergic reaction, lip and tongue swelling, mouth ulcers, abdominal colic, palpitations, increased menstrual flow

  e. Sudden withdrawal may cause post-feverfew syndrome (muscle aches, pain, and stiffness); taper off to discontinue

  f. Other proven (conventional) remedies for relief of migraine should be used first

  g. May interfere with blood-clotting mechanism; not to be used with bilberry, garlic, ginger, ginkgo

  h. Discontinue use prior to surgery or dental extractions to reduce risk of bleeding

  i. Feverfew is known to cause rebound headaches

 5. Herb-to-drug interactions that increase risk of bleeding: aspirin, heparin, nonsteroidal anti-inflammatory drugs (NSAIDs), warfarin, or other anticoagulants

G. Garlic (*Allium sativum*, stinking root or rose, nectar of the gods, camphor of the poor, poor man's treacle, rustic treacle)

1. Description
   a. Empirical support for effectiveness and use; most widely researched herb
   b. Active ingredients: (23 constituents), allicin (odorless, sulfur-containing amino acid), ajoene
   c. Should be crushed or bruised to effectively convert various enzymes, protein, lipids, amino acids, and other ingredients to active ingredient, allicin
   d. Allicin and ajoene are not found in dried garlic, but may be present if dried at low temperatures or taken in enteric-coated tablets
   e. Inhibits platelet aggregation
   f. Well-documented research shows that it inhibits metabolism of cholesterol, leading to reduction of cholesterol
   g. Increases bile acid secretion

2. Uses
   a. Principle use: reduce cholesterol (decreases triglycerides, low-density lipoproteins and increases high-density lipoproteins)
   b. Principle use: treatment of mild hypertension
   c. Reduce risk of stroke
   d. Antibacterial, antiviral, antifungal
   e. Anticancer properties
   f. Lower blood glucose
   g. Lay use: antihelminthic, antispasmodic, diuretic, carminative (relieves flatulence, digestant, expectorant, topical antibiotic)

3. Dosage
   a. Available in dried powder, fresh bulb, tablets (allicin total potential, garlic extract), antiseptic oil, fresh extract, freeze-dried garlic powder, garlic oil (essential oil)
   b. Commercial preparation not standardized; should deliver minimum of 10 mg daily or 5,000 mcg of total allicin potential
   c. One clove of fresh garlic daily; mince one clove (necessary to activate the allicin), allow to stand 10–15 minutes, mix with yogurt, applesauce, honey, etc.; do not chew
   d. High dose of garlic can lead to GI problems

4. Cautions
   a. Avoid large amounts of garlic with other herbs affecting coagulation (bilberry, feverfew, ginger, ginkgo)
   b. May potentiate antidiabetic drugs
   c. Adverse effects: contact dermatitis, vertigo, garlic breath, hypothyroidism, GI irritation, nausea and vomiting with large doses
   d. Enteric-coated tablets containing powdered form may reduce bad breath, but are not as potent as raw garlic
   e. Contraindicated in pregnancy, GI (peptic ulcer disease and GERD), and bleeding disorders
   f. Chronic use may lower hemoglobin levels
   g. When used to decrease cholesterol levels, plan should be monitored by the healthcare provider

5. Herb-to-drug interactions
   a. Aspirin, NSAIDs, warfarin, or other anticoagulants (increased risk of bleeding); note: 5–20 garlic cloves equivalent to one 325-mg aspirin
   b. Insulin or oral antidiabetic agents (enhanced hypoglycemic effect)

Practice to Pass

Name three types of phytomedicines that are contraindicated in the client with a history of hemorrhagic stroke.

H. Ginger (*Zingiber officinal*, Jamaica ginger, African ginger, Cochin ginger, black ginger, race ginger)
1. Description
   a. Green-purple flower resembling the orchid
   b. Active ingredient: sesquiterpenes, aromatic ketones (gingerols), and volatile oils
   c. Inhibits thromboxane production to enhance effects of anticoagulation
   d. Inhibits leukotrienes and prostaglandins to produce anti-inflammatory and analgesic effect
2. Usage
   a. Principle use: antiemetic, improve appetite, treatment of motion sickness and vertigo
   b. Diuretic, digestion aid, dyspepsia
   c. Anti-inflammatory in treatment of rheumatoid arthritis and osteoarthritis
   d. Relief of muscle pain
   e. Antitumor, antioxidant, antimicrobial
3. Dosage
   a. Dosage depends on use—consensus varies
   b. Available in capsules, liquid, powder extract, root, chewable tablets, tea, candied form
   c. Most commonly available in 500-mg capsules of powdered form
   d. Antiemetic: 500–1,000 mg in four divided doses/day of powdered ginger
   e. Dyspepsia, diuretic, vertigo: 2–4 grams/day in divided doses or 2 cups tea with 1 tsp fresh ginger root each or 0.5 tsp ground ginger or two 1-inch squares of candied ginger that may be repeated every 4 hours as needed
   f. Antiemetic: 1–2 grams in two divided doses
   g. Motion sickness: 1 gram 30 minutes before traveling and 0.5–1 gram every 4 hours as needed during trip (most effective when regimen started several days before traveling)
4. Cautions
   a. Adverse effects: headache, anxiety, insomnia, elevated blood pressure, tachycardia, asthma attack, postmenopausal bleeding
   b. Contraindicated in postoperative nausea caused by increased risk of bleeding
   c. Not to be used concomitantly with bilberry, feverfew, garlic, or ginkgo (increased risk of bleeding)
   d. Severe overdose: possible CNS depression and cardiac arrhythmias
   e. Dose in excess of 6 grams/day results in gastric irritation and ulcer formation
   f. Conflicting data related to safe use during pregnancy (relatively safe according to FDA); contraindicated in treatment of hyperemesis gravidarum
   g. Discontinue use 2 weeks before surgery or dental extractions
5. Herb-to-drug interactions (increased risk of bleeding): aspirin, heparin, NSAIDs, warfarin, or other anticoagulants

I. Ginkgo (*Ginkgo biloba*)
1. Description
   a. Active ingredients: flavone glycosides, flavonoids, terpene lactones (such as ginkgolides and bilobalide)
   b. Ginkgo biloba extract referred to as GBE
   c. Flavonoids act as antioxidants by destroying lipid layer of cell membrane
   d. Flavone glycosides produce mild platelet aggregation inhibition
   e. Ginkgolides antagonize platelet-activating factor to decrease coagulation
   f. Bilobalide increases cerebral circulation to improve tissue perfusion and increase memory
   g. Protects brain from effects of hypoxia

2. Uses
   a. Cerebrovascular insufficiency and symptomatic relief of organic brain dysfunction to improve short-term memory loss
   b. Peripheral vascular disease (e.g., Raynaud disease, intermittent claudication), varicosities
   c. Senile macular degeneration
   d. Treatment of age-related mental decline related to short-term memory loss, poor concentration
   e. Treatment of depression-related cognitive disorders
   f. Treatment of depression in older adults particularly related to chronic cerebrovascular deficiency not responding to standard drug therapy
   g. Tinnitus, vertigo
   h. Improvement of symptoms of early-stage senility of Alzheimer's type
   i. Reduces asthma symptoms by reducing platelet-activating factor

3. Dosage
   a. Standardization should contain 24% flavonoids and 6% terpenes
   b. Available in capsule or tablet form containing 40 mg GBE, nutrition bars, sublingual sprays, tablets, concentrated alcohol extract of fresh leaf
   c. Treatment of vascular disorders, tinnitus, or vertigo: 120–160 mg/day in two or three divided doses
   d. Treatment of dementia: 120–240 mg/day in two or three divided doses

4. Cautions
   a. Effects may not be apparent for 4–8 weeks
   b. Not to be used concomitantly with bilberry, feverfew, garlic, ginger, or other anticoagulants, such as ASA (aspirin) or warfarin
   c. Avoid use of unprocessed ginkgo leaves that contain allergens related to urushiol, the chemical responsible for the itch in poison ivy
   d. Crude, dried leaf or tea may not contain sufficient active ingredients to be effective
   e. Large doses may cause restlessness, headache, nausea and vomiting, diarrhea
   f. Edible solid form sold in Asian shops should be kept out of reach of children as seeds may cause seizures
   g. Avoid use in pregnancy, lactation, children

5. Herb-to-drug interactions
   a. Aspirin or NSAIDs
   b. Heparin, warfarin, or other anticoagulant
   c. Monoamine oxidase inhibitors (MAOIs)
   d. Tricyclic antidepressants (TCAs)

J. **Ginseng, Korean** (*Panax ginseng*, American ginseng)
   1. Description
      a. Active ingredients: triterpenoid saponin glycosides (ginsenosides, panaxosides)
      b. Possible effect on pituitary gland with action similar to corticosteroids
      c. Improves glycosylated hemoglobin (HbA1c) and amino terminal propeptide (PIIINP) concentrations
      d. Hypertensive effect with low doses, hypotensive effect with higher doses
      e. Improves serum cholesterol and triglyceride levels
   2. Uses
      a. Most common: counteract effects of physical and mental fatigue
      b. Improve stamina and concentration in healthy individuals
      c. Treatment of chronic hepatotoxicity related to alcohol and drug ingestion
      d. Improve body's ability to resist stress and disease, increase vitality
      e. Regulation of blood pressure
      f. Improve psychomotor performance (attention, auditory reaction time)

Practice to Pass

A college student asks the nurse about the use of gingko biloba during exam week to enhance performance on exams. What client education is necessary?

       g. Reduce serum cholesterol and triglyceride levels

       h. Regulation of blood glucose levels in type 2 diabetes mellitus

       i. Aphrodisiac

       j. Adjunct in cancer chemotherapy or radiation therapy

  3. Dosage

       a. Depends on species and strength

       b. Confirmation of standards varies according to source

       c. Available in capsule, extract, root powder, tea, cream, eye gel, nutrition bar, oil, **bulk** (unpackaged, loose body of plant used for tea or decoction); a **decoction** is a term referring to a liquid form of herb brewed from seeds, bark, and root; herb is covered with boiling water, and covered, boiled, simmered, and then strained with water added for consumption

       d. Little consensus on dosing with wide variations, but universal acceptance of ginseng-free period; dosing should be spaced at intervals (e.g., 2–3 weeks on, 12 weeks off)

       e. 0.5–1 gram in two divided doses for 2–3 weeks, 1–2 weeks off

       f. Best taken in morning, 2 hours before meal, not less than 2 hours after meal

  4. Cautions

       a. Most side effects reported related to excessive or inappropriate use

       b. Avoid concomitant use with stimulants (e.g., coffee, tea, cola)

       c. May potentiate MAOI actions

       d. Adverse effects: insomnia, palpitations, pruritus

  5. Herb-to-drug interactions

       a. CNS depressants

       b. Digoxin

       c. Diuretics

       d. Insulin or oral antidiabetic agents

       e. MAOIs

       f. Warfarin or other anticoagulants

K. Ginseng, Siberian (*Eleutherococcus senticosus*, five fingers, tartar root, Western ginseng, seng and sang, Asian ginseng)

  1. Description

       a. Active ingredients: eutherosides

       b. Pharmacological actions not well understood

       c. Elevates lymphocyte count (T cells), boosts immune system

  2. Uses

       a. Enhances physical and mental performance under stress

       b. Improves athletic performance

       c. Increases oxygen metabolism, work capacity, and exhaustion time in variety of illnesses (e.g., atherosclerosis, diabetes, chronic bronchitis)

       d. Stimulates WBC production in clients undergoing antineoplastic therapy

  3. Dosage

       a. Little consensus on dosing with wide variations, but general consensus on ginseng-free period of 2–3 weeks every 4–8 weeks

       b. 0.6–3 grams daily

  4. Cautions

       a. Adverse reactions: hypertension, tachycardia, insomnia, and irritability

       b. Contraindicated in pregnancy, lactation, premenopausal women, hypertension, CNS stimulants, or antipsychotic medications

L. Glucosamine and **chondroitin** (glucosamine extracted from skeletons of crustaceans and other arthropods and synthetically; chondroitin extracted from shark or beef cartilage, bovine trachea, or synthetic)

1. Description
   a. Compounds found in healthy cartilage and synovial fluid
   b. Ingredients may be taken separately but most often used jointly
   c. Helps slow cartilage degradation in osteoarthritis
   d. Improves pain and movement in osteoarthritis and temporomandibular joint (TMJ)
2. Uses
   a. Osteoarthritis, TMJ
   b. Venous insufficiency, leg pain
   c. Inflammatory bowel disease, rheumatoid arthritis
   d. Chondroitin used to help with bladder control in interstitial cystitis, overactive bladder, and unstable bladder
3. Dosage
   a. Glucosamine—1,000–1,500 mg/day
   b. Chondroitin—800–1,200 mg/day
4. Cautions
   a. Avoid use in pregnancy and lactation
   b. Higher doses of glucosamine may be needed if taking diuretics
   c. Use with caution in kidney disease, diabetes, bleeding disorders, or if taking drugs that affect bleeding times
   d. Adverse effects: well tolerated; may cause GI upset, drowsiness, or insomnia

M. **Hawthorn** (*Crataegus oxyacantha*, Mayblossom, Maybush, whitehorn, LI 132)

1. Description
   a. Small to medium tree of several species; leaves, flowers, berries (fruit) are used in standardized extracts
   b. Active ingredients: flavonoids, primarily procyanidins and proanthocyanidins
   c. Acts as antioxidant that decreases damage by free radicals to cardiovascular system by increasing levels of vitamin C intracellularly
   d. Increases coronary and myocardial circulation
   e. Decreases peripheral vascular resistance to decrease blood pressure
   f. Increases strength of myocardial contraction (positive inotropic effect) and decreases heart rate (negative chronotropic effect)
   g. Angiotensin-converting enzyme (ACE) activity that prevents conversion of angiotensin I to angiotensin II, a potent vasoconstrictor
   h. Decreases total plasma cholesterol and low-density lipoprotein (LDL) levels
   i. Improves cardiac function in clients with chronic angina and those with early congestive heart failure
2. Uses
   a. Treatment of mild hypertension
   b. Treatment of athero- and arteriosclerosis
   c. Treatment (prevention) of chronic angina; not intended for acute angina
   d. Treatment of early congestive heart failure
3. Dosage
   a. Standardized preparation should contain 18.75% oligomeric procyanidins and 2.2% flavonoids
   b. Available in extract, berry capsule, leaf capsule, extended-release capsule, dried fruit, tincture
   c. Dried fruit: 0.2–1 gram tid
   d. Liquid extract (1:1 in 25% alcohol): 0.5–1 mL tid
   e. Tincture (1:5 in 45% alcohol): 1–2 mL tid or 20–40 drops tid
4. Cautions
   a. Contraindicated with concomitant use of prescription antihypertensives or nitrates

        b. Supervision of healthcare provider necessary for those with existing cardiac disease

        c. May interfere with digoxin pharmacodynamics and monitoring

        d. Adverse effects: nausea, fatigue, perspiration and cutaneous eruption of the hands, increased CNS depression and sedation

        e. Contraindicated in pregnancy and lactation

    5. Herb-to-drug interactions (drug effect)

        a. Digoxin additive

        b. ACE inhibitors

N. Milk thistle (*Silybum marianum*, Mary thistle, Marian thistle, Lady's thistle, Holy thistle, silymarin, the "liver herb")

    1. Description

        a. Tall plant, prickly leaves, milky sap, member of daisy family

        b. Active ingredients: silymarin and its component silybinin to act as hepatoprotectant

        c. Promotes glutathione production, a powerful endogenous antioxidant

        d. Binds to hepatocyte membrane to block uptake of toxins into liver cell

        e. Stimulates nucleolar polymerase A activity to promote new liver cell growth

        f. Stimulates regeneration of liver by stimulating protein synthesis

        g. Inhibits action of leukotriene by Kupffer cells

        h. Binds to site on liver cell membrane, blocking availability for attack from phalloidin, the toxin in death cap mushroom

        i. Stabilizes liver cell membrane by decreasing turnover rate of phospholipids

    2. Uses

        a. Reduces hepatotoxicity related to psychoactive drugs such as phenothiazines

        b. Adjunct therapy in liver inflammation related to cirrhosis, hepatitis, and fatty infiltrate related to alcohol or other toxins

        c. Treatment of overdose of death cap mushroom

    3. Dosage

        a. Available in capsule, tablet, extract, and 200 mg concentrated seed extract equal to 140 mg silymarin

        b. 140 mg tid (dosage varies according to source)

        c. Standardization should contain at least 70–80% silymarin

    4. Cautions

        a. Insoluble in water, not to be taken in tea form

        b. Avoid alcohol-based extract in decompensated cirrhosis

        c. Cross allergy to ragweed

        d. Adverse effects: loose stools, diarrhea in high doses

        e. Contraindicated in pregnancy and lactation

        f. Close monitoring by healthcare provider in presence of active liver disease

O. Saw palmetto (*Serenoa repens*, sabal, American dwarf palm tree, LSESR)

    1. Description

        a. Shrublike palm tree with red-brown/black berries

        b. Active ingredients: saturated and unsaturated fatty acids and sterols from berries (liposterolic acid)

        c. Reduces action of 5-alpha-reductase enzyme that converts testosterone to dihydrotestosterone (DHT) in aging (effects similar to finasteride with fewer side effects)

        d. No effect on prostatic-specific antigen

        e. May reverse testicular and mammary gland atrophy

        f. May increase sperm production and increase sexual vigor

2. Uses
   a. Symptomatic treatment of benign prostatic hyperplasia (BPH)
   b. Helps initiate urine stream, decreases urinary frequency, residual volumes, nocturia, dysuria; unclear whether actual prostatic size is reduced
   c. Lay uses: treatment of asthma, bronchitis, treatment of gynecomastia
3. Dosage
   a. Standardized extract should contain 85–95% fatty acids and sterols
   b. Mild to moderate BPH: 160 mg standardized liposterolic acid twice/day with meals to decrease GI distress OR 1–2 grams fresh berry decoction OR 0.5–1 gram dried berry PO tid
4. Cautions
   a. Long-term use with approximately 6 weeks for initial effects
   b. Insoluble in water, not to be taken in tea form
   c. Adverse effects: nausea, abdominal pain, hypertension, headache, diarrhea with large doses
   d. May interfere with iron absorption
   e. Supervision by healthcare provider necessary for diagnosed BPH
   f. Do not take with estrogen or hormone replacement
5. Herb-to-drug information: finasteride (enhanced effect)

P. Turmeric (Indian saffron, curcuma, red valerian)
1. Description
   a. Turmeric is derived from rhizome of plant *curcuma longa*
   b. Active ingredients: curcumin, sesquiterpene ketones, tumerin, oleo-resins
   c. Appears to inhibit carcinogenesis in all steps of cancer formation
   d. By inhibiting lipid peroxidation and sensitizing cortisol receptors, it has anti-inflammatory and antiarthritic activity
   e. Strong antihepatotoxic properties
   f. Reduces muscle injury after trauma
   g. Interferes with viral replication and may increase CD4 counts
   h. Increases immune function by increasing WBC and macrophage phagocytic activity
   i. Cholagogue activity promotes bile and intestinal motility
2. Uses
   a. Cancer prevention and adjuvant therapy
   b. Inflammatory conditions, including osteo- and rheumatoid arthritis, irritable bowel syndrome, gastric ulcers
   c. Flatulence, cholelithiasis, and colic
   d. Antioxidant
   e. Hepatoprotective
   f. Reduction of cholesterol and triglyceride levels
3. Dosage
   a. 1.5–4 grams of powdered resin
   b. Standardized extract (curcumin 95%): 350 mg twice daily
   c. Fresh tincture: 40–80 gtt (2–4 mL) two to three times a day
4. Cautions
   a. Isolated curcumin is poorly absorbed, so when taken for systemic effects, must have piperine added to promote absorption
   b. Avoid use in pregnancy (abortifacient effects) or breastfeeding
   c. Contraindicated in biliary obstruction
   d. Avoid large doses concurrently with anticoagulants; may increase bleeding risk
   e. High dose may inhibit fertility
   f. May decrease effect of immunosuppressants

Q. Red yeast rice (fermented rice, which obtains its color from cultivation with the mold *Monascus purpureus*)

1. Description
   a. Inhibits action of HMG CoA reductase in liver
   b. Lowers total cholesterol, low-density lipid (LDL) cholesterol, and triglycerides; increases high-density lipid (HDL) cholesterol
   c. Contains the substance monacolin K, the same substance contained in prescription drug lovastatin

Practice to Pass

What phytomedicine is known as the liver herb? Why?

2. Uses
   a. Hyperlipidemia, elevated cholesterol and triglyceride levels
   b. Coronary heart disease, circulation
   c. Diabetes mellitus
3. Dosage: 1,200 mg twice a day with food
4. Cautions
   a. Do not take in conjunction with prescription cholesterol-lowering medications
   b. Contraindicated in liver disease
   c. Grapefruit juice may elevate drug levels
   d. Adverse effects: gastritis, abdominal pain, headache, muscle pain
   e. Increased risk of rhabdomyolysis if taken with cyclosporine, ranitidine, and some antibiotics
5. Herb-to-drug interactions (drug effect)
   a. Additive effect may occur with benzodiazepines and barbiturates
   b. Altered drug levels can occur with thyroid medications, digoxin, St. John's wort, vitamin A, and coenzyme Q10

R. St. John's wort (*Hypericum perforatum*, amber, goat weed, touch-and-heal, St. John's wort, witch's herb, klamath weed, chasse-diable, devil's scourge)

1. Description
   a. Yellow perennial flower with red pigmented leaves containing small black dots
   b. Active ingredient: hypericin from red pigment leaves, pseudohypericin and flavonoids, tannin, and others
   c. Inhibits reuptake of serotonin
   d. Low MAOI
   e. Actions not well determined or understood
   f. Effects comparable to imipramine
   g. Produces fewer side effects than prescription antidepressants
2. Uses
   a. Treatment of mild to moderate depression
   b. Not intended for treatment of suicidal ideation, psychotic behavior, or severe depression
   c. Possible antibacterial, antiviral, wound-healing properties
   d. Topical application of *Hypericum* tincture or oil effective for herpetic lesions and shingles; topical oil useful for neuralgias, sunburn, shingles and nerve pain
3. Dosage
   a. Standardization should contain 0.14–0.3% hypericin
   b. Available in capsule, sublingual, dried plant, oil, tea, liquid tincture, topical cream
   c. Depression: capsules—300 mg tid; tincture—40–80 drops tid; tea—1–2 cups a.m. and p.m. with 1–2 heaping tsp dried herb per cup (steeped for 10 minutes); therapy should continue for 4–6 weeks
4. Cautions
   a. Not to be used concomitantly with prescription antidepressants, especially selective serotonin reuptake inhibitors (SSRI) or MAOIs or foods containing tyramine (such as aged cheese, smoked meats, liver, figs, dried or cured fish, yeast, beer, Chianti wine)

   b. Not to be used concomitantly with opioids, amphetamines, OTC cold and flu preparations

   c. May inhibit absorption of iron

   d. Adverse effects (may continue for 2–4 weeks): GI distress, emotional vulnerability, fatigue, pruritus, weight gain, headache, dizziness, restlessness

   e. May cause photosensitivity; avoid sun exposure, especially if fair-skinned

   f. May decrease digoxin levels

   g. Contraindicated in pregnancy, lactation, and children

5. Herb-to-drug interactions

   a. CNS depressants or opioid analgesics

   b. Cyclosporine

   c. MAOIs

   d. Efavirenz or protease inhibitors (antivirals)

   e. Antidepressants: TCAs or SSRIs

   f. Reserpine

   g. Theophylline

   h. Warfarin or other anticoagulants

S. Valerian root (*valeriana officinalis*, wild valerian, garden heliotrope, setwall, capon's tail, all-heal, Amantilla, Baldrian wurzel, benedicta)

1. Description

   a. Tall perennial with hollow stem, leaves, and white or red flowers

   b. Active ingredients: valepotriates and sesquiterpene derivatives, valeric acid, valeranone, and others

   c. Binds weakly to gamma aminobutyric acid (GABA) receptor sites to decrease CNS activity, causing sedation with decreased side effects

   d. Action similar to benzodiazepines, but does not lead to dependence, and does not cause morning hangover

2. Uses

   a. Sedative, reduction of anxiety, restlessness, tension

   b. Treatment of insomnia

   c. Adjunct therapy for benzodiazepine withdrawal

   d. Possible antispasmodic

3. Dosage

   a. Standardization should contain minimum of 0.5–0.8 valerenic acid or 0.8% valeric acid; tincture should contain 2% essential oils

   b. Available in capsule, tablet tincture, tea

   c. Composition and purity vary widely

   d. Insomnia: 150–500 mg of root extract one-half hour before bedtime or as tea with 1 tsp dried root per cup; repeat dose two to three times if needed

   e. Anxiety: 200–300 mg each a.m.

4. Cautions

   a. Valepotriate (which may be carcinogenic) should be removed from final product

   b. Not to be used concomitantly with other sedative/hypnotics, anxiolytics, or antidepressants

   c. May be used safely while operating machinery or car, although CNS effects should be monitored

   d. Sedation not increased with alcohol use, although caution should be exercised

   e. Adverse effects: headache; mild, temporary upset stomach

   f. Adverse effects with overdose or long-term use (overdose with 2.5 grams): excitability, insomnia, cardiac dysfunction, blurred vision, hepatotoxicity, severe headache, morning headache, nausea

Practice to Pass

What are some other names used to identify St. John's wort?

   !   **g.** May cause hepatotoxicity; monitor liver function and avoid use in hepatic
                dysfunction
          h. Extract contains 40–60% alcohol; avoid use in those with alcoholism
          i. Contraindicated in pregnancy and lactation
       5. Herb-to-drug interactions (additive sedation): barbiturates, benzodiazepines, and
              CNS depressants

III. NURSING MANAGEMENT

   ### A. General assessment
   !   **1.** Physical exam
          a. Vital signs, height, weight, lung sounds
          b. Depending on herb, liver and kidney function status
   !   **2.** History
          a. Age
          b. Comorbid diseases
          c. Allergies, including food and others
          d. Use of prescription, over-the-counter medications, and phytomedicines, all to be
                entered into client's health record
          e. Cultural beliefs that may be related to race or ethnicity
          f. Pregnancy (or potential) and lactation

   ### B. Principles of herbal administration
       1. General use
   !   **a.** Not intended for acute illness episodes or long-term therapy
          b. Appropriate as adjunct to conventional Western therapies
   !   **c.** Therapeutic effectiveness is slower than prescription medications; may take as
                long as several weeks, depending on herb
          d. Many herbs available in multiple forms, including teas, extracts, tinctures, capsules
                or tablets containing powdered or freeze-dried forms of herb
          e. Most herbs possess multiple uses, such as skin wash, gargle, compress, lotion, and
                eye bath
   !   **f.** They are not intended to replace healthy lifestyle
          g. Safe use in pregnancy and lactation is either contraindicated or unknown and
                may dry up breast milk during lactation
          h. Although they may be effective in children, phytomedicines should be avoided in
                acute, sudden-onset illness
   !   **i.** Many interact with other herbs, food, and prescription medications
       2. Government regulation
          a. Dietary Supplement Health and Education Act (DSHEA) of 1994 defines herbs
                as dietary supplements
          b. Not defined as medicines, herbs cannot make therapeutic claims, only how they
                affect structure and function of human body
   !   **c.** Food and Drug Administration (FDA) does not regulate use of phytomedicines in
                United States but approves certain ones for their action on body (how they affect
                structure and function)
          d. FDA does not monitor herbs for their quality, composition, or preparation
          e. Formulations vary in their potency and recommended dosage with frequent lack
                of consensus on dosing
          f. The National Center for Complementary and Alternative Medicine (NCCAM),
                under the National Institutes of Health (NIH), is the main research component in
                the government on phytomedicine

Practice to Pass

The client asks the nurse about safe use of phytomedicines. What should the nurse tell the client regarding what to look for on the container label?

3. Safety, labeling, and purity
   a. Container labels must carry a disclaimer stating FDA does not evaluate product for treating, curing, or preventing disease
   b. Labels should contain specific directions for dosing and use
   c. Only the standardized extract, when available, should be used
   d. Not all phytomedicines have empirical support for their safety and efficacy
   e. Much of the research and standardization originates in Europe, where use of phytomedicine is popular, particularly in Germany
   f. Many herbs contain toxic substances (e.g., arnica, belladonna, hemlock, lily of the valley, and sassafras)
   g. Healthcare providers should report all adverse effects of phytomedicines to the FDA's Med-Watch (online or 888-463-6332)

C. **Client education**
   1. Need for a complete history and physical before starting any therapy with herbs
   2. Phytomedicines are not effective for or to be used for acute illness or episodes
   3. Phytomedicines take longer to work than prescription medications, usually weeks
   4. Report use of all herbs to healthcare provider
   5. Start with one herb at a time, at lower than recommended doses, and closely monitor response
   6. Know particular use, dosing, and safe administration of each herb and take only as directed
   7. Herbs may cause allergic reactions and adverse effects; if these occur, discontinue herb and report symptoms to healthcare provider
   8. Become familiar with all herb–herb, herb–drug, and herb–food interactions
   9. Purchase herbs from a reputable source and be aware of where and how herb was processed
   10. Purchase standardized form of herbs, if possible
   11. "Natural" or "all natural" does not equate with herb safety or efficacy
   12. Become familiar with many various names by which particular herbs are identified
   13. Avoid use of phytomedicines in pregnancy (potential for pregnancy), lactation, and in children
   14. Accurately assess advertising claims; provide reputable sources of information, including referrals to the following resources on the Internet: American Botanical Council, Herb Research Foundation, National Center for Complementary and Alternative Therapy, and Natural Standard

Case Study

A client has been taking St. John's wort 300 mg tid for treatment of depression with good success. He also takes garlic (one to two cloves) daily to help keep his cholesterol levels low and ginkgo biloba, 40 mg daily, for improvement of memory. He is scheduled for an elective surgery.

1. What are possible unintended effects of St. John's wort, garlic, and ginkgo biloba?

2. Do you have any concerns with the client's use of the combination of these herbs?

3. What precautions should he take prior to surgery?

4. What teaching is indicated for his postoperative recovery?

For suggested responses, see page 538.

POSTTEST

1. A client with a history of chronic urinary tract infections (UTIs) has started taking cranberry capsule supplements in hopes of preventing the UTIs. Which statement is most appropriate for the nurse to make to the client?

   1. "These supplements may cause constipation."
   2. "Take at least 300–500 mg twice/day."
   3. "Always take the capsules with a full glass of milk."
   4. "Avoid taking capsules in the evening."

2. The nurse should interpret that glucosamine and chondroitin have met the intended therapeutic effect after assessing which outcome in a client?

   1. Relief of signs and symptoms of osteoarthritis
   2. Reduced severity of GI disturbances such as nausea and vomiting and bloating
   3. Reduction of hair loss and constipation
   4. Decreased manifestations of anxiety disorder

3. A client who uses fresh ginger for nausea does not like using kitchen spoons because they are not universal in size. The nurse provides the client with a medicine cup and instructs the client to fill to which mL line for a single dose of ginger? Record your answer rounding to a whole number.

   _____ mL

4. Which appropriate information should the home health nurse include in the health record of a client ingesting ginkgo biloba? Select all that apply.

   1. Client was instructed to be alert for unexpected bleeding.
   2. Client was informed that ibuprofen decreases ginkgo biloba's effects.
   3. Depression has improved since ingestion of ginkgo was initiated.
   4. Client was instructed to inform surgeon of long-term ingestion of the drug.
   5. Client was informed that drug is a potent enhancer of platelet-activating factor.

5. The nurse should document which statement as an appropriate outcome of teaching for a client using St. John's wort?

   1. Client is aware of the need to cease bowling activities.
   2. Client demonstrated knowledge of the need to wear protective clothing and apply sunscreen.
   3. Client able to select foods high in tyramine from a list as preferred to foods low in tyramine.
   4. Client aware of need to select a designated driver when ingesting non-alcoholic beverages at same time as herb.

6. Which client behavior most clearly indicates a client's acceptance of the nurse's instructions before beginning use of saw palmetto?

   1. Requests that the assigned healthcare provider prescribe liver function tests
   2. Agrees not to ingest ibuprofen or aspirin concurrently
   3. Agrees not to ingest laxatives or stool softeners concurrently
   4. Requests that the assigned healthcare provider prescribe a prostate-specific antigen (PSA) test

7 Because a client is ingesting red yeast rice, the nurse should perform which follow-up activity?

1. Assess the client for heavy menstrual bleeding.
2. Make sure drug has been discontinued because of abortifacient properties.
3. Monitor the client for excessive bruising or bleeding.
4. Determine that the client is not taking any prescription cholesterol-lowering medications.

8 The nurse should instruct the client not to use valerian root if the client has been prescribed which medication?

1. Estrogen
2. Alprazolam
3. Digoxin
4. Aspirin

9 The nurse informs a client diagnosed with increased intraocular pressure (IOP) that use of which phyto-medicine may decrease IOP?

1. Glucosamine/chondroitin
2. Black cohosh
3. Aloe
4. Bilberry

10 Which priority nursing concern is most appropriate for the client ingesting chamomile?

1. Constipation
2. Interruptions in sleep pattern
3. Changes in breathing pattern
4. Reduced gas exchange

➤ *See pages 45–46 for Answers and Rationales.*

ANSWERS & RATIONALES

Pretest

1 **Answer: 1 Rationale:** Because the herbal industry is not as highly regulated as traditional remedies, the focus should be on the client's ability to assess the reliability of the information source. Inability to use discretion could place the client at risk. The ability to make appropriate decisions about resources would include examining the author, the type of magazine, and the client's level of education. **Cognitive Level:** Analyzing **Client Need:** Pharmacological and Parenteral Therapies **Integrated Process:** Nursing Process: Assessment **Content Area:** Pharmacology **Strategy:** The wording of the question tells you that the correct option is likely to be one that is a broad statement rather than one that is narrow in focus. Evaluate each option, choosing the one that encompasses the other options within it. **Reference:** Smith, S. F., Duell, D. J., & Martin, B. C., Aebersold, M. L., Gonzalez, L. (2017). *Clinical nursing skills: Basic to advanced skills* (9th ed.). New York, NY: Pearson, pp. 551–553.

2 **Answer: 1 Rationale:** Regardless of the drug, avoiding the use of chemicals of any kind is a common underlying principle of management of the pregnant client.

Reducing the dosage is insufficient. The client should not take any further doses of the herb unless it is determined that the client is not pregnant. Consulting a healthcare provider is of lesser priority than immediately discontinuing the herb. **Cognitive Level:** Applying **Client Need:** Pharmacological and Parenteral Therapies **Integrated Process:** Nursing Process: Implementation **Content Area:** Pharmacology **Strategy:** The core issue of the question is knowledge that the use of the herb could be hazardous to the fetus during pregnancy. Consider that the primary concern is for the safety of the fetus to guide your selection. **Reference:** Adams, M. P., Holland, N., & Urban, C. (2017). *Pharmacology for nurses: A pathophysiologic approach* (5th ed.). New York, NY: Pearson, p. 109.

3 **Answer: 2 Rationale:** Since valerian root actions are similar to that of a benzodiazepine and lorazepam is a benzodiazepine derivative, they should not be taken together. There is no evidence supporting the herb's safe use in children or a relationship between the form of the herb and its effectiveness. It is not necessary to take it on an empty stomach. **Cognitive Level:** Applying **Client Need:** Pharmacological and Parenteral Therapies **Integrated Process:** Nursing Process: Evaluation **Content**

Area: Pharmacology **Strategy:** Consider that medications and herbs should not be combined to eliminate one option. Next, eliminate a second option because the literature does not provide evidence of safe use of this herb in children. Apply knowledge of safe use of this herb to choose between the remaining options. **Reference:** Adams, M. P., Holland, N., & Urban, C. (2017). *Pharmacology for nurses: A pathophysiologic approach* (5th ed.). New York, NY: Pearson, p. 109.

4 **Answer: 1,020 Rationale:** First convert the client's weight in pounds to kilograms by dividing 150 by 2.2 = 68 kg. Then multiply 68 by 1.5 grams to equal 1,020 grams. **Cognitive Level:** Applying **Client Need:** Pharmacological and Parenteral Therapies **Integrated Process:** Nursing Process: Planning **Content Area:** Pharmacology **Strategy:** First convert the client's weight to kilograms and then multiply it by the upper safe dose. **Reference:** Smith, S. F., Duell, D. J., Martin, B. C., Aebersold, M. L., & Gonzalez, L. (2017). *Clinical nursing skills: Basic to advanced skills* (9th ed.). New York, NY: Pearson, pp. 576, 634.

5 **Answer: 2 Rationale:** One of the major uses of black cohosh is the treatment of postmenopausal symptoms, which include hot flashes and night sweats. Echinacea is commonly utilized to boost the immune response. Bilberry is commonly utilized to treat acute diarrhea. Valerian has been used to aid in sleep. **Cognitive Level:** Analyzing **Client Need:** Pharmacological and Parenteral Therapies **Integrated Process:** Nursing Process: Implementation **Content Area:** Pharmacology **Strategy:** Most menopausal signs and symptoms occur at night. Associate *black* with *night* to help make a connection between the client's symptoms and this herbal agent. **Reference:** Smith, S. F., Duell, D. J., Martin, B. C., Aebersold, M. L., & Gonzalez, L. (2017). *Clinical nursing skills: Basic to advanced skills* (9th ed.). New York, NY: Pearson, p. 553.

6 **Answer: 1 Rationale:** The effectiveness of garlic is based on scientific evidence and clinical trials. Garlic has the ability to affect bleeding times and should not be taken with other herbs or over-the-counter medications, such as aspirin and ibuprofen, which also prolong bleeding times. Garlic is available in enteric-coated tablets, which is effective in reducing bad breath associated with the plant. **Cognitive Level:** Applying **Client Need:** Pharmacological and Parenteral Therapies **Integrated Process:** Nursing Process: Evaluation **Content Area:** Pharmacology **Strategy:** Specific knowledge is needed to answer the question. Apply information gleaned from current research regarding the herb to make a selection. **Reference:** Smith, S. F., Duell, D. J., Martin, B. C., Aebersold, M. L., & Gonzalez, L. (2017). *Clinical nursing skills: Basic to advanced skills* (9th ed.). New York, NY: Pearson, p. 553.

7 **Answer: 3 Rationale:** Hawthorn has an action that is similar to the action of angiotensin-converting enzyme (ACE) inhibitors, which reduce blood pressure by blocking the conversion of angiotensin I to angiotensin II, a potent vasoconstrictor. Its use should be restricted to chronic, self-limiting conditions and not for acute episodes of any nature. Hawthorn has a negative chronotropic effect resulting in a decreased heart rate rather than an increased one. Verapamil is a calcium channel blocker that decreases blood pressure by blocking the influx of calcium ions across the cardiac and arterial muscle cell membrane. **Cognitive Level:** Analyzing **Client Need:** Pharmacological and Parenteral Therapies **Integrated Process:** Nursing Process: Planning **Content Area:** Pharmacology **Strategy:** Associate the drug with the angiotensins and the relationship to vasoconstriction and blood pressure. **Reference:** Smith, S. F., Duell, D. J., Martin, B. C., Aebersold, M. L., & Gonzalez, L. (2017). *Clinical nursing skills: Basic to advanced skills* (9th ed.). New York, NY: Pearson, p. 553.

8 **Answer: 3 Rationale:** Because ginseng is a stimulant, it should not be used in combination with coffee, tea, or colas. There is no evidence that the herb affects the ability to drive a car or operate machinery, or that it is related to increased incidence of adverse effects. A ginseng-free period is recommended, usually 2–3 weeks on and 1–2 weeks off. **Cognitive Level:** Applying **Client Need:** Pharmacological and Parenteral Therapies **Integrated Process:** Nursing Process: Implementation **Content Area:** Pharmacology **Strategy:** Associate the herb with stimulation. This will assist you to eliminate each incorrect option systematically. **Reference:** Smith, S. F., Duell, D. J., Martin, B. C., Aebersold, M. L., & Gonzalez, L. (2017). *Clinical nursing skills: Basic to advanced skills* (9th ed.). New York, NY: Pearson, p. 553.

9 **Answer: 2, 3, 4 Rationale:** The drug has a half-life of 24 hours so St. John's wort may take several weeks before the effects are evident. The effectiveness of almost all phytomedicines is slower than prescribed medications; however, many antidepressants have long onset time periods as well. The drug also has anti-inflammatory actions so it might be useful in managing arthritis. The time period does not correlate with the drug's characteristics. St. John's wort is appropriate for the treatment of mild to moderate depression. **Cognitive Level:** Applying **Client Need:** Pharmacological and Parenteral Therapies **Integrated Process:** Teaching and Learning **Content Area:** Pharmacology **Strategy:** Associate the herb with long onset and antidepressants and then use the process of elimination to make a selection. **Reference:** Smith, S. F., Duell, D. J., Martin, B. C., Aebersold, M. L., & Gonzalez, L. (2017). *Clinical nursing skills: Basic to advanced skills* (9th ed.). New York, NY: Pearson, p. 553.

10 **Answer: 2 Rationale:** Seizures are a side effect of evening primrose so assessing for a history of seizures would be of key importance. The ability to swallow is an appropriate assessment prior to drug administration but is not unique to this drug. Determining the credibility of resources is an appropriate assessment for planning client care but is not unique to this particular herb. Immunosuppression is a more likely side effect than altered

ANSWERS & RATIONALES

red blood cell count. **Cognitive Level:** Applying **Client Need:** Pharmacological and Parenteral Therapies **Integrated Process:** Nursing Process: Assessment **Content Area:** Pharmacology **Strategy:** Associate the drug with epilepsy and match the herb with the critical word *seizure* in the correct option. **Reference:** Wilson, B. A., Shannon, M. T., & Shields, K. M. (2016). *Pearson nurse's drug guide 2016.* New York, NY: Pearson, p. 1740.

Posttest

1 **Answer: 2 Rationale:** The recommended dose for cranberry capsules is 300–500 mg twice daily. Cranberry taken in high doses may cause diarrhea, not constipation. It is not necessary to take the capsules with milk, although fluid, especially water, should be taken in liberal amounts when dealing with chronic UTIs. It is not necessary to avoid taking the capsules in the evening. **Cognitive Level:** Applying **Client Need:** Pharmacological and Parenteral Therapies **Integrated Process:** Nursing Process: Implementation **Content Area:** Pharmacology **Strategy:** Recall recommended dosing and common side effects of cranberry capsules. **Reference:** Wilson, B. A., Shannon, M. T., & Shields, K. M. (2016). *Pearson nurse's drug guide 2016.* New York, NY: Pearson, p. 1740.

2 **Answer: 1 Rationale:** The drug combination results in replacement of mucopolysaccharides, an element necessary for maintenance of joints, tendons, and cartilages. GI disturbances, alopecia, and constipation are side effects of the drug. Anxiolytic properties are more commonly associated with kava kava. **Cognitive Level:** Analyzing **Client Need:** Pharmacological and Parenteral Therapies **Integrated Process:** Nursing Process: Planning **Content Area:** Pharmacology **Strategy:** Associate glucosamine and chondroitin with the musculoskeletal system. **Reference:** Adams, M., Holland, L., & Urban, C. (2017). *Pharmacology for nurses: A pathophysiologic approach* (5th ed.). New York, NY: Pearson, p. 834.

3 **Answer: 5 Rationale:** The recommended dose of ginger is 1 teaspoon, which is equivalent to 5 mL. **Cognitive Level:** Applying **Client Need:** Pharmacological and Parenteral Therapies **Integrated Process:** Nursing Process: Planning **Content Area:** Pharmacology **Strategy:** Recall the recommended dose of ginger and then apply household-to-metric conversions to calculate correct answer. **Reference:** Smith, S. F., Duell, D. J., Martin, B. C., Aebersold, M. L., & Gonzalez, L. (2017). *Clinical nursing skills: Basic to advanced skills* (9th ed.). New York, NY: Pearson, p. 553.

4 **Answer: 1, 4, 5 Rationale:** Since ginkgo biloba can inhibit platelet-activating factor, it can contribute to an increase in bleeding. Because of the risk of bleeding, the client should discontinue the drug until after any surgery. Nonsteroidal anti-inflammatory drugs (NSAIDs) such as ibuprofen are more likely to increase the risk of bleeding also. The drug is a potent inhibitor of platelet-activating factor. Gingko is not indicated for use in

treating depression. **Cognitive Level:** Applying **Client Need:** Pharmacological and Parenteral Therapies **Integrated Process:** Communication and Documentation **Content Area:** Pharmacology **Strategy:** Evaluate the increased risk to clients with serious side effects associated with the drug. Specific knowledge of gingko biloba is needed to choose correctly. **Reference:.** Adams, M. P., & Urban, C. (2016). *Pharmacology: Connections to nursing practice* (3rd ed.). New York, NY: Pearson, pp. 62, 86.

5 **Answer: 2 Rationale:** One of the side effects of St. John's wort is photosensitivity, requiring the client to avoid direct exposure to sunlight, especially if fair-skinned. Because it may increase the toxic effects of monoamine oxidase inhibitors (MAOIs), foods high in tyramine should be avoided. The drug's effect should not interfere with bowling. The client should utilize a designated driver when ingesting alcoholic beverages. **Cognitive Level:** Applying **Client Need:** Pharmacological and Parenteral Therapies **Integrated Process:** Communication and Documentation **Content Area:** Pharmacology **Strategy:** Associate the side effects of the drug with risks to the client. **Reference:** Adams, M. P., & Urban, C. (2016). *Pharmacology: Connections to nursing practice* (3rd ed.). New York, NY: Pearson, p. 254.

6 **Answer: 4 Rationale:** Saw palmetto is used primarily in the treatment of benign prostatic hyperplasia (BPH) and male-pattern hair loss. Because the drug may cause a false-positive prostate-specific antigen (PSA), the test should be done before starting the drug. Additive bleeding risks can occur with concurrent ingestion of nonsteroidal anti-inflammatory drugs (NSAIDs) and ginger, gingko, and some other herbs, but not saw palmetto. The client may take laxatives or stool softeners. Liver function tests are unnecessary. **Cognitive Level:** Applying **Client Need:** Pharmacological and Parenteral Therapies **Integrated Process:** Nursing Process: Evaluation **Content Area:** Pharmacology **Strategy:** Apply knowledge of proper protocol associated with saw palmetto. **Reference:** Adams, M. P., & Urban, C. (2016). *Pharmacology: Connections to nursing practice* (3rd ed.). New York, NY: Pearson, p. 1221.

7 **Answer: 4 Rationale:** Red yeast rice inhibits HMG CoA reductase, leading to a decrease in total cholesterol, low-density lipoprotein, and triglyceride levels. Clients using this herbal supplement should avoid concurrent use of prescription drugs given to reduce these elements. There is no increased risk of bleeding or bruising. Red yeast rice is not an abortifacient. **Cognitive Level:** Applying **Client Need:** Pharmacological and Parenteral Therapies **Integrated Process:** Nursing Process: Implementation **Content Area:** Pharmacology **Strategy:** Associate the drug with reduced immunity. **Reference:** Adams, M., Holland, L., & Urban, C. (2017). *Pharmacology for nurses: A pathophysiologic approach* (5th ed.). New York, NY: Pearson, p. 105.

8 **Answer: 2 Rationale:** Alprazolam is a short- to intermediate-acting benzodiazepine. Concomitant use of this drug with valerian root should be avoided since their actions are similar and the herb may potentiate the action of the alprazolam. Valerian root may interact negatively with sedatives, narcotics, selective serotonin reuptake inhibitors (SSRIs), tranquilizers, and St. John's wort. Estrogen should be avoided with saw palmetto. Digoxin should be avoided with St. John's wort. Aspirin should be avoided with milk thistle. **Cognitive Level:** Applying **Client Need:** Pharmacological and Parenteral Therapies **Integrated Process:** Teaching and Learning **Content Area:** Pharmacology **Strategy:** Associate valerian root with Valium, a benzodiazepine that has diazepam as the generic name. **Reference:** Adams, M. P., & Urban, C. (2016). *Pharmacology: Connections to nursing practice* (3rd ed.). New York, NY: Pearson, pp. 86, 227.

9 **Answer: 4 Rationale:** Increased intraocular pressure (IOP) is symptomatic of glaucoma. Bilberry is useful in the treatment of this and other eye disorders, such as diabetic retinopathy, night blindness, macular degeneration, and cataracts. Glucosamine chondroitin is used in the treatment of osteoarthritis. Black cohosh is used for the relief of postmenstrual symptoms, such as hot flashes and insomnia. Aloe is used for skin ulcerations and GI disturbances. **Cognitive Level:** Analyzing **Client Need:** Pharmacological and Parenteral Therapies **Integrated Process:** Nursing Process: Planning **Content Area:** Pharmacology **Strategy:** Associate bilberry with glaucoma. **Reference:** Smith, S. F., Duell, D. J., Martin, B. C., Aebersold, M. L., & Gonzalez, L. (2017). *Clinical nursing skills: Basic to advanced skills* (9th ed.). New York, NY: Pearson, p. 553.

10 **Answer: 2 Rationale:** Chamomile has a variety of properties and is indicated for the treatment of GI spasms, insomnia or difficulty falling asleep, mouth ulcers, anxiety, and infant colic. It reduces flatulence but does not treat constipation. It does not change the breathing pattern. It does not affect gas exchange. **Cognitive Level:** Applying **Client Need:** Pharmacological and Parenteral Therapies **Integrated Process:** Nursing Process: Diagnosis **Content Area:** Pharmacology **Strategy:** Associate this drug with calming and sedative properties. **Reference:** Smith, S. F., Duell, D. J., Martin, B. C., Aebersold, M. L., & Gonzalez, L. (2017). *Clinical nursing skills: Basic to advanced skills* (9th ed.). New York, NY: Pearson, p. 553.

References

Adams, M. P., Holland, N., & Urban, C. (2017). *Pharmacology for nurses: A pathophysiologic approach* (5th ed.). New York, NY: Pearson.

Adams, M. P., & Urban, C. (2016). *Pharmacology: Connections to nursing practice* (3rd ed.). New York, NY: Pearson.

Burchum, J., & Rosenthal, L. (2016). *Lehne's pharmacology for nursing care* (9th ed.). St. Louis, MO: Mosby.

Drug Facts & Comparisons (Updated monthly). St. Louis, MO: Wolters Kluwer.

Fontaine, K. L. (2015). *Complementary and alternative therapies for nursing practice* (4th ed.). Upper Saddle River, NJ: Pearson.

Karch, A. M. (2017). *Focus on nursing pharmacology* (7th ed.). Philadelphia, PA: Lippincott Williams & Wilkins.

Kee, J. L. (2017). *Pearson's handbook of laboratory and diagnostic tests with nursing implications* (8th ed.). New York, NY: Pearson.

Kuhn, M., & Winston, D. (2013). *Winston and Kuhn's herbal therapy and supplements: A scientific and traditional approach* (3rd ed.). Philadelphia, PA: Lippincott.

LeMone, P. T., Burke, K. M., Bauldoff, G., & Gubrud, P. (2015). *Medical surgical nursing: Clinical reasoning in patient care* (6th ed.). New York, NY: Pearson.

Lilley, L. L., Rainforth Collins, S., et al. (2017). *Pharmacology and the nursing practice* (8th ed.). St. Louis, MO: Mosby.

Smith, S. F., Duell, D. J., Martin, B. C., Aebersold, M. L., & Gonzalez, L. (2017). *Clinical nursing skills: Basic to advanced skills* (9th ed.). New York, NY: Pearson.

Wilson, B. A., Shannon, M. T., & Shields, K. M. (2016). *Pearson nurse's drug guide 2016*. New York, NY: Pearson.

Neurologic and Musculoskeletal System Medications

3

Chapter Outline

Analgesics
Antiepileptics
Central Nervous System (CNS)
Stimulants

Medications to Treat Parkinson
Disease
Medications to Treat Alzheimer
Disease

Centrally Acting Skeletal
Muscle Relaxants
Anti-anxiety, Sedative, and
Hypnotics

Objectives

➤ Describe general goals of therapy when administering neurologic
and musculoskeletal system medications.
➤ Identify significant nursing considerations related to administering
opioid analgesics.
➤ Explain side effects and adverse effects of acetylsalicylic acid
(aspirin), acetaminophen, and nonsteroidal anti-inflammatory drugs
(NSAIDs).
➤ Identify major antiepileptic medication classifications.
➤ Describe significant client education points related to the
administration of antiepileptics.
➤ Explain nursing considerations related to the administration of
central nervous system (CNS) stimulants.
➤ Explain nursing considerations related to the administration of
medications commonly used to treat Parkinson disease, Alzheimer
disease, narcolepsy, and attention-deficit/hyperactivity disorder.
➤ Identify primary uses, interactions, major side effects, and adverse
or toxic effects of the most commonly prescribed musculoskeletal
relaxants.
➤ List significant client education points related to neurologic and
musculoskeletal system medications.

NCLEX-RN® Test Prep

Access the NEW Web-based app
that provides students with additional
practice questions in preparation
for the NCLEX experience.

Review at a Glance

anorexia loss of appetite
**attention-deficit/hyperactivity
disorder** also called ADHD; a condition in which a person demonstrates
inattention, impulsivity, and possibly
hyperactivity in a persistent pattern for
more than a 6-month period
diplopia double vision

epilepsy a chronic disorder characterized by recurring seizures in which there
is a disturbance in some type of behavior
(i.e., motor, sensory, autonomic, consciousness, or mentation)
**gamma-aminobutyric acid
(GABA)** an excitatory neurotransmitter
that is one of the amino acids

gingival hyperplasia increased
growth of gum tissue; an adverse effect
of antiepileptics, especially phenytoin
hepatotoxicity a state in which liver
damage has occurred; symptoms include
dark urine, clay-colored stools, yellowing
of skin, sclera, itching, abdominal pain,
fever, and diarrhea

intracranial pressure pressure inside skull; when increased may cause serious to disastrous sequelae

level of consciousness state of awareness that includes orientation (arousal and wakefulness) and cognition (sum of cerebral mental functions)

narcolepsy inability to stay awake during the day, regardless of amount of sleep or stimulation

nystagmus involuntary oscillation of eyes

paresthesias abnormal sensations, whether spontaneous or evoked

psychomotor seizures a term referring to complex partial (focal) seizures that cause client to lose consciousness or black out for a few seconds; characteristic behavior may include lip smacking, patting, and picking at clothes

reticular activating system a diffuse system that extends from lower brainstem to cerebral cortex; controls sleep–wake cycle, consciousness, focused attention, and sensory perceptions

spasms involuntary contractions of large muscle groups (arms, legs, neck)

spasticity increased resistance to passive movement, often more pronounced at extremes of range of motion and followed by a sudden or gradual release of resistance

status epilepticus a true neurologic emergency in which a seizure lasts more than 4 minutes or seizures are so frequently repeated or prolonged that they created a lasting condition (more than 30 minutes)

Stevens–Johnson syndrome an acute inflammatory disorder of the skin and mucous membranes (toxic epidermal necrolysis)

tonic–clonic seizures formerly grand mal seizures; tonic phase begins with a sudden loss of consciousness and a major tonic contraction (stiffening of body and extremities) that lasts for about 1 minute; clonic phase is characterized by violent, rhythmic, muscular contractions and hyperventilation that lasts from 30 seconds to a minute; postictal phase is a deep sleep followed by a period of confusion and lethargy that can last minutes to hours

PRETEST

1 Methylphenidate is newly prescribed for a client with narcolepsy. The nurse should report which priority health history component to the prescriber?

1. Congestive heart failure (CHF)
2. Diabetes mellitus
3. Irritable bowel syndrome
4. Anemia

2 A medication regimen that includes phenytoin has controlled the seizures of an adult client for several days. Prior to discharge, the nurse should place highest priority on including which information in the teaching plan? Select all that apply.

1. Many seizure disorders will eventually stop on their own.
2. Adherence to medication therapy is essential to avoid recurrence of seizures.
3. Side effects may include confusion and headache.
4. The client cannot drive a vehicle permanently.
5. Labwork for drug levels will need to be done routinely.

3 The nurse should include which instruction when teaching a client prescribed ergotamine tartrate for treatment of cluster headaches?

1. "Take the medication every 4 hours."
2. "Take the medication with plenty of water."
3. "You will feel energetic and warm after taking the medication."
4. "Lie down in a darkened room after taking the medication."

4 Because a client with a spinal cord injury has developed spasticity, the nurse should prepare to teach the client about which newly prescribed medication?

1. Dexamethasone
2. Dantrolene
3. Donepezil
4. Dobutamine

5 An opioid analgesic has been administered to a client postoperatively. The nurse should make which priority follow-up assessments? Select all that apply.

1. Respiratory rate and level of consciousness
2. Blood pressure and heart rate
3. Interactions with foods and other prescribed drugs
4. History of drug abuse and pain management history
5. Pain level

6 The nurse should include which precaution when teaching a client with liver disease about the use of over-the-counter (OTC) acetaminophen, aspirin, or nonsteroidal anti-inflammatory drugs (NSAIDs)?

1. "Take your temperature before taking one of these drugs."
2. "Consult your healthcare provider before taking one of these medications."
3. "You should have your cholesterol level measured before using these medications."
4. "Taper the discontinuance of any of these medications over a 3-day period."

7 Because phenytoin was prescribed STAT for a client who was just admitted to the nursing unit from the emergency department, which set of assessments is of highest priority for the nurse to perform?

1. Hydration status and emotional response to seizures
2. Blood urea nitrogen, creatinine, and urine output
3. Seizure activity, mental status, and respiratory status
4. Electrolytes, serum osmolality, and leg edema

8 A client with chronic depression has a new medication prescription for phenelzine. The nurse calls the prescriber to clarify the prescription if the client is already taking which medications? Select all that apply.

1. Propranolol
2. Meperidine
3. Glucagon
4. Carbamazepine
5. Dicyclomine

9 The nurse should include in a teaching plan for a client diagnosed with seizure disorder that which drug groups can potentiate the effects of the prescribed carbamazepine?

1. Nonsteroidal anti-inflammatory drugs (NSAIDs)
2. Anorexiants and amphetamines
3. Anticholinergics
4. Hydantoins and benzodiazepines

10 The client with a spinal cord injury is taking dantrolene for spasticity. The nurse should instruct the client to notify the healthcare provider immediately if which adverse effects occur? Select all that apply.

1. Persistent diarrhea
2. Change in blood or urine glucose levels
3. Abdominal pain, scleral jaundice
4. Painful urination and urinary frequency
5. Change in hearing or smell

➤ *See pages 80–81 for Answers and Rationales.*

I. ANALGESICS

A. Opioids

1. Action and use
   a. Symptomatic relief of severe acute and chronic pain
   b. Most commonly used in postoperative settings and to treat pain caused by malignancy
   c. Produce effects by binding to opioid receptors throughout central nervous system (CNS) and peripheral tissues
   d. Considered controlled substances by Food and Drug Administration (FDA)

      e. Classified by their ability to stimulate or block opioid receptors or by the severity of pain for which they are used

      f. Onset of action is immediate if given by intravenous (IV) route and rapid if given by intramuscular (IM) route, subcutaneously (subQ), or by mouth (PO)

      g. Peak action is from 1–2 hours and duration up to 12 hours depending on formulation

      h. These agents cross the blood–brain and placental barriers and also into breast milk

2. Common opioid analgesic medications (Table 3-1)

3. Administration considerations

      a. Check respiratory rate prior to administration due to CNS depressant effects

      b. May increase **intracranial pressure** (ICP; pressure inside skull); never administer an opioid to a client with a traumatic brain injury because it could mask symptoms of deteriorating level of consciousness (LOC)

      c. Opioids may be given short term for acute pain, or on a long-term basis for chronic pain; tolerance should not be confused with addiction in clients requiring long-term pain management therapy

      d. Clients with severe heart, liver, or kidney disease or respiratory or seizure disorders should be closely monitored

      e. Initial therapy begins with decreased dosages for older adults or debilitated clients

      f. Double-check dosages for neonates, infants, and children with prescriber or pharmacist

      g. Use caution if given to clients more prone to addiction because of possibility of dependence; however, do not withhold if client is experiencing pain

      h. Determine client's pattern of use if long term; be aware that some opioids, such as oxycodone, are used as street drugs

4. Contraindications

      a. Hypersensitivity reactions occur frequently

      b. Check for sensitivity prior to administration

Table 3-1 Common Opioid Analgesics

Type	Generic Name	Route
Pure agonists (No ceiling effect, increase in analgesia by increase in dose)	Codeine	IM, PO
	Hydrocodone bitartrate	PO, subcutaneous
	Oxycodone	PO
	Propoxyphene	PO
	Morphine sulfate	PO, IV
	Fentanyl citrate	IM, transdermal patch
	Oxymorphone	Subcutaneous, IM, IV
	Hydromorphone hydrochloride	PO, IM, IV, subcutaneous
	Meperidine	PO, IM, IV, subcutaneous
	Methadone hydrochloride	PO, IM, subcutaneous
	Levorphanal tartrate	PO, subcutaneous
Mixed agonists–antagonists (Have ceiling effect)	Pentazocine hydrochloride	PO, IM, IV, subcutaneous
	Butorphanol tartrate	IM, IV
	Dezocine	IM, IV
	Nalbuphine hydrochloride	Subcutaneous, IM, IV

c. Do not use with clients who have acute bronchial asthma or upper airway obstruction, increased ICP, seizure disorders, pancreatitis, acute ulcerative colitis, or severe liver or kidney insufficiency; traumatic brain injury

5. Significant drug interactions
    a. Barbiturates, other narcotics, hypnotics, antipsychotics, or alcohol can increase CNS depression when combined with opiates
    b. Combined use with monoamine oxidase inhibitors (MAOIs) may precipitate hypertensive crisis
    c. Analgesia may be inhibited if used with phenothiazines
6. Significant food interactions: alcohol may have additive effect
7. Significant laboratory studies: monitor liver and kidney function to determine ability to excrete medication and metabolites
8. Side effects
    a. Nausea and vomiting, **anorexia** or loss of appetite
    b. Sedation, light-headedness, dizziness
    c. Constipation, gastrointestinal (GI) cramps, urinary retention, oliguria
    d. Pruritus (these effects decrease over time)
9. Adverse effects/toxicity
    a. Respiratory depression, respiratory arrest
    b. Circulatory depression
    c. Increased ICP
10. Client-centered nursing care
    a. Assess pain for type, intensity, and location prior to administration (use pain scale)
    b. Assess for respiratory rate, depth, and rhythm; if less than 12 breaths/minute, withhold medication and notify prescriber
    c. Assess for central nervous system (CNS) changes including **level of consciousness (LOC)**, which is the state of awareness, as well as dizziness, drowsiness, hallucinations, and pupil size
    d. Assess client for allergic reactions such as rash or urticaria
    e. Administer opiate for pain and antiemetic for nausea and vomiting
    f. Evaluate the therapeutic response and maintain comfort
    g. Monitor vital signs regularly
    h. Assess older adults frequently because of possible slower biotransformation and sensitivity to CNS drugs
    i. Note that there are multiple formulations and strengths of most opioids; double-check prescriptions and medication before administration
11. Client education
    a. Avoid alcohol and other CNS depressants while using opioids
    b. Do not take over-the-counter (OTC) medications without approval by prescriber
    c. Avoid ambulation, smoking, driving, or other activities without assistance after administration of medication until drug response is known
    d. Report any CNS changes, allergic reactions, or shortness of breath
    e. Long-term use can lead to withdrawal symptoms with termination of use, including nausea and vomiting, cramps, fever, faintness, and anorexia; considered dependence, not addiction

B. Opioid antagonists

1. Actions and use
    a. Include naloxone and naltrexone
    b. Compete with opioids at opiate receptor sites, blocking effects of opioids
    c. Used to reverse respiratory depression and sedation induced by overdose of opioids, pentazocine, and propoxyphene
    d. Onset of effect 1–2 minutes; duration 45 minutes

Practice to Pass

You are caring for a client with a patient-controlled analgesia (PCA) pump that has morphine sulfate as the medication. The client has been out of surgery for 1½ hours. He reports that his hands itch and he has a rash. What would you do first?

2. Side effects

   a. Reversal of analgesia

   b. Increased blood pressure (BP)

   c. Tremors, hyperventilation, drowsiness, nervousness, rapid pulse

   d. Hyperpnea and nausea and vomiting

3. Adverse effects/toxicity

   a. Hypotension

   b. Ventricular tachycardia and fibrillation

   c. Seizures

   d. Hepatitis

   e. Pulmonary edema

4. Client-centered nursing care

   a. Assess vital signs every 3 to 5 minutes

   b. Assess arterial blood gases (ABGs)

   c. Assess cardiac status: tachycardia, hypertension

   d. Monitor electrocardiogram (ECG)

   e. Assess respiratory function (rate, rhythm) and LOC

   f. Administer only with resuscitative equipment nearby

   g. Evaluate therapeutic response, LOC, and need for reversal of respiratory depression

   h. In clients with physical dependence on narcotics, administration of naloxone may precipitate symptoms of withdrawal

C. Nonopioids

   1. Acetylsalicylic acid (aspirin)

     a. Action and use

       1) A salicylate medication

       2) Inhibits prostaglandins involved in production of inflammation, pain, and fever

       3) Blocks pain impulses in CNS

       4) Antipyretic action results from vasodilation of peripheral vessels

       5) Powerfully inhibits platelet aggregation

       6) Relieves mild to moderate pain, including pain caused by rheumatoid arthritis, osteoarthritis, acute rheumatic fever, systemic lupus erythematosus (SLE), bursitis, transient ischemic attacks (TIA), post–myocardial infarction (MI), prophylaxis of MI, stroke, and angina

     b. Administration considerations

       1) Dosage varies depending on age of client and condition being treated

       2) Gastric irritation may be decreased by administering with full glass of water, milk or food

       3) Pills can be crushed or chewed, but do not crush enteric-coated preparations

       4) Give 30 minutes prior to or 2 hours following meals

       5) Administer at least 30 minutes prior to physical therapy or planned activity to minimize discomfort

     c. Contraindications

       1) History of hypersensitivity to salicylates or other nonsteroidal anti-inflammatory drugs (NSAIDs), gastrointestinal bleeding, bleeding disorders

       2) Contraindicated in children younger than 12 years old because of risk of Reye syndrome, children or teenagers with chickenpox or flulike symptoms, third-trimester pregnancy, lactation

       3) Contraindicated with vitamin K deficiency, peptic ulcer disease, anemia, renal or hepatic dysfunction

        d. Significant drug interactions

            1) Decreased effects of aspirin (ASA) with antacids (high-dose) and urinary alkalizers

            2) Increased bleeding with anticoagulants and alcohol

            3) Increased gastrointestinal bleeding when taken concurrently with corticosteroids

            4) Increased effects of warfarin, insulin, thrombolytic agents, penicillins, phenytoin, valproic acid, oral hypoglycemics, and sulfonamides

            5) Increased salicylate levels (leads to toxicity) with ammonium chloride, urinary acidifiers, and nizatidine

            6) Decreased effects of probenecid, spironolactone, sulfinpyrazone, sulfonamides, NSAIDs, beta blockers

        e. Significant food interactions: increased risk of bleeding with horse chestnut, kelpware, dong quai, feverfew, red clover, and ginger; caffeine may increase absorption of aspirin

        f. Significant laboratory studies

            1) Increases coagulation studies, liver function studies, serum uric acid, amylase, CO_2, and urinary protein

            2) Decreases serum potassium, cholesterol, and T_3 and T_4 concentrations

            3) Interference with urine catecholamines, pregnancy test, and urine glucose tests

        g. Side effects

            1) Increased prothrombin time (PT), activated partial thromboplastin time (APTT), bleeding time

            2) Stimulation, drowsiness, dizziness, confusion, headache, hallucinations

            3) Diarrhea, heartburn, anorexia, and nausea and vomiting

            4) Rash, urticaria, bruising

            5) Tinnitus

        h. Adverse effects/toxicity

            1) Hematologic: thrombocytopenia, agranulocytosis, leukopenia, neutropenia, and hemolytic anemia

            2) Seizures, coma

            3) Gastrointestinal bleeding, hepatitis

            4) Reye syndrome (children), characterized by encephalopathy and fatty liver degeneration

        i. Client-centered nursing care

            1) Assess for allergy to salicylates prior to administration

            2) Assess liver function tests, renal function tests (BUN, creatinine), and blood studies including complete blood count (CBC), hematocrit (Hct), hemoglobin (Hgb), prothrombin time (PT) if on long-term therapy

            3) Assess for **hepatotoxicity** (state of liver damage): dark urine, clay-colored stools, yellowing of skin, sclera, itching

            4) Abdominal pain, fever, diarrhea, especially if on long-term therapy

            5) Evaluate for therapeutic responses such as decreased pain, inflammation, and fever

            6) Assess for aspirin toxicity when administered with ammonium chloride

        j. Client education

            1) Report any symptoms of hepatotoxicity or renal toxicity

            2) Report visual changes, tinnitus, allergic reactions, and bleeding

            3) Take medication with 8 oz water, milk, or food, and sit upright for 30 minutes following dose

            4) Do not exceed recommended dose; acute salicylate poisoning may result

            5) Do not combine with other OTC medications that also contain ASA

6) Therapeutic response can take up to 2 weeks

7) Avoid alcohol ingestion to decrease chance of GI bleeding

8) This medication should not be given to children or teens with flulike or chickenpox symptoms (risk of Reye syndrome)

9) May need to be discontinued 7–10 days prior to surgery to reduce risk for excessive bleeding

2. Acetaminophen

  a. Action and use

    1) May block pain impulses peripherally that occur in response to inhibition of prostaglandin synthesis

    2) Possesses weak anti-inflammatory properties

    3) Antipyretic action results from inhibition of prostaglandins in the CNS resulting in peripheral vasodilation, sweating, and dissipation of heat

    4) Used for mild to moderate pain or fever, especially when ASA or NSAIDs are not tolerated

  b. Administration considerations

    1) Usual dose is 325–600 mg q4–6h by mouth or by rectum; maximum dose is 4 grams per day

    2) Oral forms may be crushed or given as whole or chewable tablets

    3) May give with food or milk to increase gastric tolerance

    4) Co-administration with high-carbohydrate meal may significantly retard absorption rate

    5) Intravenous use: only one formulation available; administered via a 15-minute infusion for mild to moderate postsurgical pain management

  c. Contraindications

    1) Hypersensitivity to acetaminophen or phenacetin

    2) In children younger than 3 years unless directed by prescriber

    3) Repeated administration to clients with anemia or hepatic diseases, including alcoholism, malnutrition, or thrombocytopenia

  d. Significant drug interactions

    1) Decreased effect and increased hepatotoxicity with barbiturates, alcohol, carbamazepine, hydantoins, rifampin, sulfinpyrazone

    2) Cholestyramine decreases absorption

    3) Hypoprothrombinemia may occur when used concurrently with warfarin

    4) Bone marrow suppression may occur with zidovudine

  e. Significant food interactions: caffeine enhances analgesic effect; alcohol increases risk of liver damage

  f. Significant laboratory studies: interference with Chemstrip G, Dextrostix, Visidex II (false increases in urinary glucose), 5-HIAA (false increases), blood glucose (false decreases), serum uric acid (false increases)

  g. Side effects: rash; otherwise negligible with recommended dosage

  h. Adverse effects/toxicity

    1) Anaphylaxis

    2) Hematology: leukopenia, neutropenia, hemolytic anemia, thrombocytopenia, pancytopenia

    3) GI: hepatotoxicity with hepatic necrosis

    4) Angioedema

    5) Toxicity: cyanosis, anemia, neutropenia, jaundice, pancytopenia, CNS stimulation, delirium followed by vascular collapse, seizures, coma, and death

  i. Client-centered nursing care

    1) Assess liver function tests, BUN and creatinine, and CBC and PT if on long-term therapy

2) May cause hepatotoxicity at doses greater than 4 grams/day with chronic use; recommendations for older adults are no more than 3 grams/day

3) Assess client for chronic poisoning; signs including rapid, weak pulse, dyspnea, cold, clammy extremities; report them immediately to prescriber

4) Assess for hepatotoxicity: dark urine, clay-colored stools, yellowing of skin, sclera, itching, abdominal pain, fever, diarrhea, especially if on long-term therapy

5) Be prepared to administer acetylcysteine as antidote for acetaminophen poisoning

6) Evaluate client for therapeutic response, such as decreased pain or fever

j. Client education

1) Do not exceed recommended dose; acute poisoning with liver damage may result

2) Be aware of acute toxicity symptoms such as nausea and vomiting, abdominal pain; notify prescriber of these immediately

3) Do not combine with other OTC medications that also contain acetaminophen

4) Recognize signs of chronic overdose such as bleeding, bruising, malaise, fever, and sore throat

5) Notify prescriber of pain or fever lasting longer than 3 days

3. Nonsteroidal anti-inflammatory drugs (NSAIDs)

a. Action and use

1) Inhibit cyclooxygenase and decrease prostaglandins and thromboxane

2) Used to treat mild to moderate pain, osteoarthritis, rheumatoid arthritis, and dysmenorrhea

b. Common nonsteroidal anti-inflammatory medications (Table 3-2)

c. Administration considerations

1) Gastric irritation may be decreased by administering with full glass of water, milk, or food

2) Pills can be crushed or chewed; capsules should not be crushed, dissolved, or chewed

3) Give 30 minutes before or 2 hours after meals for best absorption

4) Administer at least 30 minutes prior to physical therapy or planned activity to minimize discomfort

Practice to Pass

A client comes to the ambulatory care center reporting nausea and vomiting and abdominal pain. He has been taking acetaminophen for a headache (two extra-strength) every 4 hours, as well as DayQuil and NyQuil every 4 hours for several days. What is the probable source of his nausea and vomiting?

Table 3-2	**Common Nonsteroidal Anti-Inflammatory Agents**	
Medication	**Route**	**Significant Drug Interactions**
Celecoxib	PO	↑ effect of anticoagulants ↓ effect of ASA, ACE inhibitors, and diuretics ↑ adverse reactions of glucocorticoids, NSAIDs, and ASA ↑ toxicity: lithium, antineoplastics
Diclofenac sodium	PO	↓ effect of beta blockers, diuretics ↑ effect of anticoagulants, digoxin; toxicity of phenytoin, lithium, cyclosporine, methotrexate, and ASA Hyperkalemia with potassium-sparing diuretics
Etodolac	PO	↓ effect of beta blockers, diuretics, and antacids ↑ effect of anticoagulants, digoxin ↑ toxicity of phenytoin, lithium, cyclosporine, methotrexate, and ASA
Fenoprofen	PO	Phenobarbital ↓ effect of fenoprofen ↓ effect of diuretics ↑ effects of oral anticoagulants and sulfonylureas ↑ GI toxicity with ASA ↑ GI reactions with corticosteroids, alcohol (ETOH)

(*continued*)

Table 3-2	Common Nonsteroidal Anti-Inflammatory Agents (*continued*)	
Medication	**Route**	**Significant Drug Interactions**
Flurbiprofen	PO	↑ effects of oral anticoagulants, heparin, phenytoin, sulfonylureas, and sulfonamides ↑ effect of flurbiprofen: phenytoin, sulfonylureas, and sulfonamides
Ibuprofen	PO	↓ effect of antihypertensives, thiazides, and furosemide ↑ reactions: corticosteroids, ASA ↑ toxicity: digoxin, lithium, oral anticoagulants, and cyclosporine
Indomethacin	PO	↓ effect of antihypertensives ↑ effect of digoxin, penicillamine, and phenytoin ↑ toxicity: lithium, methotrexate, cyclosporine, aminoglycosides, ASA, corticosteroids, triamterene, and ETOH ↑ risk of bleeding with anticoagulants
Ketoprofen	PO	↑ toxicity: lithium, methotrexate, cyclosporine, phenytoin, and alcohol ↑ risk of bleeding: warfarin ↑ effects of ketoprofen with ASA and probenecid ↑ GI reactions: corticosteroids, ASA ↓ effect of diuretics, antihypertensives
Ketorolac	IV, IM, PO	↑ toxicity: lithium, methotrexate ↑ risk of bleeding: anticoagulants, salicylates ↑ renal impairment: ACE inhibitors ↓ effect of diuretics, antihypertensives
Mefenemic acid	PO	↑ toxicity: lithium, sulfonylureas, sulfonamides, phenytoin, and warfarin ↑ risk of bleeding: anticoagulants, heparin
Nabumetone	PO	↓ effect of diuretics, antihypertensives ↑ risk of bleeding: anticoagulants, thrombolytics, valproic acid, cefamandole, cefotetan, and cefoperazone ↑ risk of hematologic reactions: antineoplastics, radiation ↑ GI reactions: salicylates, NSAIDs, ETOH, potassium, and corticosteroids
Naproxen	PO	↑ toxicity: methotrexate, oral anticoagulants, sulfonylureas, probenecid, and lithium ↓ effect of diuretics, antihypertensives ↑ GI reactions: ASA, ETOH, and corticosteroids Possible renal impairment: ACE inhibitors ↑ risk of bleeding: oral anticoagulants, heparin
Oxaprozin	PO	↓ effect of antihypertensives, diuretics ↑ risk of adverse effects with corticosteroids
Piroxicam	PO	↑ toxicity: cyclosporine, methotrexate, lithium, alcohol, oral anticoagulants, ASA, and corticosteroids ↓ effects of antihypertensives, diuretics Hypoglycemia: oral antidiabetics ↑ risk of bleeding: oral anticoagulants, heparin ↑ GI reactions: ASA, ETOH
Sulindac	PO	↑ risk of bleeding: oral anticoagulants ↑ nephrotoxicity: cyclosporine ↓ sulindac effect with use of diflunisal—**do not use together** ↑ toxicity: methotrexate, sulfonamides, sulfonylureas, probenecid, and lithium ↑ GI reactions: ASA, NSAIDs

      d. Contraindications
        1) Hypersensitivity
        2) Contraindicated with asthma, severe renal or hepatic disease, GI bleeding, bleeding disorders, peptic ulcer disease, or anemia
      e. Significant drug interactions: see Table 3-2 for specific interactions for each medication
      f. Significant food interactions: food may increase absorption of NSAIDs; increased risk of bleeding with dong quai, feverfew, garlic, ginger, horse chestnut, and red clover; increased risk of photosensitivity with St. John's wort
      g. Significant laboratory studies
        1) Liver function tests
        2) Serum uric acid
        3) Urinary bilirubin, urinalysis, BUN, creatinine
        4) Bleeding time, PT, CBC
      h. Side effects
        1) Nausea, abdominal pain, anorexia
        2) Dizziness, drowsiness
      i. Adverse effects/toxicity
        1) FDA has recommended that NSAID product manufacturers include a boxed warning, highlighting possible increased risk of cardiovascular events and serious risk for GI bleeding associated with their use
        2) Nephrotoxicity including dysuria, hematuria, oliguria, azotemia
        3) Blood dyscrasias, cholestatic hepatitis
      j. Client-centered nursing care
        1) Assess lab tests for renal, hepatic, and hematologic function before treatment begins and periodically thereafter
        2) Audiometric and ophthalmic exam may be done before, during, and after treatment
        3) Assess for ear and eye problems; blurred vision and tinnitus may indicate toxicity
        4) Evaluate for therapeutic response including decreased pain, stiffness in joints, decreased swelling in joints, ability to move more easily
        5) Client may need to refrain from administration for several days before surgery to reduce risk of operative bleeding
      k. Client education
        1) Take drug with food or fluids to reduce GI irritation
        2) Report blurred vision, ringing, and roaring in ears, which may indicate toxicity
        3) Avoid driving or other hazardous activities if dizziness and drowsiness occur, especially in older adults
        4) Report changes in urine pattern, increased weight, edema, increased pain in joints, fever, or blood in urine indicating nephrotoxicity
        5) Therapeutic effects may take up to 1 month, depending on formulation

D. Medications to treat headaches
    1. Action and use: serotonin-selective drugs (known as *triptans*) relieve pain and inflammation associated with migraine headaches; aimed at prevention with prophylactic therapy and acute symptomatic treatment during an attack
      a. Migraine headaches
        1) Acute therapy directed toward abolishing or limiting headache as it begins
        2) Ergot preparations are alpha-adrenergic agonists or antagonists that cause vasoconstriction or vasodilation, depending on state of vessel; they also block uptake of serotonin by platelets that can cause precipitous decline of serotonin, leading to migraine attack
        3) Prophylaxis medications are beta-adrenergic blockers, serotonin antagonists, and antiepileptics

        b. Tension-type headaches

          1) Therapy is directed toward rapid treatment of pain

          2) Prevention and reduction of occurrence is also a goal

          3) Mild analgesics and muscle relaxants are first-line agents; antidepressants may be used with counseling; ASA, acetaminophen, ibuprofen are used for pain; amitriptyline is helpful for muscle contraction pain

        c. Cluster headaches

          1) Treatment is directed at elimination of triggers

          2) Preventative therapies used may include high-dose calcium channel blockers, lithium, methysergide, or corticosteroids

    2. Common medications to treat headaches (Table 3-3)

    3. Administration considerations

        a. For abortive treatment medications, taking early in headache is imperative

        b. Dose that was effective for last headache should be starting dosage for this headache

    4. Contraindications

        a. Hypersensitivity to ergot alkaloids, pregnancy, cardiac disease, hypertension, sepsis, or severe pruritus

        b. Triptans: contraindicated in clients with history of acute myocardial infarction (MI), uncontrolled hypertension, and cerebrovascular diseases such as stroke

    5. Significant drug interactions

        a. Beta blockers and calcium channel blockers are additive in effects with these medications

        b. Ergot toxicity can occur if ergot is given with erythromycin or other macrolides

        c. Serotonin-selective drugs have many interactions; see product literature

        d. Triptans should be given cautiously if ergotamine has been taken within the previous 24 hours

    6. Significant food interactions: none reported

    7. Significant laboratory studies: see specific medications

    8. Side effects: see Table 3-3

    9. Adverse effects/toxicity: see Table 3-3

Table 3-3   **Medications Used to Treat Headaches**

Medication	Route	Therapeutic Indications	Adverse Effects
Ergots			
Ergotamine tartrate	PO	Abort headache unresponsive to non-narcotic treatment; cluster headaches	Nausea and vomiting, weakness, numbness, tingling of fingers and toes; possible throat or nasal irritation, altered taste; delirium, seizures, cerebral hemorrhage, intermittent claudication
Dihydroergotamine	IM, IV, intranasal	Parenteral treatment for established headache	
Serotonin receptor agonists			
Sumatriptan	subQ, PO, intranasal	Migraine or cluster headaches	Dizziness, vertigo, fatigue, anxiety, warming sensation, coronary artery vasospasm, dysrhythmias, transient myocardial ischemia, myocardial infarction, cardiac arrest
Almotriptan	PO	Acute migraine headache with or without aura	
Eletriptan	PO		
Frovatriptan	PO		
Naratriptan	PO		
Rizatriptan	PO, SL		
Zolmitriptan	PO, SL, intranasal		

10. Client-centered nursing care
    a. Assess for medication-specific side effects as well as efficacy of treatment
    b. Planning for care must begin with careful history, including treatments that have been effective in past
    c. Provide a quiet and low-light environment for client to relax
    d. Obtain an accurate dietary history from client to determine if a relationship exists between onset of headache and certain foods
    e. Avoid prolonged use of medication
    f. When administering triptans, do not break oral disintegrating tablets
    g. Beware of ergotamine rebound or an increase in frequency and duration of headache
11. Client education
    a. How to identify type of headache: migraine, cluster, or tension
    b. Identify triggers for headaches and how to ameliorate them
    c. Keep a headache diary
    d. Stress reduction, stress management and lifestyle changes, including diet, to minimize headaches
    e. Do not eat, drink, or smoke while tablet is dissolving (if using sublingual tablet)
    f. Avoid exposure to cold weather for a prolonged period; cold may increase adverse reactions to drug
    g. Do not increase dose without consulting prescriber
    h. Use comfort measures during attack, such as lying in darkened, quiet room with cold compresses applied to head

II. ANTIEPILEPTICS

A. Hydantoins

1. Action and use
   a. Suppress sodium influx across neuronal cell membranes
   b. Inhibit spread of seizure activity in motor cortex
   c. Used in general **tonic–clonic seizures** (grand mal seizures), **status epilepticus** (seizures that last longer than 4 minutes), and **psychomotor seizures** (complex focal seizures)
2. Common antiepileptic medications (Table 3-4)
3. Administration considerations
   a. Fosphenytoin should only be given IV for status epilepticus in emergency department or critical care area; respiratory rate, BP, and ECG should be monitored
   b. Do not interchange chewable phenytoin products with capsules
   c. Phenytoin readily binds with protein so should not be given with gastric feedings, which inhibit uptake
   d. Phenytoin metabolism varies greatly among people, and thus drug levels should be monitored and maintained at 10–20 mcg/mL
   e. Carbamazepine given via nasogastric tube should be mixed with D_5W or NS and flush with at least 100 mL solution afterward
   f. Give ethosuximide, diazepam, and carbamazepine with food or milk to reduce GI symptoms
4. Contraindications
   a. Hypersensitivity
   b. Contraindicated with psychiatric condition, pregnancy, bradycardia, SA and AV node block, Stokes–Adams syndrome, hepatic failure
5. Significant drug interactions: see Table 3-4
6. Significant food interactions: phenytoin absorption is decreased by enteral nutrition products; withhold feedings 30–60 minutes before and after medication

Table 3-4   **Antiepileptics**

Generic Name	Route	Therapeutic Indications	Drug-to-Drug Interactions
Hydantoins			
Fosphenytoin	PO	Grand mal seizures, complex partial seizures, status epilepticus	Many drugs may either ↑ or ↓ fosphenytoin levels: see product literature Tricyclic antidepressants lower the seizure threshold
Phenytoin	PO, IV	Grand mal, psychomotor, tonic–clonic, nonepileptic seizures, seizures following head injury, prevention of seizures during and after surgery	Antiepileptics may ↑ or ↓ phenytoin levels Phenytoin may ↓ absorption and ↑ metabolism of oral anticoagulants Phenytoin ↑ metabolism of oral contraceptives, corticosteroids Amiodarone, chloramphenicol, omeprazole, and ticlopidine ↑ phenytoin levels Antituberculosis agents ↓ phenytoin levels Gingko may ↓ antiepileptic effectiveness
Iminostilbenes			
Carbamazepine	PO	Partial or generalized tonic–clonic seizures	Many drug interactions; see product literature
Oxcarbazepine	PO	Partial seizures	
Barbiturates			
Mephobarbital	PO	Grand mal, petit mal seizures; used in combination with other antiepileptics to manage delirium tremens	↓ metabolism of anticoagulants, corticosteroids ↓ effectiveness with digoxin Griseofulvin ↓ mephobarbital absorption Kava kava and valerian may potentiate sedation
Phenobarbital	PO, IV	Grand mal, partial seizures, status epilepticus	
Succinimides			
Ethosuximide	PO	Petit mal and myoclonic seizures	↓ ethosuximide levels with carbamazepine ↑ ethosuximide levels with isoniazid Phenobarbital and ethosuximide levels may be altered with ↑ seizure frequency Gingko may ↓ antiseizure effectiveness
Methsuxmide	PO	Petit mal seizures when refractory to other drugs	Lamotrigine concentrations may be ↓ ↓ serum levels along with therapeutic effects of primidone
Benzodiazepines (Anxiolytics)			
Clonazepam	PO	Myoclonus, status epilepticus, petit mal seizures refractory to succinimides or valproic acid	↑ effect with cimetidine, disulfiram, omeprazole, and hormonal contraceptives ↓ effectiveness with theophylline ↑ digoxin level and toxicity
Clorazepate	PO	Adjunctive therapy for partial seizures	↑ effect with cimetidine, disulfiram, omeprazole, and hormonal contraceptives ↓ effectiveness with theophylline ↑ digoxin level and toxicity
Diazepam	IV, PR	Adjunct therapy for status epilepticus Severe recurrent seizures	↑ effect with cimetidine, disulfiram, omeprazole, and hormonal contraceptives ↓ effectiveness with theophylline, ranitidine

Table 3-4 Antiepileptics (*continued*)

Generic Name	Route	Therapeutic Indications	Drug-to-Drug Interactions
Lorazepam	IV	Status epilepticus	↑ CNS depression with barbiturates, opioids ↓ effectiveness with theophylline Risk of toxicity with probenecid, valproate Kava kava ↑ sedation effect

Others

Generic Name	Route	Therapeutic Indications	Drug-to-Drug Interactions
Ezogabine	PO	Adjunct treatment of partial-onset seizures (adults)	↓ serum levels with carbamazepine, phenytoin ↑ serum digoxin concentration
Felbamate	PO	Partial and secondary seizures	Use limited to clients with poor control on other antiseizure medications
Gabapentin	PO	Adjunctive therapy for partial seizures	↓ serum levels when administered with antacids
Lamotrigine	PO	Partial seizures and adjunctive antiseizure therapy	↓ serum levels with acetaminophen, carbamazepine, phenobarbital, phenytoin, primidone, and hormonal contraceptives ↑ serum levels with folate ↓ seizure threshold with oil of primrose
Levetiracetam	PO	Complex partial seizures	↓ sedation when combined with antihistamines, benzodiazepines, opioids, and tricyclic antidepressants Do not administer with carbamazepine, clozapine, and drugs that cause leucopenia or neutropenia
Magnesium sulfate	IM, IV infusion	Seizures related to toxemia	Neuromuscular relaxants such as tubocurarine, atracurium, pancuronium, and vecuronium
Pregbalin	PO	Adjunct therapy for partial-onset seizures in adults	↑ CNS depression when given with other CNS depressants Fewer drug–drug interactions than many antiepileptic drugs
Tiagabine hydrochloride	PO	Adjunctive therapy for partial seizures	↑ serum levels with carbamazepine, phenytoin, and primidone Possible interaction with valproate CNS depressants can ↑ sedation
Topiramate	PO	Partial seizures, generalized tonic–clonic seizures	↑ serum levels when given with drugs that inhibit cytochrome such as fluoxetine
Valproate Sodium	PO	Grand mal seizures, petit mal seizures, psychomotor seizures, myoclonic seizures	↑ sedation with CNS depressants ↑ serum levels with salicylates, cimetidine, chlorpromazine, erythromycin, and felbamate ↑ effects (more rapid drug metabolism) with carbamazepine, phenobarbital, and phenytoin
Zonisamide	PO	Adjunctive therapy for partial seizures	Should not be administered with sulfonamides Rapid elimination of zonisamide with carbamazepine, phenytoin, phenobarbital, and primidone

administration or per institutional policy and procedure manual; folic acid, calcium, and vitamin D absorption may be decreased by phenytoin

    7. Significant laboratory studies: therapeutic phenytoin level of 10–20 mcg/mL

    8. Side effects

        a. Drowsiness, dizziness, insomnia, **paresthesias** (abnormal sensations), depression, suicidal tendencies, aggression, headache, confusion, slurred speech

    b. Hypotension

    c. Nystagmus (involuntary oscillation of eye), **diplopia** (double vision), blurred vision

    d. Constipation, nausea and vomiting, anorexia, weight loss, hepatitis, jaundice, **gingival hyperplasia** (increased growth of gum tissue)

    e. Urine discoloration

    f. Rash, lupus erythematosus, hirsutism

    g. Hypocalcemia

9. Adverse effects/toxicity

    a. Ventricular fibrillation

    b. Hepatitis or nephritis

    c. Agranulocytosis, leukopenia, aplastic anemia, thrombocytopenia, megaloblastic anemia

    d. Lupus erythematosus, **Stevens–Johnson syndrome** (an acute inflammatory disorder of the skin)

    e. Toxicity: bone marrow suppression, nausea and vomiting, ataxia, diplopia, cardiovascular collapse, slurred speech, confusion

10. Client-centered nursing care

    a. Assess for seizure activity including type, location, duration, and character; provide seizure precautions

    b. Rapid administration of phenytoin can cause cardiac arrest; be sure to use infusion pump

    c. Assess for mental status, mood, sensorium, affect, and memory (short and long term)

    d. Assess for respiratory depression, rate, depth, and character of respirations

    e. Assess for blood dyscrasias, fever, sore throat, bruising, rash, and jaundice

    f. Evaluate client for therapeutic responses such as decreases in severity of seizures and decreased ventricular dysrhythmias

    g. Administer dose with food to reduce risk of GI upset

11. Client education

    a. Medication regimen including name, dose, schedule, side effects, and possible adverse effects

    b. Urine may turn pink

    c. Do not discontinue medication abruptly or without consulting prescriber; emphasize that abrupt discontinuation may precipitate seizures

    d. Brush teeth with soft-bristle toothbrush and do proper flossing to prevent gingival hyperplasia; more frequent visits to dentist may be needed

    e. Carry medic alert identification stating medication use

    f. Avoid heavy use of alcohol as it may decrease effectiveness of medication

    g. Do not change brands of medication once seizure activity has stabilized; bioavailability differs among formulations

    h. Hydantoins decrease effectiveness of oral contraceptives; phenytoin has teratogenic effects

B. Barbiturates

1. Action and use

    a. Decrease impulse transmission to cerebral cortex

    b. Used in all forms of **epilepsy**, a chronic disorder characterized by recurring seizures

2. Common medications (Table 3-4)

3. Administration considerations

    a. Administer IM injection into large muscle mass to prevent tissue sloughing

    b. Use less than 5 mL/site

Practice to Pass

Your client is receiving continuous gastric feeding and receiving phenytoin IV for seizures. The healthcare provider decides to change the phenytoin to oral suspension to be administered via the feeding tube. What precautions must you take to ensure that the client's level of antiepileptic does not diminish due to the change in administration method?

    c. When prescribed IV, give slowly (after dilution) at a rate of 65 mg or less per minute

    d. Give oral dose on empty stomach to increase absorption

  4. Contraindications: hypersensitivity, pregnancy, porphyria, and liver disease

  5. Significant drug interactions: see Table 3-4

  6. Significant food interactions: none reported

  7. Significant laboratory studies

    a. Increases serum phosphatase

    b. Affects bromsulphthalein retention test, which enhances hepatic uptake and excretion of dye

  8. Side effects

    a. Paradoxical excitement (older adults), drowsiness, lethargy, hangover headache, flushing, hallucinations

    b. Possible confusion, depression, or irritability in children or older adults with high doses

    c. Nausea and vomiting, diarrhea, constipation

    d. Rash, urticaria, local pain, swelling, necrosis

  9. Adverse effects/toxicity

    a. Coma

    b. Stevens–Johnson syndrome, angioedema, thrombophlebitis

  10. Client-centered nursing care

    a. Assess for mental status changes such as mood, sensorium, affect, and memory (long and short term)

    b. Assess for respiratory status or depression including rate, rhythm, and depth

    c. Assess for blood dyscrasias, fever, sore throat, bruising, rash, and jaundice

    d. Assess for seizure activity including type, duration, and precipitating factors

    e. Blood studies and liver function tests are done routinely during long-term treatment

    f. Evaluate client for therapeutic responses such as decreased seizures or increased sedation

  11. Client education

    a. Medication regimen including name, dose, schedule, side effects, and possible adverse effects

    b. Avoid other CNS depressants including alcohol

    c. Do not discontinue medication abruptly or without consulting prescriber

    d. Avoid hazardous activities until stabilized on drug; drowsiness may occur

    e. Carry medic alert bracelet stating medication use

    f. Therapeutic effects may not be seen for 2–3 weeks

C. Succinimides

  1. Action and use

    a. Suppress calcium influx into neurons, increasing electrical threshold and decreasing ability to generate an action potential

    b. Inhibit spike, wave formation in absence seizures (petit mal), decrease amplitude, frequency, duration, and spread of discharges in minor motor seizures

    c. Used in absence seizures, partial seizures, and tonic–clonic seizures

  2. Common medications (Table 3-4)

  3. Administration considerations: give with food or milk to decrease GI symptoms

  4. Contraindications: hypersensitivity

  5. Significant drug interactions: see Table 3-4

  6. Significant food interactions: none reported

  7. Significant laboratory studies: increased liver function tests and false-positive direct Coombs test

   8. Side effects
      a. Drowsiness, dizziness, fatigue, euphoria, lethargy
      b. Anorexia, nausea and vomiting, heartburn
      c. Pink urine
      d. Urticaria, pruritic erythema
      e. Myopia, blurred vision
   9. Adverse effects/toxicity
      a. Agranulocytosis, aplastic anemia, thrombocytopenia, leukocytosis, eosinophilia, pancytopenia
      b. Stevens–Johnson syndrome
      c. Toxicity: bone marrow depression, nausea and vomiting, ataxia, diplopia, and cardiovascular collapse
   10. Client-centered nursing care
      a. Assess for mental status changes including mood, sensorium, affect, and behavioral changes
      b. Monitor renal studies including urinalysis, BUN, and creatinine
      c. Monitor blood studies including CBC, Hct, Hgb, reticulocyte counts every week for 4 weeks
      d. Monitor hepatic studies including AST, ALT, and bilirubin
      e. Assess for eye problems; may need regular ophthalmic exams
      f. Assess for allergic reactions such as red, raised rash or exfoliative dermatitis
      g. Assess for blood dyscrasias, fever, sore throat, bruising, rash, or jaundice
      h. Monitor weight weekly; report any signs of anorexia or weight loss
   11. Client education
      a. Carry ID card or medic alert bracelet with medication, client's name, prescriber's name, and phone number
      b. Avoid driving and other activities that require alertness as appropriate
      c. Avoid alcohol ingestion and other CNS depressants as they may increase sedation
      d. Do not discontinue medication abruptly or without consulting prescriber
      e. Continue regular dental checkups to identify gingival hyperplasia
      f. Emphasize importance of contraception, as drug therapy is a risk to fetus
D. Benzodiazepines
   1. Action and use
      a. Enhance inhibitory neurotransmitter **gamma-aminobutyric acid (GABA)** to decrease anxiety and as an adjunct for seizure activity
      b. Relief of delirium tremens
   2. Common medications (Table 3-4)
   3. Administration considerations
      a. Give with food or milk to reduce GI symptoms
      b. IV injection should be given into large vein
      c. Administer IV medication at a rate of 5 mg or less per minute
   4. Contraindications
      a. Hypersensitivity
      b. Contraindicated in acute narrow-angle glaucoma or psychosis
      c. Contraindicated in children younger than 6 months
      d. Do not give to clients with liver disease (clonazepam) or during lactation (diazepam)
   5. Significant drug interactions: see Table 3-4
   6. Significant food interactions: none reported
   7. Significant laboratory studies: increases AST and ALT, serum bilirubin levels, and 17-OHCS and decreases radioactive iodine uptake
   8. Side effects
      a. Dizziness, drowsiness, confusion, headache, fatigue

      b. Orthostatic hypotension

      c. Blurred vision

      d. Constipation, dry mouth

      e. Rash, itching

  9. Adverse effects/toxicity

      a. Neutropenia

      b. Respiratory depression

      c. ECG changes, tachycardia

  10. Client-centered nursing care

      a. Assess BP (lying, standing), pulse; if systolic BP drops 20 mmHg, withhold drug, notify prescriber because of orthostatic hypotension

      b. Assess hepatic and renal function, high-density lipoprotein, alkaline phosphatase

      c. Assess for mental status changes including mood, sensorium, affect, memory (long and short term)

      d. Assess respiratory status for depression including rate, rhythm, and depth

      e. Assess seizure activity including type, duration, and precipitating factors

      f. Evaluate client for therapeutic responses such as reduced or absent seizure activity, anxiety

  11. Client education

      a. Medication regimen including name, dose, schedule, side effects, and possible adverse effects

      b. Avoid other CNS depressants, including alcohol

      c. Do not discontinue medication abruptly or without consulting prescriber

      d. Avoid hazardous activities until stabilized on drug; drowsiness may occur

      e. Use barrier contraceptives while taking benzodiazepines

E. Other antiepileptics

  1. Carbamazepine

      a. Action and use

          1) Inhibits nerve impulses by limiting influx of sodium ions across cell membrane in motor cortex

          2) Used in tonic–clonic, complex-partial, and mixed seizures

      b. Given by oral or enteral (GI tube) route

      c. Administration considerations

          1) Give oral forms with food or milk to reduce GI symptoms

          2) Chewable pills must be chewed or crushed, should not be swallowed whole

          3) Prolonged administration produces physical dependence; withdrawal symptoms will occur if stopped suddenly

      d. Contraindications

          1) Hypersensitivity to carbamazepine or tricyclic antidepressants

          2) Contraindicated with bone marrow depression and concomitant use of MAOIs

      e. Significant drug interactions: see Table 3-4

      f. Significant food interactions: increased peak concentrations of carbamazepine with grapefruit

      g. Significant laboratory studies: increases false-negatives for pregnancy tests

      h. Side effects

          1) Increased PT

          2) Syndrome of inappropriate antidiuretic hormone (SIADH), mostly with older adults

          3) Drowsiness, dizziness, confusion

          4) Constipation, diarrhea, nausea and vomiting

          5) Rash, urticaria

          6) Tinnitus, dry mouth, blurred vision, nystagmus

       7) Hypotension

       8) Fever, dyspnea, pneumonitis

       9) Urinary frequency or retention, increased BUN

    i. Adverse effects/toxicity

       1) Thrombocytopenia, agranulocytosis, leukocytosis, neutropenia, aplastic anemia, eosinophilia

       2) Paralysis, worsening of seizures

       3) Hepatitis

       4) Stevens–Johnson syndrome

       5) Hypertension, CHF, dysrhythmias, AV block

       6) CNS toxicity with lithium

       7) Fatal reaction with MAOIs

    j. Client-centered nursing care

       1) Assess for seizure activity including type, duration, and precipitating factors

       2) Monitor blood, hepatic, and renal studies including red blood cell (RBC) count, Hct, Hgb, reticulocyte count, AST, ALT, bilirubin, urinalysis, BUN, creatinine

       3) Assess mental status including mood, sensorium, affect, and memory (long and short term)

       4) Assess for eye problems; may need regular ophthalmic exams

       5) Assess for allergic reactions including purpura or red, raised rash

       6) Assess for blood dyscrasias, fever, sore throat, bruising, rash, or jaundice

       7) Evaluate client for therapeutic response such as decreased or absent seizure activity

    k. Client education

       1) Medication regimen including name, dose, schedule, side effects, and possible adverse effects

       2) Avoid other CNS depressants including alcohol

       3) Do not discontinue medication abruptly or without consulting prescriber

       4) Avoid hazardous activities until stabilized on drug; drowsiness may occur

       5) Carry medic alert ID with name, drug, prescriber's name, phone number

       6) Urine may turn pink to brown and is harmless

2. Valproates

    a. Action and use

       1) Increases levels of GABA in brain, which decreases seizure activity

       2) Use in simple (petit mal), complex (petit mal) absence, or mixed seizures; manic episodes associated with bipolar disorder and migraine headaches

    b. Given by oral or enteral (GI tube) route

    c. Administration considerations

       1) Do not crush tablets or capsules; take them whole

       2) Elixir forms should be given alone; do not dilute with carbonated beverage

       3) May give with food or milk to decrease GI symptoms

    d. Contraindications

       1) Hypersensitivity

       2) Contraindicated during pregnancy and with hepatic disease

    e. Significant drug interactions: see Table 3-4

    f. Significant food interactions: none reported

    g. Significant laboratory studies

       1) Increase risk of false-positive for ketones

       2) Interfere with thyroid function tests

    h. Side effects

       1) Sedation, drowsiness

       2) Constipation, diarrhea, heartburn, nausea and vomiting

       3) Rash

    i. Adverse effects/toxicity

        1) Thrombocytopenia, leukopenia, lymphocytosis

        2) Hepatic failure, pancreatitis, toxic hepatitis

        3) Rare but fatal adverse effects include elevated ammonia levels with encephalopathy and liver toxicity

    j. Client-centered nursing care

        1) Assess for seizure activity including type, duration, and precipitating factors

        2) Monitor blood, hepatic, and renal studies including RBCs, Hct, Hgb, serum folate, PT, platelets, vitamin D, reticulocyte count, AST, ALT, bilirubin, urine analysis, BUN, creatinine

        3) Assess mental status such as mood, sensorium, affect, and memory (long and short term)

        4) Assess respiratory status/depression including rate, rhythm, and depth

        5) Evaluate for therapeutic response, such as decreased seizure activity

    k. Client education

        1) Medication regimen including name, dose, schedule, side effects, and possible adverse effects

        2) Avoid other CNS depressants including alcohol

        3) Do not discontinue medication abruptly or without consulting prescriber

        4) Avoid hazardous activities until stabilized on drug; drowsiness may occur

        5) Carry medic alert ID with name, drug, prescriber's name, and phone number

        6) Physical dependency may result from extended use

        7) Report visual disturbances, rash, diarrhea, light-colored stools, jaundice, or protracted vomiting to provider

III. CENTRAL NERVOUS SYSTEM (CNS) STIMULANTS

A. Anorexiants

  1. Action and use

    a. Act similar to amphetamines, as indirect sympathomimetic amines with alpha- and beta-adrenergic activity

    b. May have moderate appetite suppressant properties but have short-lived effects and have increased potential for tolerance

  2. Common medication: diethylpropion (Table 3-5)

  3. Administration considerations

    a. Anorexiant effects of diethylpropion are temporary

    b. Do not abruptly discontinue medication

    c. Should be given on empty stomach; additional dose may be given mid-evening to control nighttime hunger

  4. Contraindications

    a. Hypersensitivity

    b. Contraindicated with angle-closure glaucoma, advanced cardiac disease, hyperthyroidism, agitated states, history of drug abuse, and children under 12 years of age

  5. Significant drug interactions: see Table 3-5

  6. Significant food interactions: none reported

  7. Significant laboratory studies: none reported

  8. Side effects

    a. Restlessness, insomnia

    b. Palpitations

    c. Dysmenorrhea

Practice to Pass

A female client has started taking an anorexiant as prescribed by her healthcare provider for weight reduction. If she has multiple medical diagnoses, what types of medications might need to be adjusted because of the addition of the anorexiant?

Table 3-5	Central Nervous System (Adrenergic) Stimulants	
Generic Name	**Route**	**Significant Drug Interactions**
Anorexiant		
Diethylpropion	PO	↑ BP effects: furazolidone ↑ effects of alcohol, other CNS depressants
Amphetamine		
Amphetamine sulfate	PO	↓ elimination of amphetamine: acetazolamide, sodium bicarbonate (NaHCO₃) ↑ elimination of amphetamine: ammonium chloride, ascorbic acid ↓ effects of guanethidine, guanadrel Hypertensive crisis and intracranial hemorrhage may occur if given within 14 days of MAOIs, selegiline ↓ effectiveness of amphetamine: tricyclic antidepressants ↑ BP effects: furazolidone ↑ effects of alcohol, other CNS depressants
Methylphenidate	PO	Hypertensive crisis: MAOIs within 14 days, or vasopressor ↑ sympathomimetic effect: decongestants, vasoconstrictors ↓ effects of warfarin, tricyclics, and antiepileptics
Dextroamphetamine sulfate	PO	Hypertensive crisis: MAOIs within 14 days Delayed absorption: barbiturates, phenytoin ↑ effect of dextroamphetamine: acetazolamide, antacids, and NaHCO₃ ↑ CNS effect: haloperidol, tricyclics, and phenothiazines ↓ effect of dextroamphetamine: ascorbic acid, ammonium chloride ↓ effect of adrenergic blockers, antidiabetics
Selective Norepinephrine Reuptake Inhibitor		
Atomoxetine	PO	↑ serum levels when combined with CYP2D6 inhibitors (paroxetine, fluoxetine, and quinidine) Withhold MAOIs for 2 weeks before starting atomoxetine

9. Adverse effects/toxicity
    a. Decrease in seizure threshold in epilepsy
    b. Tachycardia
10. Client-centered nursing care
    a. Assess BP and pulse during treatment
    b. Evaluate client for therapeutic response such as decrease in weight over time
    c. Implement psychosocial interventions
11. Client education
    a. Discuss all medications currently taken (including OTC) with provider
    b. Take medications exactly as prescribed; do not use during pregnancy—alert prescriber
    c. Avoid driving or other hazardous activities until reaction to medication is determined
    d. Report palpitations, weight loss, dry mouth, and difficulty swallowing
B. **Amphetamines**
    1. Action and use
        a. Increase release of norepinephrine and dopamine in cerebral cortex to **reticular activating system**, a diffuse system that extends from lower brainstem to cerebral cortex
        b. Used in treating narcolepsy, **attention-deficit/hyperactivity disorder (ADHD)**
    2. Common medications (Table 3-5)

3. Administration considerations
   a. Give first dose on awakening and give last dose not closer than 6 hours to bedtime
   b. Administer on empty stomach 30–60 minutes prior to meal
4. Contraindications
   a. Hypersensitivity
   b. Tourette syndrome (methylphenidate), hyperthyroidism, hypertension, glaucoma, severe arteriosclerosis, drug abuse, cardiovascular disease, anxiety, or lactation
5. Significant drug interactions: see Table 3-5
6. Significant food interactions: none reported
7. Significant laboratory studies: serum thyroxine (T_4) with high amphetamine doses
8. Side effects
   a. Hyperactivity, insomnia, restlessness, talkativeness
   b. Dry mouth, nausea and vomiting
   c. Impotence, change in libido
   d. Palpitations, tachycardia
9. Adverse effects/toxicity: same as previously described
10. Client-centered nursing care
   a. Assess vital signs, especially BP, since may reverse antihypertensive medication action
   b. Monitor CBC, urinalysis, and in diabetics, monitor blood glucose levels; changes in insulin may be required
   c. Assess mental status for mood, sensorium, and affect; stimulation, insomnia, or aggressiveness may occur
   d. Assess for withdrawal symptoms including headache, nausea and vomiting, muscle pain, weakness
   e. Evaluate client for therapeutic responses such as decreased activity in ADHD or absence of sleeping during day in **narcolepsy**
11. Client education
   a. Medication regimen including name, dose, schedule, side effects, and possible adverse drug effects; if a dose is missed, do not double-dose
   b. Avoid or decrease caffeine consumption (coffee, tea, cola, chocolate), which may increase irritability or stimulation
   c. Avoid OTC preparations unless approved by prescriber and avoid alcohol consumption
   d. Do not discontinue medication abruptly or without consulting prescriber
   e. Importance of rest
   f. Seizure threshold is decreased in clients with seizure disorders

C. **Nonstimulant medication to treat ADHD**
1. Action and use: selective norepinephrine reuptake inhibitor (SNRI) increases concentration of norepinephrine in prefrontal cortex
2. Common medication: atomoxetine
3. Administration considerations: daily dose is usually weight-based in children and adolescents
4. Contraindications
   a. Hypersensitivity
   b. Concurrent use of MAOIs or MAOI use within last 2 weeks
   c. Serious cardiac or liver disease
   d. Major depressive disorder or presence of suicidal ideation
   e. Efficacy in children under 6 years of age or in older adults is not established
5. Significant drug interactions: see Table 3-5
6. Significant food interactions: increased stimulation and amine effect with caffeine
7. Significant laboratory studies: none reported

8. Side effects
 a. Hyperactivity, insomnia, restlessness, and talkativeness
 b. Dry mouth
 c. Palpitations and tachycardia
 d. Rash
 e. Nausea and vomiting, decreased appetite, and weight loss
 f. Sexual dysfunction
9. Adverse effects/toxicity
 a. Suicidal ideation
 b. Dysrhythmias and palpitations
 c. Severe liver injury
10. Client-centered nursing care
 a. Assess vital signs, especially BP, since increased BP may occur
 b. Assess for mental status changes including mood, sensorium, and affect; stimulation, insomnia, and aggressiveness may occur
 c. Assess client for changes in appetite, sleep, speech patterns
 d. Assess client for suicidal ideation
 e. Evaluate client for therapeutic responses such as decreased activity in ADHD
11. Client education
 a. Medication regimen including name, dose, schedule, side effects, and possible adverse effects
 b. Avoid or decrease caffeine consumption (coffee, tea, cola, chocolate), which may increase irritability or stimulation
 c. Avoid OTC preparations unless approved by prescriber and avoid alcohol consumption
 d. Do not discontinue medication abruptly or without consulting prescriber

IV. MEDICATIONS TO TREAT PARKINSON DISEASE

A. Anticholinergics

1. Action and use
 a. Block or compete at central acetylcholine receptor sites in autonomic nervous system
 b. Used to decrease involuntary movements and rigidity in parkinsonism
2. Common medications (Table 3-6)
3. Administration considerations
 a. Parenteral dose of trihexyphenidyl is given with client in recumbent position to prevent postural hypotension
 b. Oral form of trihexyphenidyl is given with or after food to prevent GI upset; may give with fluids other than water
 c. Parenteral dose of benztropine is given slowly; keep client under observation at least 1 hour after administering dose and monitor vital signs
 d. Monitor dosage of medication very carefully; even slight overdose can lead to toxicity
4. Contraindications: clients with narrow-angle glaucoma, myasthenia gravis, or gastrointestinal obstruction should not use
5. Significant drug interactions: see Table 3-6
6. Significant food interactions: none reported
7. Significant laboratory studies: none reported
8. Side effects
 a. Dry mouth, constipation
 b. Urinary retention or hesitancy
 c. Headache or dizziness

Table 3-6 Medications Used to Treat Parkinson Disease

Generic Name	Route	Uses	Drug-to-Drug Interactions
Dopaminergics			
Carbidopa-levodopa Levodopa	PO	Parkinson disease	Antacids may ↑ absorption of levodopa components Antihypertensives may have ↑ hypotensive effects Iron salts ↓ bioavailability MAOIs ↑ risk of severe hypertension Papaverine, phenytoin, phenothiazines, and antipsychotics may ↓ antiparkinsonism effects Kava may ↓ dopamine action
Selegiline	PO	Parkinson disease	Adrenergics ↑ pressor response Use cautiously with citalopram, fluoxetine, fluvoxamine, nefazodone, paroxetine, sertraline, venlafaxine Do not administer selegiline for at least 2 weeks after stopping MAOIs Meperidine may cause stupor and rigidity Cacao tree products may have vasopressor effects Ginseng may ↑ adverse reactions
Rasagiline	PO	Parkinson disease	Use with dextromethorphan can cause episodes of psychosis Potentiates levodopa ↑ plasma levels of opioids including meperidine and methadone
Dopamine Agonists			
Apomorphine	PO	Parkinson disease	May ↑ CNS depression with other CNS depressants; hypotension and unconsciousness with granisetron and similar drugs; multiple other drug interactions
Bromocriptine	PO	Parkinson disease, acromegaly, hyperprolactinemia	Antihypertensives will ↓ BP significantly Ergot alkaloids, estrogens, hormonal contraceptives interfere with bromocriptine Erythomycin ↑ bromocriptine Haloperidol, loxapine, MAOIs, methyldopa, metoclopramide, phenothiazines, reserpine interfere with bromocriptine Levodopa produces additive effects
Pramipexole	PO	Parkinson disease	Butyrophenones, metoclopramide, phenothiazines, thiothixenes ↓ pramipexole levels Cimetidine, diltiazem, quinidine, quinine, ranitidine, triamterene, and verapamil ↓ pramipexole clearance Levodopa ↑ adverse effects Black horehound produces ↑ dopaminergic effect
Ropinirole hydrochloride	PO	Parkinson disease	CNS depressants ↑ CNS effects Dopamine antagonists ↓ ropinirole effects Estrogens ↓ ropinirole clearance Erythromycin, fluvoxamine, diltiazem, tacrine ↓ ropinirole clearance
Anticholinergic Agents			
Atropine sulfate	PO, IM, IV	Hypersalivation and irregular movements related to Parkinson disease	↑ anticholinergic effect with phenothiazines, antidepressants, MAOIs, amantadine ↑ effects of atenolol

(*continued*)

Table 3-6 **Medications Used to Treat Parkinson Disease (*continued*)**

Generic Name	Route	Uses	Drug-to-Drug Interactions
Benztropine mesylate	PO	Hypersalivation and irregular movements related to Parkinson disease	Amantadine, phenothiazines, tricyclic anti-depressants ↑ anticholinergic effects, intolerance to heat and hyperthermia Cholinesterase inhibitors ↓ efficacy of cholinesterase inhibitors
Diphenhydramine	PO, IM, IV		CNS medications will ↑ sedation MAOIs ↑ anticholinergic effects
Glycopyrrolate	PO	Hypersalivation and irregular movements related to Parkinson disease, peptic ulcer disease, and irritable bowel syndrome	↓ effect with antipsychotic agents ↑ anticholinergic effect with tricyclic antidepressants and amantadine ↑ effect of atenolol and digoxin
Hyoscyamine sulfate	PO, SL		↑ effect with other anticholinergic agents, amantadine, haloperidol, phenothiazines, MAOIs, tricyclic antidepressants, and antihistamines ↓ absorption when given with antacids
Propantheline bromide	PO		↓ effectiveness with antipsychotic medications, particularly haloperidol ↓ effectiveness with phenothiazines
Scopolamine hydrobromide	PO, subQ, IM, IV		↓ effectiveness with antipsychotic medications, particularly haloperidol ↓ effectiveness with phenothiazines
Trihexyphenidyl	PO		↓ therapeutic effects of chlorpromazine, haloperidol, phenothiazines MAOIs potentiate drug effects ↑ bioavailability of digoxin
Antiviral			
Amantadine hydrochloride	PO	Parkinson disease and drug-induced extrapyramidal reactions	↑ atropine-like side effects when administered with anticholinergic agents ↑ effects of amantadine when administered with hydrochlorothiazide and triamterene

9. Adverse effects/toxicity: paralytic ileus
10. Client-centered nursing care
   a. Monitor intake and output (I&O); retention may cause decreased urinary output
   b. Assess client for urinary hesitancy and retention; palpate bladder if retention occurs
   c. Assess client for constipation; increase fluids, bulk, and exercise to counteract constipation; assess bowel sounds to rule out paralytic ileus
   d. Assess mental status for affect, mood, CNS depression, worsening of mental symptoms during early therapy
   e. If tolerance occurs during long-term therapy, dose may need to be increased or changed
   f. Protect client from heat
   g. Evaluate for therapeutic responses such as decreased tremors, secretions, absence of nausea and vomiting

11. Client education
    a. Void before taking dose of anticholinergic to reduce urinary retention
    b. Avoid driving or other hazardous activities; drowsiness may occur
    c. Avoid OTC medications such as cough and cold preparations with alcohol, and antihistamines unless prescribed by provider; separate antacid use from anticholinergics by 2–4 hours

B. **Medications affecting dopamine level in brain**
    1. Action and use
        a. These medications include amantadine, levodopa, dopamine agonists, and MAO type B inhibitors (MAOBIs)
        b. Amantadine (an antiviral) promotes synthesis and release of dopamine
        c. L-dopa is the immediate natural precursor of dopamine
        d. Dopamine agonists (DA) directly stimulate specific subclasses of dopamine receptors
        e. MAOBIs increase dopamine activity by an incompletely understood mechanism
        f. DAs and MAOBIs are used to enhance effects of L-dopa
        g. All are used to increase available dopamine; parkinsonism symptoms are decreased by having more dopamine available to body
    2. Common medications (Table 3-6)
    3. Administration considerations
        a. Administer medication after meals for better absorption and to decrease GI symptoms
        b. Absorption of levodopa and selegiline is decreased with high-protein meals; administer after a low-protein food or snack
    4. Contraindications
        a. Hypersensitivity
        b. Narrow-angle glaucoma
        c. Undiagnosed skin lesions
    5. Significant drug interactions: see Table 3-6
    6. Significant food interactions
        a. Decreased levodopa and selegiline absorption with high-protein foods
        b. With selegiline and rasagiline, tyramine-containing foods may increase hypertensive reactions
    7. Significant laboratory studies
        a. Bromocriptine: increases growth hormone, AST, ALT, potassium, BUN, uric acid, alkaline phosphatase
        b. Selegiline results in false-positive of urine ketones and glucose; also results in false-negative of urine glucose
    8. Side effects
        a. Nausea and vomiting, dry mouth, and constipation
        b. Dizziness, headache, and depression
        c. Cough
        d. Cardiac dysrhythmias and orthostatic hypotension
        e. Sleep disturbance, "on–off" phenomenon
    9. Adverse effects/toxicity
        a. Amantadine: seizures, CHF, leukopenia
        b. Levodopa: hemolytic anemia, leukopenia, agranulocytosis
        c. DAs: seizures, shock
        d. MAOBIs: tachycardia or sinus bradycardia
        e. Levodopa toxicity: disturbed sleep patterns, hallucinations, personality changes, increased twitching, grimacing, tongue protrusion

Practice to Pass

A client with Parkinson disease is admitted to the nursing unit after a surgical procedure. What type of medication would you be careful not to administer because he or she takes selegiline, an MAOBI?

10. Client-centered nursing care
    a. Assess BP and respirations
    b. Assess mental status for affect, mood, behavioral changes, and depression; complete a suicide assessment
    c. Monitor for involuntary movement, akinesia, tremors, staggering gait, muscle rigidity, and drooling
    d. Evaluate for therapeutic responses such as a decrease in akathisia and increased mood
11. Client education
    a. Change positions slowly to prevent orthostatic hypotension
    b. Report side effects such as twitching and eye spasm; may indicate overdose
    c. Use drugs exactly as prescribed; never discontinue them abruptly since this may precipitate parkinsonian crisis
    d. Avoid alcohol use
    e. Do not take foods high in protein with dose (decreased absorption)
    f. Quit smoking if taking ropinirole because drug clearance is increased (drug is less effective)

V. MEDICATIONS TO TREAT ALZHEIMER DISEASE

A. Action and use
   1. Cholinesterase inhibitors elevate acetylcholine concentrations in cerebral cortex
   2. Accomplish this by slowing degradation of acetylcholine released in cholinergic neurons
B. Common medications used to treat Alzheimer disease (Table 3-7)
C. Administration considerations
   1. Administer medication between meals; may be given with meal to reduce GI symptoms
   2. Use rivastigmine cautiously with NSAIDs because of increased risk for bleeding
   3. Dosage adjusted to response no more frequently than every 6 weeks
D. Contraindications
   1. Hypersensitivity to drug
   2. Development of jaundice when taking drug
E. Significant drug interactions: see Table 3-7
F. Significant food interactions: none reported
G. Significant laboratory studies: none reported
H. Side effects
   1. Insomnia, headache, dizziness, confusion, ataxia, anxiety, depression, hostility, and abnormal thinking
   2. Nausea and vomiting, diarrhea, abdominal pain, and constipation
   3. Urinary frequency and incontinence
   4. Rash
   5. Rhinitis or cough
I. Adverse effects/toxicity
   1. Seizures
   2. Hepatotoxicity
   3. Urinary tract infection (UTI)
   4. Atrial fibrillation
J. Client-centered nursing care
   1. Assess BP for hypotension or hypertension
   2. Assess mental status for affect, mood, behavioral changes, depression, hallucinations, and confusion; complete a suicide assessment
   3. Assess GI symptoms such as nausea and vomiting, anorexia, constipation, or abdominal pain

Table 3-7	Medications Used to Treat Alzheimer Disease		
Generic Name	**Route**	**Uses**	**Drug-to-Drug Interactions**
Donepezil	PO	Mild to moderate Alzheimer disease	↓ effects of anticholinergic drugs Bethanechol, succinylcholine produce additive effects Carbamazepine, dexamethasone, phenytoin, phenobarbital, and rifampin ↑ elimination of donepezil Cholinomimetics, cholinesterase inhibitors produce a synergistic effect Jaborandi tree and pill-bearing spurge may cause toxic effects of donepezil
Ergoloid mesylate	PO	Senile dementia of Alzheimer disease	No clinical significant interactions noted
Rivastigmine tartrate	PO	Mild to moderate Alzheimer disease	↓ effects of anticholinergic drugs Bethanechol, succinylcholine, and neuromuscular blockers have synergistic effects Smoking ↑ rivastigmine clearance
Memantine hydrochloride	PO	Mild to severe Alzheimer disease	Cimetidine, hydrochlorothiazide, quinidine, ranitidine, and triamterene alter drug levels Amantadine, dextromethorphan, and ketamine can interact and should be used cautiously ↑ effect and possible toxicity of memantine if administered with drugs that alkalinize urine (i.e., carbonic anhydrase inhibitors, sodium bicarbonate)
Galantamine hydrobromide	PO	Mild to moderate dementia of Alzheimer disease	Cimetidine, ketoconazole, paroxetine, erythromycin, succinylcholine, and bethanechol can produce galantamine toxicity

       4. Assess client for urinary frequency and incontinence

       5. Monitor liver function tests frequently

       6. Evaluate client for therapeutic responses such as decrease in confusion, improved mood

K. Client (and/or caregiver) education

       1. Use drug exactly as prescribed, at regular intervals, preferably between meals; may be taken with food to decrease GI upset

       2. Report side effects such as twitching, nausea and vomiting, and sweating, which might indicate overdose

       3. Notify provider of nausea and vomiting, diarrhea (dose increase or beginning treatment), or rash

       4. Do not increase or abruptly decrease dose; serious consequences may result

       5. Drug is not a cure; it only relieves symptoms

       6. Stop smoking

       7. Use of sodium bicarbonate to treat symptoms of GI upset can produce toxic levels of memantine

       8. Change position slowly to avoid orthostatic hypotension

VI. CENTRALLY ACTING SKELETAL MUSCLE RELAXANTS

    A. Medications for spasticity

       1. Action and use

          a. Decrease synaptic responses at neurotransmitters to decrease frequency, severity of spasms

          b. Used to reduce **spasticity** (increased resistance to passive movement) after spinal cord injuries, stroke, and in cerebral palsy and multiple sclerosis (MS)

2. Common skeletal muscle relaxant medications (Table 3-8)
3. Administration considerations: see Table 3-8
4. Contraindications
   a. Hypersensitivity to medication
   b. Contraindicated in compromised pulmonary function, active hepatic disease, impaired myocardial function
5. Significant drug interactions: see Table 3-8
6. Significant food interactions: none reported
7. Significant laboratory studies: baclofen increases AST, alkaline phosphatase, and blood glucose levels

Table 3-8 Skeletal Muscle Relaxants

Generic Name	Route	Therapeutic Indications	Drug-to-Drug Interactions
Baclofen	PO	Spasticity in MS and spinal cord injuries	Administration with CNS depressants ↑ CNS depression MAOIs, tricyclic antidepressants elicit respiratory depression and hypotension
Carisoprodol	PO	Relieve pain and discomfort from musculoskeletal disorders	CNS depressants may ↑ CNS depression
Cyclobenzaprine	PO	Relieve pain and discomfort from musculoskeletal disorders	CNS depressants may ↑ CNS depression Anticholinergic agents ↑ anticholinergic activity MAOIs may exacerbate CNS depression
Dantrolene hydrochloride	PO	Spasticity of neuromuscular disorders, malignant hyperthermia, metabolic acidosis, hypercarbia	CNS depressants ↑ CNS depression Estrogens ↑ risk of hepatotoxicity Verapamil IV causes cardiovascular collapse when administered to anesthetized clients
Diazepam	PO	Relieve pain and discomfort from musculoskeletal disorders Management of anxiety Acute alcohol withdrawal Treatment of tetanus Antiepileptic	↑ CNS depression with alcohol, omeprazole ↑ effect of diazepam if combined with cimetidine, disulfiram, and hormonal contraceptives ↓ effectiveness with theophylline and ranitidine
Metaxalone	PO	Relieve pain and discomfort from musculoskeletal disorders	Cimetidine, furosemide, cationic drugs such as digoxin, amiloride, and vancomycin will ↑ risk of hypoglycemia ↑ risk of lactic acidosis with glucocorticoids and ethanol ↑ risk of hypoglycemia with juniper berries, ginseng, garlic, fenugreek, coriander, dandelion root, and celery
Methocarbamol	PO	Relieve pain and discomfort from musculoskeletal disorders; spasms from black widow spider bite	↑ theophylline clearance ↓ effectiveness in hyperthyroidism ↑ anticoagulant effects Possible toxicity with digitalis glycoside, metoprolol, and propranolol
Orphenadrine citrate	PO	Relieve pain and discomfort from musculoskeletal disorders	↑ anticholinergic activity with anticholinergic medications ↑ CNS depression with CNS depressants, particularly phenothiazine Tardive dyskinesia with phenothiazines and haloperidol
Tizanidine	PO	Spasticity in clients with MS, spinal cord injury, or brain trauma	↑ depression with alcohol, baclofen, and CNS depressants ↑ effect with hormonal contraceptives Do not use alpha-2 adrenergics

8. Side effects: dizziness, weakness, fatigue, drowsiness, disorientation, nausea and vomiting
9. Adverse effects/toxicity
    a. Seizures
    b. Eosinophilia, hepatic injury
10. Client-centered nursing care
    a. Monitor BP, weight, blood glucose level, and hepatic function
    b. Assess client for increased seizure activity; drugs decrease seizure threshold
    c. Monitor I&O, check for urinary frequency, retention, or hesitancy
    d. Monitor electroencephalogram (EEG) in epileptic clients due to poor seizure control
    e. Assess client for allergic reactions, fever, rash, or respiratory distress
    f. Monitor client for severe weakness or numbness in extremities
    g. Monitor client for CNS depression, dizziness, drowsiness, or psychiatric symptoms
    h. Monitor hepatic function (AST, ALT) and renal function (BUN, creatinine, CBC)
    i. Report unusual bleeding
    j. Large doses of relaxants may lead to dependency
    k. Evaluate client for therapeutic responses such as decrease in pain and spasticity
11. Client education
    a. Do not discontinue medication quickly; hallucinations, spasticity, tachycardia will occur; it should be tapered off gradually by prescriber
    b. Notify prescriber of abdominal pain, jaundiced sclera, clay-colored stools, or change in color of urine (hepatotoxicity)
    c. Do not take alcohol or other CNS depressants
    d. Avoid using OTC medications, cough preparations, or antihistamines, unless recommended by prescriber
    e. Do not break, crush, or chew capsules

B. **Medications used for spasms**
1. Action and use
    a. Depress multisynaptic pathways in the spinal cord, causing skeletal muscle relaxation and/or sedation
    b. Used for adjunct relief of **spasms** (involuntary contractions of large muscles) and pain in musculoskeletal conditions
2. Common medications (Table 3-8)
3. Administration considerations: see Table 3-8
4. Contraindications
    a. Hypersensitivity
    b. Contraindicated in children under age 12, intermittent porphyria, acute recovery phase of MI, heart block, CHF, or thyroid disease
5. Significant drug interactions: see Table 3-8
6. Significant food interactions: none reported
7. Significant laboratory studies: methocarbamol results in false increased levels of VMA, urinary 5-HIAA
8. Side effects: dizziness, weakness, drowsiness, nausea
9. Adverse effects/toxicity
    a. Erythema multiforme
    b. Angioedema, anaphylaxis
    c. Dysrhythmias
    d. Seizures
10. Client-centered nursing care
    a. Blood studies including CBC, WBC with differentials
    b. During and after injection, assess for CNS effects, rash, conjunctivitis, and nasal congestion
    c. Liver studies including AST, ALT, alkaline phosphatase

   d. EEG in clients with seizures
   e. Assess for allergic reactions including idiosyncratic reaction, anaphylaxis, rash, fever, or respiratory distress
   f. Assess client for severe weakness or numbness in extremities
   g. Assess for CNS depression, dizziness, drowsiness, and psychiatric symptoms
   h. Monitor client for psychological dependency, increased need for drug, and increased pain
   i. Evaluate client for therapeutic responses such as decreased pain, spasm, and spasticity
11. Client education
   a. Do not discontinue medication abruptly; insomnia, nausea, headache, spasticity, tachycardia will occur
   b. Do not take with alcohol or other CNS depressants
   c. Avoid using OTC medications, cough preparations, antihistamines unless recommended by provider
   d. Avoid hazardous activities if drowsiness or dizziness occurs

VII. ANTI-ANXIETY, SEDATIVE, AND HYPNOTICS (REFER TO CHAPTER 4)

Case Study

T. P., a 48-year-old male client, is admitted to the emergency department (ED) after having a seizure while attending church. You are the admitting nurse in the ED. The client has a history of a seizure disorder. He is arousable but lethargic.

1. What questions will you ask the client or the family upon arrival?
2. What initial assessments will you make?
3. What are the priorities of care for the client while he is in the ED?
4. What education points are of highest priority prior to discharge home?
5. Give examples of medications or foods that could interfere with T. P.'s prescribed seizure medications, phenytoin, and phenobarbital.

For suggested responses, see page 538.

POSTTEST

1 Because a healthcare provider prescribed levodopa for a client newly diagnosed with Parkinson disease, the nurse should place a high priority on teaching the client which information prior to discharge?

1. Side effects include cushingoid symptoms such as moon face and weight gain.
2. Postpone vaccinations during levodopa therapy.
3. Report any ulcerations or sores in the mouth to provider immediately.
4. Avoid taking medication with high-protein foods.

2 Which statement made by the client indicates an understanding of client teaching regarding antiepileptic drug therapy?

1. "After taking the medication, I should lie down."
2. "I must be sure to have my cholesterol levels checked regularly."
3. "I need to take this medication regularly to avoid the recurrence of seizures."
4. "I probably will not need this medication very long."

3 A client suffers from migraine headaches. Which statement indicates the client knows what activity may help to reduce or eliminate the headaches?

1. "I keep a diary of my headaches so that I can see if there is a pattern."
2. "I stopped my exercise program since it has not helped my headaches."
3. "I take the pain medication every 4 hours."
4. "I have taken the bus to work instead of driving."

---

4 The provider prescribed methylphenidate for a client diagnosed with attention-deficit/hyperactivity disorder (ADHD). The nurse should question the prescription if the client has which contraindication?

1. Age less than 12 years
2. History of anemia
3. History of seizures
4. History of Tourette syndrome

---

5 A client is scheduled to take 4 mg of hydromorphone intravenously (IV). Prior to administering the drug, what should the nurse do?

1. Assist the client to the bathroom to void.
2. Obtain a baseline respiratory assessment.
3. Place a suction kit at the head of the bed.
4. Check the client's serum potassium level.

---

6 A client has begun taking an anticholinergic medication. The nurse should make it a priority to assess for which unintended manifestations?

1. Bradycardia and hypotension
2. Urinary retention, hesitancy, and constipation
3. Pain resembling the pattern associated with cholecystitis
4. Pain resembling renal colic

---

7 A client is receiving both selegiline and meperidine. What instructions should the nurse provide to the unlicensed assistive personnel (UAP)?

1. Set up infection control precautions.
2. Use automatic blood pressure (BP) machine to measure client's BP at preset frequencies.
3. Assist client with activities of daily living.
4. Place a "no visitors" sign on the door.

---

8 The healthcare provider has prescribed cyclobenzaprine for a 16-year-old football player who sustained a back injury during the first game of the season. The pediatric office nurse provides which instruction to the client and his parents?

1. Client should avoid prolonged walking while taking the medication.
2. Client should use sunscreen and protective clothing while taking the medication.
3. Client may need to take the drug for the rest of the football season.
4. Client should report edema of the tongue immediately.

---

9 A 71-year-old client in long-term care has been taking phenytoin 100 mg by mouth three times daily for some time. The nurse carries out which most important health promotion measure as prescribed?

1. Administer calcium supplements as well as vitamin D.
2. Wear dark glasses when exposed to the sun.
3. Give medication with food to prevent nausea.
4. Instruct client to massage gums every morning after brushing teeth.

---

10 A client is prescribed naproxen for the treatment of rheumatoid arthritis. The home care nurse should explain to the client that maximum relief may take up to how many weeks to occur? Provide a numeric answer.

_____ weeks

➤ *See pages 81–83 for Answers and Rationales.*

POSTTEST

ANSWERS & RATIONALES

Pretest

1 Answer: 1 Rationale: Methylphenidate is a central nervous system stimulant that results in the release of norepinephrine and dopamine, which can lead to hypertension and life-threatening dysrhythmias in the client with chronic heart failure. Methylphenidate can increase the metabolic rate, which could increase the serum glucose level, but this is not significant enough to prohibit its use in a client with diabetes mellitus. The drug can cause anorexia, nausea, and abdominal pain, which could be troublesome for the client with irritable bowel syndrome, but again the risks are not as great as in congestive heart failure (CHF). The drug can result in myelosuppression, so a history of anemia should be monitored, but again this is not as great a risk as CHF. **Cognitive Level:** Analyzing **Client Need:** Pharmacological and Parenteral Therapies **Integrated Process:** Nursing Process: Implementation **Content Area:** Pharmacology **Strategy:** Specific knowledge about how the drug acts is needed to answer the question. Nonetheless, if you know that the drug is a stimulant, you can reason that the drug action may be harmful to a client with heart disease, particularly congestive heart failure (CHF). **Reference:** Wilson, B. A., Shannon, M. T., & Shields, K. M. (2017). *Pearson nurse's drug guide 2017.* New York, NY: Pearson, p. 462.

2 Answer: 2, 3, 5 Rationale: For seizure control, medication must be taken to maintain therapeutic blood levels, even if there is no seizure activity. Seizures affecting adults usually do not resolve spontaneously in the absence of treatment. The most frequent adverse effects of phenytoin present as central nervous system symptoms. In most states driving is permitted after a client is seizure free for 6–12 months. Obtaining a therapeutic blood level between 10 and 20 mcg/mL may take time, particularly initially. **Cognitive Level:** Applying **Client Need:** Pharmacological and Parenteral Therapies **Integrated Process:** Teaching and Learning **Content Area:** Pharmacology **Strategy:** The critical words are *controlled* and *recurrence.* Note that two options are essentially providing opposite information, making it more likely that one of them is correct. Use knowledge of the principles of antiepileptic therapy to choose correctly. **Reference:** Wilson, B. A., Shannon, M. T., & Shields, K. M. (2017). *Pearson nurse's drug guide 2017.* New York, NY: Pearson, pp. 1252–1253.

3 Answer: 4 Rationale: Cluster headaches are aggravated by light. Darkening the room reduces this noxious environmental stimulus, thereby promoting maximum therapeutic effects. Ergotamine tartrate should be given orally 1–2 mg followed by 1–2 mg every 30 minutes until the headache abates or until the maximum dose of 6 mg/24 hours. It is unnecessary to drink large amounts of fluids. Tachycardia can be a side effect of this drug, but increased warmth and energy are not associated with this medication. **Cognitive Level:** Applying **Client Need:** Pharmacological and Parenteral Therapies **Integrated Process:** Communication and Documentation **Content Area:** Pharmacology **Strategy:** Associate the disease characteristics with management of cluster headaches and promotion of drug effectiveness. **Reference:** Wilson, B. A., Shannon, M. T., & Shields, K. M. (2017). *Pearson nurse's drug guide 2017.* New York, NY: Pearson, pp. 595–596.

4 Answer: 2 Rationale: Dantrolene is a central-acting skeletal muscle relaxant known to be effective in managing spasticity after spinal cord injury. Dexamethasone, a corticosteroid, decreases inflammation. Spinal cord–related spasms are not caused by inflammation. Donepezil, a cholinesterase inhibitor, slows progression of Alzheimer disease in clients. Dobutamine, a beta-adrenergic agonist, acts primarily on cardiac tissue. **Cognitive Level:** Analyzing **Client Need:** Pharmacological and Parenteral Therapies **Integrated Process:** Teaching and Learning **Content Area:** Pharmacology **Strategy:** Recall that spasticity is a condition affecting muscles. Associate the drug category (central-acting muscle relaxant) with the client need, which is to inhibit the spasm of muscles. **Reference:** Wilson, B. A., Shannon, M. T., & Shields, K. M. (2017). *Pearson nurse's drug guide 2017.* New York, NY: Pearson, pp. 425–426.

5 Answer: 1, 2, 5 Rationale: The primary purpose of administering opioid analgesics is pain relief. Side effects placing the client at greatest risk are respiratory depression and reduced level of consciousness (LOC). Blood pressure and heart rate could decrease because of diminished sympathetic nervous system stimulation following effective pain relief. Concerns about drug interactions are preadministration concerns also, and should be investigated before the dose is administered. History of drug abuse and past experiences with pain management are preadministration concerns. **Cognitive Level:** Applying **Client Need:** Pharmacological and Parenteral Therapies **Integrated Process:** Nursing Process: Evaluation **Content Area:** Pharmacology **Strategy:** Link the drug category, purpose, action, and primary side effect to nursing practice. **Reference:** Adams, M. P., Holland, N., & Urban, C. (2017). *Pharmacology for nurses: A pathophysiologic approach* (5th ed.). New York, NY: Pearson, p. 242.

6 Answer: 2 Rationale: A client with liver disease may be at risk for toxicity with acetaminophen, or at increased risk of bleeding if taking aspirin or NSAIDs. Unless temperature elevation is the reason for the prescription, it does not need to be measured. Tachycardia can occur if the drugs are combined with various cold remedies.

There is no evidence that changes in cholesterol levels influence administration of these drugs. These drugs may be abruptly withdrawn and do not need to be tapered. **Cognitive Level:** Applying **Client Need:** Pharmacological and Parenteral Therapies **Integrated Process:** Teaching and Learning **Content Area:** Pharmacology **Strategy:** The core issue of the question is the level of risk to a client with liver disease in taking medications. Recall that the liver plays a key role in the biotransformation of many drugs. Use this information and the process of elimination to consider that the client should consult the healthcare provider before taking these medications. **Reference:** Adams, M. P., Holland, N., & Urban, C. (2017). *Pharmacology for nurses: A pathophysiologic approach* (5th ed.). New York, NY: Pearson, p. 509.

7 **Answer: 3 Rationale:** Since the medication was prescribed stat, one can conclude the seizure disorder is unstable. The assessments of greatest assistance to the nurse include seizure activity, changes in mental status, and current respiratory status. To prevent toxicity, hydration needs to be attended to later along with the client's emotional needs. Although renal failure can be a side effect of the drug, impaired airway, changes in mental status, and the nature of seizure activity need to be managed first. Although altered electrolyte status and leg edema may need attention if they occur, management of the seizure activity takes priority first. **Cognitive Level:** Applying **Client Need:** Pharmacological and Parenteral Therapies **Integrated Process:** Nursing Process: Planning **Content Area:** Pharmacology **Strategy:** The critical word is *stat*, suggesting that the client's status is unstable. Recognize that phenytoin is an antiepileptic to choose the option that includes seizure activity. **Reference:** Wilson, B. A., Shannon, M. T., & Shields, K. M. (2017). *Pearson nurse's drug guide 2017.* New York, NY: Pearson, pp. 1252–1253.

8 **Answer: 1, 2, 4 Rationale:** Both propranolol, a beta blocker, and monoamine oxidase inhibitors (MAOIs) such as phenelzine have hypotensive effects and should not be administered concurrently. Hyperpyrexia may occur if meperidine and MAOIs are administered concurrently. Because carbamazepine can significantly compound the depressant and anticholinergic effects of MAOIs, it should *not* be administered within 14 days of taking MAOIs. The outcome of the interactions of the two drugs is potentially fatal. Glucagon increases glucogenesis, while MAOIs potentiate hypoglycemic activity of oral hypoglycemics, thus offsetting each other's effects. Dicyclomine is a parasympatholytic resulting in antispasmodic activity, while MAOIs are more likely to compound sympathomimetic activity. **Cognitive Level:** Analyzing **Client Need:** Pharmacological and Parenteral Therapies **Integrated Process:** Teaching and Learning **Content Area:** Pharmacology **Strategy:** Apply knowledge of the normal effect of MAOIs on neurotransmitters such as norepinephrine, serotonin, and dopamine to the

actions of the specific drugs. **References:** Wilson, B. A., Shannon, M. T., & Shields, K. M. (2017). *Pearson nurse's drug guide 2017.* New York, NY: Pearson, pp. 1242–1243.

9 **Answer: 2 Rationale:** Amphetamines and anorexiants increase the secretion of norepinephrine, resulting in a decrease in the seizure threshold. Seizures are often associated with the excessive release of acetylcholine. When these drug groups are used concurrently with antiepileptics, the seizure control is more efficient. A reduction in red blood cells may be compounded if given concurrently with nonsteroidal anti-inflammatory drugs (NSAIDs). Since anticholinergics may cause tremors and cerebral dystonia, they would be contraindicated in a client with a seizure disorder. Because of a potential increase in metabolism, administration with other antiepileptics may result in decreased serum levels. **Cognitive Level:** Applying **Client Need:** Pharmacological and Parenteral Therapies **Integrated Process:** Nursing Process: Planning **Content Area:** Pharmacology **Strategy:** The critical word in the question is *potentiate*. This tells you that the correct option is a drug or group of drugs that enhances the antiepileptic effect of carbamazepine. Use specific drug knowledge and the process of elimination to answer the question. **Reference:** Wilson, B. A., Shannon, M. T., & Shields, K. M. (2017). *Pearson nurse's drug guide 2017.* New York, NY: Pearson, p. 255.

10 **Answer: 1, 3, 4 Rationale:** Dantrolene is a skeletal muscle relaxant. Hepatotoxicity is an adverse reaction for dantrolene, which may be manifested by abdominal pain and scleral jaundice. Diarrhea is a common side effect, but persistent diarrhea may cause dehydration. Hepatic necrosis may result in changes in the serum glucose levels, but other signs are more indicative of this serious impairment. Painful urination and urinary frequency may occur and should be reported. Changes in hearing or smell are not common side effects of dantrolene. **Cognitive Level:** Applying **Client Need:** Pharmacological and Parenteral Therapies **Integrated Process:** Teaching and Learning **Content Area:** Pharmacology **Strategy:** Apply knowledge of primary side effects of the drug. **Reference:** Wilson, B. A., Shannon, M. T., & Shields, K. M. (2017). *Pearson nurse's drug guide 2017.* New York, NY: Pearson, pp. 425–426.

Posttest

1 **Answer: 4 Rationale:** High-protein foods significantly decrease absorption of levodopa. For this reason, clients are taught to take it with a low-protein food. Cushingoid symptoms are associated with ingesting cortisone derivatives. There is no need to avoid vaccinations. GI disturbances associated with the drug include anorexia and nausea and vomiting but not mouth ulcerations. **Cognitive Level:** Analyzing **Client Need:** Pharmacological and Parenteral Therapies **Integrated Process:** Teaching and Learning **Content Area:** Pharmacology **Strategy:** Associate levodopa with "leave off the protein." **Reference:** Wilson, B. A., Shannon, M. T., & Shields, K. M. (2017). *Pearson nurse's drug guide 2017.* New York, NY: Pearson, pp. 257–258.

2 **Answer: 3** **Rationale:** Doses must be taken regularly to maintain therapeutic blood levels, even without seizure activity. The side effects of antiepileptic drugs vary widely. A mild drowsiness can occur with some of them, but it should not be significant enough to require lying down. There is no evidence of an impact on serum cholesterol levels. Most common side effects involve the central nervous system and the hematologic system. Antiepileptic therapy is prescribed for long-term or lifelong use. **Cognitive Level:** Applying **Client Need:** Pharmacological and Parenteral Therapies **Integrated Process:** Nursing Process: Evaluation **Content Area:** Pharmacology **Strategy:** Apply knowledge of the relationships between therapeutic dose levels and seizure activity. **Reference:** Adams, M. P., Holland, N., & Urban, C. (2017). *Pharmacology for nurses: A pathophysiologic approach* (5th ed.). New York, NY: Pearson, pp. 181–186.

3 **Answer: 1** **Rationale:** There is evidence that certain lifestyle patterns contribute to development of migraine headaches, which cannot be completely controlled by medications. If the client can identify the triggering factors, the nurse and the client can collaborate and design a plan of care that will reduce or eliminate the headaches. The client should continue to exercise for general health and stress management. The client should take the pain medication when pain is experienced, but frequent ongoing self-administration could result in tolerance. Unless the client is continually impaired, driving is permitted. **Cognitive Level:** Applying **Client Need:** Pharmacological and Parenteral Therapies **Integrated Process:** Nursing Process: Evaluation **Content Area:** Pharmacology **Strategy:** Correlate the management of migraine headaches with "not by medicine alone." **Reference:** Adams, M. P., Holland, N., & Urban, C. (2017). *Pharmacology for nurses: A pathophysiologic approach* (5th ed.). New York, NY: Pearson, pp. 251–253.

4 **Answer: 4** **Rationale:** Since methylphenidate is a stimulant, a history of Tourette syndrome is a contraindication for its use. There are other medications that could be used for treatment of attention-deficit/hyperactivity disorder (ADHD), such as pemoline or dextroamphetamine. Methylphenidate has a calming effect on pediatric clients and is appropriate for use with this age group. Aplastic anemia is a side effect of Cylert. Because it is a stimulant, the use of methylphenidate in clients with a seizure disorder should be done so with caution. **Cognitive Level:** Applying **Client Need:** Pharmacological and Parenteral Therapies **Integrated Process:** Nursing Process: Assessment **Content Area:** Pharmacology **Strategy:** First recall that this medication is a stimulant, and then consider each option in terms of which item would be a contraindication to use of a stimulant. **References:** Wilson,

B. A., Shannon, M. T., & Shields, K. M. (2017). *Pearson nurse's drug guide 2017.* New York, NY: Pearson, pp. 1014–1015.

5 **Answer: 2** **Rationale:** A serious side effect of hydromorphone is respiratory depression, so respiratory assessment is appropriate. The client does not need to void before receiving hydromorphone. Hydromorphone does not cause airway blockage, so a suction kit is not needed. Hydromorphone is not associated with changes in potassium level. **Cognitive Level:** Applying **Client Need:** Pharmacological and Parenteral Therapies **Integrated Process:** Nursing Process: Implementation **Content Area:** Pharmacology **Strategy:** Recall that most anorexiants increase metabolism, which would increase the basal metabolic rate (BMR). Then consider that an increased BMR would increase physiological processes such as blood pressure. **Reference:** Adams, M. P., & Urban, C. (2016). *Pharmacology: Connections to nursing practice* (3rd ed.). New York, NY: Pearson, pp. 374–375, 377..

6 **Answer: 2** **Rationale:** Anticholinergic medications block the action of acetylcholine, resulting in decreased stimulation in the GI and urinary tract systems. This leads to urinary and bowel problems such as urinary retention, hesitancy, and constipation. Anticholinergic drugs stimulate the parasympathetic system and tachycardia and hypertension indicate sympathetic system stimulation. Cholinergic agonists, not anticholinergics, cause biliary contractions. Renal colic is also more commonly associated with cholinergic agonists rather than anticholinergics. **Cognitive Level:** Applying **Client Need:** Pharmacological and Parenteral Therapies **Integrated Process:** Nursing Process: Assessment **Content Area:** Pharmacology **Strategy:** Correlate the nature of the drug category with the signs and symptoms. Specific knowledge of this drug category is needed to answer this question. **Reference:** Adams, M. P., Holland, N., & Urban, C. (2017). *Pharmacology for nurses: A pathophysiologic approach* (5th ed.). New York, NY: Pearson, p. 141.

7 **Answer: 2** **Rationale:** Selegiline is a monoamine oxidase inhibitor (MAOI). Concurrent administration of meperidine, an opioid analgesic, and selegiline can lead to a life-threatening hypertensive crisis, so the blood pressure will require careful monitoring. Selegiline primarily affects the dopamine levels in the brain and has no effect on the immune system. The client will need to refrain from all activity until it is determined that there is no risk of a hypertensive crisis. Decreased stimulation will be needed if it is determined that the client's blood pressure has become significantly elevated. **Cognitive Level:** Applying **Client Need:** Pharmacological and Parenteral Therapies **Integrated Process:** Nursing Process: Planning **Content Area:** Pharmacology **Strategy:** Associate MAOIs with a hypertensive crisis as the greatest risk to the client. **References:** Wilson, B. A., Shannon, M. T., & Shields, K. M. (2017). *Pearson nurse's drug guide 2017.* New York, NY: Pearson, p. 983.

8 Answer: 4 Rationale: Cyclobenzaprine can cause edema of the tongue, which can place the client at risk for airway obstruction. Because the medication can cause drowsiness, the client should avoid driving and other activities that could lead to injury while taking the medication; however, walking should be safe. The side effects affecting the skin include pruritus and skin rash. The drug is recommended for short-term rather than long-term treatment. Cognitive Level: Applying Client Need: Pharmacological and Parenteral Therapies Integrated Process: Teaching and Learning Content Area: Pharmacology Strategy: Whenever a new medication is prescribed, an important element of client teaching is the risk of adverse effects. With this in mind, evaluate each option for the worst consequence to choose it as the answer to the question. Reference: Wilson, B. A., Shannon, M. T., & Shields, K. M. (2017). *Pearson nurse's drug guide 2017.* New York, NY: Pearson, pp. 399–400.

9 Answer: 1 Rationale: Prolonged phenytoin therapy may result in osteoporosis, especially in clients with limited sun exposure and who are more at risk of the disease. Since osteoporosis is a chronic condition, it is perceived as the greatest risk to the client. The dark glasses reduce the sensitivity occurring with photophobia but do not necessarily prevent its occurrence. Taking the dose with food may decrease the rate of absorption, but may also be effective in reducing nausea and vomiting; however, this is not the greatest health promotion concern. Massaging the gums can prevent gingival hyperplasia caused by phenytoin, but is less significant than the risk of developing osteoporosis. Cognitive Level: Applying Client Need: Pharmacological and Parenteral Therapies Integrated Process: Nursing Process: Implementation Content Area: Pharmacology Strategy: The critical words in the question are *for some time* and *most important.* This tells you that the correct option may be one that results from long-term use and also that more than one option may be technically correct. Consider the adverse effects of the drug and choose the option that counteracts the most significant one over time. Reference: Wilson, B. A., Shannon, M. T., & Shields, K. M. (2017). *Pearson nurse's drug guide 2017.* New York, NY: Pearson, pp. 1014–1015.

10 Answer: 4 Rationale: Since the joints are inflamed, it will take some time to reduce the inflammation and thereby relieve the pain. The therapeutic effect of naproxen does not occur for 3–4 weeks, making 4 the correct number of weeks to identify because of the words *up to.* Cognitive Level: Analyzing Client Need: Pharmacological and Parenteral Therapies Integrated Process: Nursing Process: Evaluation Content Area: Pharmacology Strategy: The critical words in the stem are *up to,* meaning that the number to be provided in the answer is at the top of the possible range. Associate naproxen with a long onset, but beyond that specific drug knowledge is needed to answer the question. Reference: Wilson, B. A., Shannon, M. T., & Shields, K. M. (2017). *Pearson nurse's drug guide 2017.* New York, NY: Pearson, pp. 1077–1079.

References

Adams, M. P., Holland, N., & Urban, C. (2017). *Pharmacology for nurses: A pathophysiologic approach* (5th ed.). New York, NY: Pearson.

Adams, M. P., & Urban, C. (2016). *Pharmacology: Connections to nursing practice* (3rd ed.). New York, NY: Pearson.

Burchum, J., & Rosenthal, L. (2016). *Lehne's pharmacology for nursing care* (9th ed.). St. Louis, MO: Elsevier.

Drug Facts & Comparisons. (2017; updated monthly). St. Louis, MO: A. Wolters Kluwer.

Karch, A. M. (2016). *Focus on nursing pharmacology* (7th ed.). Philadelphia, PA: Lippincott Williams & Wilkins.

Kee, J. (2017). *Handbook of laboratory and diagnostic tests and nursing implications* (8th ed.). New York, NY: Pearson.

LeMone, P. T., Burke, K. M., Bauldoff, G., & Gubrud, P. (2015). *Medical surgical nursing: Clinical reasoning in patient care* (6th ed.). New York, NY: Pearson.

Lilley, L. L., Rainforth Collins, S., & Snyder, K. M. (2017). *Pharmacology and the nursing process* (8th ed.). St. Louis, MO: Mosby.

Vallerand, A. H., Sanoski, C. A., & Deglin, J. H. (2017). *Davis's drug guide for nurses* (8th ed.). Philadelphia, PA: F.A. Davis.

Wilson, B. A., Shannon, M. T., & Shields, K. M. (2017). *Pearson nurse's drug guide 2017.* New York, NY: Pearson.

ANSWERS & RATIONALES

4 Psychiatric Medications

Chapter Outline

Antipsychotics
Antidepressants
Mood Stabilizers

Sedative–Hypnotics and
Anxiolytics

Substance Misuse

NCLEX-RN® Test Prep

Access the NEW Web-based app that provides students with additional practice questions in preparation for the NCLEX experience.

Objectives

➤ Describe the general goals of therapy when administering medications to treat psychiatric disorders.
➤ Identify the indications for use of an antipsychotic medication.
➤ Identify the signs and symptoms and nursing management of extrapyramidal adverse effects of antipsychotic medications.
➤ List the classifications of antidepressant medications.
➤ Explain dietary restrictions associated with the use of monoamine oxidase inhibitors.
➤ Identify the indications for the use of lithium.
➤ Describe the signs and symptoms and nursing management of the adverse or toxic effects associated with the use of lithium.
➤ List client teaching points related to safety and the use of sedative–hypnotics and anxiolytics.
➤ Identify the signs associated with substance misuse.
➤ Identify specific client education points related to disulfiram therapy.
➤ List significant client education points related to medications to treat psychiatric disorders.

Review at a Glance

agranulocytosis an acute disease marked by deficit or absolute lack of granulocytic white blood cells
akathisia a subjective sense of restlessness with a need to move or pace continuously
antagonists chemicals that inhibit activity at a receptor site
anticholinergic effects effects caused by drugs that block acetylcholine receptors
dystonia rigidity in muscles that control posture, gait, or ocular movements

extrapyramidal side effects (EPSEs) involuntary muscle movements resulting from effects of neuroleptic medications on extrapyramidal system; include akathisia, akinesia, dystonia, drug-induced parkinsonism, and neuroleptic malignant syndrome
metabolite results of biotransformation of a drug; most tend to be pharmacologically inactive; there are exceptions including many benzodiazepines, fluoxetine, and ethanol
neuroleptic malignant syndrome (NMS) a disorder

associated with sudden high fever, rigidity, tachycardia, hypertension, and decreased level of consciousness
neuroleptics antipsychotic medications
parkinsonism masked facies, muscle rigidity, and shuffling gait; extrapyramidal side effects related to dopamine blockade
serotonin syndrome a state (agitation, sweating, confusion, fever, hyperreflexia, tachycardia, hypotension, muscle rigidity, and ataxia) that occurs when SSRIs are given concurrently with

other serotonin-enhancing drugs, causing an excess of serotonin in the system

synesthesia a condition in which stimulation to one sense causes a reaction in another sense, such as smelling a flavor or tasting an odor

tardive dyskinesia (TD) an extrapyramidal syndrome that includes movements such as grimacing, buccolingual movements, and dystonia (impaired muscle tone); usually late-onset

side effects of antipsychotic agents; may be irreversible

tolerance need for an increased amount of an agent to achieve same effects

PRETEST

1 The psychiatrist prescribed chlorpromazine 50 mg IM as an initial dose for a client hospitalized with psychosis. The primary focus of the nursing care should include which assessment?

1. Vital signs
2. Decrease in psychotic symptoms
3. Ability to ambulate independently
4. Dietary intake

2 The home care nurse is visiting a client discharged yesterday from an inpatient unit with a prescription for a 10-day supply of olanzapine 10 mg daily. The client states a prescription refill is needed because the prescription provided yesterday is all gone. The nurse should then assess the client for which signs? Select all that apply.

1. Psychosis
2. Diarrhea
3. Nervousness
4. Hypoglycemia
5. Dizziness upon standing

3 A client reports during an initial interview that the healthcare provider prescribed trazodone 50 mg tid. The nurse assesses for which important item in the client's health history?

1. Insomnia
2. Panic attacks
3. Mania
4. Anxiety

4 A client is discharged with a prescription for phenelzine, a monoamine oxidase inhibitor (MAOI). What items of information should the nurse include during client teaching? Select all that apply.

1. Written instructions on how to take daily doses of medication
2. How family members can contact appropriate healthcare provider
3. Written and oral information about food and drug interactions
4. That family members should administer the medication to the client
5. The importance of checking blood pressure and pulse daily

5 The healthcare provider has prescribed a benzodiazepine for a 74-year-old client. The acute care nurse anticipates transcribing which medication onto the medication administration record (MAR)?

1. Diazepam
2. Chlordiazepoxide
3. Trazodone
4. Lorazepam

6 Because a client is taking a psychotropic medication, the nurse should plan to teach family members to report which signs or symptoms immediately?

1. Hyperprolactinemia, gynecomastia
2. Hyperpyrexia and muscle rigidity
3. Parkinson syndrome
4. Akathisia

7 A client enters the emergency department vomiting profusely and smelling of alcohol. The client states several times, "It's the medicine that's doing it; if I live through this I'll never drink again." The nurse should ask which priority assessment questions? Select all that apply.

1. "How much alcohol have you had to drink?"
2. "Are you taking antihypertensive medications?"
3. "Have you eaten today?"
4. "Are you taking disulfiram?"
5. "Have you had your gallbladder removed?"

8 After several days of hospitalization on a psychiatric inpatient unit for clinical depression, the client is discharged with a prescription for imipramine 75 mg by mouth daily. The nurse should include which information in client teaching? Select all that apply.

1. Change positions slowly.
2. Avoid driving until clear vision is restored.
3. Report urinary retention.
4. Cardiac dysrhythmias are uncommon.
5. Drug may decrease levels of liver enzymes.

9 After taking fluoxetine 20 mg by mouth every morning for 3 weeks, the client reports to the outpatient clinic today. The client reports a weight loss of 4.5 kg (10 lb) during the last 2 weeks. Based on this assessment data, the nurse should take which action?

1. Instruct client to suspend taking dosages of this medication.
2. Instruct client to increase the daily fluid intake.
3. Consult with prescriber regarding possible need for an antiemetic.
4. Consult with prescriber regarding need to decrease the dosage.

10 Because a client is experiencing frequent, recurrent hiccups, the nurse contacts the healthcare provider. While waiting for the prescriber to respond, the nurse should prepare for client teaching by obtaining an information sheet about which drug?

1. Risperidone
2. Lorazepam
3. Chlorpromazine
4. Thioridazine

➤ *See pages 126–128 for Answers and Rationales.*

I. ANTIPSYCHOTICS

A. Phenothiazines

1. Action and use

    a. Phenothiazines are **neuroleptics** (medications used to treat psychosis); they are also known as typical (traditional) antipsychotic agents

    b. Divided into three chemical subclasses: the aliphatics, the piperidines, and the piperazines; see Table 4-1 for a list of neuroleptic medications

    c. Typical antipsychotics are predominantly dopamine (DA) **antagonists** (produce an effect by preventing receptor activation by endogenous regulatory molecules and drugs); thus they block postsynaptic D_2 receptors in several DA tracts in brain, although they have other synaptic effects as well; their two main effects are:

    1) A decrease in positive symptoms of schizophrenia (see Box 4-1 for a listing of positive and negative symptoms of schizophrenia)

    2) Production of **extrapyramidal side effects (EPSEs)**: a variety of neurologic disturbances resulting from dysfunction of extrapyramidal system; this may occur as a reversible side effect of certain psychotropic drugs, particularly antipsychotics; see Table 4-2 for a list of EPS manifestations and their management

Table 4-1	Antipsychotic Drugs	
Chemical Class and Generic Name	**Route**	**Uses**
First-Generation Agents		
Phenothiazines		
Chlorpromazine	PO, IM, R; IV rarely	Schizophrenia, schizoaffective disorders, manic phase of bipolar disorder, preoperative restlessness, antiemetic, adjunctive therapy for tetanus, intractable hiccups
Fluphenazine	PO, IM, LA	Psychotic disorders, chronic schizophrenia, behavioral complications due to mental retardation
Perphenazine	PO, IM	Schizophrenia, severe nausea and vomiting
Thioridazine	PO	Schizophrenia when unacceptable response to other antipsychotics, psychotic disorders
Trifluoperazine	PO	Schizophrenia, psychotic disorders
Nonphenothiazines		
Haloperidol	PO, IM, LA	Tourette syndrome, chronic psychotic disorder, nonpsychotic behavioral disorder
Loxapine	PO	Schizophrenia
Pimozide	PO	Vocal and motor tics accompanying Tourette syndrome, off-label for schizophrenia
Thiothixene	PO, IM	Psychotic disorders, schizophrenia
Second-Generation (Atypical) Agents		
Aripiprazole	PO, IM	Schizophrenia, bipolar mania
Asenapine	SL	Schizophrenia, mania, or mixed episodes associated with bipolar disorder
Clozapine	PO	Schizophrenia, schizoaffective disorder, reduce risk of suicidal behavior
Iloperidone	PO	Acute schizophrenia
Lurasidone	PO	Schizophrenia
Molindone	PO	Schizophrenia
Olanzapine	PO, IM	Dementia related to Alzheimer disease, schizophrenia, acute manic episode, agitation
Paliperidone	PO, IM	Schizophrenia, schizoaffective disorder
Quetiapine	PO	Schizophrenia, acute mania accompanying bipolar disorder
Risperidone	PO, LA	Schizophrenia, mania accompanying bipolar disorder
Ziprasidone	PO	Schizophrenia, schizoaffective disorder, psychotic depression

PO, oral tablets, capsules; IM, intramuscular injection; R, rectal (suppository); L, oral liquid, suspension, concentrate; LA, long-acting injectable preparations

    d. Psychosis is a phenomenon of brain activity; therefore effects of antipsychotic medications occur in central nervous system (CNS)

    e. Selected agents are also used as antiemetics and antihistamines; chlorpromazine is also used to treat intractable hiccups

    f. Typical antipsychotics are most effective in treating "positive" symptoms of schizophrenia (behaviors and symptoms that are normally seen), but are less effective in treating "negative" symptoms of schizophrenia (symptoms that develop over an extended period of time; include an absence of behaviors or

Box 4-1	Positive Symptoms	Negative Symptoms
Positive and Negative Symptoms of Schizophrenia	Hallucinations Delusions Disordered thinking Combativeness Agitation Paranoia Grandiosity Illusions Insomnia	Social withdrawal Emotional withdrawal Lack of motivation Poverty of speech Alogia Anergia Anhedonia Attention deficits Blunted affect Poor insight or judgment Poor self-care

Table 4-2   Extrapyramidal Side Effects (EPSEs)

Side Effects	Nursing Interventions
Peripheral Nervous System Effects	
Constipation	Increase fluid intake, encourage high fiber intake, provide laxatives as needed
Dry mouth	Advise client to use sugarless hard candy or gum, sips of water frequently
Nasal congestion	Suggest over-the-counter nasal decongestants that are safe for use with antipsychotic agents
Blurred vision	Ask client to avoid dangerous tasks This symptom will usually last only a short time at the beginning of treatment Eye drops should be used for the short-term need
Mydriasis	Advise client to report any eye pain immediately
Photophobia	Advise client to wear sunglasses when in sunlight
Orthostatic hypotension	Advise client to get out of chair or bed slowly, to sit before standing, and rise slowly Observe to see if change to another antipsychotic is advisable
Tachycardia	Usually a reflex response to hypotension and decreases when intervention for hypotension is effective With clozapine, withhold dose if pulse rate is greater than 140/min
Urinary retention	Encourage client to void when urge is present and void frequently Catheterize for residual urine Client should closely monitor output Older men with benign prostatic hyperplasia are more susceptible
Urinary hesitation	Provide privacy, encourage client to take the time to void, run water in sink, or pour warm water over perineum
Sedation	Help client to get up, get dressed, and begin the day early
Weight gain	Advise client to maintain appropriate diet
Agranulocytosis	There is a high incidence in clients taking clozapine White cell counts need to be monitored weekly If the WBC is less than 3500 cells/mm^3 prior to therapy, no treatment should begin After treatment has begun, a WBC less than 3000 cells/mm^3 and a granulocyte count of less than 1500 cells/mm^3 indicate that treatment should be interrupted to monitor for infection If WBC is less than 2000 cells/mm^3 and granulocyte count is less than 1000 cells/mm^3, halt therapy and do not begin treatment with drug again If infection develops, antibiotics should be prescribed

(*continued*)

Table 4-2 Extrapyramidal Side Effects (EPSEs) (continued)	
Side Effects	**Nursing Interventions**
Central Nervous System Effects	
Akathisia	Usually develops within the first 2 months There is an uncontrollable need to move Occurs most often with high-potency antipsychotics Treatment is usually with beta blockers, benzodiazepines, and anticholinergic drugs The antipsychotic agent should be changed to a lower-potency agent It is important to distinguish between akathisia and exacerbation of psychosis If akathisia is confused with anxiety or psychotic agitation, the antipsychotic dosage would likely be increased, thereby making akathisia more intense
Dystonias	Acute: Usually occur early in treatment and are dangerous and severe Oculogyric crisis or torticollis is the most common occurrence Treatment includes antiparkinson drug or antihistamine immediately and offer reassurance Obtain a prescription for IM administration when client begins treatment with antipsychotics or if in acute state of dystonia, call prescriber immediately For less acute dystonias, notify prescriber when a prescription for an antiparkinson drug is warranted
Drug-induced parkinsonism	A chronic nervous disease characterized by a fine, slowly spreading tremor, muscular weakness and rigidity, and a peculiar gait induced by some antipsychotic medications Assess for three major symptoms: tremors, rigidity, and bradykinesia Report to prescriber immediately Antiparkinson drugs will be indicated
Tardive dyskinesia (TD)	Develops in 15–20% of clients during long-term therapy The risk is related to duration of treatment and dosage For many clients symptoms are irreversible Assess for signs using the Abnormal Inventory Movement Scale (AIMS) Anticholinergic agents will worsen TD, so use is contraindicated
Neuroleptic malignant syndrome	This is a potentially fatal side effect of antipsychotic medications Monitor for hyperthermia; routinely take client's temperature and encourage adequate water intake Also routinely assess for rigidity, tremor, and similar symptoms
Seizures	Occur in approximately 1% of clients taking antipsychotic medications Clozapine causes a higher rate, up to 5% of clients taking 600–900 mg/day For clozapine doses greater than 600 mg/day, a normal EEG should be performed If a seizure occurs, clozapine may need to be discontinued

features usually seen); refer again to Box 4-1 for positive and negative symptoms of schizophrenia

g. Typical antipsychotics are not different from each other in overall clinical response at equivalent doses; thus selection of a drug is determined by extent, type, and severity of side effects produced, as well as effect of drug in a first-degree relative (see Box 4-2 for a list of antipsychotics by potency classification)

   1) A low-potency drug such as chlorpromazine can reduce risk of EPS, while a high-potency drug such as haloperidol can minimize postural hypotension, sedation, and anticholinergic effects

   2) These drugs are equally effective in treating positive symptoms of schizophrenia but are less effective in treating negative symptoms

h. Tolerance to antipsychotic medications is very uncommon; they are also the most toxic drugs used in psychiatry

Box 4-2	**High-Potency Antipsychotic Drugs**

Classification of Traditional Antipsychotics by Potency

High-Potency Antipsychotic Drugs

- Fluphenazine
- Haloperidol
- Pimozide
- Thiothixene
- Trifluoperazine

Moderate-Potency Antipsychotic Drugs

- Loxapine
- Perphenazine

Low-Potency Antipsychotic Drugs

- Chlorpromazine
- Thioridazine

2. Common medications (refer again to Table 4-1)
   a. Chlorpromazine and other antipsychotics are used primarily to treat psychotic disorders, specifically schizophrenia and other chronic mental illnesses; treatment of schizophrenia has three goals:
      1) Suppression of acute episodes
      2) Prevention of acute exacerbations
      3) Maintenance of highest possible level of functioning
   b. Selection of traditional antipsychotic drugs is based largely on side effect profile
   c. Client should not receive a drug that, because of its side effects, is likely to cause discomfort, inconvenience, or harm; for example, if a client has a history of prostatic hyperplasia or glaucoma, or is sensitive to anticholinergic drugs, a low-potency neuroleptic should not be prescribed
3. Administration considerations
   a. Typical antipsychotics effectively suppress symptoms during acute psychotic episodes and, when taken long term, can greatly reduce incidence of relapse (a major risk in treatment of schizophrenia); but since etiology of psychotic illness is entirely unknown, the relationship of receptor blockade to therapeutic effects can only be estimated
   b. Medication effects can usually be seen in 1–2 days, but substantial improvement usually takes 2–4 weeks and full effects may not develop for several months
   c. Dosage requirements vary considerably for each client and must be adjusted as target symptoms change and side effects are monitored; initially, depending on dosage, a client receives several doses per day and total daily dose can be titrated slowly until a safe, effective dose is reached
   d. The half-life of antipsychotic drugs is more than 24 hours, so client usually can be dosed once a day after safe, effective dose is reached
   e. Dosing for older adults requires small doses, typically 30–50% of those taken by younger clients; also poorly responsive clients may need larger doses than highly responsive clients (although very large doses are generally avoided)
   f. Positive symptoms of schizophrenia respond better than negative symptoms
   g. Antipsychotic drugs do not alter underlying pathology of schizophrenia; treatment is not curative; it offers only symptomatic relief
   h. A thorough baseline evaluation should be done, including laboratory tests and electrocardiogram (ECG), for clients beginning treatment

> i. Antipsychotic medications can also be used for clients with bipolar disorder (used to reduce acute symptoms of psychosis) and for clients who have Tourette syndrome (specifically, haloperidol can reduce severe symptoms of disease); neuroleptics suppress emesis in clients by blocking dopamine receptors in chemo-receptor trigger zone of medulla

> j. Depot antipsychotic preparations such as haloperidol and fluphenazine are long-acting injectable preparations used for long-term maintenance therapy of schizo-phrenia; with this form of treatment, relapse rate is usually reduced and thus is more favorable if a client needs long-term therapy; dosage should be reduced in older adults

4. Contraindications

   a. Hypersensitivity

   b. Cross-sensitivity may exist among phenothiazines

   c. Use with caution in clients with narrow-angle glaucoma, adynamic ileus, prostatic hyperplasia, cardiovascular disease, hepatic or renal dysfunction, and seizure disorders

   d. Should not be used in clients who have CNS depression

   e. Contraindicated for comatose or severely depressed clients

   f. Also contraindicated in Parkinson disease, prolactin-dependent carcinoma of the breast, bone marrow depression, and severe hypotension or hypertension

5. Significant drug interactions

   a. May decrease therapeutic response to levodopa

   b. May be at increased risk for **agranulocytosis**, a low white blood cell (WBC) count, when also taking antithyroid agents

   c. See Table 4-3 for additional adverse drug–drug interactions and effects

6. Significant food interactions: use of nutmeg is contraindicated with haloperidol; dong quai and St. John's wort increase photosensitivity; evening primrose decreases seizure threshold; kava kava increases dystonia

7. Significant laboratory studies

   a. Before treatment is started, clients should have a complete evaluation including ECG, blood profile that includes WBC, hemoglobin, and hematocrit

   b. Ongoing monitoring is indicated to assess for decreases in WBC counts

   c. Assess liver function

8. Side effects (refer back to Table 4-2)

   a. D_2-receptor blockade is known to be responsible for many side effects of typical antipsychotics

   b. Dopamine blockade can lead to gynecomastia, galactorrhea, amenorrhea (occa-sionally), and weight gain

9. Adverse effects/toxicity (refer back to Table 4-2)

   a. Most common adverse effects are sedation, orthostatic hypotension, and **anticho-linergic effects** (dry mouth, blurred vision, urinary retention, photophobia, consti-pation, tachycardia); others include **akathisia** (uncontrollable need to move) and **parkinsonism** (set of symptoms that resembles Parkinson disease)

   b. Photosensitivity occurs; clients should take measures to protect eyes when exposed to sunlight

   c. Agranulocytosis, which is an acute deficit or absolute lack of granulocytic white blood cells (neutrophils, basophils, and eosinophils)

   d. **Neuroleptic malignant syndrome (NMS)** is characterized by catatonia, rigidity, stupor, unstable BP, hyperthermia, profuse sweating, dyspnea, and incontinence; it sometimes occurs as a toxic reaction to use of potent neuroleptic agents in thera-peutic doses and may last 5–10 days after drug is discontinued; mortality rate may be as high as 20%; bromocriptine and dantrolene have been used to treat NMS if

Practice to Pass

A client taking an anti-psychotic medication asks, "What is neuro-leptic malignant syn-drome?" How would the nurse describe the syndrome and its management?

Table 4-3	Adverse Interactions of Antipsychotics with Other Drugs
Drug	**Effect of Interaction**
Alcohol, antihistamines, opioids, antidepressants, sedative–hypnotics, analgesics	Additive CNS depression with other CNS depressants
Alcohol, nitrates, or antihypertensives	Additive hypotension with acute ingestion
Amoxapine, fluoxetine	↑ extrapyramidal side effects
Amphetamines	↓ antipsychotic effect
Antacids	May ↓ absorption
Anticholinergic or antiparkinson drugs	↑ anticholinergic effects; delayed onset of effects of oral doses of antipsychotics; potentially ↑ risk of hyperthermia
Barbiturates, nonbarbiturate hypnotics	Respiratory depression and ↑ sedation; ↓ antipsychotic serum levels; hypotension
Benzodiazepines	↑ sedation; respiratory depression with lorazepam and loxapine
Beta-adrenergic blocking agents (propranolol)	Effects of either or both drugs increased
Cimetidine	Chlorpromazine absorption decreased; increased sedation with chlorpromazine
Diazoxide	Can cause severe hyperglycemia
Dopaminergic antiparkinson drugs (e.g., bromocriptine)	Antagonizes the antipsychotic effect
Guanethidine	Control of hypertension is decreased
Insulin, oral hypoglycemics	Control of diabetes is weakened
L-dopa	↓ antiparkinson effect; may exacerbate psychosis
Lithium	May ↓ blood levels and effectiveness of phenothiazines
Phenobarbital	May ↑ metabolism and ↓ the effectiveness of the drug
Phenytoin	May ↑ phenytoin toxicity; ↓ antipsychotic blood serum levels
Trazodone	Additive hypotension with phenothiazines
Tricyclics	Possible ventricular dysrhythmias with thioridazine; possible ↑ blood serum levels of both; hypotension; sedation; anticholinergic effect; ↑ risk of seizures

usual treatment for hyperthermia is ineffective; antipsychotic drug withdrawal is mandatory

    e. Low-potency drugs are more likely to cause sedation and hypotension, while high-potency drugs cause more EPS

    f. Overdoses of antipsychotic drugs are not usually fatal and treatment for attempted overdose is supportive (e.g., gastric lavage to empty stomach); it can cause severe CNS depression (somnolence to coma, hypotension, EPS); also reported are restlessness or agitation, seizures (lowered seizure threshold), hyperthermia, increased anticholinergic symptoms, and dysrhythmias

10. Client-centered nursing care

    a. Observe hospitalized clients take their medication so that they swallow medications and do not "cheek" them; clients may have a difficult time with "clouding" and sedating effects of antipsychotic drugs

    b. Client teaching (see following section) is a major aspect of nursing care

    c. Refer once more to Table 4-2 for more specific nursing care and teaching considerations

Box 4-3	**Anticholinergics**
Medications Used to Treat Extrapyramidal Side Effects	• Benztropine • Trihexyphenidyl
	Antihistamine
	• Diphenhydramine
	Dopamine Agonist
	• Amantadine

11. Client education

! **a.** Take medication as prescribed; the major relapse factor for clients with schizophrenia is discontinuing medications, which then leads to relapse and rehospitalization

  b. Take PO meds with food, milk, or a full glass of water to decrease gastric irritation

! **c.** Dilute most concentrates in 120 mL of distilled or acidified tap water or fruit juice just before administration

  d. Be aware of other medications that may be prescribed to treat EPS (see Box 4-3)

  e. Include family members involved in client's care and teach at a level that client or family can grasp and demonstrate knowledge acquired; provide written instructions and information about other resources, including phone contacts, if problems should arise

  f. Be aware that anticholinergic medications may decrease effectiveness of typical antipsychotics

B. Atypical antipsychotic drugs

  1. Action and use

  a. The atypical antipsychotics exert both dopamine receptor subtype 2 (D_2) and serotonin receptor subtype 2 ($5HT_2$) receptor-blocking action (are DA and 5HT antagonists)

  b. Blockage of serotonin receptors is thought to liberate dopamine in cortex and may explain some reduction in negative symptoms

! **c.** Atypical agents cause few or no extrapyramidal symptoms, including **tardive dyskinesia (TD)** (dyskinesia is difficulty performing voluntary movement, while tardive indicates late onset—usually seen as a serious side effect of antipsychotic agents)

! **d.** Used to treat positive and negative symptoms of schizophrenia and other mental illnesses with psychotic features and to treat mood symptoms, hostility, violence, suicidal behavior, and cognitive impairment seen in schizophrenia

  e. Provide new hope for clients with psychosis, particularly during first episode, for those who have not responded well to typical antipsychotics, or for those with dose-limiting side effects from traditional neuroleptics

  2. Common medications (refer back to Table 4-1 for drug names and routes)

  a. The following are some atypical antipsychotic medications commonly used at present: clozapine, risperidone, and olanzapine

  b. Clozapine

  1) Because of its serious side effect, agranulocytosis, it was released with a very rigid set of protocols including weekly blood analysis

    2) Clients are not prescribed more than a 1-week supply of medication to enforce compliance with weekly blood analysis

    3) Beneficial effects of clozapine are usually very positive for most and remarkable for others

    4) Clozapine has a greater affinity for dopamine-D_1, dopamine-D_4, and serotonin ($5HT_2$), as well as dopamine D_2 receptors

  c. Risperidone

    1) Has a greater affinity for dopamine D_2 receptors and a similar antagonism of serotonin $5HT_2$

    2) Lack of serious side effects makes it a very well-tolerated agent

    3) Has little affinity for muscarinic (i.e., cholinergic receptors), so anticholinergic side effects are minimized; neither does it appear to cause agranulocytosis, EPSEs, tardive dyskinesia, or NMS

    4) Side effects include orthostatic hypotension, insomnia, agitation, headache, anxiety, and rhinitis

  d. Olanzapine

    1) Comparable to risperidone in efficacy of treating both positive and negative symptoms and has a comparable side effects profile

    2) Does not cause agranulocytosis; early clinical trials indicate few incidents of EPSE

  e. Newer antipsychotic medications such as paliperidone and aripiprazole reduce extrapyramidal symptoms such as tardive dyskinesia, thus improving client use of medications while improving behavioral and cognitive symptoms

3. Administration considerations

  a. Clozapine is usually given one to two times daily and should not exceed 900 mg/day; because of the strict protocol, blood testing is done weekly; *if client does not comply, the drug will not be continued*

  b. Risperidone is usually administered PO in one to two daily doses; for debilitated or older clients or for those with renal or hepatic impairment, dosage should be reduced at onset of treatment

  c. Olanzapine is usually administered PO as well; dosage should not exceed 15 mg/day; for debilitated or nonsmoking female clients greater than 65 years, therapy should be initiated at 5 mg/day

  d. Refer back to Table 4-1 for generic and trade names and general information about administration of antipsychotics

4. Contraindications

  a. Clozapine, risperidone, and olanzapine are all contraindicated for clients with hypersensitivity to drug; other considerations include cautious use in bone marrow depression, during severe CNS depression or coma, and during lactation

  b. Clozapine should be used cautiously with clients who have a depressed bone marrow, prostatic enlargement, narrow-angle glaucoma, malnourished state, diabetes mellitus, seizure disorder, or in clients with cardiovascular, hepatic, or renal disease; it should also be used cautiously in children less than age 16 years (safety is not yet established)

  c. Risperidone should be used cautiously for older adults, debilitated clients, and those with renal or hepatic impairment, cardiovascular disease, or history of seizures, suicide attempts, or drug abuse; safety has not been established for use during pregnancy or lactation, or for use with children

  d. Olanzapine should be used cautiously with clients with liver disease or during pregnancy or lactation; safety for use with children has not yet been established

!   e. For older adults or debilitated clients or clients with known liver, renal, or cardiovascular disease, initial dosing should be lowered and ongoing monitoring should be emphasized

5. Significant drug interactions
   a. Clozapine may be decreased by concurrent use of carbamazepine, omeprazole, or rifampin; additive hypotension may occur with concurrent use of antihypertensives or benzodiazepines, additive CNS depression may occur with concurrent use of alcohol or other CNS depressants; atypical antipsychotics may decrease effects of levodopa or other dopamine agonists
   b. Risperidone may decrease the antiparkinson effects of levodopa or other dopamine agonists; carbamazepine increases metabolism and may decrease effectiveness of risperidone; clozapine decreases metabolism and may increase effects of risperidone; additive CNS depression may occur with other CNS depressants including alcohol, antihistamines, sedative–hypnotics, or opioids
   c. Olanzapine effects may be decreased by concurrent use of carbamazepine, omeprazole, or rifampin; additive CNS depression occurs with concurrent use of alcohol or other CNS depressants; olanzapine may also antagonize effects of levodopa or other dopamine agonists

6. Significant food interactions: none

!   7. Significant laboratory studies: for clients prescribed clozapine, there is a mandatory need for weekly blood tests (WBC counts) to prevent or detect agranulocytosis

8. Side effects
   a. Seizure incidence for clients taking clozapine is 3%; this is one reason that maximum dose should not exceed 900 mg/day
   b. See Table 4-4 for common side effects of atypical antipsychotics

9. Adverse effects/toxicity
   a. Some of the more serious adverse or toxic effects listed for clozapine have been discussed in previous section on side effects; other considerations include neuroleptic malignant syndrome (NMS)
   b. For clients prescribed risperidone, monitor for NMS
   c. For clients taking olanzapine, monitor for NMS and seizures

10. Client-centered nursing care

!   a. Because of risk of fatal agranulocytosis, clozapine is reserved for clients with severe schizophrenia who have not responded to traditional antipsychotic drugs (40–60% success rate for treatment in this group)
   b. Assist clients to adjust to changes experienced (improvement in positive and negative symptoms, ability to become more animated, and to have behavior that is more socially acceptable)

Table 4-4 **Common Side Effects of Atypical Antipsychotics**

	Clozapine	Risperidone	Olanzapine
Extrapyramidal	None	+	+
Cardiac	+++	++	+
Sedation	++++	++	+
Anticholinergic	++++	+	++
Weight gain	+++	++	++++

Occurrence: +, least; ++++, greatest

c. Usually with clients who respond well to clozapine, there is a decreased need for rehospitalization as well

d. Encourage client to void prior to administering olanzapine

11. Client education: clients will still need help with psychoeducation, social skills training, group support, and other rehabilitative interventions to improve overall level of functioning and quality of life while incorporating atypical antipsychotic drugs into life pattern

II. ANTIDEPRESSANTS

A. Tricyclics

1. Action and use

   a. Imipramine was the first antidepressant drug used to treat depression (1950s) and is still used effectively today

   b. Tricyclic antidepressants (TCAs) such as imipramine block monoamine reuptake, which indicates that TCAs intensify effects of norepinephrine and serotonin; TCAs can elevate mood, increase activity and alertness, decrease a client's preoccupation with morbidity, improve appetite, and regulate sleep patterns

   c. Initial mechanism of TCAs takes about 1–3 weeks to develop while a maximum response is achieved in approximately 6–8 weeks

   d. Other uses for TCAs are to treat clients with chronic insomnia, attention-deficit/hyperactivity disorder, obsessive–compulsive disorder (OCD), neuropathic pain, panic disorder, and as an adjunct in treatment of enuresis

2. Common antidepressant medications (Table 4-5)

   a. Several TCAs are available that are equally effective; major differences can be found in side effects

   b. For example, doxepin has sedative effects and could be more effectively used with clients who experience insomnia

   c. Older adults and clients with glaucoma, constipation, or prostatic hyperplasia can be especially sensitive to anticholinergic effects of TCAs; therefore, a TCA such as desipramine with weak anticholinergic effects would be more appropriate with these clients

3. Administration considerations

   a. Dosing with TCAs is individualized and based on clinical response or plasma drug levels (which must be above 225 ng/mL for antidepressant effects to occur)

   b. TCAs are normally given by mouth; amitriptyline and imipramine may be given by intramuscular (IM) injection; intravenous (IV) administration is not usually used

   c. TCAs have long half-lives, so they can be taken daily in a single dose; because the half-life of individual drugs varies, client dosing is also individualized

   d. Once-a-day dosing at bedtime has several advantages, such as ease of taking as part of daily routine, promoting sleep by its sedative effect, and reducing intensity of daytime side effects

   e. They can lower seizure threshold and should be used cautiously in persons with a history of seizures or conditions predisposing to seizures

4. Contraindications

   a. Hypersensitivity to TCAs

   b. Myocardial infarction

   c. Cerebrovascular disease

   d. Clients at risk for suicide who are taking TCAs should not have access to a large quantity of the drug and should be hospitalized until risk of suicide has passed

Table 4-5	Medications Commonly Used to Treat Depression
Drug Class and Generic Name	**Nursing Responsibilities**
Tricyclic Antidepressants (TCAs)	
Amitriptyline Clomipramine Desipramine Doxepin Imipramine Maprotiline Nortriptyline Protriptyline Trimipramine	• Educate the client early about potential side effects • Inform client that side effects will diminish with time and if necessary there are management alternatives that can be implemented • Advise client that response will take some time and continued use is essential • Inform client that first-time treatment for major depression should continue for 6–12 months • Warn client of a possible significant weight gain • Monitor for improvement; if minimal or no change after 2–4 weeks, it may be necessary to change drug • Educate client and family to report changes in behavior or suicidal ideation immediately
Selective Serotonin Reuptake Inhibitors (SSRIs)	
Citalopram Escitalopram Fluoxetine Fluvoxamine Paroxetine Sertraline	• Inform client to take medication as prescribed; abrupt discontinuation of the drug is contraindicated • Continuously monitor client for side effects or adverse effects, particularly in the area of sexual dysfunction; client may be reluctant to discuss • Immediately report worsening of symptoms or suicidal ideation
Serotonin Norepinephrine Reuptake Inhibitor (SNRI)	
Desvenlafaxine Duloxetine Levomilnacipran Milnacipran Venlafaxine	• Similar to SSRI, do not begin therapy within 14 days of an MAOI • Numerous drug–drug interactions • Educate client and family to report suicidal ideation or changes in behavior immediately • Educate client not to discontinue the medication abruptly
Monoamine Oxidase Inhibitors (MAOIs)	
Isocarboxazid Phenelzine Selegiline Tranylcypromine	• Educate client about the need to eat a tyramine-restricted diet • Caution client about side effects and adverse effects of MAOIs • Educate client about careful use of over-the-counter or other prescription medications and be sure client understands the seriousness of the effects • Monitor efficacy of drugs and continuously reeducate client to avoid abruptly discontinuing medication or not taking medications as prescribed
Atypical Antidepressants	
Amoxapine Bupropion Mirtazapine Nefazodone Trazodone Vilazodone	• Instruct client about the side effects and adverse effect of the medication, especially seizure risks at higher drug doses • Instruct client concerning the importance of taking this and all medication as prescribed • Instruct client to take medication as prescribed and monitor for any adverse or side effects • Instruct client to report any signs of sexual dysfunction, especially priapism, immediately

5. Significant drug interactions
   a. Combination of TCAs and a MAOI can lead to hypertensive crisis from excessive adrenergic stimulation of heart and blood vessels
   b. TCAs potentiate responses to direct-acting sympathomimetics (i.e., drugs such as epinephrine and norepinephrine); sympathetic nervous system (SNS) stimulation by these drugs can be increased because TCAs block reuptake of these drugs into adrenergic terminals, which prolongs their presence in synaptic spaces
   c. TCAs decrease responses to indirect-acting sympathomimetics (i.e., drugs such as ephedrine and amphetamine that promote release of transmitter from adrenergic nerves) because TCAs block uptake of these agents into adrenergic

nerves, which prevents them from reaching their site of action within nerve terminals

   d. TCAs exert anticholinergic actions of their own; therefore, TCAs will intensify effects of other drugs with anticholinergic actions, such as antihistamines and certain over-the-counter (OTC) sleep aids; these products should be avoided while taking TCAs

   e. CNS depression caused by TCAs will add to CNS depression caused by other drugs; therefore clients taking TCAs should avoid CNS depressants, including alcohol, antihistamines, opioids, and barbiturates

   f. Increased TCA levels occur when combined with cimetidine, fluoxetine, phenothiazines, or hormonal contraceptives

6. Significant food interactions: St. John's wort is contraindicated with TCAs

7. Significant laboratory studies: assess AST, ALT levels; monitor serum drug levels to ensure they remain within therapeutic range

8. Side effects

   a. Most common undesirable effects of the TCAs are orthostatic hypotension, sedation, and anticholinergic effects

   b. Instruct client to move slowly when changing position (lying to sitting, sitting to standing, or turning) to avoid injury; monitor BP both lying and sitting if client is hospitalized

9. Adverse effects/toxicity

   a. Most serious adverse effect of TCAs is cardiac toxicity; in the absence of overdose or preexisting cardiac impairment, serious cardiotoxicity is rare

   b. To avoid adverse cardiac effects, clients over age 40 and those with heart disease should undergo baseline ECG and then every 6 months

   c. Adverse effects of each drug are indicated in Table 4-6

10. Client-centered nursing care

   a. Advise clients of potential side effects and that therapeutic response will take some weeks to be established once therapy has begun; clients and families often become impatient when client is experiencing drug side effects while still having original symptoms

Table 4-6 **Most Common Adverse Effects from Antidepressant Medications**

Effect	Manifestations
Orthostatic hypotension	Major decrease in blood pressure with body position changes
Anticholinergic	Blocks muscarinic cholinergic receptors, which produces dry mouth, blurred vision, photophobia, constipation, urinary hesitancy, and tachycardia
Sedation	Sleepiness and difficulty maintaining arousal are common responses to TCAs because of blockade of histamine receptors in CNS
Cardiac toxicity	TCAs can adversely affect the heart's function by decreasing vagal influence (secondary to muscarinic blockade) and acting directly on bundle of His to slow conduction
Seizures	Lower seizure threshold
Hypomania	Mild mania can occur
Sexual dysfunction	Anorgasmia, delayed ejaculation, and decreased libido
Hypertensive crisis from dietary tyramine	Although MAOIs normally produce hypotension, these drugs can cause severe hypertension if client eats tyramine-rich foods
Drug interactions	Always teach clients the importance of preventing adverse drug effects and drug interactions; see individual classifications for specific nursing responsibilities

      b. Clients taking TCAs have highest rate of suicide after therapeutic levels achieved as compared to clients taking other types of antidepressants; family and client education about this effect should be included

      c. Refer back to Table 4-5 for nursing responsibilities with TCAs and see Table 4-6 for manifestations of common adverse effects

    11. Client education

      a. Use measures to prevent orthostatic hypotension

      b. Side effects will diminish with time and symptoms will be lessened as medication regimen is followed (this knowledge may enhance compliance)

      c. Utilize other available therapies as well as medications as appropriate

      d. Refer back to Tables 4-5 and 4-6 for specific teaching points

B. Monoamine oxidase inhibitors (MAOIs)

    1. Action and use

      a. Because of potentially fatal food and drug interactions, this class of antidepressant is usually not a first choice to treat clients with depression unless client has atypical depression

      b. Monoamine oxidase (MAO) is an enzyme present in liver, intestinal wall, and terminals of monoamine-containing neurons; the function of MAO in neurons is to convert monoamine transmitters (norepinephrine, serotonin, and dopamine) into inactive products; in the liver and intestine, MAO serves to inactivate tyramine and other biogenic amines in food

      c. MAOIs decrease amount of monoamine oxidase in liver that breaks down amino acids tyramine and tryptophan

      d. There is an antidepressant effect of MAOIs because of MAO-A in nerve terminals along with other enzymatic and chemical actions; MAOI biochemical action takes place rapidly, whereas clinical response (relief of depression) develops slowly

      e. MAOIs have been used with some success to treat bulimia and obsessive–compulsive disorders and to treat panic attacks in clients with panic disorder

    2. Common medications: refer again to Tables 4-5 and 4-6 for MAOIs commonly used

    3. Administration considerations: route is usually PO; see Table 4-5 for details

    4. Contraindications: clients over age 60 or those with pheochromocytoma, heart failure, liver disease, severe renal impairment, cerebrovascular defect, cardiovascular disease, or hypertension

    5. Significant drug interactions

      a. Use with caution for clients taking other TCAs

      b. Taking SSRIs with MAOIs can cause **serotonin syndrome** (agitation, sweating, confusion, fever, hyperreflexia, tachycardia, hypotension, muscle rigidity, and ataxia); avoid this combination

      c. Antihypertensive drugs will potentiate hypotensive effects of MAOIs

      d. Meperidine can produce hyperthermia in clients taking MAOIs and should be avoided

      e. Instruct client to avoid all medications (prescription and nonprescription) that have not been specifically approved by healthcare provider

    6. Significant food interactions

      a. Dietary tyramine, some other dietary constituents, and indirect-acting sympathomimetics (e.g., amphetamine, methylphenidate, ephedrine, cocaine) can precipitate a hypertensive crisis in clients taking MAOIs

      b. See Box 4-4 for lists of foods and drugs to avoid and to use cautiously while taking an MAOI

    7. Significant laboratory studies: in prescription for antidepressant effects to occur, serum drug levels need to be maintained within a specified therapeutic range

Box 4-4	**Foods and Drugs to Avoid**
Foods to Avoid with Monoamine Oxidase Inhibitors	• All strong or aged cheeses • Meats and fish: aged or cured • Fruits and vegetables: broad bean pods, tofu, soy bean extracts • Alcohol: draft beer • Other: sauerkraut, soy sauce, yeast extracts, soups (especially miso), and any non-fresh foods • Drugs: other antidepressant drugs, nasal and sinus decongestants, allergy, hay fever and asthma remedies, narcotics (especially meperidine), epinephrine, stimulants, cocaine, amphetamines **Consume with Caution** • Cheeses made from pasteurized milk (e.g., cottage, ricotta, cream) • Meats and fish: chicken liver, meats, liver, herring • Fruits and vegetables: raspberries, bananas, small amounts only of avocado, spinach • Alcohol: wine • Other: monosodium glutamate, pizza, only small amounts of chocolate, caffeine, nuts, dairy products • Drugs: insulin, oral hypoglycemics, oral anticoagulants, thiazide diuretics, anticholinergic agents, muscle relaxants

8. Side effects
   a. Orthostatic hypotension is a common initial and sometimes persistent side effect of MAOIs
   b. Edema, sexual dysfunction, and weight gain are also common and can lead to drug discontinuation
   c. Complaints of insomnia occur with all MAOIs
9. Adverse effects/toxicity: in contrast to TCAs, MAOIs cause direct CNS stimulation, which in excess can produce anxiety, agitation, hypomania, and even mania
10. Client-centered nursing care
    a. Provide oral and written instructions of how to avoid adverse effects of MAOIs; there are many factors to consider with client's safe use of drug because of side effects and adverse effects of MAOIs
    b. Assess client for ability to adhere to a strict dietary regimen
    c. Consult with prescriber about changes in vital signs to avoid potentially fatal hypertensive crisis
    d. Instruct client not to take any prescribed or OTC medication without first consulting or notifying prescriber
11. Client education
    a. Familiarize client with symptoms of orthostatic hypotension and how to avoid injury when rising from bed or chair slowly
    b. If client is hospitalized, BP needs to be monitored regularly
    c. Educate client orally and in writing or provide a dietary consultation if appropriate for client and family in order to avoid hypertensive crisis
    d. Teach client to avoid all medications (prescribed or OTC) that have not been specifically approved by prescriber

C. **Selective serotonin reuptake inhibitors (SSRIs)**
   1. Action and use
      a. Block reuptake of serotonin and intensify transmission at serotonergic synapses; effects can usually be seen after 1–3 weeks and are equivalent to those produced from TCAs

     b. SSRIs have same efficacy as TCAs, exhibit fewer side effects than either TCAs or MAOIs, and have a decreased time between initial dose and beginning of reduced signs and symptoms of depression

     c. All SSRIs are effective in treating obsessive–compulsive disorder (OCD), panic disorder, and bulimia nervosa

2. Common medications (refer again to Table 4-5)

3. Administration considerations

     a. SSRIs are administered orally in liquid or pulvules; older adults or those with impaired renal function should be given a low dosage with increases made cautiously

     b. Evaluate client frequently for safety and desired effects of drug

4. Contraindications

     a. Most SSRIs should not be prescribed for clients with a hypersensitivity to drug or those with severe hepatic or renal disease

     b. Caution should be used for debilitated clients or those with a history of seizure disorder or diabetes mellitus

     c. Lowered drug doses or longer dosing interval may be needed in clients with impaired hepatic function, older adults, or those receiving multiple drug therapy

5. Significant drug interactions

     a. SSRIs should not be administered with MAOIs to prevent serotonin syndrome, a hyperserotonergic state (confusion, autonomic dysfunction, muscle rigidity, ataxia) that occurs when an SSRI is given concurrently with other serotonin-enhancing drugs, causing an excess of serotonin in system (see Box 4-5)

     b. If a client is on an MAOI and is changed to fluoxetine, at least 5 weeks should elapse before beginning fluoxetine; to change from fluoxetine to MAOIs, at least 2 weeks should elapse before beginning MAOI

     c. A client who is taking fluoxetine and warfarin should have warfarin level monitored closely because fluoxetine is highly bound to plasma proteins and may displace other highly bound drugs such as warfarin

     d. Fluoxetine can elevate plasma levels of TCAs and lithium and should be given cautiously when prescribed along with these other agents

Box 4-5 **Medications that Contribute to Risk for Serotonin Syndrome**	• Selective serotonin reuptake inhibitors (SSRIs) (e.g., citalopram, fluoxetine) • Serotonin and norepinephrine reuptake inhibitors (SNRIs) (e.g., trazodone, duloxetine, venlafaxine) • Bupropion • Tricyclic antidepressants (e.g., amitriptyline, nortriptyline) • Monoamine oxidase inhibitors (MAOIs) (e.g., isocarboxazid, phenelzine) • Drugs to treat HIV and AIDS • Antimigraine medications (e.g., triptans, carbamazepine, valproic acid) • Opioid pain medications: (e.g., codeine, fentanyl, hydrocodone, meperidine, oxycodone, tramadol) • Illicit drugs: (e.g., LSD, Ecstasy, cocaine, amphetamines) • Herbal supplements: St. John's wort, ginseng, nutmeg • Dextromethorphan in OTC cough and cold medications • Antinausea medications (e.g., granisetron, metoclopramide, droperidol, ondansetron) • Miscellaneous medications (e.g., linezolid, lithium, ritonavir)

Data from www.mayoclinic.org/diseases/serotonin-syndrome/home/ovc-2030566; http://www.healthline.com/health/serotonin-syndrome#Symptoms2; www.medscape.com/viewarticle/733706_2

6. Significant food interactions
   a. Each SSRI is individual for effect with food; fluoxetine, paroxetine, and fluvoxamine can be taken with or without food, while sertraline is slowly absorbed following oral administration; food increases extent of absorption for sertraline; yet, if there is gastric upset, drug literature recommends administration of paroxetine with food
   b. When administering a newer SSRI, consult individual drug literature
7. Significant laboratory studies
   a. Serum drug levels are not clinically useful to determine dose or monitor for toxicity
   b. Monitor CBC, differential, and bleeding time periodically throughout treatment for signs of leukopenia, anemia, or thrombocytopenia or for increased bleeding time
8. Side effects
   a. Side effect profile of SSRIs is relatively mild compared with other antidepressants; there is minimal cardiac toxicity, eliminating need for ECGs
   b. Common initial side effects of SSRIs include nausea, drowsiness, dizziness, headache, sweating, anxiety, insomnia, anorexia, and nervousness; these are generally milder and better tolerated than side effects of TCAs
9. Adverse effects/toxicity
   a. Most SSRIs are relatively safe in overdose; when taken as a single agent, SSRI overdoses are serious and can cause seizures, but complete recovery is common
   b. Sexual dysfunction, experienced by 20–40% of clients taking SSRIs, is an adverse effect that needs to be discussed with client by prescriber
10. Client-centered nursing care
    a. Monitor mood changes; notify prescriber if client demonstrates an increase in anxiety, nervousness, or insomnia
    b. Assess for suicidal tendencies, especially during early drug therapy
    c. Restrict amount of drug available to client to prevent overdose
    d. Monitor appetite, nutritional intake, and weight
11. Client education
    a. Encourage client to comply with diet recommendations of healthcare professionals; give written and oral instructions to client and family
    b. Instruct client to notify prescriber if a rash occurs, which may indicate hypersensitivity
    c. Emphasize importance of follow-up exams to evaluate progress
    d. See also Tables 4-5 and 4-6 for points on specific SSRIs

D. Other antidepressants
1. Action and use
   a. Trazodone and bupropion are newer antidepressant agents that have varied chemical structures and modes of action; they are not easily collapsed into a group and are thus discussed individually here
   b. Bupropion
      1) Similar in structure to amphetamines and can suppress appetite; it does not have cardiotoxic, anticholinergic, and antiadrenergic side effects and can therefore be used more readily with older adults; it can also be used for smoking cessation
      2) Blocks reuptake of dopamine while having only minimal reuptake effects on norepinephrine
   c. Trazodone
      1) A second-line agent for treatment of depression; usually used in combination with another antidepressant and usually prescribed to treat insomnia because of its very pronounced sedative effect
      2) Trazodone alters effects of serotonin in CNS; its antidepressant action may develop only over several weeks

    d. Venlafaxine and duloxetine are serotonin and norepinephrine reuptake inhibitors (SNRIs); treat depression, fibromyalgia, and diabetic peripheral neuropathy.

2. Common medications: refer to Table 4-5

3. Administration considerations

    a. Starting dose of bupropion should be no greater than 75 mg tid; because of dose-related seizure risk, never give more than 150 mg at one time; when maximum dose is required, the recommended regimen is 150 mg tid

    b. Initial dose of trazodone is usually 150 mg/day in two or three divided doses, and may be gradually increased to a maximum of 400 mg/day (outpatients) and 600 mg/day (hospitalized clients); also, a majority of drug dose may be given at bedtime to decrease daytime drowsiness and dizziness

    c. Dosages may be increased gradually for SNRIs; when taken for more than 1 week, tapering is recommended if drug needs to be discontinued

4. Contraindications

    a. Bupropion can cause dose-related seizures

    b. Trazodone is contraindicated for clients with hypersensitivity, those recovering from myocardial infarction, or those who are using concurrent electroconvulsive therapy; it should be used cautiously in clients with cardiovascular disease or who exhibit suicidal behavior; dosage should be reduced in older adults or those who have severe hepatic or renal disease

    c. Recent (within 14 days) use of MAOI is a contraindication for SNRIs

5. Significant drug interactions

    a. With bupropion there is an increased risk of adverse reactions when used with levodopa or MAOIs, and an increased risk of seizures with phenothiazines, antidepressants, theophylline, corticosteroids, OTC stimulants or anorexiants, or cessation of alcohol or benzodiazepines

    b. Trazodone may increase digoxin or phenytoin serum levels; additive CNS depression can occur with alcohol, opioids, and sedative–hypnotics; additive hypotension can occur with antihypertensive agents, acute ingestion of alcohol, or use of nitrates; concurrent use with fluoxetine increases levels and risk of toxicity from trazodone

6. Significant food interactions: do not combine with alcohol; severe reaction can occur if administered with St. John's wort

7. Significant laboratory studies

    a. Monitor hepatic and renal function closely in clients with kidney or liver impairment to prevent elevated serum and tissue bupropion concentrations

    b. For trazodone, assess CBC and renal and hepatic functioning before and periodically during treatment; slight, clinically insignificant decrease in leukocyte and neutrophil counts may occur

    c. Monitor liver function tests for SNRIs on a periodic basis or with symptoms of liver problems

8. Side effects (refer again to Tables 4-5 and 4-6)

    a. Most common side effects of bupropion are agitation and insomnia

    b. Common side effects of trazodone are sedation, orthostatic hypotension, and nausea and vomiting (N/V); in contrast to TCAs, it lacks anticholinergic actions and is not cardiotoxic; it may cause priapism (prolonged erection)

    c. SNRIs may cause sustained elevation of blood pressure; generally dose related

9. Adverse effects/toxicity

    a. Major adverse effect of bupropion is seizure activity; other adverse effects include headache, mania, psychoses, dry mouth, nausea and vomiting, change in appetite, weight gain, weight loss, photosensitivity, hyperglycemia, hypoglycemia, and syndrome of inappropriate ADH secretion (SIADH)

Practice to Pass

Describe the most common adverse effects that should be discussed with a client taking fluoxetine.

    b. Overdose with trazodone is considered safer than with TCAs or MAOIs; death from overdose with trazodone alone has not been reported; adverse effects include drowsiness, confusion, dizziness, fatigue, hallucinations, headache, insomnia, nightmares, slurred speech, syncope, weakness, blurred vision, and tinnitus; also reported are hypotension, arrhythmias, chest pain, hypertension, palpitations, tachycardia, dry mouth, altered taste, constipation, diarrhea, excess salivation, flatulence, nausea and vomiting, rash, hematuria, impotence, priapism, urinary frequency, anemia, leukopenia, myalgia, and tremors

10. Client-centered nursing care

    a. Individuals with a history of bipolar disorder taking bupropion need to be assessed for symptoms of mania

    b. Monitor BP and pulse rate before and during initial therapy with trazodone; clients with preexisting cardiac disease should have ECG monitored before and periodically during therapy to detect dysrhythmias

    c. Assess mental status and mood changes frequently; assess for suicidal tendencies, especially during early therapy; restrict amount of drug available to client

    d. Give bupropion with food to decrease GI side effects; give trazodone immediately after meals to minimize side effects (nausea, dizziness) and allow for maximum absorption

    e. Ensure that client has not taken an MAOI in last 14 days before initiating any medications in this category

11. Client education: as described in Tables 4-5 and 4-6

III. MOOD STABILIZERS

A. Lithium

1. Action and use

    a. Drug of choice for controlling manic episodes in clients with bipolar disorder and is also used for long-term prophylaxis against recurrent mania and depression

    b. Lithium is an inorganic ion that carries a single positive charge; it occurs naturally in animal tissue but has no known physiological function; it is well absorbed following oral administration and is distributed evenly to all tissue and body fluids

    c. Exact mechanism of action is not fully understood, but it alters many neurotransmitter functions; it may correct an ion exchange abnormality in neurons and/or may play a role in normalizing neurotransmission of norepinephrine, serotonin, dopamine, and acetylcholine

    d. Lithium is used to treat a variety of psychiatric disorders, particularly to treat effects of bipolar disorders (treatment of acute manic episodes and prophylaxis against recurrence)

2. Common mood-stabilizing medications: see Table 4-7

3. Administration considerations

    a. Precise dosing is based on serum lithium levels; 300 mg lithium carbonate contains 8–12 mEq lithium; follow prescriber instructions for dosing ranges of adults and children

    b. Lithium reduces euphoria, hyperactivity, and other symptoms of mania but does not cause sedation; mood-stabilizing effects are usually seen in 5–7 days after initial doses, but full effect does not usually occur for 2–3 weeks

    c. For many clients using lithium, adjunctive therapy with a benzodiazepine can be used to provide the sedation clients need

    d. Antipsychotic medications can also be used short term to rapidly decrease symptoms of psychoses

Table 4-7	Commonly Used Mood-Stabilizing Drugs
Generic Names	**Uses**
Lithium carbonate	Manic-depressive episodes, maintenance therapy for manic-depression, improvement of neutrophil counts in client receiving chemotherapy, prophylaxis of cluster headaches, hypothyroidism
Carbamazepine	Seizure disorders, trigeminal neuralgia, chronic pain
Valproic acid	Seizure disorders, bipolar mania, prophylaxis for migraine headaches, schizophrenia, aggressive outbursts, attention-deficit disorder, organic brain syndrome

4. Contraindications
   a. Hypersensitivity to drug, dehydration, and severe cardiovascular or renal disease; should only be used where therapy (including blood levels) may be closely monitored; some products contain alcohol or tartrazine and should be avoided in clients with known hypersensitivity or intolerance
   b. Use cautiously in older adults or debilitated clients (decrease initial dose); also use cautiously with clients with cardiac, renal, or thyroid disease or diabetes mellitus
5. Significant drug interactions
   a. Lithium may prolong action of neuromuscular blocking agents
   b. Neurologic toxicity may occur with haloperidol or molindone
   c. Diuretics, methyldopa, probenecid, fluoxetine, and NSAIDs may increase risk of toxicity
   d. Blood levels may be increased by angiotensin-converting enzyme (ACE) inhibitors
   e. Lithium may decrease effects of chlorpromazine, and chlorpromazine may mask early signs of lithium toxicity
   f. Hypothyroid effects may be additive with potassium iodide or antithyroid agents
   g. Aminophylline, phenothiazines, and drugs containing large amounts of sodium increase renal elimination and may decrease effectiveness
6. Significant food interactions: large changes in sodium intake may alter renal elimination of lithium; increasing sodium intake will increase renal excretion
7. Significant laboratory studies
   a. Monitor serum lithium levels frequently because of danger of lithium toxicity, especially since therapeutic level and toxic level are very close; therapeutic range is 0.8–1.4 mEq/L, while toxic level is 1.5 mEq/L or greater
   b. Pre-lithium workup
      1) Renal: urinalysis, blood urea nitrogen (BUN), creatinine, electrolytes, 24-hour creatinine clearance
      2) Thyroid: thyroid-stimulating hormone (TSH), T_4 (thyroxine), T_3 resin uptake, T_4I (free thyroxine index)
      3) Other: fasting blood glucose, complete blood count (CBC), ECG
   c. Maintenance lithium dosing: lithium level every 3 months (for first 6 months); every 6 months reassess thyroid function and ECG; assess more often if client is symptomatic
8. Side effects
   a. Seizures, fatigue, headache, impaired memory, ataxia, confusion, dizziness, drowsiness, psychomotor retardation, restlessness, stupor
   b. Also aphasia, blurred vision, dysarthria, tinnitus, dysrhythmias, ECG changes, edema, hypotension

    c. Others include abdominal pain, anorexia, bloating, diarrhea, nausea, dry mouth, and metallic taste in the mouth; also polyuria, glycosuria, nephrogenic diabetes insipidus, and renal toxicity

    d. Dermatologic signs include alopecia, diminished sensation, and pruritis

    e. Also reported are hypothyroidism, goiter, hyperglycemia, hyperthyroidism, hyponatremia, leukocytosis, weight gain, muscle weakness, hyperirritability, rigidity, and tremors

9. Adverse effects/toxicity

    a. Lithium has a short half-life and high toxicity; excreted by kidneys; sodium depletion will decrease renal excretion of lithium, which in turn will cause drug to accumulate and lead to lithium toxicity; toxicity is dose related: the higher the circulating blood level, the greater the risk for adverse effects and toxicity

    b. Other adverse effects with therapeutic doses include fine hand tremors, GI upset, thirst, muscle weakness; at toxic levels more adverse effects are seen, such as persistent GI upset, coarse hand tremor, confusion, hyperirritability of muscles, ECG changes, sedation, incoordination; at serum levels greater than 2.5 mEq/L, seizures, coma, dysrhythmias, and death may result

10. Client-centered nursing care

    a. Assess mood, ideation, and behaviors frequently; initiate suicide precautions if indicated

    b. Monitor intake and output ratios; report significant changes in totals

    c. Unless contraindicated, provide fluid intake of at least 2,000–3,000 mL/day

    d. Monitor weight at least every 3 months

    e. Assess client for signs and symptoms of lithium toxicity (vomiting, diarrhea, slurred speech, decreased coordination, drowsiness, muscle weakness, or twitching); if these occur, report before giving next dose

11. Client education

    a. Take medication exactly as directed, even if feeling well; take a missed dose as soon as remembered unless within 2 hours of next dose (6 hours if extended-release preparation used)

    b. Medication may cause dizziness or drowsiness; avoid driving, operating heavy machinery, or other activities requiring alertness until response to medication is known

    c. Low sodium levels may predispose client to toxicity; drink 2,000–3,000 mL fluid each day and eat a diet with consistent and moderate sodium intake to keep lithium levels stable

    d. Avoid excessive amounts of coffee, tea, and cola (because of diuretic effect); avoid activities that cause excess sodium loss; notify prescriber of fever, vomiting, and diarrhea, which also cause sodium loss, and correct dehydration quickly

    e. Advise client that weight gain may occur; review principles of a low-calorie diet with client

    f. Consult with prescriber before taking any OTC medications, before use of contraception, or if pregnancy is suspected

    g. Review side effects and toxicity effects of medication and instruct client to report any of these to a prescriber promptly

    h. Explain to clients with cardiovascular disease or over age 40 the need for an ECG evaluation before and periodically during therapy; report any irregular pulse, difficulty breathing, or if fainting occurs

B. Other mood-stabilizing medications

  1. Action and use

    a. A variety of antiepileptic drugs have beneficial effects in treating bipolar disorder when lithium is ineffective, although they do not have FDA approval for this use

   b. The two such medications presented here include carbamazepine and valproic acid; have acute antimanic and long-term mood-stabilizing effects in some clients with bipolar disorder; are also better than lithium in treating mixed or dysphoric bipolar states and in clients who are rapid cyclers

   c. When given to clients who have failed to respond to lithium, carbamazepine has had a success rate of about 60%; for treatment of acute manic episodes the mechanism by which carbamazepine stabilizes mood is unknown

   d. Clinical studies indicate that valproic acid can control symptoms in acute manic episodes of mania and depression; it alters GABA-mediated neurotransmission, and this action may underlie the drug's mood-stabilizing effects

2. Common medications (refer again to Table 4-7)

3. Administration considerations

   a. Carbamazepine should be started using low initial dose and then gradually increased

   b. Valproic acid for treatment of acute mania is given in two to four divided doses initially

4. Contraindications

   a. Carbamazepine is contraindicated with hypersensitivity to drug or bone marrow depression; it should be used only in pregnancy if potential benefits outweigh risks to fetus; it should be used cautiously in clients with cardiac or hepatic disease, prostatic hyperplasia, or increased intraocular pressure

   b. Valproic acid is contraindicated in clients with hypersensitivity or with hepatic impairment; it should not be used with products containing tartrazine; it should be used cautiously in clients with bleeding disorders, history of liver disease, organic brain disease, bone marrow depression, renal impairment, and by children (increased risk of hepatotoxicity); safe use in pregnancy has not been established

5. Significant drug interactions

   a. Carbamazepine may decrease levels and effectiveness of corticosteroids, doxycycline, felbamate, quinidine, warfarin, oral contraceptives, barbiturates, cyclosporine, benzodiazepines, theophylline, lamotrigine, valproic acid, bupropion, and haloperidol; danazol increases blood levels; concurrent use (within 2 weeks) of MAOIs may result in hyperpyrexia, hypertension, seizures, and death; verapamil, diltiazem, propoxyphene, erythromycin (should not be prescribed), clarithromycin, SSRI antidepressants, or cimetidine increases levels and may cause toxicity; may increase risk of hepatotoxicity from isoniazid; felbamate decreases carbamazepine levels but increases levels of active metabolite

   b. Carbamazepine may decrease effectiveness and increase risk of toxicity from acetaminophen, increase risk of CNS toxicity from lithium, and decrease duration of action of nondepolarizing neuromuscular blocking agents

   c. Significant drug–drug interactions for valproic acid include an increased risk of bleeding with antiplatelet agents (including aspirin, NSAIDs, tirofiban, eptifibatide, and abciximab), cefamandole, cefoperazone, cefotetan, heparin and heparin-like agents, thrombolytic agents, or warfarin; there is a decreased metabolism of barbiturates and primidone, which increases the risk for toxicity; blood levels and toxicity may be increased by carbamazepine, cimetidine, erythromycin, or felbamate; additive CNS depression with other CNS depressants, including alcohol, antihistamines, antidepressants, opioids, MAOIs, and sedative–hypnotics

   d. Large doses of salicylates (in children) increase effects of valproic acid; it may also increase or decrease effects and toxicity of phenytoin; MAOIs and other antidepressants may also lower seizure threshold and decrease effectiveness of valproates

   e. Carbamazepine, rifampin, or lamotrigine may decrease valproic acid blood levels; valproic acid may increase toxicity of carbamazepine, ethosuximide, lamotrigine, or zidovudine

6. Significant food interactions: none reported for either agent
7. Significant laboratory studies
   a. For clients receiving carbamazepine, target trough plasma levels are 6–12 mcg/mL
   b. Routine CBC, including platelet count, reticulocyte count, and serum iron should be checked weekly during first 2 months and yearly thereafter for evidence of potentially fatal blood cell abnormalities; drug should be discontinued if bone marrow depression occurs
   c. Target plasma drug level of valproic acid is 50–125 mcg/mL; clients receiving near the maximum recommended 60 mg/kg/day should be monitored for toxicity
   d. Also monitor hepatic function (LDH, AST, ALT, and bilirubin) and serum ammonia concentrations prior to and periodically during therapy with valproic acid (drug may cause hepatotoxicity); therapy should be discontinued if ammonia level becomes elevated
8. Side effects
   a. Common side effects for carbamazepine include sedation, GI disturbance, tremor, leukopenia, and hepatotoxicity
   b. Reported side effects for valproic acid include sedation, nausea, tremor, hepatotoxicity, and hair loss; nausea can be reduced by using delayed-release tablets or by applying "sprinkle" formulation to food
9. Adverse effects/toxicity
   a. Some adverse effects for carbamazepine include ataxia, drowsiness, agranulocytosis, aplastic anemia, thrombocytopenia, chills, fever, and lymphadenopathy
   b. For valproic acid some reported adverse effects include confusion, dizziness, headache, hepatotoxicity, indigestion, nausea and vomiting, prolonged bleeding time, thrombocytopenia, ataxia, and paresthesia
10. Client-centered nursing care
    a. Assess client frequently for seizure activity when taking carbamazepine and assess for facial pain because of possibility of trigeminal neuralgia
    b. Perform liver function tests, urinalysis, and BUN routinely and measure serum ionized calcium levels at least every 6 months or if seizure frequency increases
    c. Implement seizure precautions as indicated; administer dose with food to minimize gastric irritation; tablets may be crushed if client has difficulty swallowing — except for extended-release tablets
11. Client education
    a. Take carbamazepine around the clock, exactly as directed; if a dose is missed, take as soon as possible but not just before next dose is due; drug should be gradually decreased to prevent seizures
    b. Report fever, sore throat, mouth ulcers, easy bruising, petechiae, unusual bleeding, abdominal pain, chills, rash, pale stools, dark urine, or jaundice to prescriber immediately
    c. Use sunscreen and protective clothing to prevent photosensitivity reactions with carbamazepine
    d. Female clients should use a nonhormonal form of contraception while taking carbamazepine
    e. Avoid activities requiring alertness; carbamazepine and valproic acid may cause dizziness or drowsiness
    f. Do not concurrently use alcohol, other CNS depressants, or OTC drugs with either of these drugs without consulting prescriber first
    g. Carry information (such as a medic alert tag or bracelet) describing disease and medication regimen at all times
    h. Notify healthcare professional of drug regimen before any treatment or surgery

Practice to Pass

The client is being discharged on lithium carbonate. What would be included in the teaching plan related to the client's medication regimen when at home?

    i. Compliance with follow-up lab tests, eye exams, and ECGs is important

    j. Take valproic acid exactly as directed; if a dose is missed on a once-a-day schedule, take it as soon as remembered that day; if on a multiple-dose schedule, take it within 6 hours of scheduled time, then space remaining doses throughout remainder of the day; abrupt withdrawal may lead to seizures

    k. For clients taking valproic acid, notify prescriber if anorexia, severe nausea and vomiting, yellow skin or eyes, fever, sore throat, malaise, weakness, facial edema, lethargy, unusual bleeding or bruising, pregnancy, or loss of seizure control occur; children less than age 2 years are especially at risk for fatal hepatotoxicity

IV. SEDATIVE–HYPNOTICS AND ANXIOLYTICS

A. Benzodiazepines

    1. Action and use

        a. Benzodiazepines (BZ) are thought to reduce anxiety because they are powerful potentiators (receptor agonists) of inhibitory neurotransmitter GABA

        b. A postsynaptic receptor site specific for BZ molecule is located next to GABA receptor; BZ molecule and GABA bind to each other at GABA receptor site, resulting in an *inhibition* of neurotransmission that results in a clinical decrease in anxiety level

        c. Most BZs are well absorbed following oral administration; because of their high lipid solubility, BZs readily cross blood–brain barrier to reach sites within CNS; most BZs undergo extensive metabolic alterations; with few exceptions, drug **metabolites** (result of drug biotransformation) are pharmacologically active so drug effects persist long after parent drug is gone from plasma (thus there may be poor correlation between plasma half-life of parent drug and duration of pharmacological effect)

        d. Major indications for use of BZs are anxiety, insomnia (sedative–hypnotic effect), and seizure disorders

        e. Other uses include alcohol withdrawal, anxiety associated with medical disease, skeletal muscle relaxation, preoperative anxiety and apprehension, substance-induced (except for amphetamines) and psychotic agitation in emergency departments or in other crisis situations; in higher doses alprazolam and clonazepam may effectively treat panic disorder and social phobia; other uses are to induce general anesthesia and to manage seizure disorders and muscle spasm

    2. Common sedative-hypnotic and anxiolytic medications: see Table 4-8 for generic names, dosage form, half-life, speed of onset, and approved use indications

        a. Benzodiazepines differ significantly with regard to course of action; specifically, they differ in onset of action, duration of action, and tendency to accumulate with repeated dosing

        b. Because all BZs have essentially equivalent pharmacological actions, selection is based in large part on differences in pharmacokinetics

    3. Administration considerations

        a. Benzodiazepines should be started at low doses and gradually increased as needed to achieve desired clinical response; there is a rapid onset of clinical action once an appropriate dose is achieved

        b. In anxiety disorders, some anxiety reduction may be apparent almost immediately; anti-anxiety effect with initial dosing may not last as long as serum half-life would suggest because of drug redistributing out of the brain; with continued dosing, steady-state brain levels and sustained efficacy are achieved; for treatment of anxiety, BZs are usually dosed at bedtime or bid; only occasionally is tid dosing required

Table 4-8	Sedative–Hypnotic and Anxiolytic Medications			
Drug Class Generic and Name	**Dosage Forms**	**Half-Life (hr)**	**Speed of Onset (PO)**	**Approved Use Indication**
Barbiturates				
Butabarbital	C	34–42	Short to intermediate	Hypnotic
Pentobarbital	C	15–48	Long-acting	Hypnotic
Phenobarbital	C	80–120	Long-acting	Hypnotic
Secobarbital	C	15–40	Short to intermediate	Hypnotic
Benzodiazepines				
Alprazolam	T	12–15	Intermediate	A, AD, P
Chlordiazepoxide	C, T, I	5–30	Intermediate	A, AW, PS
Clonazepam	T	20–50	Intermediate	LGS
Clorazepate	C, T, T-SR	20–80	Fast	A
Diazepam	C-SR, T, L, I	20–80	Very fast	A, PS, SE
Lorazepam	T, I	10–20	Intermediate	A, PS
Oxazepam	C, T	5–20	Intermediate to slow	A, AD, AW
Nonbarbiturate/Nondiazepines				
Buspirone	T	2–4	Intermediate	A
Eszopiclone	T	5–6	Fast	Insomnia
Zaleplon	T	2–4	Fast	Insomnia
Zolpidem	T	1.5–4	Fast	Hypnotic
Benzodiazepine Antagonist				
Flumazenil	I	—	Fast	R
Melatonin Agonist				
Ramelteon	T	1–2.6	Fast	Insomnia

Approved Use Indicators: A, anxiety; AD, anxiety associated with depression; AW, alcohol withdrawal; LGS, Lennox-Gastaut syndrome/seizures; P, panic disorder; PS, psychotic disorder; R, reverse moderate sedation or general anesthesia; SE, status epilepticus

Dosage Forms: C, capsule; C-SR, capsule, sustained-release; I, injection; L, oral, liquid; T, tablet; T-SR, tablet, sustained-release

    c. For use as a hypnotic, BZs are rapidly absorbed, have a short onset of action, and have a short elimination half-life, so that next-day sedation and impaired cognition are minimized (although clients may experience some sedation or "hangover effect" the next day)

    d. Treatment for insomnia should occur for as short a time as possible (not longer than 7–10 days) and should be used as an adjunct to help clients establish a regular sleep pattern along with improved sleep hygiene techniques; clients are at risk for rebound insomnia and anxiety if drugs are used for longer periods of time

4. Contraindications

    a. BZs are contraindicated with drug sensitivity or during pregnancy or lactation because they cross blood–brain barrier and enter breast milk with ease (and develop quickly to toxic levels)

    b. BZs should not be used with clients with preexisting CNS depression, severe uncontrolled pain, or for clients with narrow-angle glaucoma

    c. BZs are readily absorbed after oral ingestion; however, intramuscular (IM) injection produces slow and inconsistent absorption for most of these drugs

    d. A convenient way of categorizing BZs is to divide them into those with short half-lives (less than 20 hours) and long half-lives (more than 20 hours) (see Table 4-8 for details); BZs with short half-life are usually preferable for use with older adult clients

    e. Because hepatic metabolism is primary mechanism for drug disposition, drugs that interfere with liver metabolism (e.g., alcohol) dangerously compound the effect of BZs

5. Significant drug interactions

    a. CNS depressant actions of BZs are additive to those of other CNS depressants (e.g., alcohol, barbiturates, opioids), so although BZs are very safe when used alone, they can be extremely hazardous in combination with other depressants

        1) A combined overdose of a benzodiazepine with another CNS depressant can lead to profound respiratory depression, coma, and death

        2) Clients should be warned against use of alcohol and all other CNS depressants

    b. BZs are poorly absorbed when taken with antacids; disulfiram and cimetidine use increases plasma level of BZs that are oxidized; befazodone inhibits metabolism of alprazolam and triazolam while phenytoin increases anticonvulsant serum level; use of BZs with TCAs increases sedation, confusion, and impairs motor function; when used with MAOIs, CNS depression occurs; succinylcholine decreases neuromuscular blockade

    c. With prolonged use of benzodiazepines, **tolerance** (increased need of drug to achieve the same effect) develops to some effects but not to others

        1) No tolerance develops to anxiolytic effects, and tolerance to hypnotic effects is generally low

        2) In contrast, significant tolerance develops to antiseizure effects

        3) Clients tolerant to barbiturates, alcohol, and other general CNS depressants show some cross-tolerance to benzodiazepines

        4) BZs can cause physical dependence, but incidence of substantial dependence is low (especially for clients taking alprazolam)

6. Significant food interactions: none

7. Significant laboratory studies: none unless a client is on long-term therapy with BZs; then CBC, liver, and renal function should be monitored

8. Side effects

    a. Most common side effect is decreased mental alertness; caution clients against driving or using heavy or hazardous equipment

    b. Tolerance to most side effects quickly develops

    c. Monitor BP of inpatients routinely; withhold dose and report to prescriber a drop of 20 mmHg (systolic) while standing

    d. Other side effects include dry mouth, ataxia, dizziness, drowsiness, nausea, and withdrawal symptoms (increased anxiety, flulike symptoms, tremors)

9. Adverse effects/toxicity: as stated earlier, use of BZs with other CNS depressants can cause fatal results; signs of overdose include somnolence, confusion, coma, diminished reflexes, and hypotension

10. Client-centered nursing care

    a. Assess degree and manifestation of anxiety before client begins therapy

    b. Assess client for drowsiness, light-headedness, and dizziness periodically during treatment; usually disappear as therapy progresses

    c. Always caution client about driving or operating hazardous machinery, especially in early treatment with BZs

    d. Monitor BP, pulse, and respirations and provide supportive care as indicated

e. Prolonged therapy may lead to psychological or physical dependence; risk is greater with larger drug doses; restrict amount of drug available to client

f. Most BZs can be taken with food or crushed and put in food if client has difficulty swallowing

11. Client education

a. Take medications exactly as prescribed and do not skip or double up on missed doses; if a dose is missed, take within 1 hour or skip the dose and return to regular schedule

b. If medication is less effective after a few weeks, check with prescriber; do not increase dose

c. Abrupt drug withdrawal may cause sweating, vomiting, muscle cramps, tremors, and seizures

d. Avoid use of alcohol or other CNS depressants concurrently with BZ therapy

B. **Benzodiazepine antagonist**

1. Action and use

a. Flumazenil is a BZ antagonist (receptor blocker); it selectively blocks BZ receptors but does not block adrenergic or cholinergic receptors

b. In other words, it can reverse the *sedative* effects of BZs but may not reverse BZ-induced *respiratory depression*

c. Because it does not stimulate CNS and does not block other receptors, it can be given when BZ overdose is suspected and can also be used to reverse effects of BZs following general anesthesia

d. A reaction occurs within 30–60 seconds after administration

2. Common medications: flumazenil is the only drug in this class

3. Administration considerations

a. Does not speed up the metabolism or excretion of BZs and has a short duration of action, which poses a clinical management problem; if client responds to flumazenil, then BZs are present, but client may need vigilant, ongoing dosing and monitoring as body eliminates BZs

b. Administration is IV: inject dose slowly over 30 seconds and repeat every minute as needed; first dose is 0.2 mg, second is 0.3 mg, and all subsequent doses are 0.5 mg; effects fade in approximately 1 hour, so additional dosing may be needed

c. In children, 0.01 mg/kg (up to 0.2 mg); if desired level of consciousness (LOC) is not obtained after waiting an additional 45 seconds, further injections of 0.01 mg/kg can be given and repeated at 60-second intervals when necessary (up to a maximum of four additional times)

4. Contraindications

a. Hypersensitivity; clients receiving BZs for life-threatening medical problems, including status epilepticus or increased intracranial pressure; clients with serious TCA overdose

b. Use cautiously in clients with mixed CNS depressant overdose, with history of seizures, or clients with head injury; safety has not been established for use during pregnancy, lactation, or in children less than 2 years old

5. Significant drug interactions: none noted

6. Significant food interactions: none noted

7. Significant laboratory studies: none

8. Side effects: minor side and adverse effects include dizziness, agitation, confusion, nausea and vomiting, hiccups, paresthesia, rigors, and shivering

9. Adverse effects/toxicity: principle adverse effect is precipitation of seizures, which is most likely to occur in clients taking BZs to treat epilepsy or who are physically dependent on BZs

10. Client-centered nursing care
  a. Assess LOC and respiratory status before and throughout therapy
  b. Establish that client has a patent airway before administering flumazenil
  c. Observe IV site frequently for redness or irritation; give drug through a free-flowing IV infusion into a large vein to minimize pain at injection site
  d. Institute seizure precautions; seizures are more likely to occur in clients experiencing sedative–hypnotic withdrawal, who have recently received repeated doses of BZs, or who have a previous history of seizure activity; seizures may be treated with BZs, barbiturates, or phenytoin (larger than normal doses of BZs may be required)
  e. For suspected BZ overdose: if no effects are seen after giving flumazenil, consider other causes of decreased LOC (alcohol, barbiturates, opioid analgesics)
  f. Observe client for at least 2 hours after giving last dose for reappearance of sedation; hypoventilation may occur

11. Client education
  a. Flumazenil does not consistently reverse amnesic effects of BZs; provide client and family with written instructions for postprocedure care
  b. Client may appear alert at time of discharge but sedative effects of BZs may reoccur; avoid driving or other activities requiring alertness for at least 24 hours after discharge
  c. Do not take *any* alcohol or nonprescription drugs for at least 18–24 hours after discharge
  d. Resume usual activities only when no residual effects of BZs remain

C. Barbiturates

1. Action and use
  a. Like BZs, barbiturates bind to GABA receptor–chloride channel complex to enhance inhibitory actions of GABA and directly mimic actions of GABA; since barbiturates can directly mimic GABA, there is no ceiling to degree of CNS depression they can produce and, unlike BZs, they can readily cause death when taken in overdose
  b. Barbiturates cause relatively nonselective depression of CNS function and are prototypes of general CNS depressants; because they depress multiple aspects of CNS function, they can be used for daytime sedation, induction of sleep, suppression of seizures, and general anesthesia
  c. Barbiturates can cause tolerance and dependence, have a high abuse potential, and are subject to multiple drug interactions; they are powerful respiratory depressants that can readily prove fatal in overdose as well; because of these effects, they have often been replaced by safer drugs such as BZs
  d. Barbiturates can be grouped into three classes, based on duration of action: (1) ultrashort-acting agents, (2) short- to intermediate-acting agents, and (3) long-acting agents; duration of action is inversely related to their lipid solubility; barbiturates with highest lipid solubility have shortest duration of action; conversely, barbiturates with lowest lipid solubility have longest duration

2. Common medications (see Table 4-8)

3. Administration considerations
  a. Barbiturates are administered orally usually for daytime sedation and to treat insomnia; for general anesthesia and emergency treatment of seizures, they are usually given by IV injection; barbiturate solutions are highly alkaline and can cause pain and necrosis when injected IM, so this route is generally avoided
  b. Ability to cause generalized CNS depression underlies both therapeutic and adverse effects; as dosage is increased, responses progress from *sedation* to *sleep* to *general anesthesia*

    c. Most barbiturates can be considered nonselective CNS depressants; exceptions are phenobarbital and other barbiturates used to control seizures

    d. At hypnotic doses, barbiturates may reduce BP and heart rate; by contrast, toxic doses can cause profound hypotension and shock (from direct depressant effects on both myocardium and vascular smooth muscle)

    e. Barbiturates stimulate synthesis of hepatic microsomal enzymes (principal drug-metabolizing enzymes of liver); as a result, barbiturates can accelerate their own metabolism as well as metabolism of many other drugs

    f. Tolerance develops with repeated drug use; when taken regularly, tolerance develops to many (but not all) CNS effects; specifically, tolerance develops to sedative and hypnotic effects and to other effects that underlie barbiturate abuse

4. Contraindications: hypersensitivity, clients with overt or latent porphyria, severe hepatic/renal/respiratory dysfunction, or previous addiction to sedative–hypnotics

5. Significant drug interactions

    a. Drugs with CNS-depressant properties (e.g., barbiturates, benzodiazepines, alcohol, opioids, antihistamines) intensify each other's effects; if these drugs are combined, additive CNS depression can be hazardous or even fatal; warn clients emphatically not to combine barbiturates with alcohol and other CNS depressants

    b. Because barbiturates stimulate synthesis of hepatic drug-metabolizing enzymes and accelerate metabolism of other drugs, doses of *warfarin* (an anticoagulant), *oral contraceptives*, and *phenytoin* (an antiseizure agent) should be increased to account for accelerated degradation; once drug dosages are increased, they need to be gradually reregulated once barbiturate treatment ends to their previous amounts; barbiturates must be tapered and not stopped abruptly

6. Significant food interactions: none

7. Significant laboratory studies: clients on prolonged therapy (e.g., antiseizure therapy) should have hepatic and renal function and CBC evaluated periodically; also see individual agents for specific laboratory tests

8. Side effects

    a. Barbiturates have long half-lives and therefore can produce residual effects (hangover) when taken to treat insomnia; hangover can manifest as sedation, impaired judgment, and reduced motor skills; another possible effect is paradoxical excitement (especially in older adult and debilitated clients); the mechanism of this response is not known

    b. Barbiturates can intensify sensitivity to pain and may cause pain directly; their use has produced muscle pain, joint pain, and pain along nerves

9. Adverse effects/toxicity

    a. Acute intoxication with barbiturates is a medical emergency; left untreated, overdose can be fatal; poisoning often results from attempted suicide, although it can occur by accident (usually in children or drug abusers)

    b. Acute barbiturate overdose produces a classic triad of symptoms: *respiratory depression*, *coma*, and *pinpoint pupils*, which are frequently accompanied by *hypotension* and *hypothermia*; death is likely to result from pulmonary complications and renal failure

    c. Proper management usually requires admission to an intensive care unit; barbiturate poisoning has no specific antidote, so treatment usually includes gastric lavage, induction of emesis, and use of a cathartic (to reduce absorption by accelerating drug transit through intestine); hemodialysis can remove drug that is already absorbed; forced diuresis and alkalinization of urine may facilitate drug removal via kidneys

10. Client-centered nursing care
    a. With clients taking barbiturates, *always monitor respiratory status, pulse, and BP frequently*
    b. Prolonged therapy may lead to psychological or physical dependence; restrict amount of drug available to client, especially if depressed, suicidal, or with a history of addiction
    c. Always monitor client for safety, alertness, and need for help with ambulation or self-care
11. Client education
    a. Take drug exactly as prescribed and do not discontinue without consulting prescriber
    b. May cause daytime drowsiness; avoid driving and other activities requiring alertness until response to drug is known
    c. Female clients using oral contraceptives should use an additional nonhormonal contraceptive during therapy
    d. Contact prescriber immediately if adverse or toxic signs or symptoms occur

D. **Other sedative–hypnotics and anxiolytics**
1. Action and use
   a. Buspirone and zolpidem are two sedative–hypnotics/anxiolytics that are not barbiturates or BZs
   b. Buspirone is indicated for management of anxiety; it binds to serotonin and dopamine receptors in brain and increases norepinephrine metabolism in brain; 95% of drug is bound to plasma proteins; it is extensively metabolized by liver and 20–40% is excreted in feces
   c. Buspirone differs from other anxiolytics because it reduces anxiety while producing even less sedation than BZs; its mechanism of action is unknown; major advantages are that it does not cause sedation, has no abuse potential, and does not enhance CNS depression caused by BZs, alcohol, barbiturates, and related drugs; its major disadvantage is that onset of anxiolytic effects is delayed
   d. Zolpidem is used for the short-term treatment of insomnia; produces CNS depression by binding to GABA receptors; has no analgesic properties, but produces sedation and induction of sleep; rapidly absorbed following oral administration and 92% binds to protein; converted to inactive metabolites that are excreted by kidneys
   e. Zaleplon interacts with the GABA receptors to produce CNS depression; has a very short half-life and is useful for sleep disorders associated with early awakening as a dose can be given during the night, provided it is at least 4 hours before planning to arise
   f. Ramelteon is a melatonin receptor agonist that binds with the melatonin receptors M1 and M2, inducing sleep
2. Common medications (refer again to Table 4-8)
3. Administration considerations
   a. Buspirone is well absorbed following oral dosing but undergoes extensive first-pass metabolism in liver; giving it with food delays absorption but enhances bioavailability (by reducing first-pass metabolism)
   b. Zolpidem is rapidly absorbed following oral administration and is usually given orally just before bedtime because of its rapid onset of action
   c. Ramelteon and zaleplon are rapidly absorbed; avoid giving with high-fat food content, which could delay absorption
4. Contraindications
   a. Buspirone and zolpidem are contraindicated for clients with a hypersensitivity to drug

    b. Buspirone is also contraindicated in severe hepatic or renal impairment and should be used cautiously in clients receiving other anti-anxiety agents; slowly withdraw other agents to prevent rebound phenomenon; use cautiously for clients receiving other psychoactive drugs or who are pregnant or lactating; also use cautiously with children because safety has not yet been established

    c. Zolpidem should not be used for clients with apnea; it should be used cautiously in clients with a history of previous psychiatric illness, suicide attempt, drug or alcohol abuse, impaired hepatic function or pulmonary disease, older adults, pregnant or lactating women, and children (safety has not yet been established)

    d. Zaleplon is contraindicated in hepatic impairment; dosage adjustment is indicated

    e. Ramelteon should be avoided with severe liver impairment and should be used cautiously in severe COPD, sleep apnea, or depression

5. Significant drug interactions

    a. Buspirone interacts with MAOIs, which may result in hypertension; there may be an increased risk for hepatic effects when used with trazodone; blood levels are increased with concurrent use with itraconazole or erythromycin; avoid concurrent use with alcohol

    b. For zolpidem, additive CNS depression can occur with concurrent use of other sedative–hypnotics, alcohol, phenothiazines, TCAs, opioids, or antihistamines

    c. For zaleplon, additive CNS depression can occur with use of other sedative–hypnotic medications and alcohol; significant interactions can occur with cariprazine, leading to increased risk of psychomotor impairment; dosage adjustments of both drugs recommended if given concurrently

    d. Ramelteon is contraindicated with fluvoxamine, which could lead to risk of adverse effects

6. Significant food interactions: none reported with buspirone while food decreases and delays absorption of zolpidem; avoid administering ramelteon and zaleplon with high-fat food/meals

7. Significant laboratory studies: none since they are indicated for short-term use only

8. Side effects

    a. Buspirone is generally well tolerated; most common reactions are dizziness, nausea, headache, nervousness, light-headedness, and excitement

    b. Zolpidem has a side effect profile similar to BZs; daytime drowsiness and dizziness are most common, but only occur in about 1–2% of clients

    c. Zaleplon is generally well tolerated; most common reactions include nausea, dizziness, headache

    d. Common side effects of ramelteon include headache, somnolence, fatigue, taste changes, nausea, diarrhea, and dizziness

9. Adverse effects/toxicity

    a. Buspirone is nonsedating and does not interfere with daytime activities and poses little to no risk of suicide; does not enhance depressant effects of alcohol, barbiturates, and other general CNS depressants

    b. Zolpidem is not usually associated with tolerance, dependence, or abuse because it is used for short-term treatment only, but (like other sedative–hypnotics) it can intensify effects of CNS depressants; warn clients not to combine zolpidem with alcohol or other CNS depressants

    c. Signs of toxicity with zaleplon include hallucinations, suicidal ideation, amnesia, and aggressive behavior

10. Client-centered nursing care

    a. Assess degree and manifestations of anxiety before and periodically during therapy with buspirone

!

Practice to Pass

A 72-year-old client is in the clinic today with his daughter because his wife died 1 month ago and he must move to an assisted-living apartment, being unable to live alone. The healthcare provider prescribes lorazepam 0.5 mg bid in the morning and at bedtime. Identify at least three side effects of this drug that require client teaching.

b. Buspirone does not appear to cause physical or psychological dependence or tolerance; however, clients with a history of drug abuse should be assessed for tolerance or dependence—amount of drug available to these clients should be restricted

c. Clients changing from other anti-anxiety agents should receive gradually decreasing doses; buspirone will not prevent withdrawal symptoms

! d. With zolpidem, there may be a potential for physical or psychological dependence if used longer than 7–10 days; limit amount of drug available to client

e. For clients taking zolpidem, assess alertness at time of peak effect; notify prescriber if desired sedation does not occur

f. Assess client who has pain and medicate as needed; untreated pain decreases sedative effects of zolpidem

g. Avoid abrupt withdrawal with prolonged use of zaleplon and use cautiously in older adults

11. Client education

a. As with all medications, take exactly as prescribed

! b. Buspirone and zolpidem may cause dizziness or drowsiness; avoid driving or other activities requiring alertness until response to medication is known

c. Avoid concurrent use of buspirone and zolpidem and alcohol or other CNS depressants

d. Do not take OTC medications without consulting prescriber

! e. With buspirone, report any chronic abnormal movements such as **dystonia** (muscle rigidity), motor restlessness, involuntary movements of facial or cervical muscles, or if pregnancy is suspected

! f. With zolpidem, go to bed immediately after taking dose because of rapid onset of action

g. Follow-up exams are important to determine drug effectiveness

h. Teach to only take a dose of zaleplon during the night if at least 4 more hours of sleep are planned

V. SUBSTANCE MISUSE

A. Alcohol

1. Action and use

a. Alcohol is a CNS depressant and, like barbiturates, it causes general (relatively nonselective) depression of CNS function

b. Alcohol appears to affect CNS primarily by enhancing actions of GABA

c. Effect of alcohol on CNS is dose dependent

1) When dosage is low, higher brain centers (cortical areas) are primarily affected

2) As dosage is increased, more primitive brain areas (e.g., medulla) become depressed

3) With depression of cortical function, thought processes and learned behaviors are altered, inhibitions are released, and self-restraint is replaced by increased sociability and expansiveness; cortical depression also results in significant impairment of motor function; as CNS depression deepens, reflexes diminish greatly and consciousness becomes impaired

4) At very high doses, alcohol produces a state of general anesthesia

d. Tolerance to alcohol increases with alcohol use; abuse and addiction progress over time

e. Management of withdrawal depends on degree of alcohol dependence; when dependence is mild, withdrawal can be accomplished on an outpatient basis; when dependence is great, risks of withdrawal can be fatal if medical intervention is not carried out

Practice to Pass

The client is admitted to the unit for detoxification from alcohol. He states that his last drink was 12 hours ago. What are four major nursing priorities related to withdrawal from alcohol for the client?

 f. The major objective of medically supervised withdrawal is safe and effective removal of alcohol and/or other drugs; most medical treatment includes use of BZs—chlordiazepoxide, diazepam, and lorazepam have been used safely; a regimen of atenolol (a beta-adrenergic blocking agent) used in conjunction with BZs decreases dose of BZs necessary for safe detoxification

 g. Disulfiram is an inhibitor of enzyme *alcohol dehydrogenase*, which catalyzes a major step in breakdown of alcohol

  1) When enzyme is inhibited and client drinks alcohol, blood concentrations of toxic metabolite *acetaldehyde* increase significantly

  2) Acetaldehyde produces unpleasant symptoms of flushing, tachycardia, nausea and vomiting, and hypotension

  3) In medically fragile clients, these symptoms may rarely prove life-threatening; because of associated risks, disulfiram is used only with highly selected clients in good physical health

 h. Acamprosate interacts with CNS glutamate and GABA neurotransmitter systems to restore normal balance between excitation and inhibition of neurons

  1) Reduces alcohol cravings but without disulfiram-like reaction or alcohol aversion

  2) Used to maintain abstinence from alcohol in clients with alcoholism

2. Common medications: disulfiram is the only alcohol antagonist in use; acamprosate balances neurotransmitters to lessen alcohol craving

3. Administration considerations

 a. Disulfiram

  1) Disulfiram maintenance can significantly reduce drinking; dose is typically 500 mg daily for 1–2 weeks; maintenance dosages range from 125 to 500 mg a day, usually taken as a single dose in the morning

  2) At least 12 hours should elapse from time of last alcohol intake and initial dose of disulfiram

  3) The relatively long half-life of disulfiram ensures that several days must elapse between stopping drug and safely drinking alcohol; this long half-life probably decreases likelihood of impulsive relapse

 b. Acamprosate

  1) Indicated for clients with alcohol dependence but who are abstinent when treatment begins

  2) Intended to decrease alcohol cravings and significantly lower rate of relapse

4. Contraindications: because of severity of acetaldehyde syndrome, candidates for therapy must be carefully chosen; those who lack determination to stop drinking should not be given disulfiram

5. Significant drug interactions

 a. Disulfiram causes irreversible inhibition of aldehyde dehydrogenase, the enzyme that converts acetaldehyde to acetic acid; adverse effects caused by alcohol plus disulfiram are collectively known as the *acetaldehyde syndrome*

 b. Acamprosate has no known drug interactions

6. Significant food interactions: none

7. Significant laboratory studies: obtain creatinine clearance before initiating acamprosate

8. Side effects: in absence of alcohol, disulfiram rarely causes significant effects; drowsiness and skin eruptions may occur during initial use but diminish with time

9. Adverse effects/toxicity: acetaldehyde syndrome is manifested by marked respiratory depression, cardiovascular collapse, cardiac dysrhythmias, myocardial infarction, acute congestive heart failure, seizures, and death

10. Client-centered nursing care
    a. As with all medications, advise client to take medication as prescribed
    b. Advise client that simultaneous use with alcohol can precipitate acetaldehyde syndrome
    c. Advise client that effects of disulfiram may persist for about 2 weeks after last dose is taken; alcohol must not be consumed until this interval is over
    d. Notify prescriber of alcohol use while taking acamprosate
11. Client education
    a. Avoid all forms of alcohol, including alcohol found in sauces and cough and cold syrups and in after-shave lotions, colognes, and liniments
    b. Adhere to all forms of self-help groups (individual and group therapies) while using therapy to establish a recovery program

B. **Opioids**
   1. Opioids (e.g., morphine, heroin) are major drugs of abuse and are usually Schedule II substances
   2. Opioid abuse may be found in all segments of American society
   3. For most abusers, initial exposure to opioids occurs either socially (illicitly) or in the context of pain management in a medical setting; only a very small percentage of those who develop an addictive pattern begin use therapeutically
   4. Opioid abuse by healthcare providers deserves special consideration; healthcare providers, nurses, and pharmacists, as a group, abuse opioids to a greater extent than all other groups with similar educational backgrounds, and this is believed to be primarily the result of drug access
   5. Tolerance develops with prolonged opioid use; persons tolerant to one opioid are cross-tolerant to other opioids; however, there is no cross-tolerance between opioids and general CNS depressants (e.g., barbiturates, benzodiazepines, alcohol)
   6. Physical dependence is substantial with long-term use, but although opioid withdrawal syndrome can be extremely unpleasant, it is rarely dangerous
   7. Opioid toxicity produces a classic triad of symptoms: respiratory depression, coma, and pinpoint pupils; withdrawal symptoms begin 6–8 hours after last dose and reach peak intensity within 48–72 hours, including craving, chills, sweating and piloerection (gooseflesh), abdominal pain and cramps, diarrhea, runny nose, and irritability
   8. Naloxone, an opioid antagonist, is the treatment of choice; it rapidly reverses all signs of opioid poisoning; dosage must be titrated carefully because excess dose can move client from a state of intoxication to one of withdrawal; because of its short half-life, naloxone must be given again every few hours until opioid has dropped to a nontoxic level
   9. Nalmefene, a long-acting opioid antagonist, is an alternative to naloxone; because of its long half-life, nalmefene does not require repeated dosing; however, if dose is excessive in an opioid-dependent person, then nalmefene will put client into prolonged withdrawal
   10. Methadone, an oral opioid with a long duration of action, is most commonly used agent for easing opioid withdrawal and preventing abstinence syndrome; once stabilized on methadone, withdrawal is accomplished by administering it in gradually smaller doses; the resultant abstinence syndrome is mild, with symptoms resembling those of moderate influenza; entire process of methadone substitution and withdrawal takes about 10 days; objective of maintenance therapy is to avoid withdrawal and need to procure illicit drugs; methadone maintenance is most effective when done in conjunction with nondrug measures directed at altering patterns of drug use

C. Cocaine

1. Cocaine, extracted from coca plant, is a fine, white, odorless powder; cocaine and its offspring, crack, have caused major drug problems in the United States
2. Cocaine crosses blood–brain barrier readily, which causes an instantaneous high; when administered IV (mainlining) it is rapidly metabolized by liver, so the exhilarating "rush" does not last long; cocaine exerts both CNS and peripheral nervous system (PNS) effects because of its ability to block norepinephrine and dopamine reuptake into presynaptic neurons; depletes these neurotransmitters
3. Cocaine can be taken orally but is poorly absorbed and has little effect by this route; also "snorted" (absorbed through nasal mucosa) or mixed with baking soda and ether and smoked (called *freebasing*, probably the most dangerous method of ingesting cocaine); crack is a less expensive way of using cocaine than snorting or mainlining, primarily because it is sold and marketed in smaller packages ($10 or $20 "rocks"); crack is used at every level in society, reported to be the most addictive street drug today, and risk for overdose is extremely high; although physical dependence is less than with opioid abuse, psychological dependence is intense
4. Death from cocaine is linked to metabolic and respiratory acidosis and hyperthermia associated with prolonged seizures; tachydysrhythmias have also led to death
5. Although cocaine is highly addictive, physical withdrawal is relatively mild; psychological withdrawal is severe because drug is so pleasurable and causes an intense craving for drug; treatment is aimed at restoring depleted neurotransmitters; amino acid catecholamine precursors (such as tyrosine and phenylalanine), TCAs, and the dopamine agonist bromocriptine are three approaches used to increase availability of neurotransmitters

D. Cannabis (marijuana/hashish)

1. Marijuana (perhaps most widely used drug in United States) is derived from Indian hemp plant *Cannabis sativa*, which has separate male and female forms; two most common cannabis derivatives are marijuana and hashish; major psychoactive substance in *Cannabis sativa* is delta-9-tetrahydrocannabinol (THC), which is an oily chemical with high lipid solubility
2. THC has several possible mechanisms, including activation of specific cannabinoid receptors found in various brain regions; when marijuana or hashish is smoked, about 60% of THC content is absorbed; absorption from lungs is rapid; subjective effects begin in minutes and peak in 20–30 minutes; effects from a single marijuana cigarette may persist 2–3 hours; with oral administration, absorption is only 6–20%
3. Marijuana produces three principal subjective effects: euphoria, sedation, and hallucinations; no other psychoactive drug produces all three of these; because of this singular pattern of effects, marijuana is in a class by itself
   a. Responses to low doses of THC are variable and depend on several factors including dosage size, route of administration, setting of drug use, and expectations and previous experience of user
   b. More common effects of low-dose THC include euphoria and relaxation; gaiety and a heightened sense of humor; an increased sensitivity to visual and auditory stimuli; enhanced sense of touch, taste, and smell; increased appetite and a more intense appreciation of flavor of food; distortion of time (seems to pass more slowly)
   c. Some undesirable effects of low-dose THC include impairment of short-term memory; decreased capacity to perform multiple tasks; decreased ability to drive or operate machinery; inability to distinguish time (past, present, and future); depersonalization (a sense of feeling strange about self); a decreased ability to distinguish emotions of others; and reduced interpersonal interactions

        d. In higher doses, marijuana can have serious adverse psychological effects including hallucinations, delusions, and paranoia; euphoria may be replaced by intense anxiety and a dissociative state in which user feels "outside of him- or herself"

        e. In extremely high doses, marijuana can produce a state resembling toxic psychosis, which may persist for weeks; also dangerous is the use of marijuana with alcohol or other CNS depressants

    4. Chronic marijuana use can produce a syndrome known as *amotivational syndrome*, characterized by apathy, dullness, poor grooming, reduced interest in achievement, and disinterest in pursuit of conventional goals

    5. Other effects of marijuana include change in heart rate, orthostatic hypotension, pronounced reddening of conjunctivae, and—when used acutely—respiratory bronchodilation; when smoked chronically, effects such as bronchitis, sinusitis, and asthma can be seen; scientists believe carcinogens in marijuana smoke are more potent than tar from cigarettes

    6. When used in extremely high doses, marijuana is able to produce tolerance and physical dependence; abrupt discontinuation of marijuana can lead to irritability, restlessness, nervousness, insomnia, reduced appetite, and weight loss; tremor, hyperthermia, and chills may also occur but these symptoms usually subside in 4–5 days and no symptoms of withdrawal are noted

    7. Cannabinoids are sometimes used to treat nausea and vomiting (more effectively than traditional antiemetics) that occur as severe side effects of cancer chemotherapy; THC has been approved for stimulating appetite in clients with AIDS

E. Hallucinogens

    1. Use of hallucinogens, also called psychedelics or psychotomimetics, is rising again, especially among young people; these drugs alter perception; there are two basic groups of hallucinogens—natural and synthetic; see Table 4-9 for examples

    2. Hallucinogens can heighten awareness of reality or cause a terrifying psychosis-like reaction; users report distortions in body image, a sense of depersonalization, and/or a frightening loss of sense of reality; they have also reported seeing grotesque creatures; emotional consequences are panic, anxiety, confusion, and paranoid reactions; users have experienced frank psychotic reactions after minimal use,

Table 4-9	Categories and Examples of Drugs of Abuse
Category	**Examples**
General CNS depressants	Alcohol, barbiturates (three most widely abused are *secobarbital*, *pentobarbital*, and *amobarbital*), benzodiazepines (diazepam [Valium] is most widely abused)
Opioids	Heroin, morphine, meperidine, hydromorphone
Stimulants	Cocaine, amphetamines, nicotine
Marijuana/hashish	Can sometimes be classified with hallucinogens because of hallucination effect but is in a class by itself
Hallucinogens	LSD (lysergic acid diethylamide-25), PCP (phencyclidine), mescaline (peyote from cactus), MDA (3,4-methylenedioxyamphetamine)
Inhalants	Anesthetics (nitrous oxide, ether), nitrites (amyl nitrite, butyl nitrite, isobutyl nitrite), organic solvents (toluene, gasoline, lighter fluid, paint thinner, nail-polish remover, benzene, acetone, chloroform, and model-airplane glue)
Anabolic (androgenic) steroids	Testosterone, nandrolone decanoate, stanozolol

sometimes referred to as a "bad trip"; two most commonly used hallucinogens are LSD and PCP

   a. LSD causes a phenomenon known as **synesthesia**, a blending of senses (such as smelling a color or tasting a sound); it can cause increases in BP, tachycardia, trembling, and dilated pupils; CNS effects include a sense of unreality, perceptual alteration, distortions, and impaired judgment

   b. LSD users can experience flashbacks (frightening episodes that can heighten a sense of "going crazy"); bad trips from LSD cause anxiety, paranoia, and acute panic; some clients who have experienced psychotic "breaks" from LSD have never fully recovered and a number of people have killed themselves while under influence of LSD

   c. PCP, a synthetic drug, traditionally has been used as an animal tranquilizer; the main safety risk for users is unpredictable behavior (progressing from coma to violent behavior without warning); can be taken orally, IV, smoked, or snorted; it is well absorbed by all routes and effects last 6–8 hours

   d. With PCP the user experiences a high; euphoria and peaceful feelings are the effects sought after; undesired effects of PCP can be serious; BP and heart rate are elevated; other peripheral nervous system effects include ataxia, salivation, and vomiting; a catatonic type of muscular rigidity alternating with violent out-bursts may be frightening to others; psychological symptoms include hostile and bizarre behavior, a blank stare, and agitation

   e. LSD and PCP deaths may be caused by overdose but are more likely to be linked to perceptual disorientation and unresponsiveness to environmental stimuli; hallucinogens do not produce physical dependence, so there are no withdrawal symptoms

   f. The nurse should provide a safe, calm, reassuring environment for clients detoxifying from hallucinogens

F. Inhalants

   1. Inhalants are a varied group of drugs that are inhaled; they can be divided into three classes: anesthetics, volatile nitrites, and organic solvents (see Table 4-9 for examples)

   2. Anesthetics produce subjective effects similar to alcohol—euphoria, exhilaration, and loss of inhibitions; the anesthetics most abused are nitrous oxide—"laughing gas"—and ether; these drugs may be popular because of ease of administration (neither requires difficult-to-obtain equipment); for nitrous oxide, ready availability also promotes use (small cylinders of drug, marketed for aerating whipping cream, can be purchased without restrictions)

   3. Nitrites (refer again to Table 4-9) are subject to abuse because of an ability to relax the anal sphincter and a reputed ability to prolong and intensify sexual orgasm; venodilation is a pronounced effect, which in turn causes a profound drop in systolic BP, leading to dizziness, light-headedness, palpitations, and possibly pulsatile headache; drug effect begins seconds after inhalation and fades rapidly; the primary toxicity is methemoglobinemia, which can be treated with methylene blue and supplemental oxygen

   4. A wide assortment of organic solvents have been inhaled to induce intoxication (see Table 4-9 for examples); used primarily by children and the very poor; administered by three processes

      a. "Bagging": pouring solvent into a plastic bag and inhaling vapor

      b. "Huffing": pouring solvent on a rag and inhaling vapor

      c. "Sniffing": inhaling solvent directly from its container

5. Acute effects of organic solvents are similar to those of alcohol (euphoria, impaired judgment, slurred speech, flushing, and CNS depression); they can also cause visual hallucinations and disorientation to time and place; high doses can cause sudden death, possibly from anoxia, respiratory depression, vagal stimulation (slows heart rate), and dysrhythmias; prolonged use can cause multiple toxicities; gasoline can cause lead poisoning; chloroform is toxic to heart, liver, and kidneys; and toluene can cause severe brain damage and bone marrow depression; many solvents can cause damage to heart

6. Management of acute toxicity is strictly supportive; objective is to stabilize vital signs because there are no antidotes for these agents

G. Anabolic (androgenic) steroids

1. Androgens are frequently abused to enhance athletic performance; most are now regulated by Controlled Substances Act; the most widely used androgen is testosterone; there are substantial benefits for athletes as well as many risks

2. Steroids increase muscle mass in young males and in females of all ages and significantly increase muscle mass and strength in sexually mature males; the potential for adverse effects of androgens is significant; salt and water retention can lead to hypertension; when athletes take high doses there can be an increase in luteinizing hormone (LH) and follicle-stimulating hormone (FSH), resulting in testicular shrinkage and sterility; acne is common; reduction of HDL-cholesterol and elevation of LDL-cholesterol may accelerate development of atherosclerosis; there are potentially harmful effects to liver as well; in females, androgens can cause menstrual irregularities and virilization (growth of facial hair, deepening of the voice, decreased breast size, uterine atrophy, clitoral enlargement, and male-pattern baldness); hair loss; and irreversible voice change

3. Long-term androgen use can lead to abuse or "addiction" syndrome; characteristics include preoccupation with androgen use and difficulty in stopping use; when it is discontinued an abstinence syndrome can develop similar to that produced by withdrawal from alcohol, opioids, and cocaine

H. CNS depressants

1. Refer back to previous section on sedative–hypnotic and anxiolytic medications

2. Benzodiazepines are not likely to produce abuse in clients who do not have a history of substance dependence; usually abused in combination with alcohol and/or barbiturates, which leads to CNS depression and may cause death; tolerance in those with substance dependence is rapid for sedative and euphoric effects and negligible for anti-anxiety effects

3. Barbiturates are frequently abused drugs among young or middle-aged users who abuse prescription drugs because they are legitimately manufactured and are available in many forms; usual route of administration is oral or IV; barbiturates have a cross-tolerance to other chemically similar drugs, including alcohol, BZs, and heroin; IV users experience a sudden warm "rush," followed by a prolonged drowsy feeling

4. Mild barbiturate intoxication is exhibited by sluggishness in coordination, emotional lability, aggressive impulses, slowness of speech, thought disorders, and faulty judgment; neurologic signs include nystagmus (involuntary eye oscillations), diplopia (double vision), strabismus (deviation of the eye), ataxic gait, positive Romberg sign (swaying of body when standing with feet close together and eyes closed), hypotonia, dysmetria (disturbance to control range of movement in muscular acts), and decreased superficial reflexes; intoxication with barbiturates is confirmed by blood tests

5. Barbiturates have potentially fatal effects; they are used frequently in accidental overdose and suicide attempts; death occurs as a result of deep coma, which progresses to respiratory arrest and cardiovascular failure; lethal doses vary widely from person to person; there is a narrow therapeutic index for sedative effects with the therapeutic dose being very close to lethal dose

6. Tolerance and withdrawal are similar to alcohol (both are CNS depressants)

I. **Central nervous system stimulants**

1. Amphetamines are CNS stimulants discussed here; discussion of cocaine, another CNS stimulant, can be found in a previous section

2. Amphetamines are also discussed in Chapter 3; family of amphetamines includes dextroamphetamine, methamphetamine; when used for abuse, they are usually taken by mouth or IV; in addition, a form of dextroamphetamine known as "ice" or "crystal meth" can be smoked

3. Effects from amphetamine abuse include arousal and elevation of mood, euphoria, talkativeness, a sense of increased physical strength and mental capacity, increased self-confidence, and little or no desire for food or sleep (thus the term "uppers"); sexual orgasm is delayed, intensified, and more pleasurable

4. Some adverse effects of amphetamines can be fatal, including production of a psychotic state characterized by hallucinations and paranoid ideation; they can cause vasoconstriction and excessive stimulation of heart (sympathomimetic actions), leading to hypertension, angina pectoris, and dysrhythmias; overdose may also cause cerebral and systemic vasculitis and renal failure; vasoconstriction can be relieved by phentolamine (alpha-adrenergic blocker); cardiac stimulation can be reduced with a beta blocker (e.g., labetalol); drug elimination can be accelerated by giving ammonium chloride to acidify urine

5. Extended use of amphetamines produces a tolerance to mood elevation, appetite suppression, and cardiovascular effects; physical dependence is moderate while psychological addiction is intense; amphetamine withdrawal can produce dysphoria and a strong sense of craving; other symptoms include fatigue, prolonged sleep, excessive eating, and depression

6. A stimulant drug that is becoming less acceptable is nicotine; the only pharmacologically active drug in tobacco smoke other than carcinogenic tars; exerts powerful effects on brain, spinal cord, peripheral nervous system, heart, and various other body structures; nicotine stimulates specific acetylcholine receptors in CNS including cerebral cortex, producing increases in psychomotor activity, cognitive function, sensorimotor performance, attention, and memory consolidation; as with all stimulant drugs, a period of depression follows withdrawal

7. Nicotine does not appear to induce any pronounced degree of biological tolerance; smokers seem to learn how to dose themselves so as to maintain a blood level of nicotine within a reasonably narrow range; nicotine induces both physiological and psychological dependence

8. Nicotine exerts a potent reinforcing action, especially in early phases of drug use; in the veteran smoker, the reinforcing action of repeated smoking is primarily to relieve or avoid withdrawal symptoms; in addition to CNS effects, normal doses of nicotine can increase heart rate, BP, and cardiac contractility; withdrawal from cigarettes is characterized by an abstinence syndrome, including a craving for nicotine, irritability, anxiety, anger, difficulty concentrating, restlessness, impatience, increased appetite, and insomnia; the period of withdrawal may last many months

9. See Chapter 3 for discussion of other specific CNS stimulants

Case Study

A 46-year-old female with bipolar disorder has been stable with her symptoms for the past 6 months on a dose of lithium 600 mg bid. She comes in for an office visit and informs her primary healthcare provider she is planning a 2-month camping trip to a remote location in the Southwest. She wants to be sure she has a sufficient supply of her medication as she will not have quick access to healthcare facilities.

1. What concerns might there be regarding this trip?

2. What nutritional advice would you want to give this client?

3. What signs and symptoms of adverse effects should the client watch for and be prepared to address?

4. What signs and symptoms of toxicity should be reviewed with the client?

5. What other teaching should be included?

For suggested responses, see pages 538–539.

POSTTEST

1 Because a client is taking prescribed risperidone tid, the nurse provides which instructions to the unlicensed assistive personnel (UAP)? Select all that apply.

1. Set the room up for bleeding precautions.
2. Set the room up for seizure precautions.
3. Set the room up for fall precautions.
4. Report signs or symptoms of a psychotic break.
5. Monitor sleeping respiratory rate.

2 When a client taking bupropion 100 mg twice daily for 2 weeks returns to the clinic, the nurse should have which priority communication with the client?

1. "You may now have a martini with your evening meal."
2. "I need to listen to your heart with a stethoscope."
3. "Has the number of your mood swings decreased?"
4. "Are you still hearing voices?"

3 Because a prescriber needed to change the antipsychotic drug for a client diagnosed with schizophrenia, the nurse should monitor for which intended outcome?

1. The new drug is likely to be more effective in controlling symptoms of schizophrenia.
2. The new drug is likely to become effective at a more rapid rate.
3. There should be a reduction in severity and type of side effects experienced.
4. Client should find drug easier to take and better tasting.

4 A client taking lithium carbonate is confused, agitated, has blurred vision, and is having difficulty walking. The nurse should expect the lithium level drawn earlier in the day to be within which range?

1. 0.5–0.8 mEq/L
2. 1.2–1.5 mEq/L
3. 1.5–1.8 mEq/L
4. 2–3 mEq/L

5 A home health nurse is most likely to request that a prescriber consider discontinuing a phenothiazine prescribed for a client with psychosis after assessing which client data?

1. Urinary hesitation
2. White blood cell (WBC) count <3000 cells/mm^3
3. Blurred vision
4. Photophobia

6 A nurse working on an inpatient psychiatric unit would plan to monitor which client closely for neuroleptic malignant syndrome (NMS)?

1. 76-year-old female who has a typical psychotic clinical profile
2. 30-year-old male presenting with a very complex clinical profile
3. Native American who has been taking antipsychotic drugs for several months
4. Male client who has type 1 diabetes mellitus

7 Two months after beginning drug therapy with alprazolam 2 mg PO bid for generalized anxiety, an adult client states, "I feel much better, but I can't believe how dry my mouth gets and how dizzy and light-headed I get." Which would be the priority response by the nurse?

1. "You can use gum or candy that is sugarless to relieve some of those symptoms."
2. "The dosage of the medication will be lowered to decrease the side effects."
3. "Because dizziness and light-headedness are drug side effects, avoid dangerous activities."
4. "You will need to take this medication with food from now on."

8 Because there is a higher risk of successful suicide in clients receiving selected antidepressant drugs, the nurse should plan to instruct the nursing staff to monitor clients receiving which type of antidepressant drug?

1. Selective serotonin reuptake inhibitors (SSRIs)
2. Monoamine oxidase inhibitors (MAOIs)
3. Tricyclic antidepressants (TCAs)
4. Anxiolytics

9 A 46-year-old client newly diagnosed with schizophrenia will be discharged in 5 days. The client lives in a two-bedroom apartment with his older adult mother who is frail but self-sufficient. To promote adherence to medication therapy, the nurse should include which item in the teaching plan?

1. Teach the client and his mother how adherence to drug therapy contributes to the client's ongoing recovery process.
2. Teach the client's mother the importance of regular meals so the client can take his medication after meals.
3. Instruct the mother to be sure that the client is taking his medication daily as prescribed.
4. Teach the client that the medication regimen will help him remain symptom-free indefinitely.

10 Because a client is being discharged today with a prescription for lithium the nurse should collaborate with the interdisciplinary team to prevent which occurrences that would most likely result in readmission to an inpatient unit? Select all that apply.

1. Development of a family crisis
2. Diet regimen to lose weight
3. Nonadherence to lithium therapy
4. Development of serious illness in the family
5. Viral illness with symptoms of diarrhea and vomiting

➤ See pages 128–130 for Answers and Rationales.

ANSWERS & RATIONALES

Pretest

1 **Answer: 2 Rationale:** Clients are admitted to the hospital because of the level of acuity of the psychosis. The primary focus of the nursing care should include reduction in the signs and symptoms of the psychosis. Monitoring for drug side effects such as tachycardia and hypotension is part of the health maintenance but is not the focus of the nursing care. Because sedation and dizziness are common side effects of chlorpromazine, the nurse determines the safety risks to the client's health and should possibly not allow the client to ambulate alone. Appetite and food intake should improve as medication therapy takes effect and the client is better able to respond meaningfully with the environment; however, this is an indirect assessment rather than the primary focus. **Cognitive Level:** Analyzing **Client Need:** Pharmacological and Parenteral Therapies **Integrated Process:** Nursing Process: Planning **Content Area:** Pharmacology **Strategy:** Determine the relationship between the purpose of prescribing the drug and the setting. The critical words *primary focus* imply that more than one option may be of interest to the nurse and that the priority option must be selected. **Reference:** Wilson, B. A., Shannon, M. T., & Shields, K. M. (2016). *Pearson nurse's drug guide 2016.* New York, NY: Pearson, pp. 331–332.

2 **Answer: 3, 5 Rationale:** The nurse expects the primary possible side effects of nervousness, somnolence, dizziness, or insomnia, to be compounded with excessive ingestion. Olanzapine is a newer drug approved for schizophrenia and other psychotic disorders. With ingestion of an appropriate therapeutic dose, this agent is generally well tolerated and appears devoid of serious adverse effects. Psychosis is not expected to increase in intensity. Constipation is more likely to occur than diarrhea. Fluid retention and hyperglycemia are more likely to occur. Orthostatic hypotension is an increased risk during the initial dosing period; possible overdose would increase this risk. **Cognitive Level:** Applying **Client Need:** Pharmacological and Parenteral Therapies **Integrated Process:** Nursing Process: Assessment **Content Area:** Pharmacology **Strategy:** Consider that the client is at risk for toxicity because of ingestion of a 10-day dose. Use knowledge of the adverse or toxic effects of this medication to make your selection. **Reference:** Wilson, B. A., Shannon, M. T., & Shields, K. M. (2016). *Pearson nurse's drug guide 2016.* New York, NY: Pearson, pp. 1137–1138.

3 **Answer: 1 Rationale:** Trazodone is an atypical antidepressant. Because of the sedative effect, it is often used more for insomnia than for depression. Alprazolam and diazepam and beta-adrenergic blocking agents such as propranolol are used for panic attacks. Divalproex, lithium, or lamotrigine are more appropriate for mania. The same drugs used for panic attacks can be used for anxiety. **Cognitive Level:** Applying **Client Need:** Pharmacological and Parenteral Therapies **Integrated Process:** Nursing Process: Assessment **Content Area:** Pharmacology **Strategy:** First determine the possible uses for this drug. Then for this question, associate the common use of the drug with the most common side effect. **Reference:** Wilson, B. A., Shannon, M. T., & Shields, K. M. (2016). *Pearson nurse's drug guide 2016.* New York, NY: Pearson, p. 1597.

4 **Answer: 1, 2, 3, 5 Rationale:** Client instructions should be both written and oral. Management of most clients with mental health problems includes teaching family members when and how to notify healthcare providers. Monoamine oxidase inhibitors (MAOIs) such as phenelzine can interact negatively with a large number of drugs and foods, which can then place the client at great risk. For example, MAOIs taken with tricyclic antidepressants can result in seizures and hyperthermia. MAOIs taken with sympathomimetics or tyramine-containing foods such as aged cheese, avocado, and

chocolate can lead to a life-threatening hypertensive crisis. Blood pressure and pulse should be monitored closely during initial period of administration. Depending on the degree of impairment, the family may need to assist with the drug therapy, but there is not enough information to know if this applies to this question. Thus, this option is not the priority when considering the risks inherent with use of this medication. **Cognitive Level:** Analyzing **Client Need:** Pharmacological and Parenteral Therapies **Integrated Process:** Teaching and Learning **Content Area:** Pharmacology **Strategy:** Categorize the drug group as high drug–drug interactionist as well as high drug–food interactionist. This will help you to eliminate incorrect options easily and focus on the options that address the risks to use of this medication. **Reference:** Wilson, B. A., Shannon, M. T., & Shields, K. M. (2016). *Pearson nurse's drug guide 2016.* New York, NY: Pearson, p. 1242.

5 **Answer: 4 Rationale:** Because it has a shorter half-life (10–20 hours) and is not metabolized by the liver, lorazepam is most appropriate for use in older adults. Since diazepam and chlordiazepoxide are metabolized by the liver and have longer half-lives (20–50 hours and 5–30 hours, respectively) they are contraindicated for use in older adults. Trazodone is an atypical antidepressant, not a benzodiazepine. **Cognitive Level:** Analyzing **Client Need:** Pharmacological and Parenteral Therapies **Integrated Process:** Nursing Process: Planning **Content Area:** Pharmacology **Strategy:** First eliminate trazodone since it is not a benzodiazepine. Then apply knowledge of the drug profiles to the age of the client listed in the question. **Reference:** Wilson, B. A., Shannon, M. T., & Shields, K. M. (2016). *Pearson nurse's drug guide 2016.* New York, NY: Pearson, pp. 324–325, 470–471, 942, 1597.

6 **Answer: 2 Rationale:** Hyperpyrexia, muscle rigidity, and altered consciousness level are indicative of a life-threatening side effect called *neuroleptic malignant syndrome.* Immediate medical intervention is warranted. Excessive production of prolactin can result in osteoporosis over a long period of time but is not an urgent priority. Gynecomastia is without threats but may affect the client's self-esteem. Parkinson syndrome can occur because of the blockade of dopamine but is reversible and nonurgent. Akathisia, a strong urge to pace, needs to be reported but is nonurgent. **Cognitive Level:** Applying **Client Need:** Pharmacological and Parenteral Therapies **Integrated Process:** Nursing Process: Implementation **Content Area:** Mental Health **Strategy:** Select the option containing elements with the threat on immediate onset as well as the greatest magnitude. **Reference:** Potter, M., & Moller, M. (2016). *Psychiatric-mental health nursing: From suffering to hope.* New York, NY: Pearson, p. 372.

7 **Answer: 1, 2, 4 Rationale:** Because disulfiram causes the adverse reactions noted when alcohol is ingested simultaneously, the nurse should ask if the client is taking the drug. Intensity of reaction to disulfiram is generally proportional to the amount of alcohol ingested. A major life-threatening response to simultaneous ingestion of disulfiram and an alcoholic beverage includes hypotension. Ingestion of antihypertensive at the same time could compound the problem, making this a good follow-up question. Since the client is vomiting continuously, whether or not the client has eaten would not assist the nurse in managing the client's current condition. A prior history of cholecystectomy is not relevant. The client is experiencing a disulfiram reaction, not cholecystitis. **Cognitive Level:** Analyzing **Client Need:** Pharmacological and Parenteral Therapies **Integrated Process:** Nursing Process: Assessment **Content Area:** Pharmacology **Strategy:** Apply knowledge of a drug that may cause the signs and symptoms when alcohol is ingested. **Reference:** Wilson, B. A., Shannon, M. T., & Shields, K. M. (2016). *Pearson nurse's drug guide 2016.* New York, NY: Pearson, p. 509.

8 **Answer: 1, 2, 3 Rationale:** Orthostatic hypotension, blurred vision, and urinary retention are common side effects of imipramine. Dysrhythmias are a common side effect rather than an uncommon one. Imipramine is more likely to increase liver enzymes rather than decrease them. **Cognitive Level:** Analyzing **Client Need:** Pharmacological and Parenteral Therapies **Integrated Process:** Teaching and Learning **Content Area:** Pharmacology **Strategy:** Specific medication knowledge is needed to answer the question. Recall that this drug is an antidepressant and consider the typical side effects to make the correct selection. **Reference:** Wilson, B. A., Shannon, M. T., & Shields, K. M. (2016). *Pearson nurse's drug guide 2016.* New York, NY: Pearson, p. 805.

9 **Answer: 3 Rationale:** Because fluoxetine increases the level of serotonin, clients experience diarrhea and nausea resulting in decreased intake as well as decreased absorption of nutrients. Management of the side effects can prevent the weight loss. Abrupt discontinuance of the drug is discouraged. The client will need to increase the caloric intake but not necessarily fluid intake. The dosage should be related more to the therapeutic effect rather than the appearance of side effects. **Cognitive Level:** Applying **Client Need:** Pharmacological and Parenteral Therapies **Integrated Process:** Nursing Process: Planning **Content Area:** Pharmacology **Strategy:** Use knowledge of side effects to determine appropriate remedy. Consider that the therapeutic effect should drive decisions regarding dosage decisions to help make the correct selection. **Reference:** Wilson, B. A., Shannon, M. T., & Shields, K. M. (2016). *Pearson nurse's drug guide 2016.* New York, NY: Pearson, pp. 692–694.

10 **Answer: 3 Rationale:** Chlorpromazine is not only the oldest of the antipsychotic medications; it can also be used for relief of intractable hiccups. Risperidone is a benzisoxazole derivative that would not relieve hiccups. There is also no evidence that lorazepam or thioridazine reduces or relieves intractable hiccups. **Cognitive Level:** Applying

Client Need: Pharmacological and Parenteral Therapies **Integrated Process:** Nursing Process: Planning **Content Area:** Pharmacology **Strategy:** Specific drug knowledge is needed to answer the question. Take time to learn this information if the question was difficult. **Reference:** Wilson, B. A., Shannon, M. T., & Shields, K. M. (2016). *Pearson nurse's drug guide 2016.* New York, NY: Pearson, pp. 331–335, 942–944, 1398–1400, 1541–1543.

Posttest

1 **Answer: 2, 5 Rationale:** Seizures are a primary side effect of this drug, so seizure precautions should be put in place. Respiratory depression and laryngospasms are side effects, so monitoring respiratory rate (while awake and asleep) would be beneficial. The client would be prone to leukopenia and risk for infection rather than decreased platelets and risk for bleeding. Fall precautions are designed for disoriented clients or for clients who have limited mobility and are not needed by the client with the information given. Reporting signs or symptoms of a psychotic break are beyond the expected competencies of UAP. **Cognitive Level:** Applying **Client Need:** Pharmacological and Parenteral Therapies **Integrated Process:** Nursing Process: Planning **Content Area:** Pharmacology **Strategy:** Note the drug in the question and determine the expected outcomes of the drug and the side or adverse effects of the drug. With the wording of the question, focus on side effects or adverse effects as being the focus of the correct option(s). **Reference:** Wilson, B. A., Shannon, M. T., & Shields, K. M. (2016). *Pearson nurse's drug guide 2016.* New York, NY: Pearson, pp. 1398–1400.

2 **Answer: 2 Rationale:** One of the primary side effects of bupropion includes dysrhythmias, making assessment of the cardiac rate and rhythm most important. Ingesting alcohol with the drug may increase the development of seizures so drinking is not recommended. Bupropion is utilized for anxiety and not for depression (mood swings). Antipsychotics such as clozapine are prescribed for clients with hallucinations; bupropion is prescribed for anxiety. **Cognitive Level:** Applying **Client Need:** Pharmacological and Parenteral Therapies **Integrated Process:** Nursing Process: Assessment **Content Area:** Pharmacology **Strategy:** When responding to priority questions, select the option presenting the greatest risk along with the risk with the most rapid onset. **Reference:** Wilson, B. A., Shannon, M. T., & Shields, K. M. (2016). *Pearson nurse's drug guide 2016.* New York, NY: Pearson, pp. 218–219.

3 **Answer: 3 Rationale:** Changing the prescription is more likely related to the type, severity, and extent of the side effects. Clinical effectiveness of most antipsychotic drugs at equivalent dosages is typically the same. The onset may be more rapid, but this is not the primary predicted outcome the nurse should monitor. Although ease of use and taste may be a factor in compliance, they would not be the primary rationale for a change in prescription. **Cognitive Level:** Applying **Client Need:** Pharmacological and Parenteral Therapies **Integrated Process:** Nursing Process: Evaluation **Content Area:** Pharmacology **Strategy:** Use principles of pharmacology related to mental health problems. Consider the common rationale for changing drugs prescribed for clients with schizophrenia. **Reference:** Adams, M. P., Holland, N., & Urban, C. (2017). *Pharmacology for nurses: A pathophysiologic approach* (5th ed.). New York, NY: Pearson, pp. 228–229.

4 **Answer: 4 Rationale:** The symptoms listed are those of lithium toxicity that are seen when the serum level is 2–3 mEq/L. The therapeutic dose level is 1.2–1.5 mEq/L. A low dosage level of 0.5–0.8 mEq/L would not be effective in controlling manifestations of bipolar disorder but would not be an indicator of toxicity. A level of 1.5–1.8 mEq/L is slightly elevated but would not produce the manifestations listed. **Cognitive Level:** Analyzing **Client Need:** Pharmacological and Parenteral Therapies **Integrated Process:** Nursing Process: Assessment **Content Area:** Pharmacology **Strategy:** Select the option that is most representative of the level in which clients are likely to experience signs or symptoms of toxicity. **Reference:** Wilson, B. A., Shannon, M. T., & Shields, K. M. (2016). *Pearson nurse's drug guide 2016.* New York, NY: Pearson, pp. 934–936.

5 **Answer: 2 Rationale:** Agranulocytosis is a common side effect of phenothiazines and a WBC count of <3,000 (normal 5,000–10,000) could place the client at risk for infection. Discontinuance of the drug is recommended and the client should be changed to a different drug. Since urinary hesitation is a treatable side effect, drug therapy would not need to be interrupted. Blurred vision could be managed with safety instructions and this side effect actually resolves after a short period of time. Wearing dark glasses when in sunlight will reduce the discomfort from photophobia. **Cognitive Level:** Analyzing **Client Need:** Pharmacological and Parenteral Therapies **Integrated Process:** Nursing Process: Planning **Content Area:** Pharmacology **Strategy:** Note the critical word *discontinuing* in the stem of the question. This implies a severe adverse medication effect. Look at the various options and use nursing knowledge to select the low WBC count as placing the client at greatest risk. **Reference:** Adams, M., Holland, L., & Urban, C. (2017). *Pharmacology for nurses: A pathophysiologic approach* (5th ed.). New York, NY: Pearson, p. 229.

6 **Answer: 2 Rationale:** Younger male clients presenting with complex clinical profiles are more prone to neuroleptic malignant syndrome (NMS). The complexity makes it difficult to separate the syndrome from the mental health alteration. Clinical profiles are generally variable. Being female is not one of the demographic factors associated with NMS. There is no evidence that the Native American population taking antipsychotic drugs over a long period of time is more likely to develop

NMS. Diabetes mellitus is associated with male schizophrenic clients who take antipsychotic drugs, but it is not necessarily associated with NMS. **Cognitive Level:** Analyzing **Client Need:** Pharmacological and Parenteral Therapies **Integrated Process:** Nursing Process: Assessment **Content Area:** Mental Health **Strategy:** The core issue of the question is what client demographics correlate most frequently with NMS. Use specific knowledge of risk factors for NMS and the process of elimination to make a selection. **Reference:** Potter, M., & Moller, M. (2016). *Psychiatric-mental health nursing: From suffering to hope.* New York, NY: Pearson, p. 372.

7 **Answer: 3 Rationale:** Without proper instructions the client may perform activities such as driving or using equipment that could lead to injury if the client was experiencing dizziness or light-headedness. Dry mouth is an uncomfortable side effect, but if unresolved would not place the client at the greatest risk. Side effects may be dose-related during early high-dose therapy, but client has been taking the drug for 2 months and "high dosage" is 8 mg/day. The medication has no known GI effects so it does not need to be taken with food. **Cognitive Level:** Analyzing **Client Need:** Pharmacological and Parenteral Therapies **Integrated Process:** Communication and Documentation **Content Area:** Pharmacology **Strategy:** Determine first that the issue of dizziness and light-headedness is more serious than dry mouth. Then compare each of the options to find the statement that provides guidance to the client to maintain safety. Another way to approach this question would be to ask, "The client would be at greatest risk if which intervention was not initiated?" **Reference:** Wilson, B. A., Shannon, M. T., & Shields, K. M. (2016). *Pearson nurse's drug guide 2016.* New York, NY: Pearson, pp. 51–53.

8 **Answer: 3 Rationale:** Tricyclic antidepressants (TCAs) account for 70% of all deaths from intentional drug overdose. Selective serotonin reuptake inhibitor (SSRI) overdoses are serious and result in seizures, but most clients recover and these drugs are not commonly utilized for suicide. Life-threatening risks associated with monoamine oxidase inhibitors (MAOIs) include interaction with foods containing tyramine, which results in a hypertensive crisis. Anxiolytics are not a class of antidepressants; rather, they are a class of medications used to treat anxiety. **Cognitive Level:** Applying **Client Need:** Pharmacological and Parenteral Therapies **Integrated Process:** Nursing Process: Assessment **Content Area:** Pharmacology **Strategy:** Use knowledge of which drug groups clients tend to utilize most to attempt or commit suicide. **Reference:** Wilson, B. A., Shannon, M. T., & Shields, K. M. (2016). *Pearson nurse's drug guide 2016.* New York, NY: Pearson, pp. 77–78.

9 **Answer: 1 Rationale:** Clients with schizophrenia are at high risk for nonadherence to drug therapy. Factors contributing to nonadherence include drug side effects, nonsupportive environment, lack of understanding, and numerous other factors. Because discontinuation of medications is the primary reason for relapse and rehospitalization, it is essential for the nurse to teach both the client and his mother the importance of adhering to the medication schedule. Timing of meals is not an important factor. The relationship for mental health maintenance should be a shared activity, rather than placing the burden primarily on the mother. Various factors can override drug effectiveness so this statement could provide false assurance to the client. **Cognitive Level:** Applying **Client Need:** Pharmacological and Parenteral Therapies **Integrated Process:** Teaching and Learning **Content Area:** Mental Health **Strategy:** Select the option that contributes most to maintaining the client's health. First eliminate the options that focus on the mother rather than the client. Then eliminate another option because of the unrealistic words *symptom-free indefinitely*. **Reference:** Potter, M., & Moller, M. (2016). *Psychiatric-mental health nursing: From suffering to hope.* New York, NY: Pearson, pp. 372–373.

10 Answer: 3, 5 Rationale: Lithium is very effective in managing bipolar disorder. Rehospitalization of a client with bipolar disorder who has the drug prescribed generally indicates the client has stopped taking the medication. Clients often do not associate "feeling better" with the drug actions, and thus think they do not need to continue the medication. A viral illness that results in dehydration from vomiting and diarrhea can cause renal toxicity and lithium toxicity, which could require rehospitalization. A family crisis or having a seriously ill family member could impact the stability of the client's mental status; however, with appropriate counseling and drug therapy, the client should be able to cope without requiring rehospitalization. A weight loss regimen would not require hospitalization. Serious illness in the family would not cause readmission. One side effect of lithium includes altered renal function that could lead to fluid retention; however, this would be more likely to cause readmission to a medical–surgical unit rather than a psychiatric unit. **Cognitive Level:** Applying **Client Need:** Pharmacological and Parenteral Therapies **Integrated Process:** Nursing Process: Planning **Content Area:** Pharmacology **Strategy:** Eliminate the options related to family crises first because they are similar. Then associate the characteristics of the health problem with the ability to comply with a drug regimen. Noting the critical words *most likely*, recognize that clients with mental health problems may interpret feelings of wellness with a cure and thus terminate drug therapy independently. **Reference:** Wilson, B. A., Shannon, M. T., & Shields, K. M. (2016). *Pearson nurse's drug guide 2016.* New York, NY: Pearson, pp. 890–893.

References

Adams, M. P., Holland, N., & Urban, C. (2017). *Pharmacology for nurses: A pathophysiologic approach* (5th ed.). New York, NY: Pearson.

Adams, M. P., & Urban, C. (2016). *Pharmacology: Connections to nursing practice* (3rd ed.). New York, NY: Pearson.

Burchum, J., & Rosenthal, L. (2016). *Lehne's pharmacology for nursing care* (9th ed.). St. Louis, MO: Elsevier.

Drug Facts & Comparisons (2017; Updated monthly). St. Louis, MO: Wolters Kluwer.

Karch, A. M. (2016). *Focus on nursing pharmacology* (7th ed.). Philadelphia, PA: Lippincott Williams & Wilkins.

Kee, J. (2015). *Laboratory and diagnostic tests and nursing implications* (9th ed.). Upper Saddle River, NJ: Pearson.

Kee, J. L. (2017). *Pearson's handbook of laboratory and diagnostic tests* (8th ed.). New York, NY: Pearson.

Lewis, S., Dirksen, S., Heitkemper, M., & Bucher, L. (2017). *Medical-surgical nursing: Assessment and management of clinical problems* (10th ed.). St. Louis, MO: Elsevier.

Potter, M., & Moller, D. (2016). *Psychiatric-mental health nursing: From suffering to hope.* New York, NY: Pearson.

Smith, S. F., Duell, D. J., Martin, B. C., Gonzalez, L., & Aebersold, M. (2017). *Clinical nursing skills: Basic to advanced skills* (9th ed.). New York, NY: Pearson.

Vallerand, A. H., Sanoski, C. A., & Deglin, J. H. (2017). *Davis's drug guide for nurses* (8th ed.). Philadelphia, PA: F.A. Davis.

Wilson, B. A., Shannon, M. T., & Shields, K. M. (2016). *Pearson nurse's drug guide 2016.* New York, NY: Pearson.

Respiratory System Medications

5

Chapter Outline

Bronchodilators
Inhaled Corticosteroids
Inhaled Nonsteroidals

Leukotriene Modifiers
Antihistamines
Drugs to Control Secretions

Monoclonal Antibodies
Oxygen

Objectives

➤ Describe general goals of therapy when administering respiratory system medications.

➤ Explain action, contraindications, side effects, and adverse/toxic effects of bronchodilators.

➤ Identify client teaching points related to the administration of inhaled respiratory medications.

➤ Identify nursing considerations related to the administration of intravenous bronchodilators.

➤ Describe client-centered nursing care when administering antihistamines, decongestants, expectorants, antitussives, and mucolytics.

➤ Identify signs and symptoms of oxygen toxicity.

➤ Describe nursing considerations related to the administration of oxygen.

➤ Identify client education points related to safety and home care use of oxygen.

➤ List significant client education points related to respiratory system medications.

NCLEX-RN® Test Prep

Access the NEW Web-based app that provides students with additional practice questions in preparation for the NCLEX experience.

Review at a Glance

acute asthma attack bronchospasm with shortness of breath, wheezing, and cough

adrenergic agonist medication that exerts same effects as sympathetic nervous system

anticholinergic effect caused by blockade of acetylcholine receptors that inhibits transmission of parasympathetic nervous system impulses

antihistamine a medication used to treat allergic symptoms that competes with histamine for receptor sites to block action of histamine; result is to inhibit smooth muscle contraction,

decrease capillary permeability, decrease salivation and tear formation, and inhibit vascular permeability and edema formation

antitussive a medication that aids in quieting a nonproductive, ineffective cough

atelectasis incomplete lung expansion or collapse of alveoli

catecholamine an agent released from adrenal medulla in response to sympathetic nervous system stimulation

decongestant medication that relieves nasal stuffiness by shrinking swollen nasal mucous membranes

expectorant a medication used to aid clients with sputum production during cough

histamine substance released from mast cells and basophils in response to stimuli, such as in allergic reactions or cellular injury; effects of histamine include bronchoconstriction

hypoxemia deficiency of oxygen in arterial blood

hypoxia a state in which insufficient oxygen is available to meet needs of body cells and tissues

inhaler device used for administration of a medication by inhalation

interleukin plasma protein that increases during inflammatory process

lacrimal a term referring to glands or ducts involved with secretion of tears

leukotrienes substances released when client is exposed to an allergen and experiences an allergic response; cause inflammation, bronchoconstriction, and mucus production

mast cell type of cell involved in hypersensitivity reactions; many are found in skin, nasal region, and lungs; contain histamine, kinins, chemotactic factors, leukotrienes, prostaglandins, and thromboxanes; irritants or allergens cause breakdown of mast cells, causing release of bronchoconstrictive and inflammatory substances, resulting in airway edema, bronchospasm, and excess mucus production

mucolytic a medication administered by inhalation to liquefy respiratory secretions

nebulizer a device used for inhalation medications that produces a fine spray or mist

neutrophils white blood cells that increase in concentration in response to inflammation or infection

noncatecholamine not from sympathetic nervous system

opioid narcotic agent that acts on central nervous system to reduce pain perception

rhinitis inflammation of nasal mucous membrane

status asthmaticus severe asthma that cannot be controlled with typical medications; symptoms persist in spite of treatment efforts

sympathomimetic medication that mimics effect of sympathetic nervous system

xanthines medications that lead to bronchodilation by inhibiting the enzyme phosphodiesterase (PDE) and thereby increasing cyclic adenosine monophosphate

PRETEST

1 After the nurse administers albuterol to a 24-year-old client with symptoms of an acute asthma attack, which of the following outcomes is best?

1. Relief of wheezing
2. Respiratory rate decreased from 34 to 22
3. Dyspnea rating scale decreased from 9 to 6
4. Oxygen saturation of 82%

2 The nurse should question a prescription for epinephrine for the treatment of acute bronchitis when the client has which health problem?

1. Asthma
2. Coronary artery disease
3. Hypotension
4. Bradycardia

3 A client receiving theophylline asks the nurse why a specific item was removed from the food tray. Which response is most appropriate?

1. "Peas contain a chemical that can reduce the effects of the drug."
2. "Brown beans are high in protein and can increase the effects of the drug."
3. "Milk is high in calcium and increases the cardiac rate."
4. "Coffee contains caffeine, which can increase the drug level more quickly."

4 After assessing a client with chronic obstructive pulmonary disease (COPD) who is being treated with beclomethasone dipropionate via oral inhaler, which clinical manifestations should the nurse conclude are medication side effects? Select all that apply.

1. Excess salivation
2. Delayed healing
3. Oral fungal infection
4. Fluid retention with weight gain
5. Decreased respiratory rate

5 A client on the inpatient unit is having an acute asthma attack. The nurse is most likely to administer which medication with an appropriate prescription?

1. Aminophylline
2. Albuterol
3. Cromolyn disodium
4. Salmeterol

6 The nurse is evaluating the effectiveness of client teaching about self-administration of zafirlukast. Which statement by the client indicates that further instruction is needed?

1. "I will take the drug a few weeks before I expect to notice an improvement in my symptoms."
2. "I will use this medication when I have the symptoms of an acute asthma attack."
3. "I will increase my fluid intake while I am taking this medication."
4. "I will plan to take my medicine one hour before meals."

7 Which statement should the nurse include when teaching a client about loratadine?

1. "This medication may make you feel nervous."
2. "It will take this medication a few hours before it becomes effective."
3. "This medication will help in an acute asthma attack."
4. "Be sure to take this medication on an empty stomach."

8 Under which circumstance should the nurse suspend intravenous administration of phenylephrine and consult with the healthcare provider?

1. After 3 days of continuous use
2. If client develops hypertension or tachycardia
3. If client develops a dry, irritated oral cavity
4. If client develops rebound congestion

9 Because of a potential side effect of guaifenesin, the nurse at the outpatient clinic should provide which instruction to the client?

1. Consider using over-the-counter (OTC) antiemetic.
2. Report increased production of respiratory secretions.
3. Follow medication with a sip of water.
4. Take aspirin 625 mg for temperature elevation.

10 A client with acute bronchitis is apprehensive because the flaps on the nonrebreather oxygen mask close during exhalation. The nurse should make which adjustment?

1. None, because the mask is functioning properly.
2. Change client to a nasal cannula.
3. Replace nonrebreather mask with a new one.
4. Call the respiratory therapist.

➤ *See pages 160–162 for Answers and Rationales.*

I. BRONCHODILATORS

A. Beta adrenergics

1. Action and use
   a. Act as sympathetic nervous system (SNS) **adrenergic agonists**; raise intracellular levels of cAMP (cyclic adenosine monophosphate), which dilates constricted bronchi and bronchioles by relaxing smooth muscle
   b. Medications that lead to bronchodilation stimulate beta$_2$-adrenergic receptors in smooth muscle of bronchi and bronchioles
   c. Medications can have alpha, beta$_1$, or beta$_2$ activity; beta$_1$-adrenergic receptors increase heart rate and force of myocardial contraction
   d. Used during an **acute asthma attack**, which is characterized as bronchospasm with shortness of breath and wheezing, for quick airway dilation; used also for emphysema, acute and chronic bronchitis, and relief of bronchospasm; alpha-adrenergic stimulators can act as a decongestant due to constriction of blood vessels in nasal cavity

e. Beta adrenergic agents can be classified as **catecholamines** released from adrenal medulla in response to stimulation of SNS or **noncatecholamines**, which are not released by SNS; all beta adrenergic agents stimulate beta$_2$ receptors; catecholamines affect both alpha and beta receptors and cause cardiovascular effects

2. Common beta-adrenergic medications (Table 5-1)

a. Selective beta$_2$ agonists are preferred drugs for bronchial smooth muscle dilation as they produce fewer cardiac side effects

b. Albuterol: predominantly a beta$_2$ stimulator; given PO or by inhalation; not as likely to cause cardiac side effects and is used for prevention and treatment of bronchoconstriction

c. Ipratroprium bromide: has **anticholinergic** (parasympatholytic) effect or sympathomimetic effect; given by inhalation

d. Levalbuterol: short-acting beta$_2$ agonist used for prevention and treatment of bronchoconstriction; given by nebulizer and is not as likely to cause cardiac side effects

e. Ephedrine: alpha and beta stimulant and therefore causes nasal decongestion; given by mouth, intramuscularly, intravenously, or subcutaneously

f. Epinephrine alpha and beta stimulant; given by subcutaneous or intramuscular injection or by inhalation; epinephrine has beta$_1$-adrenergic action causing increased heart rate and increased force of myocardial contraction

g. Ethylnorepinephrine: alpha and beta stimulant, given by intramuscular or subcutaneous injection

h. Isoetharine: beta$_1$ and beta$_2$ stimulant; given by inhalation

Table 5-1	**Common Beta-Adrenergic Agents**		
Generic Name	**Route**	**Therapeutic Indications**	**Adverse Effects**
Albuterol sulfate	Inhalation Nebulizer PO	Relief of bronchospasm, asthma, exercise-induced bronchospasm	Nervousness, restlessness, tremors, pain, bronchospasm, chest pain, angina, palpitations, hypertension, hypokalemia, hyperglycemia
Arformoterol	Nebulizer	COPD including chronic bronchitis and emphysema	
Formoterol	Inhalation Nebulizer	Asthma prophylaxis, relief of bronchospasm	
Indacaterol	Inhalation	COPD including chronic bronchitis and emphysema	
Levalbuterol	Nebulizer Inhalation	Bronchospasm in reversible obstructive pulmonary disease	Increased cough, dyspepsia, hyperglycemia, anxiety, dizziness, headache
Metaproterenol	Inhalation	Bronchial asthma, emphysema	Nervousness, anxiety, tremors, headache, insomnia, dysrhythmias, angina, hypertension, bronchospasm
Olodaterol	Inhalation	Bronchospasm, asthma	
Salmeterol	Inhalation	Bronchospasm, asthma	
Terbutaline	PO	Bronchospasm, bronchial asthma	Angina, tremors, dysrhythmias, nervousness, tachycardia, nausea and vomiting, hyperglycemia
Ipratropium tiotropium (anticholinergic effects)	Inhalation or nebulizer	Bronchospasm related to chronic obstructive pulmonary disease, chronic bronchitis, emphysema	Bitter taste, dry oropharyngeal membranes, cough, urinary retention, headache, paradoxical bronchospasm

      i. Isoproterenol; beta$_1$ and beta$_2$ stimulant; given IV, sublingual, or by inhalation; used for short-acting bronchodilation effect but also has cardiac stimulant effects

      j. Metaproterenol: beta$_2$ stimulant; given PO or by inhalation; causes cardiac and CNS stimulation in higher doses

      k. Pirbuterol: beta$_2$ stimulant; given by inhalation; short-acting beta$_2$ agonist used for prevention and treatment of bronchoconstriction; not as likely to cause cardiac side effects

      l. Salmeterol: beta$_2$ stimulant; given by inhalation; used very commonly because of 12-hour duration of action; used for prophylaxis of acute bronchoconstriction

      m. Terbutaline: beta$_2$-adrenergic agonist; long-acting bronchodilator; administered PO, subcutaneously, or by inhalation

      n. Ipratroprium bromide/albuterol sulfate: combination product

  3. Administration considerations

      a. May see adverse effects with albuterol, bitolterol, levalbuterol, and pirbuterol if used too frequently because they lose beta$_2$ specific actions at larger doses (so beta$_1$ receptors are stimulated and the result can be elevated heart rate, nausea, anxiety, palpitations, and tremors)

      b. Epinephrine, ephedrine, and ethylnorepinephrine can be used as a nasal decongestant due to alpha stimulation

      c. Use with caution in young children and monitor for tremors, restlessness, hallucinations, dizziness, palpitations, tachycardia, and gastrointestinal (GI) difficulties

      d. Epinephrine is given subcutaneously for bronchoconstriction; effects are usually seen in 5 minutes and may last up to 4 hours

      e. Salmeterol is not used in an acute asthma attack because of slow onset of action (20 minutes); not to be dosed more often than every 12 hours due to 12-hour duration of action

  4. Contraindications

      a. Albuterol is contraindicated in clients with hypersensitivity to drug as well as those with tachydysrhythmias and severe coronary artery disease

      b. Contraindicated with hypersensitivity to **sympathomimetics**, which mimic effect of SNS

      c. Sympathomimetics are used with caution in clients with cardiovascular disease because of potential for increasing myocardial oxygen demand

      d. Use caution in clients with hypertension, diabetes mellitus, seizures, and hypothyroidism

      e. Avoid use with monoamine oxidase (MAO) inhibitors and sympathomimetics

      f. Children under age 12 should not use inhalations of albuterol, bitolterol, metaproterenol, and terbutaline

      g. Avoid use of extended-release albuterol in children under age 12

      h. Catecholamines should not be used in clients with tachydysrhythmias

  5. Significant drug interactions

      a. Concurrent use of MAO inhibitors may lead to hypertensive crisis

      b. Use with other sympathomimetics may cause additive adrenergic effects

      c. The action of beta agonists is antagonized by beta-adrenergic blocking agents and therefore therapeutic effects may be minimized

      d. Potassium-losing diuretics may increase risk of hypokalemia

      e. Cardiac glycoside toxicity may occur with concurrent use of cardiac glycosides and beta-adrenergic agents, especially in presence of hypokalemia

      f. These drugs can potentiate therapeutic and adverse effects of other bronchodilators

      g. Use with digoxin may lead to decreased digoxin levels

      h. Effects of sympathomimetics can be intensified by thyroid hormone, decongestants, and some antihistamines

  6. Significant food interactions: none reported

  7. Significant laboratory studies

      a. Blood glucose (liver production of glucose increases)

      b. Liver function tests (results may be elevated)

  8. Side effects

      a. When beta$_1$ receptors are stimulated, client may experience nervousness, tremors, increased heart rate, and increased blood pressure

      b. With alpha- and beta-adrenergic stimulation, client may experience insomnia, restlessness, anorexia, tremors, cardiac stimulation, and vascular headache

      c. With nonselective beta agonists, client may experience cardiac stimulation, tremors, anginal pain, and vascular headache

      d. With beta$_2$-adrenergic agents, client may experience hypotension, vascular headache, and tremors

      e. Muscle tremors are most frequent side effect of terbutaline

      f. Additional side effects may include hypokalemia, hyperglycemia, nausea and vomiting, chest pain, and dysrhythmias

      g. Paradoxic bronchospasm and urinary retention may also occur

  9. Adverse effects/toxicity

      a. CV: tachydysrhythmias, chest pain

      b. CNS: restlessness, agitation, nervousness, and insomnia

  10. Client-centered nursing care

      a. Monitor older adult clients carefully

      b. Monitor vital signs, especially heart rate and blood pressure when administering beta agonists (because of cardiovascular effects)

      c. Ensure proper use of metered-dose inhaler (MDI) for maximum benefit

      d. Use appropriate diluent when giving medications

      e. If prescribed, ensure that chest physiotherapy and postural drainage are done after client has received dose of expectorant, bronchodilator, mucolytic, or anti-inflammatory drug and that client is having intended response of expectorating mucus

      f. Ask client about current medications (including OTC and herbal products) and about any history of drug allergies

      g. At times, use of multiple drugs is effective and dosages of each can be reduced

      h. Note amount, color, and character of sputum

      i. Monitor baseline pulmonary function tests periodically throughout drug therapy to determine effectiveness of therapy

      j. Administer oral medications with meals to decrease GI irritation

      k. Solutions may remain diluted for 24–48 hours

      l. Monitor blood glucose levels in diabetic clients

      m. Avoid intramuscular (IM) injections

  11. Client education

      a. Monitor blood glucose level closely in diabetic clients because some medications, especially epinephrine, may elevate blood glucose levels; an adjustment in maintenance doses of antidiabetic agents may be indicated

      b. Contact prescriber prior to taking OTC drugs to ensure there is no potential interaction

      c. Report chest pain, palpitations, seizures, headaches, hallucinations, or blurred vision to prescriber

Box 5-1	The correct steps in administering medication with a metered-dose inhaler (MDI) are:

Client Education About the Use and Care of Metered-Dose Inhalers

- Insert the medication firmly into the inhaler.
- Remove the cap and hold the inhaler upright.
- Shake the inhaler for 3–5 seconds to ensure even mixing of medication in propellant.
- Tilt the head back slightly and hold the inhaler upright.
- Position the inhaler 1–2 inches away from the open mouth or attach it to a spacer or holding chamber. If a medicine chamber is used, seal the lips around the mouthpiece.
- Press on the inhaler while beginning to breathe in slowly through mouth.
- Breathe in slowly and deeply for 3–5 seconds.
- Hold the breath for 8–10 seconds as able to allow the medication to move down into airways.
- Wait 1–3 minutes as per product directions before the next inhalation if another inhalation is prescribed.
- Rinse the mouth with water and blow the nose.
- Use mild soap and water to clean the mouthpiece. Allow to air dry.
- Store the inhaler at room temperature.

   d. Do not take more than prescribed dose because of risk of hypertension, tachycardia, dysrhythmias, and angina

    e. Record prn use of these drugs, noting date, time, symptoms, and whether or not symptoms subsided

    f. Use inhaled preparations properly; have client give a return demonstration; see Box 5-1 and Figure 5-1

    g. Using a spacer enables more medication to reach site of drug action in lungs, and less is deposited in mouth and throat; assists pediatric clients and those without the manual dexterity to use the metered-dose inhaler alone

    h. Care of nebulizer and/or inhaler
      1) Wash and dry inhaler and nebulizer tubing and apparatus daily
      2) White vinegar can be used to rinse nebulizer tubing
      3) Read and follow manufacturer's instructions about use, storage, and cleaning of equipment

    i. Wait 1–3 minutes (some references suggest 3–5 minutes) between inhalations of aerosol medications

j. Avoid eye contact with inhaler spray

    k. Anticipated response to a nebulizer or inhalation treatment is absence of wheezing and dyspnea

    l. Take medication exactly as prescribed; do not double dosage or increase frequency of doses

Figure 5-1	

Proper use of a metered-dose inhaler

A

B

C

D

m. Avoid contact with an allergen that tends to cause bronchoconstriction; avoid contact with smoke and other irritants, such as aerosol hairspray, perfumes, and cleaning products

n. Increase fluid intake if not contraindicated by other diseases

o. Recognize symptoms of respiratory difficulty (such as activity intolerance and waking at night with asthma symptoms) so that intervention can begin as soon as possible

p. Avoid caffeine as this may increase nervousness and insomnia of bronchodilating drugs

q. An inhaled bronchodilator is the treatment of choice in an acute asthma attack

r. Do not break, chew, or crush extended-release tablets

s. Nervousness and tremors may be experienced when a medication is newly administered but frequently decrease over time

B. Xanthines

1. Action and use

a. **Xanthines** inhibit enzyme phosphodiesterase (PDE), which breaks down cAMP (cyclic adenosine monophosphate), and thereby increases amounts of cAMP, leading to bronchial dilation due to smooth muscle relaxation

b. Increase catecholamine levels, inhibiting calcium ion movement into smooth muscle, inhibiting prostaglandin synthesis, and inhibiting release of bronchoconstrictive substances from leukocytes and **mast cells** (which contain histamine, prostaglandins, and thromboxanes)

c. Cause bronchodilation and thereby increase ability of cilia to clear mucus from airways

d. Now infrequently used because of a narrow safety margin; used to treat bronchoconstriction associated with COPD (diseases such as chronic bronchitis, asthma, and emphysema) and other chronic respiratory disorders

e. Have a slow onset of action and therefore are utilized to prevent asthma attacks rather than treat them; can be used during an asthma attack if it is mild to moderate

f. Can be used as an additional treatment in pulmonary edema by decreasing vascular permeability and paroxysmal nocturnal dyspnea (PND)

g. Useful for symptom control of clients with asthma and reversible bronchospasm (may occur in clients with chronic bronchitis and emphysema)

h. Used to treat **status asthmaticus**, which is characterized by severe asthma that cannot be controlled with typical medications (use IV theophylline if client has not responded to faster-acting beta agonist)

2. Common xanthine medications (see Table 5-2)

3. Administration considerations

a. Administer cautiously to older adults because of potential for increased sensitivity

b. Administer xanthines cautiously to children over 6 months of age because direct stimulating effect on CNS may be enhanced in children

Practice to Pass

A client is admitted to the emergency department with inspiratory and expiratory wheezes, dusky color, and pulse oximetry of 88%. What is the appropriate action of the nurse in the emergency department?

Table 5-2	Common Xanthines			
Generic Name	**Route**	**Uses**		**Adverse Effects**
Aminophylline	PO, IV	Bronchial asthma, Cheyne-Stokes respirations		Nausea and vomiting, diarrhea, dizziness, restlessness, depression, unresponsiveness, proteinuria, increased AST, tachycardia, hyperglycemia, hypotension
Dyphylline	PO	Acute bronchospasm with asthma and COPD		
Theophylline	PO, IV	Bronchial asthma		

c. Monitor carefully blood levels and therapeutic response to medication to avoid potential toxicity

d. Therapeutic range of theophylline is 10 to 20 mcg/mL

e. Use correct diluent and proper time of administration when giving parenterally

f. Use cautiously in clients with cardiovascular disorders

g. Theophylline is metabolized in liver; some excretion occurs via kidneys

h. Theophylline dosages should be based on lean body weight because it does not enter adipose tissue

i. Theophylline can enter breast milk and cross placenta

j. Children metabolize drug faster than adults

k. Aminophylline is administered at a rate no faster than 25 mg/min because of potential for cardiovascular collapse

l. Dosages are often started low and titrated up as needed for relief of symptoms

m. Adults who smoke cigarettes and children metabolize these medications more quickly and therefore may need higher doses for therapeutic effects

n. Theophylline levels may be increased in liver disease, congestive heart failure (CHF), and acute viral infections because of impaired metabolism

4. Contraindications

a. Avoid use when there is known hypersensitivity to xanthines

b. Avoid use in clients with tachydysrhythmias

c. Contraindicated in clients with a history of peptic ulcer disease and GI disorders including acute gastritis because of increased gastric acid secretion

d. Contraindicated in clients with hyperthyroidism because it can exacerbate the disease

e. Theophylline can cause seizures and is therefore not given to clients with seizure disorders unless bronchospasm is unresponsive to other treatments

f. Use cautiously in clients with cardiovascular disorders

5. Significant drug interactions

a. Levels of xanthines increase if taken with allopurinol, cimetidine, erythromycin, flu vaccine, and oral contraceptives

b. Sympathomimetics can intensify cardiac and CNS stimulation

c. Metabolism of theophylline is increased with smoking

d. Phenytoin, rifampin, barbiturates, carbamazepine, phenytoin, and phenobarbital increase metabolism of theophylline

6. Significant food interactions: limit drinks and foods containing caffeine because of increased drug levels

7. Significant laboratory studies

a. Adverse effects are more severe with drug levels of 20 to 25 mcg/mL

b. Adverse cardiac effects are more frequently seen with drug levels above 30 mcg/mL

c. Seizures may be seen with drug levels above 40 mcg/mL

8. Side effects

a. Nausea and vomiting, anorexia, and gastroesophageal reflux during sleep

b. Sinus tachycardia, extrasystoles, palpitations, and ventricular dysrhythmias

c. Hyperglycemia and transient increased urination

9. Adverse effects/toxicity

a. CNS: tremors, dizziness, hallucinations, restlessness, agitation, headache, and insomnia

b. GI: nausea and vomiting

c. CV: palpitations, tachydysrhythmias, chest pain, and tachycardia

Practice to Pass

A client comes to the clinic with results of labwork that was drawn earlier that day. The theophylline level is 25 mcg/mL. The client has diabetes and his BUN is 52 mg/dL and creatinine level is 2.1 mg/dL. What actions should the nurse take?

10. Client-centered nursing care

▶ **a.** Assess for toxicity; note symptoms of restlessness, insomnia, irritability, tremors, and nausea and vomiting

▶ **b.** Restlessness is a symptom of a toxic reaction; however, it could signal hypoxia, and nurse should assess client for this

c. Monitor for adverse effects (tremors, restlessness, hallucinations, and dizziness) in all clients, especially in children

d. Monitor for cardiovascular side effects of palpitations and tachycardia

e. Carefully monitor clients with a history of cardiac disorder

f. Do not crush or allow client to chew sustained-release forms

g. Refrigerate suppository forms

▶ **h.** Use appropriate diluent when administering medications

▶ **i.** Ask client about current medications (including OTC and herbal products) and history of any allergies

j. Children may exhibit hyperactive behavior with administration of theophylline because of CNS stimulation

11. Client education

a. Do not chew or crush sustained-release forms (irritating to gastric mucosa)

b. Mechanism of drug action, usage, and side effects

▶ **c.** Do not omit or double-up on doses; take exactly as prescribed

d. Suppository forms should be refrigerated

e. Notify prescriber if suppositories cause rectal burning, itching, or irritation

▶ **f.** Notify prescriber if palpitations, nausea and vomiting, weakness, dizziness, chest pain, or seizures occur

g. Monitor blood levels

▶ **h.** Avoid use of caffeine as this could lead to an additive effect with xanthines

▶ **i.** Avoid contact with allergen that tends to cause allergic response, if possible; avoid contact with smoke and other respiratory irritants such as aerosol hairspray, perfumes, and cleaning products

j. Increase fluid intake if no contraindication with other disease process

▶ **k.** Take medications even when there are no symptoms of asthma

l. Inform prescriber prior to taking OTC medication

m. Take medications with food if GI symptoms develop

II. INHALED CORTICOSTEROIDS

A. Action and use

1. Exact mechanism of action is unknown; however, it is thought that inhaled corticosteroids stabilize membranes of cells that release bronchoconstricting substances such as **histamine** and thereby decrease release of these substances

2. Cell membranes of **neutrophils** (white blood cells that increase in concentration in response to inflammation) are stabilized and therefore inflammation-causing substances are not released; the result is decreased inflammation and bronchodilation

3. Reducing inflammation decreases mucosal edema and mucous secretions and thereby decreases bronchoconstriction

4. Inhaled corticosteroids may have a role in increasing responsiveness of bronchial smooth muscle to beta-agonist drugs

5. These agents appear to be involved in inhibiting movement of fluid and protein into tissues as well as inhibiting production of prostaglandins, **leukotrienes** (substances released after exposure to an allergen), and **interleukins** (plasma proteins that increase during inflammatory process)

6. These agents also promote mobilization of mucus by increasing mucociliary action

7. Used in chronic asthma to decrease inflammation and therefore decrease airway obstruction and are used prophylactically, not during acute attack
8. Aid in treatment of bronchospastic disorders when bronchodilators are not completely effective; not used to treat acute bronchospasm
9. Used to treat chronic bronchitis, COPD, and cystic fibrosis

B. **Common inhaled corticosteroid medications (Table 5-3)**

C. **Administration considerations**

1. Proper technique is essential when administering medications by inhalation route
2. Chemical structures of inhaled corticosteroids have been slightly altered so there is not as much systemic absorption and therefore less likelihood of systemic side effects
3. Beclomethasone has greater anti-inflammatory action and causes fewer side effects than dexamethasone
4. If client is also taking a systemic corticosteroid, dose may need to be decreased with addition of inhaled corticosteroids
5. Beclomethasone, flunisolide, and fluticasone are available as nasal solutions for treatment of allergic rhinitis
6. Monitor for impaired bone growth in children receiving inhaled corticosteroids

D. **Contraindications**

1. Clients with known allergy
2. Clients with psychosis, fungal infection, acquired immunodeficiency syndrome (AIDS), tuberculosis, and idiopathic thrombocytopenia
3. Children under age 2 years
4. Use cautiously in clients with diabetes, glaucoma, osteoporosis, ulcers, renal disease, CHF, myasthenia gravis, seizure disorders, inflammatory bowel disease, hypertension, thromboembolic disorders, or esophagitis
5. Use with caution in clients with infections due to potential for suppressed immune system

E. **Significant drug interactions**

1. There are relatively few drug interactions because these inhalers work locally rather than systemically
2. May need to adjust dose of antidiabetic agents secondary to potential for elevation of blood glucose levels when corticosteroids are administered orally
3. Rifampin, barbiturates, and phenytoin cause a decreased corticosteroid effect

F. **Significant food interaction**: none reported

Table 5-3   Inhaled Corticosteroid Medications

Generic Name	Route	Uses	Adverse Effects
Beclomethasone	Inhalation Intranasal	Bronchial asthma, allergic rhinitis	Dry mouth, sore throat, cough, hoarse voice, candidiasis of mouth or throat, hypersensitivity, Cushing syndrome with overdose (hypercorticism)
Budesonide	Dry powder inhaler	Asthma, allergic rhinitis	
Ciclesonide	Inhalation Intranasal	Allergic rhinitis	
Flunisolide	Intranasal	Allergic rhinitis	
Fluticasone	Inhalation Intranasal	Asthma	
Mometasone	Dry powder inhaler	Asthma	
Triamcinolone acetonide	Inhalation Intranasal	Pulmonary emphysema, pulmonary fibrosis, bronchial asthma, allergic rhinitis	

G. Significant laboratory studies
1. There may be a decreased response to skin test antigens
2. Skin testing should be postponed if possible until after corticosteroid therapy

H. Side effects
1. Pharyngeal irritation and sore throat
2. Coughing
3. Dry mouth
4. Oral fungal infections
5. Sinusitis

I. Adverse effects/toxicity
1. Adrenocortical insufficiency, fluid and electrolyte disturbances, nervous system effects, and endocrine effects if absorbed systemically
2. Increased susceptibility to infection, dermatologic effects, and osteoporosis
3. Diarrhea, nausea and vomiting, and stomach upset
4. Headache, fever, dizziness, angioedema, rash, urticaria, and paradoxical bronchospasm
5. **Rhinitis** or inflammation of mucous membranes of nose, menstrual disturbances, and palpitations

J. Client-centered nursing care
1. Ask client about current medications (including OTC and herbal products) and history of any allergies
2. Monitor respiratory status and lung sounds for effectiveness of therapy
3. Teach client to report early signs of respiratory difficulty (such as activity intolerance and awakening with asthma symptoms)
4. Monitor for hyperglycemia
5. Monitor growth in children
6. Assess for adrenal insufficiency when changing from systemic corticosteroid to inhalation route
7. Chronic use of inhaled corticosteroids can predispose client to osteoporosis
8. Rinse mouth after use of medication because oropharyngeal candidiasis and/or hoarseness can occur
9. Assess sputum color and viscosity for signs of infection

K. Client education
1. Use medications as prescribed; do not overuse
2. Use metered-dose **inhaler** or **nebulizer** as instructed and keep equipment clean and in working order per manufacturer's guidelines
3. Inhale bronchodilator drug before corticosteroid when both are prescribed; wait prescribed interval between puffs and rinse mouth after use of inhalation device
4. Pediatric clients may need a healthcare provider's prescription to keep this inhaler with them at school
5. Do not abruptly stop taking this medication; taper dose slowly over a 2-week period under direction of a prescriber
6. Wear a medic alert bracelet or necklace identifying steroid use
7. Be aware of symptoms of steroid use, including moon face, acne, increased fat pads, increased edema; notify prescriber if these symptoms arise
8. Report signs of decreased amounts of steroid levels including nausea, dyspnea, joint pain, weakness, and fatigue
9. Report weight gain of more than 2.3 kg (5 lb) in a week
10. Avoid smoking and contact with allergens that trigger allergic response, if possible
11. Learn to recognize respiratory difficulty early so treatment can begin promptly
12. Take drug at approximately same time each day for maximal effectiveness
13. Use inhaled corticosteroids as maintenance drugs; they are ineffective in acute bronchospasm or asthma attack

Practice to Pass

A client is newly diagnosed with chronic obstructive pulmonary disease (COPD). The medications that are to be taken at home include albuterol and beclomethasone dipropionate. What client teaching is needed related to these medications?

III. INHALED NONSTEROIDALS

A. Action and use

1. These agents stabilize mast cells so bronchoconstrictive and inflammatory substances are not released when stimulated with an allergen; therefore, inflammation is limited
2. Used to prevent and treat airway inflammation; reducing inflammation decreases mucosal edema and mucous secretions and thereby decreases bronchoconstriction
3. Used for prophylaxis of acute asthma attacks
4. Used also for prevention and treatment of allergic rhinitis

B. Common inhaled nonsteroidal medications (Table 5-4)

1. Cromolyn: oral spray or nebulizer solution for oral inhalation, or available as nasal spray
2. Nedocromil: no longer available by inhalation; different formulation available as ophthalmic drops

C. Administration considerations

1. Reduction in dose of bronchodilators and corticosteroids may be indicated with use of these drugs
2. Use with caution in clients with impaired hepatic or renal function
3. Administer by inhalation
4. Nasal solution is used for prevention and treatment of allergic rhinitis
5. It may take 3 weeks of daily dosing to see therapeutic effects

D. Contraindications

1. Not to be used in acute bronchospasm or status asthmaticus
2. Contraindicated in clients with hypersensitivity
3. Use with caution in clients with impaired renal or hepatic function; lower dosages may be required

E. Significant drug interactions: none reported

F. Significant food interactions: none reported

G. Significant laboratory studies: none reported

H. Side effects (see Table 5-4)

I. Adverse effects/toxicity (see Table 5-4)

J. Client-centered nursing care

1. Ask client about current medications (including OTC and herbal products) and history of any allergies
2. Coronary artery disease (CAD) and/or dysrhythmias may be aggravated by any propellants in aerosols; therefore, use with caution in clients with cardiac dysrhythmias
3. Pulmonary function testing may be ordered prior to administering these medications
4. Perform respiratory assessment to monitor effectiveness of therapy
5. If dose is prescribed intranasally, assess for rhinitis (stuffiness, rhinorrhea, or runny nose)
6. Doses of other asthma medications may be reduced after 2–4 weeks of therapy with inhaled nonsteroidal drugs

Table 5-4 Inhaled Nonsteroidal Medications: Mast Cell Stabilizers

Generic Name	Route	Therapeutic Indications	Adverse Effects
Cromolyn disodium	Inhalation Intranasal	Bronchial asthma, bronchospasm, allergic rhinitis	Headache, nasal irritation and stinging, sneezing, irritation to the throat and trachea, cough, unpleasant taste, erythema, parotitis, bronchospasm, epistaxis, flushing
Nedocromil sodium	Ophthalmic	Allergic conjunctivitis	Dizziness, headache, nausea and vomiting, cough, pharyngitis, rhinitis, fatigue, dyspepsia

    7. Client may require pretreatment with bronchodilator while using these inhalers

    8. Do not use cloudy solution

K. Client education

    1. Take medications exactly as prescribed

    2. Be familiar with drug action, usage, and side effects

    3. Proper use of inhaler ensures maximal effectiveness of medication; use spacer as appropriate

    4. Record frequency and severity of asthma attacks

    5. It may take 2–4 weeks to see results of medication

    6. Rinse mouth after taking medication to avoid dry mouth

    7. Do not take during an acute attack as symptoms may be aggravated

    8. Ideally, bronchodilator should be taken 20–30 minutes prior to taking cromolyn; see individual product literature; always wait a minimum of 3–5 minutes between inhalations

    9. Cromolyn can be administered 15–60 minutes prior to contact with known allergens to reduce reaction to allergens

    10. With intranasal drug use, clear nasal passages prior to use

IV. LEUKOTRIENE MODIFIERS

A. Action and use

    1. Leukotrienes are substances that are released when a client experiences an allergic response to an allergen

    2. Leukotrienes cause inflammation, bronchoconstriction, and mucus production that leads to coughing, sneezing, and shortness of breath

    3. Leukotriene modifiers work by blocking action of leukotrienes by preventing them from attaching to receptors in circulating cells and cells in lungs, and thus relieve symptoms caused by inflammation

    4. Bronchoconstriction is prevented by inhibition of smooth muscle contraction of bronchial airways

    5. Leukotriene modifiers are used for prophylaxis and chronic treatment of asthma in adults and children over age 12; they are not used in managing an acute asthma attack

B. Common leukotriene modifier medications (Table 5-5)

    1. Zileuton: inhibits enzyme 5-lipoxygenase and therefore blocks production of leukotrienes; given orally

    2. Zafirlukast: blocks specific leukotrienes called cysteinyl leukotrienes that are thought to be mediators of asthma; inflammation in lung is prevented; classified as a leukotriene receptor antagonist

    3. Montelukast: inhibits leukotriene receptors and is classified as a leukotriene receptor antagonist; given orally

C. Administration considerations

    1. They are used in adults and children age 12 and over

    2. It may take a week before therapeutic effects are seen

    3. They have localized effects in lungs

    4. They are used alone or in combination with corticosteroids

    5. Zafirlukast must not be taken during lactation because it is excreted in breast milk

    6. Montelukast and zafirlukast are taken orally, metabolized in liver, and excreted in feces

    7. Zileuton is metabolized by liver and excreted in urine

    8. Monitor hepatic aminotransferase enzymes when administering zileuton; discontinue medication if levels elevate to five times the norm or if liver dysfunction develops

Table 5-5	Leukotriene Modifiers		
Generic Name	**Route**	**Therapeutic Indications**	**Adverse Effects**
Montelukast sodium	PO	Asthma, allergic rhinitis	All: headache, sore throat, nausea, diarrhea, elevated AST (hepatotoxicity)
Roflumilast	PO	Asthma	Roflumilast: weight loss and psychiatric problems including risk of suicide
Zafirlukast	PO	Asthma, urticaria	
Zileuton	PO	Asthma	

D. Contraindications
   1. Zileuton is contraindicated in clients with liver disease and with elevations of transaminase (three times the norm)
   2. All are contraindicated in clients with hypersensitivity

E. Significant drug interactions
   1. Theophylline, warfarin, and propranolol levels increase when administered with zileuton
   2. Warfarin, tolbutamide, phenytoin, and carbamazepine levels increase when administered with zafirlukast
   3. Decreased levels of zafirlukast are seen with concurrent administration of erythromycin
   4. Increased levels of zafirlukast are seen with concurrent administration of aspirin
   5. Calcium channel blockers have increased effect with zafirlukast
   6. Phenobarbital and phenytoin may decrease available montelukast due to initiation of hepatic metabolism

F. Significant food interaction: food decreases absorption of zafirlukast and zileuton

G. Significant laboratory studies
   1. Monitor serum theophylline levels if used concurrently due to decreased theophylline clearance when taking zileuton
   2. Monitor prothrombin time (PT) or international normalized ratio (INR) when client on zafirlukast or zileuton and warfarin as PT/INR may be elevated

H. Side effects
   1. Headaches may occur with all drugs
   2. Zileuton may also cause dyspepsia, nausea, and insomnia
   3. Zafirlukast may cause nausea and diarrhea
   4. Zileuton and zafirlukast cause dizziness, which could increase risk of falls or other injury

I. Adverse effects/toxicity
   1. Mood or behavior changes, suicidal thoughts (zileuton)
   2. Hepatotoxicity: jaundice, dark urine, clay-colored stools (zileuton)

J. Client-centered nursing care
   1. Be sure drug is prescribed for chronic, not acute, treatment of asthma
   2. Ask client about current medications (including OTC and herbal products) and history of any allergies
   3. Caution client that it takes about a week to see improvement in symptoms
   4. Assess respiratory status to evaluate effectiveness of therapy
   5. Monitor liver function tests for elevated AST and ALT levels
   6. Singulair should be administered in evening

K. Client education
   1. Drugs may take a week before therapeutic effects are seen
   2. Mechanism of action, usage, and potential side effects of prescribed drug
   3. Take medications exactly as prescribed

4. Avoid contact with specific allergen, if possible
5. Drugs help prevent some symptoms of asthma; they are not intended to be used for acute attacks
6. Liver function studies may be needed
7. Increase fluid intake if not contraindicated because of other disease processes
8. Take zafirlukast 1 hour before or 2 hours after meals
9. Montelukast and zileuton may be taken with or without food
10. Use caution when driving or operating machinery with zafirlukast and zileuton because these drugs can cause dizziness

V. ANTIHISTAMINES

A. Action and use

1. The action of these drugs is to block or inhibit action of histamine
   a. They work best early in the response as they do not displace histamine from receptors
   b. **Antihistamines** compete with histamine for receptor sites so that action of histamine can be blocked; thus, they do not prevent histamine release or reduce amount released
2. Antihistamines reduce effects of histamine (vasodilation, contraction of smooth muscles, increased GI and respiratory secretions, increased capillary permeability, increased heart rate and CNS transmission); therefore, antihistamines inhibit smooth muscle contraction (respiratory system, blood vessels, and GI tract), decrease capillary permeability, decrease salivation and tear formation, and inhibit vascular permeability and edema formation
3. Cause bronchial smooth muscle relaxation
4. Reduce bronchial, salivary, gastric, nasal, and **lacrimal** (tear) secretions and reduce itching (urticaria)
5. Used to treat allergies, allergic rhinitis (hay fever), allergic conjunctivitis, allergic contact dermatitis, vertigo, motion sickness, insomnia, allergic reactions, cough, and sneezing and runny nose due to common cold
6. Used in treatment of anaphylactic shock
7. Can be used as prevention or treatment for allergic reactions to medications

B. Common antihistamine medications

1. Nonsedating antihistamines (Table 5-6) include azelastine, cetirizine, desloratadine, fexofenadine, levocetirizine, loratadine, and olopatadine
   a. Cetirizine is a metabolite of hydroxyzine but causes less drowsiness
   b. These second-generation antihistamines cause less sedation than first-generation antihistamines
   c. They are selective for peripheral H1 receptors and do not cross blood–brain barrier
   d. Second-generation medications have a rapid onset of action after oral administration
2. Traditional antihistamines (Table 5-7) have sedative effects because they work peripherally as well as centrally; first-generation H1 receptor antagonists bind to central and peripheral H1 receptors and can cause CNS depression (drowsiness or sedation) or stimulation (anxiety or agitation)
   a. CNS stimulation is more likely to occur in high doses and especially in children
   b. These drugs also have anticholinergic effects such as dry mouth, urinary retention, constipation, and blurred vision

Table 5-6	Second-Generation or Nonsedating Antihistamines		
Generic Name	**Route**	**Uses**	**Adverse Effects**
Azelastine	Intranasal	Rhinitis	All: dry mouth, nausea, dizziness, headache, hypersensitivity, hypotension, paradoxical excitation Drowsiness (cetirizine) Bitter taste in mouth (olopatadine)
Cetirizine	PO		
Desloratadine	PO		
Fexofenadine	PO		
Levocetirizine	PO		
Loratadine	PO		
Olopatadine	PO		

C. Administration considerations

1. Antihistamines treat symptoms but not the cause of the symptoms
2. Antihistamines may cause drowsiness
3. Antihistamines should not be used for treatment of an acute asthma attack or lower respiratory disorder
4. Most antihistamines are tolerated better when taken with meals
5. Brompheniramine, chlorpheniramine, and diphenhydramine are all available over the counter
6. Hydroxyzine is effective with pruritis
7. Most antihistamines are metabolized by liver
8. Azelastine is topically applied to nasal mucosa and action peaks in 2–3 hours; it does not tend to cause drowsiness but does leave an unpleasant taste in mouth
9. Hydroxyzine causes profound drowsiness; diphenhydramine has a high incidence of drowsiness and anticholinergic effects
10. Antihistamines may be used as a premedication prior to administration of blood products to decrease likelihood of allergic reactions
11. Oral antihistamines act in 15–60 minutes and last 4–6 hours; sustained-release medications last 8–12 hours
12. A rapid-acting agent should be used with an acute allergic reaction
13. Longer-acting agents give more consistent relief with chronic allergic conditions

D. Contraindications

1. Hypersensitivity
2. Astemizole should be used with caution in clients with liver dysfunction because of potential for elevation in blood levels and potential cardiac malfunction
3. Loratadine is contraindicated in acute asthma treatment and in conditions affecting lower respiratory tract

Table 5-7	Selected First-Generation Antihistamines		
Generic Name	**Route**	**Uses**	**Adverse Effects**
Chlorpheniramine	PO	Rhinitis	Drowsiness, sedation, dizziness, disturbed coordination, epigastric distress, thickening of bronchial excretions, tinnitus, labyrinthitis, palpitations, hypotension, hemolytic anemia
Diphenhydramine	PO		
Hydroxyzine	PO		
Meclizine	PO	Vertigo	Drowsiness, confusion, euphoria, nervousness, hypotension, urinary frequency, respiratory depression, death

    4. Diphenhydramine should not be given to nursing mothers or clients with conditions of lower respiratory tract

    5. Antihistamines should be used cautiously if clients have a history of increased intraocular pressure, cardiac or renal disease, hypertension, bronchial asthma, stenosing peptic ulcer disease, prostatic hyperplasia, convulsive disorders, or during pregnancy

    6. Promethazine should not be used in children with hepatic disease, Reye syndrome, history of sleep apnea, or family history of sudden infant death syndrome (SIDS)

    7. Diphenhydramine is not recommended for use with infants or for children with chickenpox or flulike infections

E. Significant drug interactions

    1. Astemizole should not be used concurrently with erythromycin, ketoconazole, or itraconazole as this can lead to cardiac arrest and ventricular dysrhythmias

    2. Anticholinergic effects are more pronounced if taken with tricyclic antidepressants, antipsychotic agents, and some antiparkinson agents

    3. Ethyl alcohol, anti-anxiety agents, tricyclic antidepressants, antipsychotic agents, opioid analgesics, sedative hypnotics, and MAO inhibitors increase effects of first-generation sedating antihistamines

    4. Loratadine blood levels are increased when taken with azithromycin, clarithromycin, erythromycin, fluconazole, itraconazole, ketoconazole, miconazole, and cimetidine

    5. Azelastine levels will be increased when administered with cimetidine

F. Significant food interactions

    1. Licorice and loratadine should not be taken together because of potential prolongation of QT interval

    2. Coffee and tea may reduce drowsiness caused by these medications

    3. Alcohol or other CNS depressants will reduce alertness if taking a sedating antihistamine

G. Significant laboratory studies: antihistamines can mask positive skin test results

H. Side effects

    1. Drowsiness is the main side effect; however, children can experience paradoxical excitement with antihistamines

    2. Anticholinergic side effects include dry mouth and nose, changes in vision, difficulty urinating, and constipation

    3. CNS: sedation from drowsiness to deep sleep, dizziness, syncope, muscular weakness, unsteady gait, paradoxical excitement (especially in older adults), restlessness, insomnia, and nervousness

    4. GI: anorexia, nausea and vomiting, diarrhea, constipation, and jaundice

    5. Urinary retention, impotence, vertigo, visual disturbances, blurred vision, tinnitus, hypotension, syncope, and headache

I. Adverse effects/toxicity

    1. Seizures can result from CNS effects

    2. Dysrhythmias, palpitations, and cardiac arrest

    3. Agranulocytosis, hemolytic anemia, leukopenia, thrombocytopenia, and pancytopenia

    4. Overdose in children can cause hallucinations, convulsions, and death

J. Client-centered nursing care

    1. Assess client's current medications (including OTC and herbal products) and history of any allergies

    2. Assist client to determine factors that precipitate allergic reactions and to identify symptoms caused by allergens

3. Assess client for drowsiness and dizziness, especially during first few days of therapy
4. Encourage increased fluid intake of 2,000–3,000 mL/day unless contraindicated by another condition
5. Give antihistamines prior to contact with allergen, if possible
6. Administer sedating antihistamines at bedtime to help with side effect of drowsiness
7. Administer IM antihistamines deeply into large muscles
8. IV injection should be over a few minutes
9. May cause false-negative results on allergy skin tests; client should discontinue use 72 hours prior to testing
10. Cetirizine, loratadine, and fexofenadine may be used in children over age 6

K. **Client education**
1. Take medications exactly as prescribed and contact prescriber before taking any OTC or herbal products
2. Be aware of potential side effects of specific drug
3. Avoid contact with allergen responsible for reaction, if possible; if unable, take medication prior to exposure
4. Do not crush or chew sustained-release tablets
5. Do not take more than one medication at a time
6. Do not operate heavy machinery or participate in other hazardous activities while taking a sedating antihistamine
7. Do not use alcohol or other CNS depressants while taking this type of medication
8. Contact healthcare provider if excessive sedation, confusion, dizziness, fainting, rapid heart rate, or hypotension occur
9. Rinse mouth and use hard sugarless candy to relieve dry mouth
10. Antihistamines may dry and thicken respiratory tract secretions and make them difficult to expectorate; increase fluid intake to 2 liters daily to decrease their viscosity
11. Take nonsedating antihistamines with meals to decrease stomach upset
12. Take loratadine on an empty stomach to increase absorption
13. Avoid prolonged exposure to sunlight and use sunscreen to reduce risk of sunburn
14. Take sedating medication at bedtime to reduce drowsiness, which should become less significant after repeated doses
15. Do not take antihistamines for 72 hours prior to allergen skin testing to reduce likelihood of false-negative results

Practice to Pass

A 22-year-old college student comes to the university clinic because of problems with allergies. He is started on fexofenadine. What teaching should the nurse in the clinic initiate?

VI. DRUGS TO CONTROL SECRETIONS

A. **Nasal decongestants**
1. Action and use
   a. **Decongestants** relieve nasal stuffiness by shrinking swollen nasal mucous membranes
   b. Adrenergic agents (sympathomimetics) do this by vasoconstriction, decreasing blood flow to nasal mucosa and thereby reducing swelling
   c. Nasal steroids act as anti-inflammatory agents by suppressing inflammatory response
   d. Used to relieve nasal congestion and nasal discharge caused by acute or chronic rhinitis (common cold), sinusitis, hay fever, and other allergies
   e. May be used to decrease local blood flow prior to nasal surgery
   f. May be used to aid visualization of nasal mucosa during diagnostic exams because of effect of decreasing blood flow
2. Common decongestant medications (Table 5-8)

3. Administration considerations
   a. Nasal decongestants can be applied topically (with sprays or drops) or can be administered orally
   b. Sustained use of topical decongestants (longer than 3 days or in excessive amounts) can cause rebound congestion; therefore, oral agents should be used if needed for longer than 3 days
   c. Topical decongestants are potent decongestants with prompt onset of action
   d. Topical decongestants are preferred if client has cardiovascular disease because of decreased likelihood of cardiovascular side effects
4. Contraindications
   a. Avoid use when client has known hypersensitivity
   b. Adrenergic agents are contraindicated in clients with hypertension and CAD
   c. Clients with nasal mucosal infection should not take nasal steroids
   d. Decongestants should not be taken during pregnancy or lactation
   e. Contraindicated in clients taking tricyclic antidepressants or MAO inhibitors
   f. Use cautiously in clients with cardiac dysrhythmias, hyperthyroidism, diabetes mellitus, glaucoma, prostatic hyperplasia, and insomnia
5. Significant drug interactions
   a. Possible increased toxicity with sympathomimetics
   b. Possible increased sympathetic effect when given concurrently with MAOIs (i.e., severe hypertensive crisis)
   c. Beta blockers decrease effects of decongestants
   d. Concurrent use with digoxin can cause dysrhythmias
   e. Decongestants decrease effectiveness of antihypertensive agents
   f. Increased effect of nasal decongestants is seen with use of cocaine, digoxin, general anesthetics, antihistamines, epinephrine, ergot alkaloids, methylphenidate, MAOIs, thyroid preparations, and xanthines
6. Significant food interactions: none reported
7. Significant laboratory studies: none significant
8. Side effects
   a. Local nasal mucosal irritation and dryness
   b. Rarely nervousness, insomnia, palpitations, and tremors
   c. Rebound congestion is common
9. Adverse effects/toxicity
   a. If a topical decongestant is absorbed, it can cause cardiovascular disturbances such as hypertension and tachycardia
   b. CNS disturbances can occur if topical decongestant is absorbed and these include headache, nervousness, dizziness, confusion, delirium, and insomnia
   c. Muscle tremors, nausea and vomiting, appetite loss, and urinary retention

Table 5-8 Nasal Decongestants

Generic Name	Route	Uses	Adverse Effects
Naphazoline	Intranasal	Nasal congestion	Oral: dry mouth, headache, insomnia, CNS stimulation, tremors, dysrhythmias, tachycardia, hypertension, difficulty voiding
Oxymetazoline			
Phenylephrine			Nasal: temporary nasal irritation, dryness, burning, sneezing, headache, rebound congestion
Tetrahydrozoline			
Xylometazoline			
Pseudoephedrine	PO		

10. Client-centered nursing care
    a. Ask client about current medications (including OTC and herbal products) and history of any allergies
    b. Assess client for other medical history to determine potential for possible side effects; older adults with significant cardiac disease should avoid nasal decongestants because they are at high risk for hypertension, dysrhythmias, nervousness, and insomnia
    c. Assess client for history of open-angle glaucoma
    d. For administration of nose drops, have client lie down or sit with neck hyperextended to instill medication
    e. Wash medication dropper after each use to prevent contamination
    f. Client should sit and squeeze nasal spray container once and avoid touching nares with spray dispenser; tip of dispenser should be rinsed after each use
    g. Observe client for decrease in nasal congestion
    h. Observe for tachycardia, hypertension, and cardiac dysrhythmias; also observe for rebound nasal congestion (after 3 days), chronic rhinitis, and ulceration of nasal mucosa
    i. Question prescriber about need to change from nasal decongestant to oral drug if needed for longer than 3 days (rebound congestion)
11. Client education
    a. Take medications exactly as prescribed
    b. Recognize potential side effects, especially palpitations, insomnia, restlessness, and nervousness; report these to prescriber if they occur
    c. Do not use alcohol or other CNS depressants while taking this medication
    d. Do not operate heavy machinery while taking this medication
    e. Avoid use of caffeine while taking this medication as it can cause nervousness, tremors, and insomnia
    f. Avoid smoking because it increases secretions and decreases ciliary action
    g. Avoid exposure to crowds to minimize spread of disease
    h. Increase fluid intake to 2,000–3,000 mL per day unless contraindicated by another medical condition
    i. Nasal congestion in infants can decrease ability to suck effectively; application of a nasal solution prior to feeding can increase infant's ability to feed
    j. Avoid eating or drinking for 30 minutes after topical (nasal) medication administration
    k. Practice good hand hygiene
    l. Rinse droppers and spray bottles after each use to avoid contamination

B. **Expectorants**
   1. Action and use
      a. **Expectorants** increase fluid flow in respiratory tract and reduce viscosity of secretions to aid in removal of secretions by cough reflex and ciliary action
      b. They are used for relief of nonproductive cough associated with common cold, bronchitis, laryngitis, and influenza; they also thin secretions
      c. Guaifenesin (glyceryl guaiacolate): most common oral expectorant
   2. Common expectorant medications (Table 5-9)
   3. Administration considerations
      a. Use with caution in older adults or debilitated clients
      b. Use with caution in clients with asthma and respiratory insufficiency
      c. Not used as commonly as in past because of questionable effectiveness
   4. Contraindications: iodide expectorants are contraindicated in clients with thyroid problems because of potential for altered thyroid function

Table 5-9	Expectorants			
Generic Name	**Route**	**Uses**		**Adverse Effects**
Guaifenesin	PO	Dry, nonproductive cough related to mucus in the respiratory tract		Headache, dizziness, rash, nausea and vomiting, gastrointestinal discomfort
Terpin hydrate elixir	PO	Dry, nonproductive cough related to mucus in the respiratory tract		Headache, dizziness, rash, nausea and vomiting, gastrointestinal discomfort

5. Significant drug interactions: iodinated products may produce hypothyroid effects when given with lithium
6. Significant food interactions: none significant
7. Significant laboratory studies: guaifenesin may interfere with results of color tests for 5-hydroxyindoleacetic acid and vanillylmandelic acid
8. Side effects
    a. Nausea and vomiting and gastric irritation
    b. Rash
9. Adverse effects/toxicity
    a. CNS: dizziness and headache
    b. GI: nausea and vomiting
    c. Skin: rash
10. Client-centered nursing care
    a. Ask client about current medications (including OTC and herbal products) and history of any allergies
    b. Increase fluid intake to 2–3 liters per day, if not contraindicated by another condition, to assist in liquefying secretions
    c. Assess respiratory status to evaluate medication effectiveness
11. Client education
    a. Take medications exactly as prescribed and be aware of potential side effects
    b. Use effective coughing techniques to mobilize secretions
    c. Do not drive or operate heavy machinery while taking this medication because of risk for dizziness
    d. Do not use alcohol or other CNS depressants while taking this medication
    e. Report a fever or a cough lasting longer than a week to healthcare provider
    f. Increase fluid intake if not contraindicated by other disease processes
    g. Avoid smoking as this increases secretions and decreases ciliary action
    h. Avoid drinking fluids for 30 minutes after taking this medication

C. Antitussives
1. Action and use
    a. **Opioid** (narcotic) and nonopioid **antitussives** suppress cough reflex by directly affecting cough center; nonopioid antitussives do this without CNS suppression of opioid antitussives
    b. Peripherally acting agents (glycerin, ammonium chloride) have local anesthetic effects to decrease irritation of pharyngeal mucosa; available in gargles, lozenges, and syrups; lozenges increase saliva flow and therefore suppress cough
    c. Used to stop a nonproductive cough or a dry, hacking, and nonproductive cough that interferes with rest and sleep
2. Common antitussive medications (Table 5-10)

Table 5-10	Antitussives			
Generic Name	**Route**	**Uses**	**Adverse Effects**	
Nonopioid				
Benzonatate	PO	Nonproductive cough	Sedation, headache, dizziness, hallucinations, burning of the eyes, constipation, nausea, GI upset, numbness of the chest, pruritis	
Dextromethorphan hydrobromide	PO	Nonproductive cough	Respiratory depression	
Opioid				
Guaifenesin and codeine	PO	Cough	Hypotension, bradycardia, respiratory depression	

3. Administration considerations
   a. Swallow benzonatate capsules whole
   b. There is a potential for addiction and CNS and respiratory depression with opioid antitussives
   c. Most antitussives are given in a liquid form or as oral tablets
   d. Antitussives in syrup form may soothe irritated mucosa in pharynx
   e. Dextromethorphan is preferred over codeine as it provides desired effect without use of opioids; available in many OTC products and does not require a prescription
4. Contraindications
   a. Dextromethorphan is contraindicated if client has asthma, emphysema, or consistent headaches
   b. Hypersensitivity
   c. Codeine preparations are contraindicated in clients with respiratory depression, increased intracranial pressure, severe liver or renal disease, hypothyroidism, adrenal insufficiency, or seizure disorders
   d. Cautious use of nonopioid agents is recommended for clients with seizure disorders, hypotension, glaucoma, and prostatic hyperplasia
5. Significant drug interactions
   a. Opioid antitussives may potentiate action of sedating drugs such as anesthetic agents, tranquilizers, hypnotics, alcohol, MAOIs, and tricyclic antidepressants
   b. Dextromethorphan should not be given with MAOIs
   c. Avoid use of dextromethorphan with selegiline because of risk of confusion, coma, and hyperpyrexia
   d. Medications that increase antitussive effects of codeine include CNS depressants such as alcohol, anti-anxiety agents, barbiturates, and sedative hypnotics
6. Significant food interactions: use of parsley and dextromethorphan can produce serotonin syndrome
7. Significant laboratory studies: none significant
8. Side effects
   a. Dizziness, headache, drowsiness or sedation, nausea, vomiting, constipation, pruritus, nasal congestion, dry mouth, blurred vision, and sweating
   b. Dependence and respiratory depression with codeine
   c. Dry mouth, palpitations, thickened respiratory mucus, anorexia, urinary retention or frequency, diarrhea, photosensitivity, and dysuria with nonopioids
   d. Nasal congestion and burning of eyes with benzonatate

9. Adverse effects/toxicity
   a. Opioid agents: hypotension, bradycardia, and respiratory depression
   b. CNS: dizziness, headache, and sedation
   c. GI: nausea, constipation, and GI upset
10. Client-centered nursing care
   a. Ask client about current medications (including OTC and herbal products) and history of any allergies
   b. Assess for inability to cough effectively from excessive cough suppression
   c. Monitor for listed side effects; assess for respiratory depression and possible drug dependence with opioid antitussive
   d. Cough may be a useful diagnostic tool and protective measure for client; therefore, antitussives should be used only cautiously for irritating, nonproductive, and ineffective cough
   e. Use cautiously in older adults
11. Client education
   a. Take medication exactly as prescribed
   b. Be aware of potential side effects
   c. Do not operate heavy machinery or other activities requiring alertness while using these types of medications
   d. Avoid alcohol and other CNS depressants while taking these medications
   e. Notify healthcare provider if client has a cough that lasts longer than a week, a persistent headache, fever, or rash
   f. Do not drink liquids for 30–35 minutes after taking a chewable tablet or a lozenge
   g. Avoid smoking because it increases secretions and decreases ciliary action
   h. For excessive respiratory secretions, teach client coughing, deep breathing, and benefits of ambulation
   i. Liquefy secretions with increased oral intake up to 2,000–3,000 mL/day unless contraindicated

D. **Mucolytics**
   1. Action and use
      a. **Mucolytics** are administered by inhalation to liquefy (thin) mucus in the respiratory tract
      b. They are used with sinusitis and the common cold
      c. Aid in removal of viscous secretions
      d. An oral form of acetylcysteine (Mucomyst) can be used to treat acetaminophen overdose
   2. Common mucolytic medications (Table 5-11)
   3. Administration considerations
      a. Not used as commonly anymore because of questionable effectiveness
      b. These drugs are nebulized using a face mask or a mouth piece; can be instilled into a tracheostomy
      c. Acetylcysteine is effective 1 minute after inhalation; maximal effect is in 5–10 minutes
      d. Acetylcysteine is effective immediately after direct instillation
   4. Contraindications
      a. Use with caution for asthmatic clients
      b. Proteolytic enzymes are contraindicated in asthmatic clients due to allergy potential
      c. Contraindicated in client with hypersensitivity to these agents
   5. Significant drug interactions
      a. Activated charcoal limits effectiveness of acetylcysteine
      b. Mucomyst is incompatible with tetracyclines, erythromycin, lactobionate, amphotericin B, and ampicillin sodium

Practice to Pass

An 80-year-old client is admitted to the hospital. She is lethargic with a respiratory rate of 8 breaths per minute and cyanosis around the lips. When questioning the daughter, she tells the nurse that her mother has had a nonproductive cough for about 2 weeks and has been taking brompheniramine, phenylpropanolamine, and codeine combination. What are the appropriate nursing actions?

Table 5-11	Mucolytic Medications		
Generic Name	**Route**	**Uses**	**Adverse Effects**
Acetylcysteine	Nebulizer (inhalation)	Abnormal, viscid, or viscous mucous secretions related to acute and chronic bronchopulmonary disease	Nausea, stomatitis, bronchospasm, rhinorrhea, urticaria
Dornase alfa	Nebulizer (inhalation)	Management of respiratory symptoms related to cystic fibrosis	Pharyngitis, increased cough, dyspnea, rhinitis, wheezes, conjunctivitis

6. Significant food interactions: none significant
7. Significant laboratory studies: none significant
8. Side effects
    a. Oral irritation and sore throat
    b. Cough
    c. Nausea and vomiting
    d. Headaches
9. Adverse effects/toxicity: bronchospasm
10. Client-centered nursing care
    a. Ask client about current medications (including OTC and herbal products) and history of any allergies
    b. Administer medications as prescribed
    c. May cause bronchospasm and are therefore usually given with bronchodilators
    d. Suction client if cough is ineffective
    e. Rinse mouth after therapy to decrease oropharyngeal irritation
    f. Discard unused medication after 4 days
11. Client education
    a. Take medication exactly as prescribed
    b. Be aware of potential side effects
    c. Increase fluid intake to thin secretions unless contraindicated by other disease processes
    d. Avoid smoking as this increases secretions and decreases ciliary action

VII. MONOCLONAL ANTIBODIES

A. Anti-asthmatics/monoclonal antibodies

1. Action and use
    a. Indicated for moderate to severe asthma not controlled by inhaled corticosteroids
    b. Inhibits binding of IgE to receptors on mast cells and eosinophils, preventing the release of mediators of the allergic response; also lowers amount of IgE and decreases amount of IgE receptors on basophils
    c. Decreased incidence of exacerbations of asthma
2. Common medication: omalizumab
3. Administration considerations
    a. To reconstitute, draw 1.4 mL of sterile water for injection into a 3-mL syringe with a 1-inch, 18-gauge needle; put vial upright on a flat surface and inject sterile water into vial; keep vial upright and gently swirl for approximately 1 min to evenly wet powder; do not shake; lyophilized omalizumab takes 15–20 minutes to dissolve; swirl vial gently for 5–10 seconds every 5 minutes to dissolve any remaining particles
    b. Solution should be clear or slightly opalescent and may have small bubbles or foam around edge of vial; do not use if particles are visible or if contents do not

dissolve completely within 40 minutes; invert vial for 15 seconds to allow solution to drain toward stopper; solution may be somewhat viscous

   c. Administer within 8 hours if refrigerated or within 4 hours if stored at room temperature; discard unused solution

   d. Because solution is slightly viscous, injection may take 5–10 seconds to administer

  4. Contraindications

   a. Clients with acute bronchospasm

   b. Clients with known allergy

  5. Significant drug interactions: none known

  6. Significant food interaction: none reported

  7. Significant laboratory studies

   a. Serum IgE levels will increase following administration

   b. Increased IgE levels may persist for up to 1 year following discontinuation

  8. Adverse effects/toxicity

   a. Myocardial infarction; venous thromboembolism, transient ischemic attack

   b. Local injection site reaction

   c. Anaphylaxis

   d. Increased risk of malignancy

  9. Client-centered nursing care

   a. Assess lung sounds and respiratory function during drug therapy

   b. Assess for hypersensitivity symptoms (rhinitis, conjunctivitis, hives, shortness of breath, cough, anxiety, flushing, itching) during treatment

   c. Observe client following injection

   d. Epinephrine, diphenhydramine, and corticosteroids should be available in case of anaphylaxis

  10. Client education

   a. Explain purpose of medication to client; inform client that results from omalizumab therapy may not be immediate

   b. Instruct client not to discontinue or reduce other asthma medications, especially inhaled corticosteroids, without consulting a healthcare professional

   c. Advise client to notify healthcare professional immediately if symptoms of allergic reaction occur

VIII. OXYGEN

A. Indications

  1. Hypoxia, deficiency of oxygen (O_2) in cells and tissues, and **hypoxemia**, deficiency of O_2 in arterial blood, are indications for use of supplemental oxygen

  2. Some conditions in which O_2 therapy is indicated include conditions associated with decreased arterial PO_2 levels (pulmonary edema), decreased cardiac output (myocardial infarction), decreased blood oxygen-carrying capacity (anemia), and increased O_2 demand (sepsis, sustained fever)

B. Types of delivery systems

  1. Nasal cannula (nasal prongs): most common form of O_2 delivery

   a. Two prongs go into nostrils and tubing attaches to oxygen source and flowmeter

   b. Client can eat and talk with a nasal cannula

   c. Oxygen can be administered at a rate ranging from 1 to 6 L/min

   d. Dryness of mucous membranes can occur

  2. Nasal catheter: inserted into throat through a nostril and should be changed to other nostril every 8 hours; not used frequently because of client discomfort; gastric distention sometimes occurs

3. Oxymizer: a nasal cannula with a reservoir that can deliver higher concentrations of O_2 than a regular cannula without use of a mask; delivers approximately twice the amount of O_2 of a regular cannula

4. Face mask: a mask that fits over client's mouth and nose
    a. Simple face mask: flow rate is 5–10 L/min with O_2 delivery capabilities of 40–60%
    b. Partial rebreather mask: consists of a face mask with a reservoir bag; some of the air client exhales goes into reservoir bag and is mixed with 100% O_2 for next inhalation; this system permits conservation of O_2 and can deliver 70–90% O_2 at rates of 6–15 L/min
    c. Nonrebreather mask: delivers highest concentration of O_2 by mask; no exhaled air goes into reservoir bag; reservoir bag contains O_2, which client breathes in with inspiration; exhaled air goes out through side vents and can deliver 60–100% O_2 at flow rates of 6–15 L/min
    d. Venturi mask: percentage of O_2 to be administered is adjusted by a dial at end of mask; amount of air pulled into system varies with needed amount of O_2; gives precise oxygen concentrations

C. **Oxygen toxicity**
    1. Lung tissue can be damaged from prolonged exposure to high O_2 concentrations; exact amount of O_2 and length of time required to cause O_2 toxicity varies with different clients depending on degree of underlying lung disease; some sources say that lung damage can occur with O_2 delivery of greater than 50% for longer than 24–48 hours
    2. **Atelectasis** or alveolar collapse can result with O_2 administration at rates of 60% for more than 36 hours or 90% for more than 6 hours
    3. Acute respiratory distress syndrome (ARDS) can result from breathing 80–100% oxygen for longer than 24 hours
    4. Symptoms of O_2 toxicity begin as a nonproductive cough, substernal chest pain, gastrointestinal upset, and dyspnea; as it worsens, client develops decreased vital capacity, decreased lung compliance, and hypoxemia; atelectasis, pulmonary edema, and pulmonary hemorrhage can result if problem is not reversed
    5. Oxygen should be weaned as soon as possible and according to client's SaO_2 level

D. **Administration and client-centered nursing care**
    1. Oxygen therapy can be anxiety-provoking; provide sufficient explanation and allow client to express anxieties
    2. Flow rate is measured in liters per minute; a measure of amount of O_2 delivered but is not completely accurate because there is loss of O_2 content with leaking and mixing with room air
    3. Oxygen analyzers are available to measure amount of O_2 client inhales, and this is recommended every 4 hours to provide precise measurement of percentage of O_2 client is receiving
    4. Clients with COPD should not receive O_2 at high percentages because higher levels of O_2 in bloodstream can cause hypoventilation; a COPD client's drive to breathe is from low levels of O_2 tension; a client with COPD can usually tolerate a rate of up to 2 L/min by nasal cannula
    5. Check O_2 delivery system frequently to ensure proper functioning
    6. Oxygen should be humidified when client is receiving O_2 at a rate higher than 2 L/min
    7. A face mask should fit client's face to avoid unnecessary leakage of O_2; if mask is too snug, skin irritation can occur
    8. Masks can be replaced with a nasal cannula during mealtime with a healthcare provider's prescription
    9. The reservoir bag on a partial rebreather should deflate slightly with inspiration

POSTTEST

10. Provide reassurance if client becomes claustrophobic

! ▶ 11. Flaps on sides of nonrebreather mask should be open during expiration and closed during inhalation

12. Monitor SaO_2 with pulse oximeter during oxygen administration; with healthcare provider prescription, O_2 may be titrated to achieve desired SaO_2 level

13. Assess for signs and symptoms of hypoxia and respiratory distress; also assess for changes in vital signs and color changes

14. Monitor arterial blood gases (ABGs) per healthcare provider prescription

15. Normal arterial O_2 levels decrease with age

! ▶ 16. Provide oral care for client comfort because of potential for drying of mucous membranes

17. Identify clients at high risk for development of O_2 toxicity

E. Client education

1. Prepare client for noise that occurs with flow of O_2

! ▶ 2. Avoid open flames with O_2 administration due to flammable nature of O_2

! ▶ 3. Ensure there are no frayed electrical cords near O_2 so there is no chance of a spark causing combustion

! ▶ 4. Smoking is prohibited when O_2 therapy is being utilized

5. Inform client that O_2 delivery can cause dryness of mouth and nasal mucosa

! ▶ 6. Remove O_2 when client uses an electric razor

7. Continue O_2 therapy at home as prescribed by healthcare provider

8. Keep O_2 tank in holder and away from direct sunlight to reduce effects of heat

9. Instruct client on signs of hypoxia and to report them to healthcare provider

Case Study

R. C. is a 14-year-old girl with newly diagnosed asthma. She will be using albuterol and beclomethasone inhalers. You are the nurse working in the healthcare provider's office where R. C. comes for her checkups.

1. What teaching does R. C. need about albuterol?

2. What teaching does R. C. need about beclomethasone?

3. What developmental issues related to a newly diagnosed illness should you anticipate, and how will you respond?

4. What are the anticipated effects and the side effects of the medications?

5. What assessment will you do when R. C. comes for office visits to assess how she is dealing with her disease and its treatment?

For suggested responses, see pages 539–540.

POSTTEST

❶ The mother of a 6-year-old client with asthma reports using metaproterenol more frequently. The nurse is most likely to caution the parent about which set of adverse effects?

1. Nervousness and tachycardia
2. Lethargy and bradycardia
3. Decreased blood pressure and dizziness
4. Increased blood pressure and fatigue

2 What statements best indicate to the nurse that the client understood instructions about self-administration of salmeterol? Select all that apply.

1. "I will use this medication every 6 hours."
2. "If my symptoms are not better within 20 minutes, I should notify my healthcare provider."
3. "Although it will remain regular, this medicine may decrease my heart rate."
4. "This drug is supposed to prevent an asthma attack, but is not good for treating one."
5. "I will take a dose of this medicine when I notice I am wheezing."

3 A client takes oxtriphylline for chronic obstructive pulmonary disease (COPD). Which explanation by the nurse accurately represents the drug's characteristics?

1. "The medicine increases your heart rate to increase the release of oxygen."
2. "The drug relaxes the lung tissue so that oxygen will pass across it easier."
3. "The medicine is used to dilate your airways and make it easier for you to breathe."
4. "The medicine thins the secretions in your lungs and makes it easier for you to cough."

4 A healthcare provider prescribed theophylline 0.4 mg/kg every 6 hours for a client. Which client information should lead the nurse to consult with the prescriber?

1. Concurrent history of Cushing disease
2. History of narcolepsy
3. Concurrent diagnosis of hyperthyroidism
4. Current state of hypothermia

5 Because a client with chronic obstructive pulmonary disease (COPD) had been taking triamcinolone acetamide 8 mg by mouth (four times daily) at home and is currently receiving dexamethasone 4 mg intravenously every 4 hours in the hospital, the nurse should anticipate which of the following in relation to these two medications?

1. Increase in the dose of triamcinolone
2. Scheduling the drugs so they peak at different times
3. Increase in symptoms with administration of the two drugs
4. Smaller dose of triamcinolone and/or dexamethasone

6 The nurse should withhold the currently scheduled drug dose and consult with the prescriber after noting that a client with which health problem is receiving fluticasone aerosol?

1. Acquired immune deficiency syndrome (AIDS)
2. Asthma
3. Chronic obstructive pulmonary disease
4. Systemic lupus erythematosus

7 A homebound client who has a history of asthma and was recently started on cromolyn sodium has a 3-week-old newborn at home. The case manager would give which priority instruction to the home health aide?

1. "Teach the client to pace activities of daily living (ADLs)."
2. "Encourage the client to wear a mask when mowing the lawn."
3. "Recommend that the client avoid individuals with upper respiratory infections."
4. "Report if breastfeeding is observed during your visit."

8 Which goal is *most likely* to be included by the nurse in the care plan for a client who is taking zileuton?

1. Client will manage lethargy commonly associated with drug.
2. Client will manage constipation commonly associated with the drug.
3. Client will manage headaches commonly associated with the drug.
4. Client will demonstrate ability to cope with the signs and symptoms of asthma.

9 After administering promethazine 12.5 mg intravenously to an 80-year-old client for nausea, the nurse should provide which instruction to unlicensed assistive personnel (UAP)?

1. Provide client with nonskid slippers for ambulation.
2. Teach client how to use emergency cord in the bathroom.
3. Place a chair next to client's bed to reduce potential falls.
4. Instruct client to remain in bed with top half rails up.

10 The nurse should select which of the following as the most appropriate nursing concern for a client who is receiving oxymetazoline?

1. Reduced gas exchange
2. Chronic pain
3. Alteration in tissue integrity
4. Interrupted sleep pattern

➤ *See pages 162–163 for Answers and Rationales.*

ANSWERS & RATIONALES

Pretest

1 **Answer: 1 Rationale:** The symptoms of an acute asthma attack are related to constriction of the airway, which leads to dyspnea, wheezing, increased respiratory rate, and declining oxygen saturation. Albuterol is a beta-adrenergic agent or sympathomimetic that relaxes the smooth muscles of the bronchial tree, resulting in bronchodilation and relief of wheezing. The respiratory rate should return to normal (12–20 per minute in an adult), making a respiratory rate of 34 to 22 slightly above the normal range. An intensity rating scale can be used for dyspnea, just as it is used for pain, and so a reduction from 9 to 6 is inadequate. The normal oxygen saturation level is 95–100%, making an oxygen saturation of 82% suboptimal. **Cognitive Level:** Analyzing **Client Need:** Pharmacological and Parenteral Therapies **Integrated Process:** Nursing Process: Evaluation **Content Area:** Pharmacology **Strategy:** Correlate the primary outcome of the disease process with the drug action. Because of the critical word *best* in the question, choose the option that has data that has fully returned to within normal limits. **Reference:** LeMone, P. T., Burke, K. M., Bauldoff, G., & Gubrud, P. (2015). *Medical surgical nursing: Clinical reasoning in patient care* (6th ed.). New York, NY: Pearson, pp. 1232–1238.

2 **Answer: 2 Rationale:** Because adrenergic agents such as epinephrine increase oxygen consumption as well as increase the workload on the myocardium, they are contraindicated in clients with cardiovascular disease. Because epinephrine causes arterial constriction, which results in decreased inflammation, it is often utilized during acute asthmatic attacks and would not be contraindicated in a client with asthma. Because of the sympathomimetic action, it may increase the blood pressure, which might then aid a client who has hypotension and increase the heart rate, which would be helpful to a client with bradycardia. **Cognitive Level:** Applying **Client Need:** Pharmacological and Parenteral Therapies **Integrated Process:** Nursing Process: Planning **Content Area:** Pharmacology **Strategy:** The critical words are *question a prescription*, indicating the answer represents a contraindication or hazard with the use of epinephrine. Correlate the drug category (sympathomimetic) with the various options and use the process of elimination to choose the one that could have an adverse effect because of impaired coronary circulation. **Reference:** Wilson, B. A., Shannon, M. T., & Shields, K. M. (2016). *Pearson nurse's drug guide 2016.* New York, NY: Pearson, p. 561.

3 **Answer: 4 Rationale:** The actions of theophylline are similar to the sympathetic response, which results in increased heart rate. Food items such as coffee or tea contain stimulants, such as caffeine, that can have an additive effect with theophylline. Peas, beans, and milk do not contain a chemical that could result in heightened adverse effects of the drug (as with the correct option) or result in inadequate drug action. **Cognitive Level:** Applying **Client Need:** Pharmacological and Parenteral Therapies **Integrated Process:** Teaching and Learning **Content Area:** Pharmacology **Strategy:** Questions that include a drug and one or more foods are highly likely to be looking for either an additive drug effect or a diminished drug effect when the drug and food are taken together. With this in mind, consider the elements that the foods and the drug have in common and the potentially combined outcomes. **Reference:** Wilson, B. A.,

Shannon, M. T., & Shields, K. M. (2016). *Pearson nurse's drug guide 2016*. New York, NY: Pearson, p. 1500.

4 **Answer: 2, 3 Rationale:** Delayed healing is related to the decreased inflammatory response. Because corticosteroids such as beclomethasone dipropionate reduce the immune response, a potential side effect of an inhaled corticosteroid is an oral fungal infection. Inhaled corticosteroids can cause dry mouth, not excessive salivation. Inhaled corticosteroids generally do not cause fluid retention and weight gain; these are not common side effects. Asthma is believed to be an abnormal inflammatory response to an irritant. Because the drug decreases inflammation, a decreased respiratory rate is expected. **Cognitive Level:** Applying **Client Need:** Pharmacological and Parenteral Therapies **Integrated Process:** Teaching and Learning **Content Area:** Pharmacology **Strategy:** Associate glucocorticoids with the outcomes of a reduced immune response and fluid retention. **Reference:** Wilson, B. A., Shannon, M. T., & Shields, K. M. (2016). *Pearson nurse's drug guide 2016*. New York, NY: Pearson, p. 158.

5 **Answer: 2 Rationale:** Albuterol is an adrenergic bronchodilator that generally results in immediate relief of an acute asthmatic attack. The onset of aminophylline is 15–20 minutes and could be utilized for an acute attack if albuterol was not available. Cromolyn is a mast cell stabilizer and is a prophylactic agent that inhibits the release of bronchoconstricting histamines. The onset is several days to 1 week after the first dose and would not be indicated for use in a client with a need for immediate bronchodilation. Salmeterol is used for prophylaxis of acute bronchoconstriction. **Cognitive Level:** Applying **Client Need:** Pharmacological and Parenteral Therapies **Integrated Process:** Nursing Process: Planning **Content Area:** Pharmacology **Strategy:** Select the option that identifies the drug with the most rapid onset. Eliminate two options first as not immediate acting and select one option from the remaining two choices because of the suffix *-terol*, which indicates a beta-adrenergic effect. Specific nursing knowledge of the various drugs and the time of onset is needed to answer the question. **Reference:** Wilson, B. A., Shannon, M. T., & Shields, K. M. (2016). *Pearson nurse's drug guide 2016*. New York, NY: Pearson, p. 29.

6 **Answer: 2 Rationale:** Zafirlukast is a leukotriene modifier. This class of medications is indicated for the prophylaxis and chronic treatment of asthma. Because leukotriene modifiers are not used during an acute attack, this response indicates that the client needs more teaching. "I will take the drug a few weeks before I expect to notice an improvement in my symptoms" is a correct response because the onset of action occurs at 1 week. Fluid intake should increase to liquefy secretions and assist the client with expectoration. To promote absorption, this medication should be taken 1 hour before meals or 2 hours after meals. **Cognitive Level:** Applying **Client Need:** Pharmacological and Parenteral Therapies **Integrated Process:** Nursing Process: Evaluation **Content Area:** Pharmacology **Strategy:** The wording of the question tells you that the correct option is an incorrect statement. Select the option that is most opposite the characteristics of the drug. **Reference:** Wilson, B. A., Shannon, M. T., & Shields, K. M. (2016). *Pearson nurse's drug guide 2016*. New York, NY: Pearson, p. 1619.

7 **Answer: 4 Rationale:** Loratadine should be taken on an empty stomach to increase absorption. Loratadine is more likely to cause drowsiness than nervousness. The onset of action is approximately 1 hour. It acts to reduce the inflammatory response by competing for histamine 1 (H_1) receptor sites within the mucous membranes, which would not reduce bronchoconstriction occurring with asthma. **Cognitive Level:** Applying **Client Need:** Pharmacological and Parenteral Therapies **Integrated Process:** Teaching and Learning **Content Area:** Pharmacology **Strategy:** Specific drug knowledge is needed to answer the question. Use the process of elimination to identify the option closest to appropriate administration of this drug. **Reference:** Wilson, B. A., Shannon, M. T., & Shields, K. M. (2016). *Pearson nurse's drug guide 2016*. New York, NY: Pearson, p. 921.

8 **Answer: 2 Rationale:** Because phenylephrine is a sympathomimetic, it has the potential to produce cardiovascular side effects such as sustained hypertension and tachycardia. If this occurs, the drug should be discontinued and the healthcare provider notified. Because of the risk of thinning of nasal mucous membranes due to prolonged vasoconstriction (which could result in increased risk of nosebleed), oral agents should be used for long-term therapy. Often, decongestants cause a dry mouth, but the client should use hard, sugarless candy rather than discontinuing the medication. Rebound congestion is more likely to occur with nasal spray decongestants. **Cognitive Level:** Applying **Client Need:** Pharmacological and Parenteral Therapies **Integrated Process:** Nursing Process: Planning **Content Area:** Pharmacology **Strategy:** Answer the critical thinking question, "What potential outcomes of phenylephrine are likely to place the client at the *greatest* risk?" **Reference:** Wilson, B. A., Shannon, M. T., & Shields, K. M. (2016). *Pearson nurse's drug guide 2016*. New York, NY: Pearson, p. 1232.

9 **Answer: 1 Rationale:** Guaifenesin is an expectorant with potential side effects such as nausea and vomiting, gastric irritation, rash, dizziness, and headache; an OTC antiemetic may be used. Since the drug is an expectorant, the purpose is to reduce the viscosity of respiratory secretion to increase mobilization of the secretions. The client should take the medication with a full glass of water unless contraindicated. Because the drug can potentially inhibit platelet function, aspirin may increase the risk of bleeding. **Cognitive Level:** Applying **Client Need:** Pharmacological and Parenteral Therapies **Integrated Process:** Teaching and Learning **Content Area:** Pharmacology **Strategy:** Recall that guaifenesin is an expectorant and the side effects of this drug frequently affect the GI tract. Next correlate the common side effects with the most appropriate remedy. **Reference:** Wilson, B. A., Shannon, M. T., & Shields, K. M. (2016). *Pearson nurse's drug guide 2016*. New York, NY: Pearson, pp. 734–735.

10 **Answer: 1 Rationale:** A nonrebreather mask has a one-way valve between the mask and the reservoir along with two flaps over the exhalation ports. This design allows the client to draw oxygen from the reservoir bag during inhalation and the flaps to close to prevent room air from entering during exhalation. Changing the equipment should not be done without a new prescription. A nasal cannula is utilized for clients with chronic lung disease. The nonrebreather mask is used to treat clients with unstable breathing patterns that may be in need of intubation. The mask is functioning properly so there is no need to replace it or call the respiratory therapist. **Cognitive Level:** Applying **Client Need:** Pharmacological and Parenteral Therapies **Integrated Process:** Nursing Process: Implementation **Content Area:** Pharmacology **Strategy:** Apply knowledge of the purposes of the flaps on a nonrebreather mask with the appropriate nursing intervention. **Reference:** Smith, S. F., Duell, D. J., Martin, B. C., Gonzalez, L., & Aebersold, M. (2017). *Clinical nursing skills: Basic to advanced skills* (9th ed.). New York, NY: Pearson, p. 1264.

Posttest

1 **Answer: 1 Rationale:** Potential side effects of metaproterenol are stimulation of the central nervous system (CNS) and cardiovascular (CV) system. Increased administration may result in excessive side effects. Lethargy and bradycardia may occur with increased doses, especially in a 6-year-old child, but are less likely effects. Decreased blood pressure and fatigue are not consistent with either CNS or CV stimulation. **Cognitive Level:** Applying **Client Need:** Pharmacological and Parenteral Therapies **Integrated Process:** Teaching and Learning **Content Area:** Pharmacology **Strategy:** Recall that sometimes the adverse effects of medications are too much of the action that was originally expected. Since this drug is a sympathetic nervous system stimulant, align excess sympathetic nervous system stimulation with an increased frequency in use. **Reference:** Wilson, B. A., Shannon, M. T., & Shields, K. M. (2016). *Pearson nurse's drug guide 2016*. New York, NY: Pearson, pp. 975–976.

2 **Answer: 2, 4 Rationale:** Salmeterol should begin to take effect within 20 minutes. Use of salmeterol is prophylactic. It is dosed every 12 hours because of the 12-hour duration. Although salmeterol is predominantly a beta$_2$ stimulant, occasionally it may cause tachycardia. It is not used for treatment of acute attack. **Cognitive Level:** Applying **Client Need:** Pharmacological and Parenteral Therapies **Integrated Process:** Nursing Process: Evaluation **Content Area:** Pharmacology **Strategy:** Recall first that this medication is a sympathetic nervous system stimulant. Beyond that, specific drug knowledge is needed to answer the question. Since multiple choices can be made in this question, consider that there is more than one correct option but that not all of them will apply. **Reference:** Wilson, B. A., Shannon, M. T., & Shields, K. M. (2016). *Pearson nurse's drug guide 2016*. New York, NY: Pearson, pp. 1387–1388.

3 **Answer: 3 Rationale:** Oxtriphylline is a xanthine bronchodilator, and the mechanism of action is to increase the amount of cyclic adenosine monophosphate (cAMP), which leads to bronchial dilation related to the relaxation of smooth muscle. Xanthines can increase heart rate and force of myocardial contraction, but that is not the rationale for administration of the medication. The drug does not increase permeability of lung tissue. Thinning of secretions is more commonly associated with expectorants. **Cognitive Level:** Analyzing **Client Need:** Pharmacological and Parenteral Therapies **Integrated Process:** Teaching and Learning **Content Area:** Pharmacology **Strategy:** Recall the primary outcome of chronic obstructive pulmonary disease (COPD) and the appropriate drug action needed to reduce the effects of the disease. **Reference:** Wilson, B. A., Shannon, M. T., & Shields, K. M. (2016). *Pearson nurse's drug guide 2016*. New York, NY: Pearson, pp. 1155–1166.

4 **Answer: 3 Rationale:** Because tachycardia is a common side effect of theophylline, it is *contraindicated* in clients with hyperthyroidism. Cushing disease has no overlapping signs or symptoms with the characteristics of the drug. Theophylline may stimulate the client with narcolepsy, thereby reducing the problem rather than aggravating it. Metabolic processes are likely to be below normal with hypothermia. The drug is not likely to have an adverse effect. **Cognitive Level:** Analyzing **Client Need:** Pharmacological and Parenteral Therapies **Integrated Process:** Nursing Process: Planning **Content Area:** Pharmacology **Strategy:** Correlate the drug category with possible side effects along with diseases that result in the same signs or symptoms. **Reference:** Wilson, B. A., Shannon, M. T., & Shields, K. M. (2016). *Pearson nurse's drug guide 2016*. New York, NY: Pearson, pp. 1498–1500.

5 **Answer: 4 Rationale:** Both of these medications are corticosteroids. Because of the increased risks of adverse effects such as hyperglycemia, hypertension, infection, hypervolemia, and many others, a *decrease* in the dose of one or both drugs may be needed. Because the actions and side effects could be compounded (placing the client at significant risk), the drug doses should not be increased. Since the suppressive effect by dexamethasone is 36–54 hours, and by triamcinolone is 18–36 hours, the effects of the drugs are likely to overlap. The nurse should not expect an increase in symptoms related to COPD. **Cognitive Level:** Applying **Client Need:** Pharmacological and Parenteral Therapies **Integrated Process:** Nursing Process: Planning **Content Area:** Pharmacology **Strategy:** Note first that both of the drugs in the question are corticosteroids. Recall the actions, side effects, and contraindications to compare and contrast the drugs and then reason that one or both drugs need to have a reduction in dose to avoid adverse effects. **Reference:** Wilson, B. A., Shannon, M. T., & Shields, K. M. (2016). *Pearson nurse's drug guide 2016.* New York, NY: Pearson, pp. 1560–1562.

6 **Answer: 1 Rationale:** Corticosteroids such as fluticasone aerosol suppress the immune system. The administration of these drugs is *contraindicated* in a client who has a suppressed immune system as in AIDS. Fluticasone is commonly used in the treatment of asthma. It may be used in the treatment of chronic obstructive pulmonary disease (COPD). Corticosteroids are sometimes utilized in the treatment of joint pain and stiffness associated with systemic lupus erythematosus (SLE). **Cognitive Level:** Applying **Client Need:** Pharmacological and Parenteral Therapies **Integrated Process:** Nursing Process: Planning **Content Area:** Pharmacology **Strategy:** The wording of the question tells you that the correct answer is a condition with which a corticosteroid is contraindicated. Recall that this drug class suppresses immune function and then look for an option that represents an issue with immune function. **Reference:** Wilson, B. A., Shannon, M. T., & Shields, K. M. (2016). *Pearson nurse's drug guide 2016.* New York, NY: Pearson, p. 1647.

7 **Answer: 4 Rationale:** This drug should be used with caution in lactating women. A healthcare provider should be consulted prior to the client breastfeeding while on this drug. Because of the risk to the newborn, this is the most relevant point. The client does also need to pace activities to prevent excessive oxygen demand, but this is not the priority. Reducing exposure to elements likely to cause an asthma attack is appropriate. An infectious process may increase the risk of an asthma attack. Of all the options, however, the most important instruction relates to the risks inherent in breastfeeding. **Cognitive Level:** Analyzing **Client Need:** Pharmacological and Parenteral Therapies **Integrated Process:** Communication and Documentation **Content Area:** Pharmacology **Strategy:** Note the critical terms *newborn* and *priority*. These tell you that the presence of an infant has relevance to the question and that more than one option is likely to be a correct statement. Consider the adverse effects of

the drug to choose correctly. **Reference:** Wilson, B. A., Shannon, M. T., & Shields, K. M. (2016). *Pearson nurse's drug guide 2016.* New York, NY: Pearson, p. 388.

8 **Answer: 3 Rationale:** Headache is one of the *most common* side effects associated with the drug zileuton. The client is more likely to be restless and nervous than lethargic. The client is more likely to have dyspepsia than constipation. The goal is to reduce or alleviate symptoms, rather than to help the client learn to live with them. **Cognitive Level:** Applying **Client Need:** Pharmacological and Parenteral Therapies **Integrated Process:** Nursing Process: Planning **Content Area:** Pharmacology **Strategy:** Recall that the drug causes vasodilation, which may result in conditions similar to migraine episodes. Use this information and the process of elimination to make a selection. **Reference:** Wilson, B. A., Shannon, M. T., & Shields, K. M. (2016). *Pearson nurse's drug guide 2016.* New York, NY: Pearson, p. 1626.

9 **Answer: 4 Rationale:** Promethazine is a traditional antihistamine that causes drowsiness because it works centrally as well as peripherally. The client should be in bed with half side-rails up until the effects of the drug wear off (2–8 hours) to promote client safety. The effects may be heightened by the client's age. Using nonskid slippers does not provide the greatest safety measure. The client will be impaired by the medication and less capable of understanding or remembering instructions and should not be left alone in the bathroom. A chair next to the bed is not a sufficient safety measure. The client should not get out of bed for at least 2–8 hours; this may be longer because of client's age. **Cognitive Level:** Applying **Client Need:** Pharmacological and Parenteral Therapies **Integrated Process:** Nursing Process: Planning **Content Area:** Pharmacology **Strategy:** Recall first that this drug is a traditional antihistamine that can cause drowsiness as a side effect. Note next the client's age to reason that this risk may be heightened further. Then choose the option that represents nursing care to avoid adverse drug effects. **Reference:** Wilson, B. A., Shannon, M. T., & Shields, K. M. (2016). *Pearson nurse's drug guide 2016.* New York, NY: Pearson, pp. 1300–1302.

10 **Answer: 4 Rationale:** Oxymetazoline is a nasal decongestant. Insomnia is a side effect of the drug. The nasal congestion is not significant enough to interfere with gas exchange. After administration, many clients experience pain and burning in the nasal passages, but not chronic pain. The nasal passages may be irritated because of the inflammatory response, but this is not related to the presence of the drug. **Cognitive Level:** Analyzing **Client Need:** Pharmacological and Parenteral Therapies **Integrated Process:** Nursing Process: Diagnosis **Content Area:** Pharmacology **Strategy:** Recall the specific side effects of the drug to arrive at the correct priority nursing concern. **Reference:** Wilson, B. A., Shannon, M. T., & Shields, K. M. (2016). *Pearson nurse's drug guide 2016.* New York, NY: Pearson, pp. 1159–1160.

ANSWERS & RATIONALES

References

Adams, M. P., Holland, N., & Urban, C. (2017). *Pharmacology for nurses: A pathophysiologic approach* (5th ed.). New York, NY: Pearson.

Adams, M. P., & Urban, C. (2016). *Pharmacology: Connections to nursing practice* (3rd ed.). New York, NY: Pearson.

Burchum, J., & Rosenthal, L. (2016). *Lehne's pharmacology for nursing care* (9th ed.). St. Louis, MO: Elsevier.

Drug Facts & Comparisons. (2017) (Updated monthly). St. Louis, MO: Wolters Kluwer.

Karch, A. M. (2017). *Focus on nursing pharmacology* (7th ed.). Philadelphia, PA: Lippincott Williams & Wilkins.

Kee, J. L. (2015). *Laboratory and diagnostic tests with nursing implications* (9th ed.). Upper Saddle River, NJ: Pearson.

Kee, J., Hayes, E., & McCuiston, L. (2015). *Pharmacology: A patient-centered nursing process approach* (8th ed.). St. Louis, MO: Elsevier.

LeMone, P. T., Burke, K. M., Bauldoff, G., & Gubrud, P. (2015). *Medical surgical nursing: Clinical reasoning in patient care* (6th ed.). New York, NY: Pearson.

Lewis, S., Dirksen, S., Heitkemper, M., & Bucher, L. (2017). *Medical-surgical nursing: Assessment and management of clinical problems* (10th ed.). St. Louis, MO: Elsevier.

Vallerand, A. H., Sanoski, C. A., & Deglin, J. H. (2017). *Davis's drug guide for nurses* (8th ed.). Philadelphia, PA: F.A. Davis.

Wilson, B. A., Shannon, M. T., & Shields, K. M. (2016). *Pearson nurse's drug guide 2016*. New York, NY: Pearson.

Cardiovascular Medications

6

Chapter Outline

Objectives

➤ Describe general goals of therapy when administering cardiovascular medications.
➤ Identify specific nursing interventions related to administering digoxin.
➤ Identify signs and symptoms of digitalis toxicity.
➤ Identify nursing considerations when administering angiotensin-converting enzyme (ACE) inhibitors and angiotensin II receptor blockers (ARBs).
➤ List side effects of the most commonly used antidysrhythmics.
➤ Identify the nursing considerations when administering antidysrhythmics.
➤ Describe side effects and adverse reactions of alpha-adrenergic blockers, beta-adrenergic blockers, calcium channel blockers, antihypertensives, and nitrates.
➤ Identify specific client teaching points related to the administration of nitroglycerin.
➤ List significant client education points related to the various cardiovascular medications.

NCLEX-RN® Test Prep

Access the NEW Web-based app that provides students with additional practice questions in preparation for the NCLEX experience.

Review at a Glance

afterload resistance to blood being ejected from left ventricle; resistance in great vessels that the heart pumps against

automaticity ability of heart to initiate impulses on its own without external stimulation

cardiac output amount of blood ejected in liters/minute by heart; consists of input from preload, afterload, contractility, and heart rate; heart rate × stroke volume = cardiac output

chronotropic affecting heart rate (HR); positive chronotropic medications increase HR; negative chronotropic medications decrease HR

conductivity ability of impulses to spread throughout cardiac muscle fibers despite absence of specialized conduction tissue

contractility amount of force and pressure to pump blood from ventricles; amount of or ability of ventricles to "squeeze"

dromotropic affecting speed with which impulses pass through conduction system; positive dromotropic medications increase speed of impulses, whereas negative dromotropic medications decrease speed of impulses

dysrhythmia a general term that refers to abnormalities in electrocardiogram (EKG, ECG) pattern; these refer to electrical activity and not mechanical pumping action (contraction) of heart

inotropic affecting force of contraction; positive inotropic medications increase force of contraction and therefore increase cardiac output (CO); negative inotropic medications decrease force of contraction and therefore decrease CO

irritability a state in which heart muscle responds to a variety of external stimuli, including hypoxia, ischemia, abnormal electrolyte levels, particular hormones, medications, and physical trauma

preload degree to which ventricles are filled with blood and myocardial fibers are stretched prior to contraction

refractory period either relative (able to respond only to a strong stimulus) or absolute refractory period (unable to respond even to a strong stimulus); refers to recovery period in cardiac cycle when heart varies in its depolarization (electrical activity leading to contraction)

renin-angiotensin-aldosterone system complex system in which renin (released by juxtaglomerular cells of kidney) changes angiotensinogen from liver to angiotensin I, which is then converted in lungs to angiotensin II, a powerful vasoconstrictor that increases peripheral resistance and thereby increases blood pressure

shock severe disturbance of hemodynamics in which circulatory system fails to maintain adequate perfusion of vital organs

titrate act of adjusting medication (usually intravenous) according to a predetermined parameter

vasoconstriction narrowing of blood vessels in response to an internal stimulus, such as nervous system, or an external stimulus, such as cold

PRETEST

1 A client is receiving nitroglycerin by continuous intravenous (IV) drip to control chest pain and to increase myocardial tissue perfusion. The nurse prepares this medication by taking which action?

1. Using a solution that is covered by a plastic bag.
2. Using a special tube designed for the medication.
3. Changing the bag every 2 hours because it is unstable.
4. Mixing the medication under a laminar flow hood.

2 The client states, "I always put my nitroglycerin (NTG) patch in the same place so I do not forget to take it off." Which of the following is the best response by the nurse?

1. "Change the patch every 24 hours."
2. "Take two acetaminophen tablets 30 minutes prior to applying the patch."
3. "Rotate the NTG patch to a different hairless area each day."
4. "After removing the patch, scrub the area vigorously with soap and water."

3 A client hospitalized for heart failure is receiving digoxin IV push. The nurse obtains the following data on the client. Place the data in order from that of highest concern to least concern to the nurse.

1. Potassium (K+) level is 3.2 mEq/L
2. Apical pulse is 53 beats per minute
3. Client has been taking furosemide 20 mg daily for 2 days
4. Client enjoys orange juice with breakfast

4 A client cannot remember the name of the antihypertensive medication that has been prescribed. Based on the presence of a dry, nonproductive cough, the nurse suspects that the client is most likely taking which antihypertensive drug?

1. Propranolol
2. Lisinopril
3. Nifedipine
4. Bumetanide

5 Before a client receives metoprolol as treatment for hypertension, the nurse should ask the client about a history of which health problem?

1. Asthma
2. Seizures
3. Peripheral arterial disease
4. Myasthenia gravis

6 A nurse assesses a 75-year-old client for side effects of verapamil. Which side effect would be of most concern regarding this client?

1. Hypertension
2. Angina
3. Skin rash
4. Constipation

7 A client with frequent premature ventricular contractions (PVCs) received a bolus of lidocaine 100 mg IV (1 mg/kg of body weight). The nurse should monitor the client for which of the following?

1. Signs/symptoms of systemic lupus erythematosus (SLE)
2. Electrocardiogram (ECG) changes and neurologic changes
3. Vital sign changes and blood dyscrasias
4. Visual changes (green halos around lights)

8 A client is admitted to the emergency department with an exacerbation of heart failure. Blood pressure is 116/86 mm/Hg and heart rate is 98 beats per minute. The nurse ensures that which medication is available for immediate use once it is prescribed?

1. Atropine sulfate
2. Digoxin
3. Propranolol
4. Verapamil

9 A client asks the nurse to explain why she is receiving lidocaine in her IV when her dentist uses it to numb her gums before a tooth filling. What information about lidocaine should the nurse include in a response? Select all that apply.

1. It regulates electrical activity in the heart.
2. It acts as a local anesthetic on nerve endings of the cardiac muscles.
3. It reduces irritability of the cardiac cells.
4. It increases the heart rate.
5. It primarily treats dysrhythmias originating in the ventricles.

10 The nurse provides discharge instructions to a client about the use of amiodarone. Which statement indicates that the client has the knowledge necessary for safe self-administration?

1. "As soon as my provider says I am stable on this medication, I will be able to enjoy the sun again."
2. "The side effects of this medication may not begin to show up for several weeks or even months after I start taking it."
3. "If my pulse drops below 100 beats per minute, I should call the primary care provider right away."
4. "If I miss a dose of medication I will take two pills the next day."

➤ *See pages 200–202 for Answers and Rationales.*

I. NITRATES AND NITRITES

A. Action and use

1. Increase oxygenated blood flow to myocardium by dilating coronary and systemic blood vessels to relieve chest pain
2. Prophylactic treatment of angina in clients with coronary artery disease (CAD)
3. Dilation of systemic vascular bed leads to pooling of blood in peripheral vascular system; reduces left ventricle workload by reducing both **preload** (volume in a ventricle just prior to contraction) and **afterload** (resistance to blood being ejected by a ventricle) and ultimately reducing myocardial oxygen (O_2) demand
4. Short-acting nitrates are used to treat angina episodes; long-acting nitrates are used to prevent angina and treat symptoms of heart failure

B. Common nitrate and nitrite medications (Table 6-1)

Table 6-1	Common Nitrates and Nitrites	
Generic Name	**Route**	**Uses**
Isosorbide dinitrate	PO	Prevention of angina pectoris; symptomatic treatment of heart failure
Isosorbide mononitrate	PO	Prevention of angina pectoris; symptomatic treatment of heart failure
Nitroglycerin SL	SL	Prophylaxis or treatment of angina pectoris
Nitroglycerin SR	SL	Prophylaxis or treatment of angina pectoris
Nitroglycerin topical	Topical	Prophylaxis or treatment of angina pectoris
Nitroglycerin transdermal	Topical	Prophylaxis or treatment of angina pectoris

C. Administration considerations

1. Client's mucous membranes should be moist when taking sublingual (SL) tablets
2. Intravenous (IV) nitroglycerin (NTG) must be delivered as a continuous or intermittent infusion (not IV push) and given via an infusion pump
3. NTG for IV use must be diluted in 5% dextrose or 0.9% sodium chloride (NaCl) solution
4. Intravenous NTG should be mixed in glass bottles and only manufacturer-supplied IV tubing should be used; regular IV tubing can absorb 40–80% of NTG because of polyvinyl chloride plastic; it is not necessary to cover IV bottle to reduce degradation of reconstituted nitrates due to light exposure
5. Administer regular form of isosorbide on empty stomach; if chewable form used, tell client to chew thoroughly before swallowing; do not crush sustained-release tablets
6. Nitroglycerin drips are often prescribed to control or treat client's chest pain; nurse should **titrate** (adjust medication according to a predetermined parameter) medication accordingly
7. Monitor blood pressure (BP) and heart rate (HR) every 15 minutes when using IV NTG and titrating medication; be prepared to treat hypotension by decreasing or stopping NTG infusion
8. Wear gloves or use applicator when applying NTG ointment to prevent self-administration
9. Rotate location of NTG paste or patch to reduce skin irritation and enhance absorption; place on hairless areas for predictable absorption and avoid areas with scar tissue; appropriate areas include chest, upper abdomen, anterior thigh, or upper arm
10. For a hospitalized client, keep tablets at bedside only if policy allows; instruct client to report all attacks; count tablets daily if kept at bedside
11. Dosing regimen should allow for a 6- to 8-hour nitrate-free period to prevent body's development of tolerance; NTG patch should be applied in morning and removed at 10:00 p.m.

D. Contraindications

1. Hypersensitivity to nitrates
2. Hypotension and/or hypovolemia
3. Severe bradycardia or severe tachycardia
4. Right-ventricular myocardial infarction
5. Use of sildenafil or other phosphodiesterase-5 inhibitors for erectile dysfunction within 24 hours

E. Significant drug interactions

1. Do not mix with any other medications in bottle or IV tubing
2. Use of phosphodiesterase-5 inhibitors within 24 hours can lead to life-threatening hypotension and cardiovascular collapse

3. All other antihypertensive and vasodilator medications may interact to cause profound hypotension
4. Intravenous NTG may antagonize heparin anticoagulation
5. Use with alcohol and antihypertensive drugs may cause additive hypotension

F. Significant food interactions: none reported but alcohol may enhance hypotensive effect

G. Significant laboratory studies

1. Nitroglycerin may increase urinary catecholamines
2. May cause a false report of decrease in serum cholesterol
3. Prolonged high-dose use of NTG may lead to methemoglobinemia

H. Side effects

1. Headache
2. Postural hypotension
3. Flushing
4. Local burning or tingling sensation
5. GI upset with oral form
6. Contact dermatitis with topical use

I. Adverse reactions/toxicity

1. Blurred vision and dry mouth
2. Central nervous system (CNS): weakness, dizziness, vertigo, and faintness
3. Cardiovascular (CV): severe postural hypotension with resulting tachycardia; when BP falls, heart rate increases to sustain **cardiac output** (amount of blood ejected in liters/minute by heart)
4. Gastrointestinal (GI): nausea and vomiting, fecal and urinary incontinence, abdominal pain, and dry mouth
5. Anaphylaxis; circulatory collapse due to hypotension

J. Client-centered nursing care

1. Drug forms appropriate for angina prophylaxis include NTG paste, NTG patch, spray, SL tablet, and oral sustained-release forms
2. Drug forms appropriate for acute angina include NTG spray, SL tablet, or IV infusion
3. Ensure that client is sitting or lying down when taking NTG to prevent dizziness or fainting
4. Allow tablet to dissolve naturally under tongue; if mouth is dry, instruct client to take a sip of water before placing tablet under tongue
5. If pain is not relieved after first dose, notify healthcare provider or emergency services; doses can be repeated up to three times every 5 minutes
6. Store ointment in a cool, dry place with cap attached tightly
7. Check NTG IV infusion concentration carefully, as many different dilutions are possible
8. See also previous section on administration considerations
9. Monitor vital signs closely, especially for hypotension; measure BP prior to each NTG tablet
10. Hypotension may be reversed with administration of IV normal saline

K. Client education

1. All forms of NTG might cause dizziness and headache; rest for at least 15 minutes after taking SL NTG to avoid dizziness; headaches decrease in intensity and frequency with continued therapy and respond to acetaminophen
2. Report to healthcare provider if symptoms become worse or increase in frequency when taking NTG
3. If pain is not relieved after first dose, call 911, as this could indicate an impending myocardial infarction (MI); may repeat dose up to three times while awaiting treatment

Practice to Pass

An overweight female client has just told you she is planning to take OTC diet pills to lose 23 kg (50 lb). The client is also taking transdermal nitroglycerin. How would you address this issue? What client teaching is needed related to this medication?

4. Write down emergency phone numbers and place them next to phone; tell client to sit near phone when taking NTG in case of need to call for help
5. Take a sublingual or spray NTG before an event that might cause angina, such as exercise or sexual intercourse; keep NTG on hand for prn use
6. Keep a written record for prescriber of times, dates, amount of medication required for relief of each attack, and possible precipitating factors
7. NTG tablets degrade in heat, light, or moisture, so store in original dark container in a cool, dry place; replace every 3–6 months after opening; tablets should cause tingling or slight stinging sensation under tongue if fresh (potent)
8. Change position slowly, especially older adults, to avoid postural hypotension and falls
9. Shake aerosol spray well prior to use as this affects metered dose; spray one to two sprays onto or under tongue at onset of angina; repeat as needed for a maximum of three sprays in 15 minutes
10. If wearing an NTG patch or paste and experiencing an angina attack, take an SL NTG tablet using safety measures previously outlined
11. Client may swim or bathe with an NTG patch in place
12. Frequent and prolonged use of NTG may reduce efficacy, requiring a medication adjustment
13. Avoid over-the-counter (OTC) medications or herbal products without consulting prescriber
14. Avoid alcohol use after taking nitroglycerin, as it can cause a sharp drop in blood pressure
15. Report blurred vision, dry mouth, chest pain, or fainting to provider, as these may warrant discontinuation of drug

II. BETA-ADRENERGIC BLOCKERS (ANTAGONISTS)

A. Action and use

1. Decrease effects of sympathetic nervous system by blocking action of circulating catecholamines (epinephrine and norepinephrine)
2. In therapeutic doses, block beta-adrenergic receptors (remember β_1—you have one heart) that are found chiefly in cardiac muscle; also referred to as *cardioselective*
3. In higher doses, they may block beta-adrenergic receptors in airways (remember β_2—you have two lungs) leading to increased airway resistance, especially in clients with asthma or chronic obstructive pulmonary disease (COPD); also referred to as *noncardioselective*
4. Blocking beta-adrenergic receptors leads to reduction in renin activity, with resulting suppression of **renin–angiotensin–aldosterone system**; this results in:
   a. Competition for binding of catecholamines at beta-adrenergic receptor sites
   b. Reduction in systolic and diastolic BP
   c. A negative **inotropic** (force of contraction) and **chronotropic** (heart rate) effect
5. Are used therapeutically to manage hypertension, angina pectoris, acute myocardial infarction (AMI), supraventricular tachycardia, and in some cases heart failure
6. Should be administered to all clients with suspected myocardial infarction (MI) and unstable angina if complications such as heart failure (HF) are absent; they also help prevent ventricular fibrillation
7. Block cardiac effects of beta-adrenergic stimulation, resulting in:
   a. Reductions in HR, myocardial **irritability** (cardiac muscle response to a variety of external stimuli such as hypoxia), and force of contraction
   b. Depression of **automaticity** (heart's ability to initiate impulses on its own without any external stimulation) of sinoatrial (SA) node

        c. Reduction in atrioventricular (AV) node and intraventricular **dromotropic** (conduction velocity) effect

    8. Also useful in controlling panic attacks, anxiety, and stage fright in some clients

B. Common beta-adrenergic blocker medications (Table 6-2)

C. Administration considerations

    1. Assess client before, during, and after initial dose

        a. Monitor BP, HR, and cardiac rhythm frequently during initial administration; if given orally, assess client 30 minutes before and 60 minutes after initial dose; hold if pulse is below 60 beats per minute or if client is hypotensive

        b. Subsequent to next dose, reassess BP, heart rate, and rhythm

    2. Give medication at consistent times with or without meals; it is recommended to take medication before meals and at bedtime

    3. Beta-adrenergic blockers are not the same as calcium channel blockers; simultaneous use of beta-adrenergic blockers and calcium channel blockers may increase adverse effects, including bradycardia and hypotension

    4. Tablets may be crushed as needed (prn) before administration and taken with fluid of choice

    5. Be alert for unintended drug effects precipitated by comorbid conditions, such as masking of hypoglycemia in diabetes mellitus and bronchoconstriction in asthma or COPD

    6. Do not discontinue therapy abruptly; dosage is reduced gradually over 1–2 weeks, and observe client for paradoxical reactions such as hypertension and tachycardia

D. Contraindications

    1. Greater than first-degree heart block (a consistent PR interval longer than 0.20 second)

    2. Right ventricular failure secondary to pulmonary hypertension

    3. Sinus bradycardia

    4. Cardiogenic **shock** (severe disturbance of hemodynamics in which circulatory system fails to maintain adequate perfusion of vital organs)

    5. Significant aortic or mitral valve disease

    6. Hyperreactive airway syndrome (asthma or bronchospasm)

Table 6-2   **Common Beta-Adrenergic Blocker Medications**

Generic Name	Route	Uses
Acebutolol	PO	PVCs, reduction of exercise-induced tachycardia
Atenolol	PO	Angina pectoris related to coronary atherosclerosis, hypertension, MI, migraine headache, alcohol withdrawal syndrome, ventricular and supraventricular dysrhythmias
Betaxolol	PO	Hypertension
Bisoprolol	PO	Hypertension
Metoprolol	PO	HF, hypertension, prevention of recurrent MI
Nadolol	PO	Hypertension, angina pectoris, ventricular dysrhythmias, migraine headaches, lithium-induced tremors, essential tremors
Nebivolol	PO	Hypertension
Pindolol	PO	Hypertension
Propranolol	PO	Hypertension, migraine headaches, pheochromocytoma, essential tremor, tardive dyskinesia, cardiac dysrhythmias, angina pectoris, 5–21 days post MI to prevent reinfarction
Timolol	PO	Hypertension, prevent reinfarction post MI, migraine headaches, reduce intraocular pressure in glaucoma

7. Severe seasonal allergies (allergic rhinitis during pollen season)
8. Concurrent use of psychotropic drugs that use an adrenergic augmentation or within 2 weeks of a monoamine oxidase inhibitor (MAOI)
9. Use cautiously in client with systemic allergies to insect stings and major surgery, renal or hepatic impairment, diabetes mellitus, asthma, COPD, myasthenia gravis, or Wolff–Parkinson–White (WPW) syndrome

E. Significant drug interactions

1. Phenothiazines have an additive effect, worsening hypotension
2. Beta-adrenergic agonists (e.g., albuterol) antagonize effects (cancel each other)
3. Atropine and tricyclic antidepressants block bradycardia
4. Diuretics and other antihypertensive medications increase hypotension
5. High doses of tubocurarine (a neuromuscular agent used as an adjunct to anesthesia to relax skeletal muscles) may potentiate neuromuscular blockade
6. Cimetidine decreases clearance and increases effect
7. Antacids may decrease absorption
8. Atropine or isoproterenol can be used to reverse bradycardia caused by beta blockers; hypotension can be reversed by a vasopressor

F. Significant food interactions: none reported

G. Significant laboratory studies

1. May cause false-negative test results in exercise tolerance electrocardiogram (ECG)
2. May cause false-positive test results with glucose tolerance test
3. Elevations in serum potassium, platelet count, uric acid, serum transaminase, alkaline phosphatase, lactate dehydrogenase (LDH), serum creatinine, and blood urea nitrogen (BUN)
4. Increase or decrease in blood glucose levels of diabetic clients

H. Side effects

1. Bradycardia, atrioventricular block, and hypotension
2. Bronchospasm, wheezing, dyspnea
3. Impotence
4. Weight gain or worsening HF
5. Dizziness, fatigue, and lethargy
6. GI upset
7. Masked cardiovascular signs of hypoglycemia in clients with diabetes mellitus

I. Adverse reactions/toxicity

1. CNS: sleep disturbances, depression, confusion, agitation, or psychosis
2. CV: hypotension, profound bradycardia, heart block, acute HF, and peripheral paresthesias resembling Raynaud phenomenon
3. Laryngospasm or bronchospasm
4. Dry eyes with a gritty sensation, blurred vision, tinnitus, or hearing loss
5. GI: dry mouth, nausea and vomiting, heartburn, diarrhea, constipation, abdominal cramps, and flatulence
6. Agranulocytosis, hypoglycemia, hyperglycemia, and hypocalcemia in clients with hyperthyroidism

J. Client-centered nursing care

1. Take apical pulse and BP before administering drug; evaluate client for fluid volume overload as it may indicate HF
2. Monitor intake and output (I&O) and daily weight
3. Withhold dose if HR is less than 60 beats per minute (bpm) or if systolic BP is less than 90 mmHg
4. Perform a head-to-toe physical exam and assess client thoroughly for a history of asthma, allergies, or COPD; beta blockers may lead to bronchospasm in clients with no history of pulmonary disease

5. Assess HR, BP, and respiratory status carefully during periods of dosage adjustment; maintain effective communication with prescriber

6. Most common adverse reaction is bradycardia; clients with digitalis toxicity and WPW syndrome are most at risk

7. With IV beta-blocker use, monitor client's ECG rhythm and rate, BP, and occasionally pulmonary capillary wedge pressure (left-ventricular end-diastolic pressure [LVEDP]) in intensive care unit (ICU); reduction in sympathetic stimulation may lead to cardiac standstill

8. When beginning therapy with sotalol, client should be on continuous cardiac monitoring for at least first 3 days

9. Adverse reactions are most likely to occur after IV form of beta blockers are administered, but may occur in older adults and clients with impaired renal function taking oral doses soon after therapy is initiated

10. Dietary sodium is usually restricted to prevent fluid volume overload; check with prescriber regarding sodium restriction or concurrent use of a diuretic

11. Fasting longer than 12 hours may induce hypoglycemia, which is worsened by beta-blocker therapy because signs are masked

12. Periodic evaluations of renal, hepatic, cardiac, and hematologic functions should be made in clients receiving prolonged medication therapy

K. Client education

1. How to check pulse and BP; be aware of desired range for these values and keep a record of daily measurements; call prescriber if outside prescribed parameters, such as pulse rate less than 60; teach significant others how to take a pulse/BP

2. Abrupt medication withdrawal can lead to severe paradoxical or rebound reactions, including sweating, tremulousness, severe headache, malaise, palpitations, hypertension, MI, and life-threatening heart rhythm disturbances

3. Establish a routine for taking medication and strive to comply with prescriptive plan for best results (write out a daily schedule for medication)

4. Take metoprolol with food to enhance absorption

5. Change position slowly to avoid postural hypotension

6. Notify prescriber if dizziness or lightheadedness occurs; avoid driving or operating machinery until these symptoms are relieved

7. Stop smoking as this might offset desired outcomes of controlled heart rate, BP, and prevention of angina; smoking also increases hepatic metabolism of beta blockers, leading to unpredictable or diminished drug effects

8. Avoid OTC medications or herbal supplements without consulting prescriber

9. Notify all healthcare providers regarding use of beta-adrenergic blockers

10. Notify ophthalmologist or optometrist while taking this medication as it may lower intraocular pressure

III. CALCIUM CHANNEL BLOCKERS

A. Action and use

1. Class IV antidysrhythmic drugs that inhibit calcium ion influx through slow channels into cells of myocardial and arterial smooth muscle (both cardiac and peripheral blood vessels); normal role of calcium is to activate myocardial contraction, which increases cardiac workload

2. Intracellular calcium remains below levels needed to stimulate cell

3. Dilate coronary arteries and arterioles and prevent coronary artery spasm

4. Myocardial O_2 delivery is increased, preventing angina

5. Slow conduction through SA and AV nodes, resulting in a lower heart rate and decreased strength of cardiac muscle contraction (negative inotropic effect)

Practice to Pass

Your client is taking a beta-adrenergic blocker medication. Upon auscultation of the lungs, you hear diffuse wheezing throughout the lung fields. What are the appropriate actions to take? What are your rationales for these interventions?

6. Decrease automaticity and **contractility** (amount of force and pressure to pump blood out of ventricles) by blocking flow of calcium into cell
7. Decrease systemic vascular resistance (SVR) and thus afterload by dilating peripheral arterioles
8. Reduce arterial BP (antihypertensive effect) and heart rate
9. Used for vasospastic angina (Prinzmetal, variant), angina at rest, chronic stable (classic and activity-induced) angina, and essential hypertension; IV form is useful in treating atrial fibrillation, atrial flutter, and supraventricular tachycardia

B. **Common calcium channel blocker medications (Table 6-3)**
C. **Administration considerations**
1. Administer oral diltiazem before meals and at bedtime and oral verapamil with food to reduce gastric irritation
2. Evaluate BP and ECG before initiation of therapy
3. Monitor for headache; an analgesic may be required
4. Intravenous forms of diltiazem: give undiluted IVP over 2 minutes and repeat in 15 minutes or dilute in D_5W, NS, or $D_5\frac{1}{2}$ NaCl; continuous infusion may be given via infusion pump at a rate of 5–15 mg/hr; infusions over 24 hours and greater than 15 mg/h are not recommended
5. Verapamil may be given IVP when diluted in 5 mL of sterile water for injection at a rate of 10 mg/min
6. Withhold medication if BP less than 90/60
7. Use caution when administering diltiazem to clients with HF

D. **Contraindications**
1. Avoid use when there is known hypersensitivity to drug
2. Sick sinus syndrome (unless pacemaker is in place)
3. Second- or third-degree heart blocks
   a. Second-degree Type I or Wenckebach: progressive PR prolongation until a QRS complex is dropped on ECG
   b. Second-degree Type II: P waves are constant until a QRS is dropped on electrocardiogram
   c. Third-degree heart block: no association between P waves and QRS, usually ventricular HR is usually 20–40 bpm
4. Severe hypotension, BP less than 90/60

| Table 6-3 | Common Calcium Channel Blocker Medications |

Generic Name	Route	Uses
Selective for Blood Vessels		
Amlodipine	PO	Mild to moderate hypertension or angina pectoris
Felodipine	PO	Chronic angina pectoris and hypertension
Isradipine	PO	Hypertension
Nicardipine	PO	Angina pectoris and hypertension
Nifedipine	PO	Angina pectoris and hypertension
Nisoldipine	PO	Angina pectoris and hypertension
Nonselective for Blood Vessels and the Heart		
Diltiazem	PO	Angina pectoris, hypertension, vasospastic angina, and Raynaud's phenomenon
Verapamil	PO	Angina pectoris, cardiac dysrhythmias, and hypertension

E. Significant drug interactions
   1. Beta blockers and digoxin may have an additive effect in prolonging AV node conduction
   2. May increase digoxin or quinidine levels leading to toxicity
   3. Cimetidine may increase serum levels of calcium channel blockers
   4. Calcium channel blockers may increase serum levels of cyclosporine (an immunosuppressant)
   5. Furosemide is incompatible in IV solution

 F. Significant food interactions: do not administer calcium channel blockers with grapefruit or grapefruit juice; grapefruit increases bioavailability of nifedipine

G. Significant laboratory studies
   1. Total serum calcium levels are not altered
   2. Monitor baseline and periodic lab tests of hepatic and renal function
   3. Monitor diabetics closely; may induce hyperglycemia
   4. Cyclosporine levels may become elevated
   5. Digoxin and quinidine levels may become elevated

H. Side effects
   1. Headache
   2. Fatigue
   3. Constipation (especially with oral and sustained-release forms)
   4. Postural hypotension
   5. Peripheral edema

I. Adverse effects/toxicity
   1. CNS: dizziness, nervousness, insomnia, confusion, tremor, and gait disturbance
   2. CV: heart block and profound bradycardia, HF, profound hypotension with syncope, palpitations, and fluid volume overload
   3. GI: nausea and vomiting and impaired taste
   4. Skin rash
   5. Altered liver and kidney function
   6. In high doses, nifedipine has been associated with increased incidence of sudden cardiac death

J. Client-centered nursing care
   1. Evaluate BP and ECG before beginning treatment and monitor them closely during medication adjustment; withhold dose and notify prescriber for BP less than 90/60; monitor heart rhythm for sick sinus syndrome and second- or third-degree AV block
   2. Monitor hepatic and renal lab test results
   3. Monitor for headache
   4. May induce hyperglycemia; monitor diabetic clients closely
   5. Advise client to report gradual weight gain and evidence of edema; may indicate onset of HF
   6. Avoid smoking and alcohol intake

K. Client education
   1. Important to take radial pulse before each dose (especially verapamil); an irregular pulse or one slower than baseline level (such as < 60) should be reported
   2. Withhold dose and notify prescriber if BP is less than 90 mmHg systolic or less than 60 mmHg diastolic
   3. Change position slowly to prevent postural hypotension
   4. Avoid driving if dizziness or faintness occur; report these symptoms immediately
   5. Take medication exactly as prescribed and avoid skipping or doubling doses; do not stop therapy without approval of prescriber

Practice to Pass

Your client is receiving a diltiazem infusion. The ECG technician notifies you that the PR intervals are becoming progressively longer and occasionally an entire QRS is dropped. What is the most appropriate action for you to take? What is the possible cause of the cardiac rhythm disturbance?

6. Do not crush or chew sustained-release tablets
7. Follow-up care is important to monitor drug effectiveness
8. Avoid OTC medications and herbal supplements without consulting prescriber
9. Client should stop smoking and avoid alcohol consumption
10. Client should report easy bruising, petechiae, or unexplained bleeding

IV. ANGIOTENSIN-CONVERTING ENZYME (ACE) INHIBITORS

A. Action and use
1. Inhibit renin-angiotensin-aldosterone mechanism by blocking conversion of angiotensin I to angiotensin II and prevent peripheral **vasoconstriction** (narrowing of blood vessels in response to an internal stimulus, such as nervous system, or an external stimulus, such as cold)
2. Used to treat hypertension
3. Are preferred drugs for kidney failure for hypertensive clients with diabetic nephropathy
4. Are effective alone in Caucasian clients and with administration of a diuretic in African American clients

B. Common ACE inhibitors (Table 6-4)

C. Administration considerations
1. Discontinue as soon as possible if pregnancy detected
2. Moexipril and captopril should be taken on an empty stomach due to decreased absorption with food

D. Contraindications
1. Pregnancy
2. Hypersensitivity to ACE inhibitors
3. Avoid use with potassium supplements and potassium-sparing diuretics

E. Significant drug interactions
1. Potassium-sparing diuretics or potassium supplements: hyperkalemia
2. Increased lithium concentration

Table 6-4 **Common Angiotensin-Converting Enzyme Inhibitors**

Generic Name	Route	Uses	Adverse Effects
Benazepril	PO	Hypertension	Cough, rash, dizziness, headache are common First-dose phenomenon, angioedema, acute kidney injury, fetotoxicity
Captopril	PO	Hypertension, heart failure, diabetic nephropathy, left ventricular dysfunction following MI	
Enalapril	PO	Hypertension, heart failure, asymptomatic left ventricular dysfunction	
Fosinopril	PO	Hypertension, heart failure	
Lisinopril	PO	Hypertension, heart failure, acute MI	
Moexipril	PO	Hypertension	
Perindopril	PO	Hypertension	
Quinapril	PO	Hypertension, heart failure	
Ramipril	PO	Hypertension, heart failure	
Trandolapril	PO	Hypertension, heart failure, left ventricular dysfunction following acute MI	

3. Increased risk of hypersensitivity with allopurinol
4. May increase digoxin concentration
5. Antacids may decrease absorption of captopril and fosinopril
6. Indomethacin may decrease hypotensive effect
7. Phenothiazines may increase drug effects

F. **Significant food interactions**
   1. Capsicum (in some peppers) may aggravate ACE-induced cough
   2. Licorice may cause sodium retention
   3. Salt substitutes may result in hyperkalemia
   4. Foods high in fat may impair drug absorption

G. **Significant laboratory studies**
   1. Agranulocytosis and bone marrow depression
   2. May increase serum BUN and creatinine
   3. May increase liver enzymes, serum bilirubin, uric acid, and blood glucose
   4. Captopril may cause false positive urinary acetone

H. **Side effects**
   1. Headache, dizziness, anxiety, fatigue, insomnia, nervousness, hypotension, and palpitations
   2. Abdominal pain, nausea and vomiting, constipation, persistent dry nonproductive cough, and dyspnea
   3. Rash, arthralgia, impotence, and dysgeusia (altered taste)

I. **Adverse effects/toxicity**
   1. Angioedema, leukopenia, agranulocytosis, pancytopenia, thrombocytopenia
   2. Cerebrovascular accident (CVA or stroke), MI, and hypertensive crisis

J. **Client-centered nursing care**
   1. Administer 1 hour before meals to increase absorption
   2. Tablets may be crushed
   3. Do not administer to pregnant or lactating women
   4. Monitor labs for increased potassium, liver enzymes, bilirubin, BUN, and creatinine, and decreased sodium levels
   5. Take BP before giving dose and monitor regularly
   6. Monitor for rashes or hives
   7. Assess for peripheral edema
   8. If client has renal disease, monitor urine protein on a regular basis by dipstick method
   9. Diuretics should be discontinued 2–3 days before ACE inhibitor therapy
   10. Monitor white blood cells (WBC) and differential counts periodically
   11. BP is lowered within 1 hour of fosinopril administration with peak at 2–6 hours

K. **Client education**
   1. Report peripheral edema, signs of infection, facial swelling, loss of taste, or difficulty breathing
   2. Change position slowly to prevent dizziness and falls
   3. Do not skip doses or stop taking drug; it may cause serious rebound BP
   4. Seek medical approval before taking OTC medications
   5. Notify prescriber if a persistent, dry cough occurs
   6. Take antacids 2 hours before or after dose of fosinopril and captopril
   7. Avoid potassium-containing salt substitutes
   8. Monitor for bruising, petechiae, or bleeding with captopril
   9. Taste of food may be diminished during first month of therapy
   10. Take captopril 20 minutes to 1 hour before a meal
   11. Eliminate licorice from diet

V. ANGIOTENSIN II RECEPTOR BLOCKERS (ARBs)

A. Action and use
1. Antagonist at angiotensin II receptor of vascular smooth muscle, blocking vasoconstriction and aldosterone-secreting effects
2. Used for hypertension

B. Common angiotensin II receptor blockers (Table 6-5)

C. Administration considerations: discontinue as soon as pregnancy is detected

D. Contraindications
1. Pregnancy
2. Hypersensitivity
3. Use with caution in clients with renal or hepatic disease

E. Significant drug interactions
1. Avoid use with potassium-sparing diuretics
2. Diuretics may increase risk for hypotension
3. Losartan and phenobarbital: decreased losartan levels
4. Losartan and cimetidine: increased losartan levels
5. Indomethacin may decrease hypotensive effect

F. Significant food interactions
1. Salt substitutes increase risk of hyperkalemia
2. Red yeast rice may increase risk of toxicity

G. Significant laboratory studies
1. WBC for neutropenia
2. Electrolytes for hyperkalemia

H. Side effects
1. Hypotension and dizziness
2. Cough, GI upset, insomnia, nasal congestion or pharyngitis, myalgia/arthralgia, or flulike symptoms

I. Adverse effects/toxicity
1. Angioedema
2. Hypotension
3. Tachycardia or bradycardia

J. Client-centered nursing care
1. Monitor client taking diuretics for additive hypotension
2. Regularly assess renal function
3. Do not administer to pregnant or lactating women
4. Monitor potassium levels
5. Monitor regularly BP and apical pulse
6. Monitor WBC and differential periodically

Table 6-5 Common Angiotensin II Receptor Blocker Medications

Generic Name	Route	Uses	Adverse Effects
Azilsartan	PO	Hypertension (candesartan and valsartan also used in heart failure)	Dizziness, vertigo, fatigue, postural hypotension, syncope, pharyngitis, rhinitis, sinusitis, angioedema, upper respiratory infection, cough, fetal toxicity
Candesartan			
Eprosartan			
Irbesartan			
Losartan			
Olmesartan			
Valsartan			

K. **Client education**
   1. Do not discontinue medication abruptly
   2. Avoid salt substitutes to reduce risk of hyperkalemia
   3. Notify prescriber immediately if pregnancy is suspected
   4. Use nonhormonal birth control methods
   5. Report side effects to prescriber
   6. Change positions slowly to avoid dizziness

VI. ALPHA-ADRENERGIC BLOCKERS (ANTAGONISTS)

A. **Action and use**
   1. Block effects of sympathetic nervous system to decrease vasomotor tone and cause vasodilation, thus reducing BP
   2. Alpha$_1$-adrenergic blockers are used for peripheral vascular disorders, hypertension, and benign prostatic hyperplasia (BPH)
   3. Mixed alpha$_1$ and beta blockers are useful in management of hypertension
   4. Alpha$_2$-adrenergic agonists are centrally acting drugs that lower BP
B. **Common alpha-adrenergic blocker medications (Table 6-6)**
C. **Administration considerations**
   1. Alpha blockers may cause syncope within 30 minutes to 1 hour after first dose; effect is transient and may be diminished by giving at bedtime
   2. To avoid first dose syncope, begin with a small dose
   3. Do not stop drug abruptly
D. **Contraindications:** hypersensitivity to drug
E. **Significant drug interactions**
   1. Alpha blockers
      a. Enhance hypoglycemia with insulin and oral antidiabetic agents
      b. Decrease antihypertensive effect of clonidine

Table 6-6 Common Alpha$_1$- and Alpha$_2$-Antagonist Medications

Generic Name	Route	Uses	Adverse Effects
Alpha$_1$-adrenergic antagonists			
Doxazosin	PO	Essential hypertension	Rash, pruritus, dizziness, vertigo, headache, somnolence, drowsiness, pain, hypotension, dysrhythmia, palpitations, pharyngitis, dyspnea, arthralgia, constipation
Prazosin	PO	Mild to moderate hypertension, BPH	Dizziness, first-dose syncope, palpitations, orthostatic hypotension, nausea and vomiting, diarrhea, priapism, impotence
Terazosin	PO	Hypertension, BPH	Thrombocytopenia, decreased libido, dyspnea, back pain, muscle pain, peripheral edema, atrial fibrillation, peripheral edema, nasal congestion, sinusitis, blurred vision, impotence, priapism
Mixed alpha$_1$ and beta blockers			
Carvedilol	PO	Hypertension, mild to severe heart failure, left ventricular dysfunction following myocardial infarction (MI)	Dizziness, headache, fatigue, postural hypotension, depression, cerebrovascular accident (stroke), hypotension, atrioventricular heart block, bradycardia, peripheral vascular disease, thrombocytopenia, hyperkalemia, hypoglycemia
Labetalol	PO, IV	Hypertension, severe hypertension, hypertensive emergency	Dizziness, fatigue, headache, transient scalp tingling, orthostatic hypotension, bradycardia, ventricular dysrhythmia, nausea and vomiting, diarrhea, sexual dysfunction, urinary retention, increased airway resistance

      c. Prazosin and indomethacin: decreased antihypertensive effect

      d. Prazosin and verapamil: increase serum prazosin concentration

      e. Prazosin and beta blockers: increase first dose syncope

      f. May increase digoxin level by 15%

  2. Mixed alpha and beta blockers

      a. Additive effects with other antihypertensive medications

      b. Carvedilol/digoxin: increase digoxin levels

      c. Carvedilol or labetalol/cimetidine: increase carvedilol or labetalol levels

      d. Carvedilol/rifampin: decrease carvedilol level

F. Significant food interactions

  1. Saw palmetto (herb) produces an additive effect for BPH; butcher's broom diminishes effect of terazosin

  2. Delayed absorption of carvedilol with food

G. Significant laboratory studies

  1. Alpha blockers

      a. May cause false positive urine assays for pheochromocytoma

      b. May increase BUN, creatinine, ALT/AST, alkaline phosphatase, triglycerides, uric acid

      c. May increase or decrease glucose levels

  2. Mixed alpha/beta blockers: may cause increased urine free and total catecholamines

H. Side effects

  1. Alpha blockers: first dose syncope, headache, drowsiness, hypotension, palpitations, impotence, nasal congestion, nausea and vomiting, tachycardia

  2. Mixed alpha/beta blockers: fatigue, orthostatic hypotension, dizziness, nausea and vomiting, diarrhea, bronchospasm, muscle spasm, transient scalp tingling, hyperglycemia, upper respiratory infections, impotence, and arthralgias

I. Adverse effects/toxicity

  1. Alpha blockers: leukopenia, neutropenia, thrombocytopenia, myelosuppression, anaphylaxis, bronchospasm, and dysrhythmias

  2. Mixed alpha/beta blockers: ventricular dysrhythmias, AV block, bradycardia, thrombocytopenia, and sudden death

J. Client-centered nursing care

  1. Assess client's past medical history

  2. Monitor vital signs, especially BP and heart rate

  3. Monitor for manifestations of HF such as edema

  4. Monitor peripheral circulation

  5. Monitor diabetic clients for manifestations of hypoglycemia

  6. Abrupt discontinuance of medication may exacerbate angina or precipitate MI

  7. Hypotensive effects may be more pronounced in older adults

  8. Maintain safety when client is changing positions

  9. Monitor for first-dose syncope (alpha and alpha/beta blockers); give first dose at bedtime to minimize risk

K. Client education

  1. Take drug exactly as prescribed

  2. Rationale for therapy

  3. Change position slowly to prevent dizziness and falls

  4. Report any side effects to prescriber

  5. Monitor blood glucose levels and BP more frequently if taking insulin or oral antidiabetic medications

  6. Monitor weight daily and report weight gain over 2.3 kg (5 lb) per week

7. Avoid hazardous activities at beginning of therapy
8. Do not stop medications without notifying prescriber
9. Seek medical approval before taking any OTC medications
10. Therapeutic effect may take 3–4 weeks
11. Avoid alcohol use, excessive exercise, prolonged standing and exposure to heat due to increased risk of orthostatic hypotension

VII. MISCELLANEOUS ANTIHYPERTENSIVES

A. Action and use
1. Stimulate alpha$_2$-receptors in central nervous system (CNS) to inhibit sympathetic cardio-accelerator and vasoconstrictor centers
2. Decrease sympathetic outflow from CNS resulting in decreased arterial BP

B. Common anti-adrenergic medications (Table 6-7)

C. Administration considerations
1. Abrupt discontinuance may result in rebound hypertension
2. Methyldopa: allow 2 days for maximum response before adjusting dose

D. Contraindications
1. Hypersensitivity for both drugs in this group
2. Methyldopa: active hepatitis or cirrhosis
3. Co-administration of methyldopa with monoamine oxidase (MAO)
4. If signs of HF occur, discontinue methyldopa

E. Significant drug interactions
1. Clonidine/beta blockers: paradoxical hypertension
2. Clonidine/tricyclic antidepressants: may block antihypertensive effect
3. Methyldopa may increase effects of levodopa, lithium, haloperidol, MAO inhibitors, and sympathomimetics
4. Methyldopa/propranolol: paradoxical hypertension
5. Additive sedation if administered with CNS depressants

F. Significant food interactions: capsicum and yohimbe may reduce antihypertensive effect

G. Significant laboratory studies
1. Blood glucose levels
2. A positive Coombs test (clonidine)
3. May cause nonprogressive elevation of liver enzymes
4. Methyldopa alters urine uric acid, serum creatinine, AST, and ALT; may cause falsely elevated levels of urine catecholamines, interfering with diagnosis of pheochromocytoma

H. Side effects
1. Sedation, headache, weakness, dizziness, and decreased mental acuity
2. Bradycardia, orthostatic hypotension, aggravation of angina, edema
3. GI disturbance, rash, impotence, dry mouth

Table 6-7 **Common Centrally Acting Anti-Adrenergic Medications**

Generic Name	Route	Uses	Adverse Effects
Clonidine	PO	Essential, renal, and malignant hypertension	Anxiety, confusion, somnolence, nervousness, bradycardia, severe rebound hypertension, impotence, urinary tract infection, nausea and vomiting, urinary retention, transient glucose intolerance, pruritis, dermatitis
Methyldopa	PO	Hypertension	Sedation, depression, headache, dry mouth, peripheral edema, reduced libido, bradycardia, may mask signs of hypoglycemia

I. Adverse effects/toxicity
1. Hepatotoxicity
2. Severe rebound hypertension

J. Client-centered nursing care
1. Administer orally; tablets may be crushed
2. Tablets do not need to be given with food unless GI upset occurs
3. Obtain baseline BP, apical pulse, and monitor weight regularly
4. Assess client for peripheral edema
5. Assess for persistent drowsiness
6. Dry mouth may contribute to development of dental caries, periodontal disease, oral candidiasis, and discomfort
7. Do not discontinue medication abruptly

K. Client education
1. Restrict sodium in diet if prescribed and lose weight as needed; report weight gain of greater than 2.3 kg (5 lb) per week
2. Relieve dry mouth by sipping water or chewing sugarless gum
3. Change position slowly to prevent dizziness and possible falls
4. Report mental acuity changes to prescriber
5. Do not drive a car or perform hazardous activities if drug causes drowsiness
6. Take medication as prescribed
7. Consult prescriber before taking OTC medications
8. Avoid alcohol or other CNS depressants medications
9. Do not stop taking drug abruptly

VIII. PERIPHERAL VASODILATORS

A. Action and use
1. Potent, non-nitrate hypotensive agents that reduce BP by direct effects on vascular smooth muscle of arteries (some vasodilators such as sodium nitroprusside work equally in all vessel beds)
2. Act directly on vascular smooth muscle to produce peripheral vasodilation, resulting in lowered arterial BP, increased heart rate, and increased cardiac output (CO)
3. Most commonly used to treat hypertension and as an adjunct in treating HF
4. Certain vasodilators may be prescribed to treat peripheral vascular disease (PVD) to increase blood flow to extremities, such as in Raynaud disease

B. Common peripheral vasodilator medications (Table 6-8)

C. Administration considerations
1. Take oral forms of medications with food to increase bioavailability
2. IV hydralazine may be given undiluted via direct IV push at a rate of 10 mg/min
3. IV sodium nitroprusside is diluted by dissolving 50 mg in 2–3 mL of D_5W and then diluted in 250 mL D_5W (200 mcg/mL); it should be infused cautiously through an IV pump; when mixed, it appears orange and must be covered in a foil pouch to avoid exposure to light during infusion
4. Do not mix with other IV solutions
5. All vasodilators should be discontinued slowly to avoid paradoxical hypertensive effects
6. Store medication in light-resistant container
7. Monitor HR and BP closely during administration to prevent sudden hypotension
8. Reflex tachycardia may occur as a compensatory response to sudden decrease in BP
9. Salt and water retention may occur as a compensatory increase in aldosterone secretion triggered by drop in BP

Table 6-8	Common Peripheral Vasodilator Medications	
Generic Name	**Route**	**Uses**
Diazoxide	IV	Reduce peripheral vascular resistance and blood pressure by vasodilation
Hydralazine	PO, IV, IM	Vasodilation, which reduces peripheral resistance to improve cardiac output
Minoxidil	PO Topical	Vasodilator with a greater hypotensive effect by blocking calcium uptake through cell membrane Male-pattern baldness
Nitroprusside sodium	IV	Acts on vascular smooth muscle to produce vasodilation
Combination Therapies		
Hydralazine and hydrochlorothiazide	PO	Moderate to severe hypertension
Hydralazine and isosorbide dinitrate	PO	Treatment of HF in African Americans

D. Contraindications

1. When client has a compensatory hypertension, as in an arteriovenous shunt or coarctation of aorta
2. Inadequate cerebral perfusion leading to a decreased cerebral perfusion pressure (CPP)
3. Hypovolemia
4. Clients with systemic lupus erythematosus (SLE) (hydralazine only)
5. Use cautiously with coronary heart disease (CHD); hydralazine can precipitate angina attacks

E. Significant drug interactions

1. All antihypertensive medications, vasodilators (e.g., nitroglycerine), and diuretics may interact to induce profound hypotension
2. Beta blockers and calcium channel blockers will compound hypotensive effects but may be used concurrently to prevent reflex tachycardia
3. No additional medication should be infused through same IV line if given as an infusion
4. NSAIDs may decrease hypotensive effects
5. Hawthorne may increase hypotensive effects

F. Significant food interactions: none reported

G. Significant laboratory studies

1. Various vasodilators have differing laboratory data that is significant; review product literature of individual drugs prior to administration
2. When administering hydralazine hydrochloride:
   a. Positive direct Coombs tests can reveal hydralazine-induced systemic lupus erythematosus (SLE); this condition mimics SLE and is potentially reversible if identified early
   b. Hydralazine interferes with urinary 17-OHCS (modified Glenn-Nelson techniques)
   c. Do baseline and periodic LE cell prep and antinuclear antibody (ANA) titer, BUN, creatinine, uric acid, serum potassium, and blood glucose levels
3. During administration of sodium nitroprusside
   a. Measure baseline and periodic BUN, creatinine, uric acid, serum potassium, and blood glucose levels
   b. Monitor serum thiocyanate levels with prolonged IV infusion and in clients with impaired renal function

    c. Monitor plasma cyanogen levels with prolonged infusion longer than 2 days or with impaired hepatic function

    d. Increased or decreased serum cobalamin levels

H. Side effects

  1. CNS: headache

  2. CV: palpitations and tachycardia

  3. SLE-like syndrome (with hydralazine)

  4. Salt and water retention

I. Adverse effects/toxicity

  1. CNS: dizziness, tremors, apprehension, and muscle twitching

  2. CV: angina, tachycardia or bradycardia, flushing, paradoxical pressor response (sudden unexpected elevation in BP and HR), ECG changes, profound hypotension, shock, reflex tachycardia, and dysrhythmias

  3. GI: anorexia, nausea and vomiting, constipation or diarrhea, abdominal pain, and paralytic ileus

  4. GU: difficulty urinating and glomerulonephritis

  5. Hematologic: decreased hematocrit and hemoglobin, anemia, agranulocytosis (rare)

  6. Skin: rash, irritation at IV site, urticaria, pruritus, fever, chills, arthralgia, eosinophilia, and cholangiitis

  7. SLE-like syndrome, edema

  8. When administering sodium nitroprusside, monitor for signs and symptoms of thiocyanate toxicity: profound hypotension, tinnitus, fatigue, pink skin color, metabolic acidosis, and loss of consciousness

J. Client-centered nursing care

  1. Assess carefully baseline vital signs including HR, cardiac rhythm, ECG, and neurologic status

  2. When administering IV vasodilators:

    a. Establish a large, stable IV site for infusions because they are irritating to tissue; administer using an IV infusion pump

    b. Monitor BP every 5–15 minutes with an automatic external BP machine or with an arterial line during initial infusion and during medication adjustment

    c. Monitor I&O

    d. If adverse response is noted (e.g., hypotension), decrease infusion and monitor client closely; if sudden severe hypotension occurs, discontinue medication; maintain airway, breathing, and circulation (ABCs); establish IV site; contact prescriber, and initiate emergency protocols as necessary

  3. Obtain baseline vital signs and check BP, heart rate, and cardiac rhythm before each dose when administering orally

K. Client education

  1. Monitor pulse and BP

  2. Headaches and palpitations are possible within 2–4 hours after first oral dose

  3. Follow-up care is important

  4. Write down questions to ask prescriber on each follow-up visit

  5. Avoid all OTC medications and herbal supplements unless approved by prescriber

  6. Stop smoking and avoid alcohol intake, which may negate positive drug effects

  7. Monitor weight daily and report edema; keep a journal of pulse, weight, and blood pressure

  8. Change position slowly and avoid hot tubs and hot baths that might induce profound vasodilation and hypotension

IX. CARDIAC GLYCOSIDES

A. Action and use

1. Until discovery of ACE inhibitors, cardiac glycosides were mainstay of heart failure treatment; used primarily in treatment of HF, although survival rates are not extended

2. Used for treatment of atrial **dysrhythmias** (abnormalities in electrical activity of heart), such as atrial fibrillation

3. Increase contractility and efficiency of myocardial contraction

4. Produce a positive inotropic action, which increases force of myocardial contraction

5. Decrease conduction velocity through AV node, which reduces heart rate and allows for greater efficiency of heart

B. Common cardiac glycoside medication: digoxin

C. Administration considerations

1. May be given with or without food

2. Tablet may be crushed and mixed with fluid or food as desired; pediatric elixir is also available

3. IV administration: IVP digoxin may be administered undiluted or diluted in 4 mL of sterile water, 5% dextrose, or NS; administer each direct IV dose over 5 minutes; client may receive a loading dose (digitalization) to achieve adequate serum drug levels

4. Never administer digoxin intramuscularly (IM) because it would cause tissue irritation and great variation in bioavailability

5. Infiltration into subcutaneous tissue can cause local irritation and tissue sloughing

D. Contraindications

1. Avoid use in clients with known hypersensitivity to drug

2. Full digitalizing dose should not be given if client has received digoxin in previous week

3. Presence of digoxin toxicity

4. Use cautiously with:
   a. Renal insufficiency
   b. Hypokalemia
   c. Advanced heart disease, acute MI, heart block, and cor pulmonale
   d. Hypothyroidism
   e. Lung disease
   f. Pregnant or nursing mothers
   g. Children or premature infants
   h. Older adults

E. Significant drug interactions

1. Antacids, cholestyramine, and colestipol decrease digoxin absorption

2. Diuretics, corticosteroids, amphotericin B, laxatives, and sodium polystyrene sulfonate may cause hypokalemia, which increases risk of toxicity

3. IV calcium when given with digoxin may increase risk of cardiac dysrhythmias

4. Quinidine, verapamil, alprazolam, and amiodarone significantly increase digoxin levels, and digoxin dose should be decreased by 50%

5. Erythromycin and nefazodone may increase digoxin levels

6. Succinylcholine may potentiate dysrhythmias

7. Dobutamine or doxapram should not be injected in same IV line or mixed in solution with digoxin

8. Ginseng may increase risk of toxicity; ma huang and ephedra may induce dysrhythmia

Practice to Pass

A client is receiving digoxin 0.125 mg PO every morning. Upon arrival to the office, you notice that the HR is 44 bpm. The client reports feeling weak and nauseated. Based on the clinical data, what might cause the low heart rate? What are the priority nursing assessments?

9. Concurrent use with beta blockers may result in bradycardia
10. Digoxin overdose can be treated with IV infusion of digoxin immune Fab

F. **Significant food interactions:** none reported

G. **Significant laboratory studies**

1. Before initiating cardiac glycoside therapy, baseline labs should be drawn, including potassium, magnesium, and calcium
2. Draw serum digoxin level periodically during therapy and if client develops symptoms of toxicity; draw sample at least 6 hours after daily dose and preferably just before next scheduled daily dose
3. Therapeutic range of serum digoxin is 0.8–2 ng/mL, and toxic levels are greater than 2 ng/mL
4. Closely monitor potassium levels; hypokalemia potentiates digoxin toxicity

H. **Side effects**

1. Nausea
2. Loss of "usual appetite"
3. Headache or blurred yellow vision

I. **Adverse reactions/toxicity**

1. CNS: fatigue, muscle weakness, headache, facial neuralgia, depression, paresthesias, hallucinations, confusion, drowsiness, agitation, dizziness, and malaise
2. CV: dysrhythmias, hypotension, AV heart block, and diaphoresis
3. GI: anorexia, nausea and vomiting, diarrhea, and dysphagia
4. Visual disturbances (blurred vision, green or yellow vision, or halo effect)
5. Digoxin toxicity may be unrecognized, since it may have same manifestations as a "flu"; these include anorexia, nausea and vomiting, diarrhea, or visual disturbances

J. **Client-centered nursing care**

1. Obtain baseline data and perform ongoing physical assessments, including neurologic status, HR, BP, and cardiac rhythm
2. Check baseline serum digoxin level prior to initiating digoxin therapy:
   a. Blood level is 0 if no digoxin has been taken before
   b. Therapeutic levels are 0.8–2 ng/mL
   c. Toxic levels are greater than 2 ng/mL
3. Assess baseline and ongoing laboratory values, including serum electrolytes, creatinine clearance, magnesium, and calcium
4. Monitor closely for digoxin toxicity in older adults taking digoxin and a diuretic for HF or atrial fibrillation
5. Take apical pulse for 1 full minute prior to administering digoxin, noting rate, rhythm, and quality; if any changes are noted, withhold dose and notify prescriber; an ECG will likely be prescribed
6. Withhold medication if client has symptoms of digoxin toxicity (anorexia, nausea and vomiting, diarrhea, or visual disturbances)
7. In children, early signs of toxicity include cardiac dysrhythmias; children rarely demonstrate anorexia, nausea and vomiting, diarrhea, or visual disturbances such as seeing halos, a yellow-green tinge, or blurring
8. Advise client to eat foods high in potassium such as oranges, bananas, fruit juices, vegetables, and potatoes if taking loop diuretics
9. Monitor I&O and daily weight, especially in clients with impaired renal function; auscultate breath sounds for crackles; assess extremities for edema because it indicates fluid volume overload
10. Antidote: digoxin immune Fab is used in extreme toxicity
11. Concurrent antibiotic and digoxin therapy can precipitate toxicity because of alterations in intestinal flora

12. Monitor client closely when being switched from one administration route to another; often a dose adjustment is required (if tablet form is replaced by elixir, potential for toxicity increases)

K. Client education

1. Check pulse for 1 full minute prior to taking digoxin; advise to contact prescriber before taking dose if pulse is below 60 bpm or above 110 or if skipped beats are present
2. Suspect toxicity if any of following occur: nausea and vomiting, anorexia, diarrhea, or visual disturbances (halos, yellow-green tinge, or blurriness)
3. Withhold next dose if digoxin toxicity is suspected and contact prescriber immediately
4. Weigh self daily with same clothes and at same time; report weight gain greater than 0.9 kg (2 lb)/day
5. Take digoxin as prescribed; do not skip or add additional dose if experiencing chest discomfort (a common report from clients admitted with digoxin toxicity is that they take digoxin as a "heart pill" when experiencing chest pain)
6. Do not take OTC medications or herbal supplements without consulting prescriber because they might have direct adverse effects on absorption of digoxin
7. Insist on original brand of digoxin prescribed to avoid errors in dosing; bioavailability may differ between brands

X. PHOSPHODIESTERASE III INHIBITORS

A. Action and use

1. Block enzyme phosphodiesterase III in cardiac and smooth muscle, leading to increased amounts of calcium available for cardiac contraction; a positive inotropic action and vasodilation occur and cardiac output is increased; cardiac output is improved because of increased contractility and decreased left ventricular afterload
2. Used to treat acute HF resistant to treatment with ACE inhibitors, digoxin and other therapies, and short-term therapy of serious and decompensated HF; phosphodiesterase inhibitors have serious toxicity that limits their use to clients with resistant HF who have not responded to ACE inhibitors, digoxin, or other therapies

B. Common phosphodiesterase III inhibitor medications (Table 6-9)

C. Administration considerations

1. Continuous monitoring for ventricular dysrhythmias is necessary
2. Therapy is limited to 2–3 days
3. Peak effects can occur within 2–3 minutes of IV administration
4. Overdose of milrinone may cause hypotension, which can be treated with normal saline or a vasopressor
5. Hypovolemia or electrolyte imbalances should be corrected before initiating infusion
6. Dosage should be reduced in client with renal impairment
7. Use requires caution

D. Contraindications

1. Severe valvular heart disease (milrinone)
2. Use with caution with preexisting dysrhythmias
3. Known drug allergy

Table 6-9 Phosphodiesterase III Inhibitors

Generic Name	Route	Uses
Inamrinone	IV	Short-term treatment of acute decompensated heart failure (HF)
Milrinone	IV	

E. Significant drug interactions

1. Additive effects may be seen when given with digoxin, dobutamine, or other inotropic drugs
2. Concurrent use of diuretics can cause significant hypotension
3. Concurrent administration with furosemide will form a precipitate

F. Significant food interactions: ginger may contribute to cardiac actions of milrinone

G. Significant laboratory studies: complete blood count (CBC), electrolytes, renal function tests

H. Side effects

1. Hypotension, angina
2. Headache, nausea and vomiting
3. Hypokalemia, tremor

I. Adverse reactions/toxicity

1. Severe hypotension
2. Ventricular dysrhythmias

J. Client-centered nursing care

1. Assess client before, during, and after initial dose
   a. Monitor BP and HR frequently during initial administration
   b. Cardiac monitoring is necessary throughout treatment
2. Slow or stop infusion if severe hypotension develops
3. Check for hypokalemia and notify provider if present

K. Client education: instruct client to immediately report chest pain should it occur during infusion

XI. ATRIAL NATRIURETIC PEPTIDE HORMONE

A. Action and use

1. A small peptide hormone produced through recombinant DNA technology
2. Structurally identical to endogenous beta-type natriuretic peptide (hBNP); when heart failure occurs, ventricles begin to secrete hBNP in response to increased stretch on ventricular walls; hBNP enhances diuresis and renal excretion of sodium
3. Promotes diuresis by inhibiting ADH and vasodilation and reducing preload
4. Should be reserved for treatment of acutely decompensated HF in clients who have dyspnea at rest

B. Common atrial natriuretic peptide hormone medication: nesiritide is the first drug in this newer class

C. Administration considerations: administer by IV bolus followed by IV infusion for up to 48 hours

D. Contraindications

1. Allergy to nesiritide
2. Hypotension with systolic BP lower than 90 mmHg
3. Clients with low cardiac filling pressures

E. Significant drug interactions: possible additive hypotension if used concurrently with antihypertensives such as angiotensin-converting enzyme (ACE) inhibitors

F. Significant food interactions: none reported

G. Significant laboratory studies: baseline and periodic serum creatinine

H. Side effects

1. Lightheadedness or dizziness
2. Confusion or weakness
3. Headache, back pain, injection site pain
4. Insomnia and anxiety
5. Abdominal pain, nausea and vomiting, fever

I. Adverse reactions/toxicity

1. Hypotension
2. Chest pain
3. Dysrhythmias

! J. **Client-centered nursing care**
1. Monitor IV infusion frequently
2. Monitor BP and other hemodynamic parameters closely and be aware that if hypotension occurs, it may persist for several hours after drug is discontinued
3. Monitor cardiac rhythm during administration
4. Observe for intended drug effects of improvement in heart failure and increased diuresis

K. **Client education:** drug is for short-term IV use (up to 48 hours) and client will be monitored closely throughout therapy

XII. ANTIDYSRHYTHMICS

A. **Class I-A (fast sodium channel blockers)**
1. Action and use
   a. Used to treat both atrial and ventricular dysrhythmias; prevent recurrence of premature ventricular contractions (PVCs) and ventricular tachycardia that are not severe enough to require cardioversion
   b. The sodium channel blockers are similar in structure and action to local anesthetics, this anesthetic-like action slows impulse conduction across heart; sodium channel blockers depress myocardial contractility and excitability and prolong **refractory period** (ability to respond only to a strong stimulus)
   c. Reduce rate of spontaneous diastolic depolarization in pacemaker cells, thereby suppressing ectopic focal activity
   d. Disopyramide shortens sinus node recovery time and increases atrial and ventricular effective refractory period
   e. Quinidine is classified as a chemical cardioversion agent useful to convert atrial fibrillation to normal sinus rhythm
2. Common antidysrhythmic medications (Table 6-10)
3. Administration considerations
   a. Give first dose of disopyramide 6–12 hours after last quinidine dose and 3–6 hours after last procainamide dose
   b. Do not administer controlled-release capsules when giving a loading dose, when rapid control is required, or when creatinine clearance is less than 40 mL/min
   ! c. Do not crush or open controlled-release capsules as it may deliver a potentially toxic dose of medication
   ! d. Start controlled-release form of capsule 6 hours after last dose of conventional capsule when switching from a conventional capsule to a controlled-release form
4. Contraindications
   a. Cardiogenic shock
   b. Second- or third-degree heart block

Table 6-10	Common Antidysrhythmic Medications: Class I-A: Fast Sodium Channel Blockers		
Generic Name	**Route**	**Uses**	
Disopyramide	PO	Life-threatening ventricular dysrhythmias, paroxysmal supraventricular tachycardia (PSVT), decreases rate of diastolic repolarization, increases action potential, and prolongs refractory period	
Procainamide hydrochloride	PO, IV	Life-threatening ventricular dysrhythmias, conversion of atrial fibrillation or flutter to normal sinus rhythm	
Quinidine gluconate; Quinidine sulfate	PO, IV	Atrial dysrhythmias, chronic atrial tachycardia, life-threatening *Plasmodium falciparum* infections when IV therapy with quinidine gluconate is indicated	

    c. Severe heart failure

    d. Hypotension

    e. Blood dyscrasias

    f. Caution should be used when administering disopyramide in presence of:

        1) Sick sinus syndrome

        2) WPW syndrome

        3) Bundle branch block

        4) Myocarditis or other cardiomyopathy

        5) Hepatic or renal impairment

        6) Urinary tract disease (especially prostatic hyperplasia)

        7) Myasthenia gravis

        8) Angle-closure (narrow-angle) glaucoma

5. Significant drug interactions

    a. Do not inject quinidine with anticholinergic drugs such as tricyclic antidepressants and antihistamines

    b. Antidysrhythmics compound toxicities

    c. Phenytoin and rifampin may increase metabolism of disopyramide and decrease blood level

    d. Disopyramide may increase warfarin-induced hypoprothrombinemia

    e. Increased cardiac depressant effects may occur when combined with other antidysrhythmics

    f. Increased anticholinergic side effects may occur if procainaminde is used concurrently with anticholinergic drugs

6. Significant food interactions: drug metabolism is decreased and risk of toxic sodium channel blocker effect is increased with grapefruit juice

7. Significant laboratory studies

    a. Determine baseline hepatic and renal function and monitor periodically during therapy

    b. Assess blood glucose levels and serum potassium levels because hyperkalemia worsens toxic effects; hypokalemia and other electrolyte imbalances should be corrected before therapy is initiated

    c. Monitor ECG closely; notify prescriber immediately if these changes occur:

        1) Prolonged QT interval

        2) Worsening of dysrhythmias

        3) Widening of QRS, greater than 25%

        4) HR less than 60 bpm or greater than 120 bpm

        5) Unusual change in rate, rhythm, or quality of pulse

    d. Serum quinidine levels are inaccurate in clients taking triamterene

8. Side effects

    a. Mild hypotension

    b. Blurred vision

    c. Dry mouth

    d. Urinary hesitancy or retention

    e. Constipation

    f. Abdominal cramping, nausea and vomiting

9. Adverse effects/toxicity

    a. CNS: dizziness, headache, fatigue, muscle weakness, seizures, paresthesias, nervousness, acute psychosis, and peripheral neuropathy

    b. CV: severe hypotension, chest pain, edema, dyspnea, syncope, bradycardia, tachycardia, increased dysrhythmias, HF, cardiogenic shock, and heart block

    c. GI: epigastric and abdominal pain, jaundice

    d. GU: profound urinary retention, frequency, urgency, and renal insufficiency

       e. Skin: pruritis, urticaria, rash, photosensitivity, and laryngospasm

       f. Drying of nose, throat, and bronchial secretions

       g. Uterine contraction during pregnancy, precipitation of myasthenia gravis, agranulocytosis (decreased granulocytes), and thrombocytopenia

   10. Client-centered nursing care

       a. Check apical pulse before administering dose

       b. Monitor ECG and report any changes to prescriber immediately

       c. Monitor BP, especially during dosage adjustment and if receiving high doses of medication

       d. Monitor I&O, especially in older adults and clients with impaired renal function, prostatic hyperplasia, and urinary retention/hesitancy

       e. Monitor labs results as appropriate

       f. Assess for peripheral neuritis

       g. In event of overdose, reverse hypotension with vasopressors

   11. Client education

       a. Measure daily weight and report weight gain greater than 0.9–1.8 kg (2–4 lb)/week

       b. Inspect ankles and tibia daily for edema

       c. Change position slowly to avoid dizziness and syncope; avoid prolonged periods of standing and lie down if feeling lightheaded; avoid driving or other hazardous activities if dizzy or lightheaded

       d. Take medication as prescribed and do not skip doses

       e. Do not stop taking medication abruptly

       f. Do not take OTC medications or drink alcohol without contacting prescriber

       g. Avoid exposure to sunlight or ultraviolet radiation

       h. Notify all other healthcare providers of medication and have regular eye exams for glaucoma

       i. Clients taking procainamide should watch for lupus-like symptoms

 B. Class I-B

   1. Action and use

       a. Decreases refractory period

       b. Suppresses automaticity in Bundle of His–Purkinje system

       c. Elevates electrical stimulation threshold of ventricle during diastole

       d. Treats or prevents ventricular dysrhythmias

   2. Common Class I-B antidysrhythmic medications (Table 6-11)

   3. Administration considerations

       a. Bolus dose of lidocaine may be given undiluted via IVP at a rate of 25–50 mg/min

       b. Add 1 gram lidocaine to 250–500 mL of D_5W for infusion; flow rate should not be more than 4 mg/mL

       c. Use microdropper and infusion pump for an infusion

Table 6-11	Common Antidysrhythmic Medications: Class I-B	
Generic Name	**Route**	**Uses**
Lidocaine	IV	Suppresses Bundle of His–Purkinje system, elevating ventricular electrical stimulation threshold during diastole, rapid control of ventricular dysrhythmias during acute MI or cardiac catheterization
Mexiletine	PO	Modest suppression of SA and AV node, acute and chronic ventricular dysrhythmias, severe tachydysrhythmias
Phenytoin	IV	Dysrhythmias (including digitalis-induced)
Tocainide	PO	Refractory ventricular dysrhythmias, prevention of ventricular tachyarrhythmia, shortens effective refractory period of atria, AV node, and ventricles without affecting AV conduction

      d. Discontinue IV infusion as soon as client's basic cardiac rhythm stabilizes

      e. Hypokalemia should be corrected prior to initiating tocainide

      f. Administer phenytoin undiluted clear without precipitate

4. Contraindications

      a. History of hypersensitivity to amide-type anesthetics

      b. Stokes-Adams syndrome

      c. Untreated sinus bradycardia

      d. Severe degrees of SA, AV, and intraventricular heart block

      e. Use cautiously with:

         1) Hepatic or renal disease

         2) HF

         3) Hypovolemia or shock

         4) Myasthenia gravis

         5) Debilitated clients or older adults

         6) Family history of malignant hyperthermia

5. Significant drug interactions

      a. Barbiturates decrease lidocaine activity

      b. Beta blockers, quinidine, phenytoin, and procainamide increase effect of lidocaine

      c. Phenytoin and cefazolin are incompatible with lidocaine infusion

      d. Decreased absorption of phenytoin and increased metabolism with concurrent oral anticoagulant use

      e. Phenytoin is incompatible with nisoldipine, amiodarone, chloramphenicol, omeprazole, and ticlopidine

6. Significant food interactions: none reported

7. Significant laboratory studies

      a. Lidocaine levels should be assessed

         1) Therapeutic level is 1.5–6 mcg/mL

         2) Potentially toxic level is greater than 7 mcg/mL

      b. Assess electrolytes and correct hypokalemia before treating with antidysrhythmics

      c. Check baseline hepatic and renal blood studies

8. Side effects

      a. Drowsiness

      b. Lightheadedness

      c. Mild hypotension

9. Adverse effects/toxicity

      a. CNS: restlessness, confusion, disorientation, irritability, apprehension, euphoria, wild excitement, numbness of lips or tongue and other paresthesias, chest heaviness, and difficulty speaking

      b. Dyspnea and difficulty swallowing, muscular twitching, tremors, psychosis, seizures, and respiratory depression with high doses

      c. CV: hypotension, bradycardia, heart block, cardiovascular collapse, and cardiac arrest

      d. Ear: tinnitus and decreased hearing

      e. Eye: severe blurred vision, double vision, and impaired color perception

      f. GI: anorexia, nausea and vomiting, and excessive perspiration

      g. Skin: urticaria, rash, edema, and anaphylactoid reactions

10. Client-centered nursing care

      a. Assess ECG for changes including prolonged PR interval, widened QRS, aggravation of dysrhythmias, and heart block

      b. Monitor BP frequently

      c. Assess CNS status at baseline and frequently during infusion

          d. Administer via infusion pump and observe rate carefully

          e. Administer oral drug with food to decrease GI upset

          f. Auscultate breath sounds for crackles and monitor respiratory rate

          g. Assess serum blood levels

   11. Client education

          a. Notify prescriber if lightheadedness, dizziness, confusion, or numbness or tingling of lips, tongue, or fingers occurs; notify for visual changes or ringing in ears

          b. Notify prescriber if unusual CNS changes occur, or nausea and vomiting, or yellowish changes in whites of eyes or skin (jaundice) when taking oral forms of medication

          c. Do not take any OTC medications or herbal supplements without consulting prescriber

          d. Take medications as prescribed without skipping doses

C. Class I-C

   1. Action and use

          a. Decrease automaticity and conductivity through AV node and ventricles

          b. Used to treat life-threatening ventricular dysrhythmias

   2. Common Class I-C antidysrhythmic medications (Table 6-12)

   3. Administration considerations

          a. Medications are available in oral forms

          b. Increasing dosages are not recommended more frequently than every 4 days, especially with older adults or clients with previous extensive myocardial damage

          c. Dosage reduction should be considered in severe liver dysfunction and with significant widening of QRS complex

   4. Contraindications

          a. Hypersensitivity to flecainide

          b. Severe degrees of heart block

          c. Intraventricular blocks

          d. Cardiogenic shock

          e. Hepatic failure

   5. Significant drug interactions

          a. Cimetidine may increase flecainide levels

          b. Flecainide may increase digoxin levels by 25%

          c. Beta blockers enhance negative inotropic effects

   6. Significant food interactions: none reported

   7. Significant laboratory studies

          a. Assess baseline electrolytes

          b. Monitor serum levels

             1) Effective trough level is 0.7 to 1 mcg/mL

             2) Toxic trough level is greater than 1 mcg/mL

          c. Monitor blood levels frequently if client is taking digoxin or has severe HF or renal failure

   8. Side effects

          a. Slight dizziness

          b. Blurred vision

          c. Nausea

Table 6-12   **Common Antidysrhythmic Medications: Class I-C**

Generic Name	Route	Uses
Flecainide	PO	Life-threatening ventricular dysrhythmias
Propafenone	PO	Ventricular tachycardia

9. Adverse effects/toxicity
   a. CNS: headache, prolonged lightheadedness, unsteadiness, paresthesias, fatigue, and fever
   b. CV: worsening dysrhythmias, chest pain, HF, edema, and dyspnea
   c. Eye: prolonged blurred vision and spots before eyes
   d. GI: prolonged nausea, constipation, and changes in taste perception
10. Client-centered nursing care
   a. Assess laboratory data and treat hypokalemia/hyperkalemia before initiating therapy
   b. Monitor ECG rhythm for changes, including worsening of dysrhythmias; client may need Holter monitoring for ambulatory assessment
   c. Determine threshold levels of pacemaker before initiating medication and at regular intervals thereafter
11. Client education
   a. Take medications as prescribed without skipping doses
   b. Report any visual changes
   c. Do not take any OTC medications or herbal supplements without consulting healthcare provider
   d. Follow-up care is important

D. **Class II (beta blockers):** see previous section II
E. **Class III (potassium channel blockers)**
   1. Action and use
      a. After action potential has passed and myocardial cell is in a depolarized state (potassium outside of cell, sodium and calcium inside cell), repolarization depends on restoring potassium ions inside cell; by blocking potassium channels, class III antidysrhythmics delay repolarization and decrease automaticity
      b. Prolongs refractory period and decreases automaticity
      c. Used to treat ventricular tachycardia and ventricular fibrillation
      d. May also be used to treat supraventricular tachycardias
   2. Common Class III antidysrhythmic medications: see Table 6-13
   3. Administration considerations
      a. Gastroenteritis symptoms may occur with high oral dose therapy and loading dose
      b. Use infusion pump when administering IV dose; central line should be used if rate exceeds 2 mg/mL
      c. Dofetilide does not have as negative an inotropic effect as amiodarone, but has significant dose-related prodysrhythmic effects including heart block, ventricular tachycardia, and *torsades de pointes*
      d. Continuously monitor ECG when infusing ibutilide and dofetilide and for at least 4 hours following infusion
      e. Correct hypokalemia and hypomagnesemia prior to initiating therapy with ibutilide and dofetilide to reduce risk for dysrhythmias
   4. Contraindications
      a. Hypersensitivity to amiodarone
      b. Cardiogenic shock

Table 6-13 **Common Antidysrhythmic Medications: Class III—Potassium Channel Blockers**

Generic Name	Route	Uses
Amiodarone	PO, IV	Atrial dysrhythmias in HF, ventricular tachycardia, atrial fibrillation, ventricular fibrillation
Dofetilide	PO	Rapid conversion of atrial flutter or fibrillation to normal sinus rhythm
Ibutilide	IV	Rapid conversion of atrial flutter or fibrillation to normal sinus rhythm

       c. Severe sinus bradycardia or severe degrees of heart block

       d. Hepatic disease

       e. Use cautiously in Hashimoto thyroiditis, goiter, hyperthyroidism or hypothyroidism, HF, electrolyte imbalance, preexisting pulmonary disease, cardiac surgery, and sensitivity to iodine

5. Significant drug interactions

       a. Increases digoxin levels

       b. Enhances effects and toxicities of disopyramide, procainamide, quinidine, flecainide, lidocaine, cyclosporine

       c. Enhances anticoagulant effects

       d. Bradycardia effects are greater when used with verapamil, diltiazem, and beta-adrenergic blockers

       e. Increases phenytoin blood levels two- to threefold

       f. Cimetidine and ritonavir may increase amiodarone levels and toxicity

       g. Cholestyramine may decrease amiodarone levels

       h. Other Class Ia and Class III antidysrhythmic drugs can increase risk for prolonged QT interval and life-threatening dysrhythmias

6. Significant food interactions: use with echinacea increases risk of hepatoxicity; aloe may cause an increased effect of amiodarone

7. Significant laboratory studies

       a. Thyroid function test abnormalities (in absence of thyroid function impairments)

       b. Baseline and periodic serum assessments of:

           1) Liver enzymes: aspartate aminotransferase (AST) and alanine aminotransferase (ALT)

           2) Lung: pulmonary function tests, ABGs

           3) Thyroid hormone levels

           4) Creatinine and electrolyte levels with dofetilide

8. Side effects

       a. Skin and corneal pigmentation (lipofuscinosis) in client receiving drug longer than 2 months; reversible in 7 months after discontinuing drug (amiodarone)

       b. Muscle weakness

       c. Hypotension, dizziness

       d. Mild anorexia, nausea, and constipation

9. Adverse reactions/toxicity

       a. CNS: peripheral neuropathy, muscle wasting, weakness, fatigue, abnormal gait, dyskinesia, dizziness, paresthesias, and headache

       b. CV: bradycardia, severe hypotension, sinus arrest, cardiogenic shock, CHF, worsening dysrhythmias, and heart block

       c. Eye: corneal microdeposits, blurred vision, optic neuritis, optic neuropathy, permanent blindness, corneal degeneration, macular degeneration, and photosensitivity

       d. Respiratory: alveolitis, pneumonitis, interstitial pulmonary fibrosis, pulmonary toxicity, pneumonia-like syndrome

       e. Skin: slate-blue pigmentation to skin and rash

       f. GI: severe anorexia, nausea and vomiting, and constipation

       g. Angioedema, hyperthyroidism or hypothyroidism, and hepatotoxicity

       h. *Torsades de pointes*, supraventricular dysrhythmias (ibutilide and dofetilide)

10. Client-centered nursing care

       a. Monitor BP during IV infusion and titrate to prevent hypotension and bradycardia

       b. Monitor client continually due to unusually long half-life of drug (10–55 days)

      c. Check laboratory and other reports for liver, lung, thyroid, GI, and neurologic dysfunction

      d. Baseline and regular ophthalmic examinations with a slit-lamp are recommended throughout therapy

      e. Report adverse reactions promptly

      f. Be alert to signs of pulmonary toxicity: dyspnea, fatigue, cough, pleuritic pain, or fever; auscultate breath sounds for adventitious sounds

      g. Monitor client for CNS changes, which generally develop within a week after amiodarone therapy begins; muscle weakness and tremors are a potential safety risk

      h. Observe client already receiving other antidysrhythmic therapy for adverse effects, especially heart block and worsening dysrhythmias

11. Client education

      a. Assess pulse daily and report HR less than 60 bpm

      b. Notify all healthcare providers of medication

      c. Have regular ophthalmic examinations

      d. Photophobia may be eased by wearing darkened glasses but some clients should avoid daylight entirely

      e. Erythema and pruritus may develop when exposed to ultraviolet radiation; avoid sunlight, tanning beds, and sunlamps

      f. Wear protective clothing and a barrier-type sunblock to avoid sun exposure (zinc-oxide or titanium-oxide preparations)

      g. Blue-gray skin pigmentation may slowly disappear after medication is stopped; may take months to resolve (amiodarone)

      h. Take medication as prescribed without skipping doses

      i. Avoid taking OTC medications or herbal supplements without consulting prescriber

      j. Follow-up care is important

      k. Instruct client to report any chest pain, cough, or shortness of breath to provider

F. Class IV (calcium channel blockers): see previous section III

G. Other antidysrhythmics (miscellaneous)

    1. Action and use

      a. Slow conduction through SA and AV nodes

      b. Interrupt reentry pathways through AV node

      c. Depress left-ventricular function (very temporary)

      d. Treat supraventricular dysrhythmias

    2. Common medication: adenosine

    3. Administration considerations

      a. Give by rapid IV bolus (over 1–2 seconds) followed by rapid normal saline flush; administer directly into vein as proximal to insertion site as possible; half-life is only 10 seconds

      b. Solution contains no preservatives so it must be clear; discard any unused portion

      c. Expect sudden slowing of HR or even asystole for a brief period of time; do not repeat dose if a high grade of AV heart block develops after first dose; have resuscitative equipment and ECG machine at bedside prior to administration

      d. Must be stored at room temperature to avoid crystallization; if crystals appear, dissolve by warming to room temperature

    4. Contraindications

      a. Severe degrees of heart block

      b. Sick sinus syndrome (without a pacemaker)

      c. Atrial fibrillation or atrial flutter

          d. Ventricular tachycardia

          e. Use cautiously with asthma, pregnancy, hepatic failure, and renal failure

     5. Significant drug interactions

          a. Dipyridamole can potentiate effects of adenosine

          b. Theophylline will block electrophysiological effects of adenosine

          c. Carbamazepine may increase risk of heart block

     6. Significant food interactions: none reported

     7. Significant laboratory studies: none reported

     8. Side effects

          a. During conversion to sinus rhythm (SR) many dysrhythmias can occur

            1) Sinus bradycardia or arrest

            2) Sinus tachycardia

            3) PVCs

            4) Premature atrial contractions (PACs)

            5) Various degrees of heart block

          b. Facial flushing

     9. Adverse effects/toxicity: transient dyspnea, dysrhythmias, hypotension

    10. Client-centered nursing care

          a. Monitor ECG continuously

          b. Evaluate baseline BP, HR, and respirations

          c. Must be administered very quickly over 1–2 seconds and followed by a rapid NS flush; if given too slowly, it will have no effect

          d. Monitor HR and BP every 15 minutes after administration until stable

          e. Monitor carefully for bronchospasm, especially in clients with asthma

    11. Client education

          a. Various forms of monitoring are needed during medication administration

          b. Transient facial flushing may occur

XIII. ANTIHYPOTENSIVES (SYMPATHOMIMETICS)

   A. Action and use

     1. Mimic fight-or-flight response of sympathetic nervous system, selectively stimulating alpha-adrenergic and beta-adrenergic receptors

     2. Stimulation of alpha-adrenergic receptors results in vasoconstriction and increased systemic BP

     3. Stimulation of beta-adrenergic receptors increases force and rate of myocardial contraction

     4. Used to treat **shock**

   B. Common sympathomimetic medications (Table 6-14)

   C. Administration considerations

     1. Drug must be diluted before administration

     2. Client should be attended constantly during drug administration

   D. Contraindications

     1. Uncorrected dysrhythmias, mesenteric or peripheral vascular thrombosis

     2. Profound hypoxia, hypercapnia, hypotension due to blood volume deficit

     3. Use with caution in clients receiving MAO inhibitors or imipramine-type antidepressants

   E. Significant drug interactions

     1. Norepinephrine interacts with general anesthesia, tricyclic antidepressants, and MAO inhibitors

     2. Beta blockers may increase potential for hypertension

     3. Diuretics decrease arterial response

Table 6-14	Common Sympathomimetic Medications		
Generic Name	**Route**	**Uses**	**Adverse Effects**
Norepinephrine	IV	Acute hypotensive state	Headache, bradycardia, hypertension, tissue sloughing with extravasation
Metaraminol	IV	Hypotension	Restlessness, bradycardia, tissue sloughing with extravasation
Dopamine	IV	Hypotension, shock	Dysrhythmias, widening QRS complex, hypotension, bradycardia, asthma attack, tissue sloughing with extravasation, anaphylaxis
Dobutamine	IV	Cardiac decompensation	Headache, increased heart rate, premature ventricular contractions, leg cramps, nonspecified chest pain, nausea and vomiting, anaphylaxis, sloughing with extravasation
Isoproterenol	IV, IM, subcutaneous	Bronchospasm, heart block, ventricular dysrhythmia, shock, bradycardia, mitral regurgitation	Headache, tremors, Stokes-Adams syndrome, cardiac arrest, bronchospasm, diaphoresis, tachycardia, palpitations, rapid rise and fall of BP

    4. Atropine and tricyclic antidepressants enhance pressor effects

    5. Metaraminol/MAO inhibitors: increase vasopressor effects

F. Significant food interactions: rue (herb) increases inotropic potential

G. Significant laboratory studies

    1. Monitor serum electrolytes

    2. Monitor blood glucose levels

    3. Isoproterenol decreases sensitivity of spirometry in diagnosis of asthma

H. Side effects

    1. Anxiety, weakness, dizziness, tremor, restlessness

    2. Bradycardia, tachycardia, palpitations

    3. Nausea and vomiting, flushing, diaphoresis, sloughing upon extravasation

    4. Azotemia, shortness of breath, and bronchospasm

I. Adverse effects/toxicity

    1. Severe hypertension, anaphylaxis

    2. Dysrhythmias, cardiac arrest, ventricular tachycardia

    3. Stokes-Adams seizures, asthmatic episodes

J. Client-centered nursing care

    1. Reevaluate if 3–5 treatments in 6–12 hours provide minimal to no relief

    2. Carefully monitor vital signs, ECG, and I&O

    3. Monitor for rebound hypertension

    4. Constant infusion pump prevents sudden infusion of excessive amounts of drugs

    5. Correct blood volume depletion first

    6. Antidote for extravasation: 5–10 mg phentolamine mesylate (Regitine) in 10–15 mL of normal saline

    7. Monitor infusion site frequently

    8. Client should be attended constantly during administration

    9. Protect solution from light

    10. Sympathomimetics are incompatible with sodium bicarbonate

K. Client education

    1. Instruct client to report adverse reactions and side effects immediately

    2. Inform client that vital signs will be monitored frequently

    3. Instruct client to report anginal pain while on dobutamine

Case Study

A 56-year-old male client is admitted to the intensive care unit with a diagnosis of acute myocardial infarction. He has a T wave inversion and elevation of the ST segment. The EKG indicates myocardial ischemia and necrosis. He is started on amiodarone hydrochloride by IV infusion. He is also given aspirin 325 mg PO, heparin subcutaneous 5,000 units bid, and atenolol 50 mg PO daily. It should be noted the client received morphine 10 mg IV to relieve chest pain in the emergency room.

1. What assessments should be made prior to administration of these medications?

2. What is the action of each of the medications listed and what is the rationale for their administration?

3. What nursing implications should be implemented with each of the medications?

4. What information about the medications should be explained to the client?

5. What adverse effects of the medications should the nurse be alert and assess for?

For suggested responses, see page 540.

POSTTEST

1 The nurse would monitor a client beginning drug therapy with sotalol for which life-threatening manifestations of an adverse drug reaction?

1. Increase in systolic blood pressure and fatigue
2. Report of blurry vision and the appearance of halos
3. Bluish discoloration of the skin
4. Bradycardia and dyspnea

2 A client with a history of mild congestive heart failure (CHF) is receiving diltiazem for hypertension. The nurse should give priority to which of the following assessments?

1. Tachycardia and rebound hypertension
2. Weight loss and euphoria
3. Bradycardia and peripheral edema
4. Improved ability to perform activities of daily living (ADLs)

3 The nurse has just administered a dose of hydralazine intravenously to a client. After the initial dose, which of the following assessments is the priority?

1. Cardiac rhythm
2. Oxygen saturation
3. Blood pressure
4. Respiratory rate

4 After initiating a continuous infusion of nitroglycerin intravenously, the nurse would use which data to conclude that the client is experiencing an unintended effect? Select all that apply.

1. Pulmonary capillary wedge pressure (PCWP) falling from 13 to 11 mmHg
2. Tachycardia
3. Heart rate (HR) falling from 96 to 78
4. Blood pressure (BP) falling from 130/80 to 90/64
5. Headache

5 A client who recently began antihypertensive drug therapy states she needs to go to the pharmacy to buy an over-the-counter (OTC) product to treat a common cold. The home health nurse should provide which most helpful instruction first?

1. "Buy a generic brand of medicine because it is more cost effective and they act in similar ways."
2. "Do not purchase a product that contains aspirin."
3. "Read the label carefully and avoid products with pseudoephedrine."
4. "Many of the common products are contraindicated if you are taking medication for high blood pressure."

6 A client taking atenolol for hypertension tells the nurse, "Since I have been taking that medicine I feel so tired." What is the most appropriate priority nursing concern?

1. Potential for reduced tolerance to activity
2. Reduced cardiac output
3. Inability to manage health maintenance
4. Inability to perform self-care

7 The nurse is scheduled to administer a dose of digoxin to an adult client with atrial fibrillation. The client has a potassium level of 4.3 mEq/L. The nurse should perform which of the following activities next?

1. Withhold dose only for that day.
2. Obtain prescription for dose of potassium before giving digoxin.
3. Withhold dose and notify prescriber.
4. Administer dose as prescribed.

8 The nurse has prepared nitroprusside 50 mg in 250 mL of 5% dextrose in water. The client is to receive 1.5 mg/min. What rate should the nurse set the infusion to administer per minute? Record your answer, rounding to one decimal place.

_____ mL

9 After a healthcare provider prescribed propranolol for a client with frequent premature ventricular contractions (PVCs), the nurse should include which of the following in the care plan?

1. Inform the client that breathing will be improved with exercise.
2. Measure heart rate daily before taking dose.
3. Monitor for client's increased resistance to infection.
4. Observe for skin rashes, a rare side effect.

10 The nurse should prepare which of the following medications for chemical cardioversion for a client in atrial fibrillation?

1. Amiodarone
2. Verapamil
3. Nifedipine
4. Lidocaine

➤ *See pages 202–204 for Answers and Rationales.*

ANSWERS & RATIONALES

Pretest

1 **Answer: 2 Rationale:** IV nitroglycerin can be absorbed through polyvinyl chloride plastic, so nonpolyvinyl chloride tubing must be used. It is not necessary to cover the infusion with a plastic bag as is done with light-sensitive medications, such as nitroprusside. Oral sublingual tablets of nitroglycerin (NTG) are kept in light-resistant bottles. The solution is stable for 24 hours in a glass bottle; it would not be necessary to change it every 2 hours. It is not necessary to mix nitroglycerin under a laminar flow hood. **Cognitive Level:** Applying **Client Need:** Pharmacological and Parenteral Therapies **Integrated Process:** Nursing Process: Planning **Content Area:** Physiological Integrity **Strategy:** Associate IV nitroglycerin with special tubing and glass containers because the medication adsorbs into polyvinyl chloride. This will easily lead you to the correct option regarding administration concerns. **Reference:** Wilson, B. A., Shannon, M. T., & Shields, K. M. (2016). *Pearson nurse's drug guide 2016*. New York, NY: Pearson, pp. 1079–1082.

2 **Answer: 3** **Rationale:** Nitroglycerin patches and ointments must be rotated daily to a hairless area to reduce skin irritation and should be removed after 12 hours (not 24) to decrease the risk of tolerance. Acetaminophen may be used if headaches develop as a side effect, but it does not need to be used prophylactically. The area should be cleansed gently after removal but does not require vigorous scrubbing. **Cognitive Level:** Applying **Client Need:** Pharmacological and Parenteral Therapies **Integrated Process:** Teaching and Learning **Content Area:** Pharmacology **Strategy:** The critical words in the question are *best response*. With this in mind, select the option that is a true statement. **Reference:** Wilson, B. A., Shannon, M. T., & Shields, K. M. (2016). *Pearson nurse's drug guide 2016*. New York, NY: Pearson, pp. 1079–1082.

3 **Answer: 2, 1, 3, 4** **Rationale:** The normal pulse for an adult is 60–100 beats per minute, and an adverse effect of digoxin is a low pulse rate. For this reason, the apical rate is assessed before each dose and the dose is withheld (and the prescriber is notified) as the first priority if the pulse rate falls below 60. A low potassium level (normal 3.5–5.1 mEq/L) increases the risk of digoxin toxicity, so this is of concern second because it increases the potential for digoxin toxicity. Although furosemide can cause hypokalemia, this would be the third concern since the other data indicate actual risk, not potential risk, to the client. Orange juice is of no concern with this medication and is therefore lowest in priority. **Cognitive Level:** Analyzing **Client Need:** Pharmacological and Parenteral Therapies **Integrated Process:** Nursing Process: Diagnosis **Content Area:** Pharmacology **Strategy:** Analyze the data and determine which element could cause the greatest harm most rapidly. Then discriminate between potential risks and normal data of no concern. **Reference:** Wilson, B. A., Shannon, M. T., & Shields, K. M. (2016). *Pearson nurse's drug guide 2016*. New York, NY: Pearson, pp. 463–465.

4 **Answer: 2** **Rationale:** A dry, persistent, tickling, and nonproductive cough is a common side effect of angiotensin-converting enzyme (ACE) inhibitors such as lisinopril. This drug side effect subsides after the drug is discontinued. Dizziness is a common side effect associated with many antihypertensive medications, including beta blockers such as propranolol (Inderal). They can also cause a reduction in pulse rate. Cough and wheezing can occur with calcium channel blockers such as nifedipine, but they are not as common as dizziness and lightheadedness. Dehydration is more common with diuretics such as bumetanide. **Cognitive Level:** Analyzing **Client Need:** Pharmacological and Parenteral Therapies **Integrated Process:** Nursing Process: Assessment **Content Area:** Pharmacology **Strategy:** Note the critical words *most likely* in the stem of the question. This tells you that

more than one option might be partially correct but one option is clearly the better answer. Select the drug category (ACE inhibitors) that is known to have a cough of unknown origin as a side effect. **Reference:** Wilson, B. A., Shannon, M. T., & Shields, K. M. (2016). *Pearson nurse's drug guide 2016*. New York, NY: Pearson, pp. 683–684.

5 **Answer: 1** **Rationale:** Metoprolol is a beta-blocking agent that blocks the effects of both beta$_1$ and beta$_2$ receptors, leading to a reduction in systemic vascular resistance. This effect also may lead to bronchospasm (from bronchoconstriction secondary to beta$_2$ blockade). Metoprolol would not be contraindicated with a history of seizures, peripheral vascular disease, or myasthenia gravis. **Cognitive Level:** Applying **Client Need:** Pharmacological and Parenteral Therapies **Integrated Process:** Nursing Process: Assessment **Content Area:** Pharmacology **Strategy:** Consider the sites of action of this drug and use this information to choose the option that matches a risk with its blockade. **Reference:** Wilson, B. A., Shannon, M. T., & Shields, K. M. (2016). *Pearson nurse's drug guide 2016*. New York, NY: Pearson, pp. 985–988.

6 **Answer: 4** **Rationale:** Verapamil is a calcium channel blocker used to treat angina. Significant constipation is a frequent complaint of clients taking the sustained-release form of verapamil. Many older adults have difficulty with this, and the nurse must anticipate the need for teaching about increasing fiber and fluid intake. Hypotension is an adverse reaction to verapamil. Since the drug dilates coronary arteries, it is not likely that angina will occur. Skin rash is not a concerning side effect. **Cognitive Level:** Applying **Client Need:** Pharmacological and Parenteral Therapies **Integrated Process:** Nursing Process: Assessment **Content Area:** Pharmacology **Strategy:** It may help to remember that verapamil causes constipation by recalling it is a calcium channel blocker (both begin with the letter *c*). Note the age of the client to further prioritize constipation as a key concern since this can be an age-related concern of older adults anyway. **Reference:** Wilson, B. A., Shannon, M. T., & Shields, K. M. (2016). *Pearson nurse's drug guide 2016*. New York, NY: Pearson, pp. 1576–1579.

7 **Answer 2** **Rationale:** The client should be monitored for a change in heart rhythm, especially heart block. Lidocaine toxicities are manifested as neurologic changes such as disorientation, euphoria, and agitation, and the client should also be monitored for these. Systemic lupus erythematosus (SLE) is associated with the antidysrhythmic drug procainamide, but not with lidocaine. Although vital signs are always closely monitored in clients receiving IV infusions of antidysrhythmic drugs, blood dyscrasias are not associated with lidocaine. Visual changes are associated with digoxin toxicity, not with lidocaine. **Cognitive Level:** Applying **Client Need:** Physiological Integrity: Pharmacological and Parenteral Therapies **Integrated Process:** Nursing Process: Assessment **Content Area:** Pharmacology **Strategy:** Recall that lidocaine is given to treat ventricular dysrhythmias and that it may cause new dysrhythmias as well. This information will help you to focus on the option that is the correct answer. Furthermore, if you recall that it causes neurologic signs at toxic levels, this will reinforce your correct choice. **Reference:** Wilson, B. A., Shannon, M. T., & Shields, K. M. (2016). *Pearson nurse's drug guide 2016.* New York, NY: Pearson, pp. 875–878.

8 **Answer: 2** **Rationale:** Because it increases contractility (inotropy) of the heart, digoxin is classified as a positive inotropic drug. Because the primary problem associated with heart failure is decreased contractility, digoxin is the drug of choice. Atropine is utilized for sinus bradycardia. Propranolol, a beta-blocker, is used for hypertension and angina. Verapamil, a calcium channel blocker, is a negative inotropic medication and is used for hypertension, tachycardia, and angina. By virtue of their action, calcium channel blockers can also cause heart failure if taken in excessive doses. **Cognitive Level:** Applying **Client Need:** Pharmacological and Parenteral Therapies **Integrated Process:** Nursing Process: Planning **Content Area:** Pharmacology **Strategy:** Correlate the altered cardiac function with the primary actions of the drug. **Reference:** Wilson, B. A., Shannon, M. T., & Shields, K. M. (2016). *Pearson nurse's drug guide 2016.* New York, NY: Pearson, pp. 134–136, 469–471, 1064–1066, 1284–1287.

9 **Answer: 1, 3, 5** **Rationale:** Intravenous lidocaine reduces dysrhythmias by raising the electrical threshold of cardiac cells, reduces the automaticity of cardiac tissue, and is used to treat ventricular dysrhythmias. Local anesthetic activity occurs when the drug is injected directly into tissue such as the skin. The drug is more likely to decrease heart rate than to increase it. **Cognitive Level:** Analyzing **Client Need:** Pharmacological and Parenteral Therapies **Integrated Process:** Teaching and Learning **Content Area:** Pharmacology **Strategy:** The wording of the question tells you the correct options are those that contain correct statements. Use the process of elimination to discard options that contain false information. **Reference:** Wilson, B. A., Shannon, M. T., & Shields, K. M. (2016). *Pearson nurse's drug guide 2016.* New York, NY: Pearson, pp. 875–878.

10 **Answer: 2** **Rationale:** The side effects of amiodarone take several weeks or longer to manifest themselves. Sometimes they persist for up to 4 months, and because photosensitivity is a continuing concern, the client should avoid tanning and excessive sunlight. The pulse should be monitored and if it remains above 100 (not below) the primary care provider should be notified. **Cognitive Level:** Analyzing **Client Need:** Pharmacological and Parenteral Therapies **Integrated Process:** Nursing Process: Evaluation **Content Area:** Pharmacology **Strategy:** Specific drug knowledge is needed to answer this question. The wording of the question tells you the correct option will be a true statement of fact. **Reference:** Wilson, B. A., Shannon, M. T., & Shields, K. M. (2016). *Pearson nurse's drug guide 2016.* New York, NY: Pearson, pp. 72–75.

Posttest

1 **Answer: 4** **Rationale:** Sotalol is a beta-adrenergic blocking agent that has negative inotropic and chronotropic effects on the heart and may block beta$_2$ receptors in the lung, resulting in side effects such as bradycardia, dyspnea, and chest pain, which can be life-threatening complications. CNS side effects are fatigue and dizziness. A decrease, not an increase, in blood pressure is caused by sotalol. Blurry vision and halos are associated with the use of digoxin. Bluish discoloration of the skin is not consistent with the use of sotalol. **Cognitive Level:** Applying **Client Need:** Pharmacological and Parenteral Therapies **Integrated Process:** Nursing Process: Assessment **Content Area:** Pharmacology **Strategy:** Note that the drug ends in *-olol*, indicating that it is a beta-adrenergic blocker. Since these drugs reduce cardiac rate, associate this with bradycardia in the correct option. As an added assurance, note that dyspnea is another sign, which can also result from blockade of the beta receptors in the lungs. **Reference:** Wilson, B. A., Shannon, M. T., & Shields, K. M. (2016). *Pearson nurse's drug guide 2016.* New York, NY: Pearson, pp. 1405–1407.

2 **Answer: 3** **Rationale:** Because calcium channel blocker agents decrease the contraction of cardiac muscle, drugs such as diltiazem should be used cautiously in clients with congestive heart failure (CHF). An excessive dosage could actually worsen the state of heart failure. Bradycardia and peripheral edema signal adverse effects of this drug group. Although reflex tachycardia could occur because of sudden hypotension, rebound hypertension is not likely. Weight gain and drowsiness may occur rather than weight loss and euphoria. Instead of improved ability to perform activities of daily living (ADLs), the client is more likely to experience fatigue, drowsiness, and weakness as side effects of this drug. **Cognitive Level:** Applying **Client Need:** Pharmacological and Parenteral Therapies **Integrated Process:** Nursing Process: Assessment **Content Area:** Pharmacology **Strategy:** Correlate the adverse effects of the drug with the primary alteration associated with congestive heart failure (CHF). Recall that the drug reduces the force of contraction and so could worsen the CHF state, making signs of CHF the answer to the question. **Reference:** Wilson, B. A., Shannon, M. T., & Shields, K. M. (2016). *Pearson nurse's drug guide 2016.* New York, NY: Pearson, pp. 1405–1407.

3 **Answer: 3** **Rationale:** Hydralazine is a powerful vasodilator that exerts its action on the smooth muscle walls of arterioles. After a parenteral dose, blood pressure is checked every 15 minutes until stable and then every hour. Normal dosage may result in tachycardia but not dysrhythmia. Decreased blood pressure could result in decreased oxygenation, but is not the primary focus of the therapy. Respiratory rate is not the primary focus. **Cognitive Level:** Applying **Client Need:** Pharmacological and Parenteral Therapies **Integrated Process:** Nursing Process: Assessment

Content Area: Pharmacology **Strategy:** To answer this question correctly, it is necessary to understand that this drug is a powerful vasodilator that exerts an antihypertensive action. With this in mind, select the option that focuses on tracking the client's blood pressure. **Reference:** Wilson, B. A., Shannon, M. T., & Shields, K. M. (2016). *Pearson nurse's drug guide 2016*. New York, NY: Pearson, pp. 733–735.

4 **Answer: 2, 4, 5** **Rationale:** Tachycardia may result because of the decreased cardiac output. Nitroglycerin (NTG) is a vasodilator resulting in redistribution of central circulating volume. A decrease in BP from 130/80 to 90/64 is excessive and warrants further assessment by the nurse to determine whether perfusion to major organs is adequate. Because of the vasodilation of blood vessels in the cranium, headache and flushing may occur. Pulmonary capillary wedge pressure (PCWP) is an indirect measurement of left-ventricular end diastolic pressure. Because nitroglycerin causes a reduction in peripheral resistance, left-ventricular preload and left-ventricular afterload are reduced. Therefore, a decrease in PCWP and central venous pressure (CVP) is expected. Heart rate would rise, not fall. **Cognitive Level:** Applying **Client Need:** Pharmacological and Parenteral Therapies **Integrated Process:** Nursing Process: Planning **Content Area:** Pharmacology **Strategy:** Recall first that this drug is a powerful vasodilator, especially when given by the IV route. Note the critical words *unintended effect* in the question. Think through the physiological effects of this drug's action, and select the options that are excessive or unexpected. **Reference:** Wilson, B. A., Shannon, M. T., & Shields, K. M. (2016). *Pearson nurse's drug guide 2016*. New York, NY: Pearson, pp. 1079–1082.

5 **Answer: 3** **Rationale:** Some clients will experience increased blood pressure with over-the-counter (OTC) cold preparations containing pseudoephedrine as this ingredient causes vasoconstriction. Therefore, clients should avoid taking these products if on antihypertensive drug therapy. Generic brands contain the same medications but generally cost less, but cost should be considered only after the proper medication is identified. Avoiding aspirin would be appropriate if allergies exist or if overlapping characteristics exist, but this information is not in the question. While it is true that many products cannot be used, the statement is vague and cannot be applied by the client without further information. **Cognitive Level:** Applying **Client Need:** Pharmacological and Parenteral Therapies **Integrated Process:** Teaching and Learning **Content Area:** Pharmacology **Strategy:** Correlate the actions of the components of most over-the-counter (OTC) cold remedies with hypertension. **Reference:** Adams, M. P., & Koch, R. W. (2016). *Pharmacology: Connections to nursing practice*. New York, NY: Pearson, pp. 567–569.

6 **Answer: 2** **Rationale:** Decreased cardiac output is an outcome of the drug therapy. Because atenolol, a beta adrenergic blocker, causes decreased heart rate, blood pressure, and cardiac output, fatigue is a most common side effect. Reduced tolerance to activity is the state in which an individual has insufficient energy to complete activities of daily living. The client reported feeling tired, but did not address being unable to perform activities. There is no evidence that the client is unable to perform health maintenance activities or is unable to perform self-care. **Cognitive Level:** Analyzing **Client Need:** Pharmacological and Parenteral Therapies **Integrated Process:** Nursing Process: Diagnosis **Content Area:** Pharmacology **Strategy:** The critical word in the question is *tired*. Consider the nature of the drug and the effect it has on the heart, and from there consider that fatigue could result from the decreased pumping action of the heart to choose correctly. **Reference:** Wilson, B. A., Shannon, M. T., & Shields, K. M. (2016). *Pearson nurse's drug guide 2016*. New York, NY: Pearson, pp. 125–126.

7 **Answer: 4** **Rationale:** Hypokalemia is a common electrolyte imbalance commonly associated with digoxin therapy. The normal adult reference range for potassium is 3.5–5.1 mEq/L. Reduced potassium levels will result in an increased risk of digitalis toxicity. The client's level is within normal limits and the dose should be administered. There is no reason to withhold the dose, administer additional potassium, or withhold the dose and notify the prescriber. **Cognitive Level:** Applying **Client Need:** Pharmacological and Parenteral Therapies **Integrated Process:** Nursing Process: Planning **Content Area:** Pharmacology **Strategy:** To answer this question correctly, it is necessary to understand the nature of the drug and the normal potassium level. Use this knowledge and the process of elimination to make a selection. **Reference:** Wilson, B. A., Shannon, M. T., & Shields, K. M. (2016). *Pearson nurse's drug guide 2016*. New York, NY: Pearson, pp. 463–465.

8 **Answer: 7.5** **Rationale:** Use the equation

$$\frac{Desired}{Have} \times Quantity\ availabe$$

$$\frac{1.5\ mg}{50\ mg} \times 250\ mL$$

$$1.5 \times 250 = 50x$$

$$375 = 50x$$

$$x = 7.5\ mL$$

Cognitive Level: Applying **Client Need:** Pharmacological and Parenteral therapies **Integrated Process:** Implementation **Content Area:** Pharmacology **Strategy:** Using the equation Desired/Have × Quantity available, calculate the correct dose. **Reference:** Wilson, B. A., Shannon, M. T., & Shields, K. M. (2016). *Pearson nurse's drug guide 2016*. New York, NY: Pearson, pp. 1082–1083.

9 **Answer: 2** **Rationale:** Because the drug is a beta-adrenergic blocker, bradycardia is a common side effect. For this reason, the client should be taught to self-monitor the heart rate daily. Exercise may make breathing harder, not easier. Agranulocytosis is a side effect that could result in decreased resistance to infection. Many serious skin eruptions are associated with the drug. **Cognitive Level:** Analyzing **Client Need:** Pharmacological and Parenteral Therapies **Integrated Process:** Nursing Process: Planning **Content Area:** Pharmacology **Strategy:** First recall that the drug is a beta-adrenergic blocking agent. Then select the option that most represents the drug characteristics. **Reference:** Wilson, B. A., Shannon, M. T., & Shields, K. M. (2016). *Pearson nurse's drug guide 2016.* New York, NY: Pearson, pp. 1284–1287.

10 **Answer: 1** **Rationale:** Amiodarone is a Class III antidysrhythmic agent that prolongs the duration of action potential and refractory period of the heart. It slows conduction through the AV node and is effective in suppressing supraventricular dysrhythmias, particularly atrial fibrillation. Verapamil is a calcium channel blocker that primarily influences the dilation of coronary arteries and has secondary effects on cardiac conduction. Although nifedipine is a calcium channel blocker, it has no effect on SA-AV node conduction. It causes greater dilation of coronary and peripheral vessels than verapamil. Lidocaine is used predominantly for treatment of ventricular dysrhythmias. **Cognitive Level:** Analyzing **Client Need:** Pharmacological and Parenteral Therapies **Integrated Process:** Nursing Process: Planning **Content Area:** Pharmacology **Strategy:** Specific drug knowledge is needed to answer the question. First consider which drug group would exert a therapeutic effect for this dysrhythmia, and then associate the electrical activity in the heart with the action of the drug. **Reference:** Wilson, B. A., Shannon, M. T., & Shields, K. M. (2016). *Pearson nurse's drug guide 2016.* New York, NY: Pearson, pp. 72–75.

References

Adams, M. P., Holland, N., & Urban, C. (2017). *Pharmacology for nurses: A pathophysiologic approach* (5th ed.). New York, NY: Pearson.

Adams, M. P., & Urban, C. (2016). *Pharmacology: Connections to nursing practice* (3rd ed.). New York, NY: Pearson.

Burchum, J., & Rosenthal, L. (2016). *Lehne's pharmacology for nursing care* (9th ed.). St. Louis, MO: Mosby.

Drug Facts & Comparisons (2017) (Updated monthly). St. Louis, MO: Wolters Kluwer.

Frandsen, G., & Pennington, S. (2017). *Abram's clinical drug therapy: Rationales for nursing practice* (10th ed.). Philadelphia, PA: Lippincott Williams & Wilkins.

Holland, L., Adams, M., & Brice, J. (2015). *Core concepts in pharmacology* (4th ed.). New York, NY: Pearson.

Ignatavicius, D. D., & Workman, M. L. (2016). *Medical-surgical nursing: Patient centered collaborative care* (8th ed.). Philadelphia, PA: Elsevier.

Karch, A. M. (2017). *Focus on nursing pharmacology* (7th ed.). Philadelphia, PA: Lippincott Williams & Wilkins.

Kee, J. (2017). *Pearson's laboratory and diagnostic tests with nursing implications* (8th ed.). New York, NY: Pearson.

LeMone, P. T., Burke, K. M., Bauldoff, G., & Gubrud, P. (2015). *Medical-surgical nursing: Clinical reasoning in patient care* (6th ed.). New York, NY: Pearson.

Lilley, L. L., Rainforth Collins, S., & Snyder, K. M. (2017). *Pharmacology and the nursing process* (8th ed.). St. Louis, MO: Mosby.

Wilson, B. A., Shannon, M. T., & Shields, K. M. (2016). *Pearson nurse's drug guide 2016.* New York, NY: Pearson.

Blood-Modifying Agents

Chapter Outline

Objectives

➤ Describe goals of therapy related to the various blood-modifying medications.
➤ Identify significant nursing interventions for the client receiving an anticoagulant, antiplatelet, or thrombolytic medication.
➤ Identify antidotes for hemorrhage caused by various anticoagulants.
➤ Identify common side effects of medications used to lower serum cholesterol.
➤ Discuss client-centered nursing care related to administration of iron, vitamin B_{12}, or folic acid.
➤ Identify dietary sources of iron, vitamin B_{12}, and folic acid.
➤ Describe the action and use of epoetin alfa.
➤ List significant client education points related to various blood-modifying medications.

NCLEX-RN® Test Prep

Access the NEW Web-based app that provides students with additional practice questions in preparation for the NCLEX experience.

Review at a Glance

activated partial thromboplastin time (APTT) a blood test used to determine intrinsic clotting response that is measured in seconds; used to monitor and evaluate a client's response to heparin

aggregation an accumulation of substances such as platelets in the blood that form a group or cluster

anticoagulants substances that prevent or delay the coagulation of blood

antithrombin III (ATIII) a specific substance in the clotting cascade that prevents the activation of three clotting factors (thrombin, activated IX, and activated X)

clotting cascade a coagulation pathway in which enzymes and specific blood factors interact to effectively maintain

normal hemostasis in the body; includes both extrinsic and intrinsic pathways and leads to conversion of prothrombin to thrombin

extrinsic pathway pathway in clotting cascade that acts within seconds to form fibrin; PT and INR measure extrinsic pathway function

fibrinolysis process whereby clot dissolution takes place utilizing specific plasminogen activators in the body to prevent excessive clotting that could lead to vascular obstruction

fibrinolytic system mechanism for releasing plasmin (through the use of plasminogen activators) to act on fibrin (blood) clot and cause it to dissolve

hemostatics substances, devices, or procedures that stop the flow of blood

heparin-induced platelet aggregation (HITT) a potentially fatal complication of heparin therapy, whereby the client develops new clot formation with severe thrombocytopenia; also called *white clot syndrome*; HITT stands for heparin-induced thrombocytopenia and thrombosis

hypercoagulation a process whereby blood coagulates faster, leading to potential problems in the coagulation cascade

International Normalized Ratio (INR) a standard reference range used to establish consistency in reporting PT levels that accounts for normal variations seen in lab testing; INR leads to a better consensus of therapeutic management and ensures that evaluation of test results are based on common standards

intrinsic pathway pathway in clotting cascade that takes several minutes to form fibrin; intrinsic pathway function is measured by the APTT

low-molecular-weight heparin (LMWH) a term that refers to a group of heparin products that are comparable in molecular weight and have a higher bioavailability than traditional heparin

pernicious anemia a specific type of megaloblastic, macrocytic anemia that is related to the lack of intrinsic factor

necessary for absorption of vitamin B_{12} in the gastrointestinal tract

pica ingestion of nonfood substances, such as chalk, dirt, or paint, that can lead to nutritional deficiency states (and sometimes potential toxicity); can be seen as a type of craving for these substances

protamine sulfate antidote used for heparin

prothrombin time (PT) a blood test used to measure in seconds extrinsic clotting response; a control level is run with

the test to determine a standard response; used to monitor and evaluate response to oral anticoagulation therapy

purple toe syndrome a complication of oral anticoagulation therapy, whereby vascular emboli are released leading to microemboli formation in the toes and disruption of circulation

thrombolytics a group of substances that break down existing clots in the vascular system to restore blood flow and circulation

PRETEST

1 A client diagnosed with iron-deficiency anemia is taking iron supplements. The nurse should instruct the client to include which of the following foods to enhance the absorption of the medication?

1. Green leafy vegetables
2. Whole-grain bread and cereals
3. Yogurt
4. Orange juice or lemonade

2 After taking an antiplatelet medication for several weeks, a client presents with a noticeable bruise on the right arm. What assessment data is most significant to managing the client's health needs?

1. Whether the bruise is the result of a specific injury
2. Whether the client is taking the medication as prescribed
3. If the client self-monitors for skin manifestations
4. If the client's response to injury is different now

3 A client has been taking iron therapy for treatment of anemia. To evaluate drug effectiveness, the nurse reviews which laboratory test result as the best verification of iron stores in the body?

1. Ferritin level
2. Transferrin level
3. Hematocrit
4. Platelet level

4 When alteplase is administered to a client diagnosed with a cerebrovascular accident (CVA or stroke) in the emergency department, the nurse determines that the priority nursing interventions in this client's care should include which of the following? Select all that apply.

1. After administration, assess vital signs every 15 minutes during the first hour.
2. Report dysrhythmias noted on the cardiac monitor.
3. Insert urinary catheter and maintain accurate hourly output measures.
4. Monitor client for hypothermia for first 8 hours after infusion.
5. Report increase in partial thromboplastin time (PTT).

5 A client is taking epoetin alfa for treatment of anemia related to chronic renal disease. The nurse uses which clinical finding as the best measure of the drug's therapeutic effectiveness?

1. The client is not experiencing any related bone pain when the medication is being administered.
2. The hemoglobin and hematocrit (H&H) levels are rising rapidly based on latest two daily blood draws.
3. The client's hemoglobin increases to 12 grams/dL.
4. The client maintains an afebrile state.

6 What information should the nurse present in an educational seminar for clients who are taking nicotinic acid for elevated cholesterol levels? Select all that apply.

1. Because niacin treatment is individualized, dose adjustments are correlated with lab values.
2. Facial flushing may occur immediately after ingesting dose.
3. Eating a diet high in niacin will ensure that the medication works effectively.
4. For maximum effect, niacin can be taken concurrently with lovastatin.
5. Taking an aspirin 30 minutes before taking niacin helps to reduce flushing.

7 A 69-year-old client, who is taking desmopressin for von Willebrand disease, asks the nurse to provide information about the drug. An appropriate response by the nurse includes which statements? Select all that apply.

1. "Desmopressin helps restore and release deficient clotting factors (vW and VIII) that are reduced in von Willebrand disease."
2. "You can ask your healthcare provider about using an intranasal preparation."
3. "You should monitor your fluid intake and output while taking this drug."
4. "Take your blood pressure every day while taking this drug."
5. "You will receive cryoprecipitate transfusions while you are taking this drug."

8 The home health nurse instructs the client to avoid taking ibuprofen after noting a decrease in which laboratory test result?

1. Ferritin level
2. Triglyceride level
3. Neutrophil count
4. Platelet count

9 The nurse is providing medication information about warfarin to a client who is being discharged following a mechanical heart valve replacement. Which items of information would provide the best protection to the client? Select all that apply.

1. "Follow-up lab testing is required every 3 months."
2. "Use an electric razor and a soft-bristle toothbrush."
3. "Take this medication upon arising in the morning on an empty stomach."
4. "If a dose is missed, take the missed dose with the next scheduled dose."
5. "Eat a diet containing consistent but not large amounts of vitamin K."

10 The nurse received a prescription to start intravenous (IV) heparin on a client admitted with deep vein thrombosis (DVT). To implement this order appropriately, what action should the nurse take?

1. Place vitamin K at the bedside.
2. Tell client about need for being NPO while the medication is infusing.
3. Use an infusion pump to administer the drug.
4. Weigh the client twice weekly.

➤ *See pages 241–242 for Answers and Rationales.*

I. ANTICOAGULANTS

A. Oral medications

1. Action and use
   a. Oral **anticoagulants**, substances that prevent or delay blood coagulation, are used both to treat and prevent thromboembolic disorders in clients who are at risk; these disorders result from increased clotting activity, increased platelets, or both
   b. Vitamin K plays an active role in **extrinsic pathway** (a pathway that forms fibrin and acts within seconds) of **clotting cascade** (a coagulation pathway)
   c. Oral anticoagulants such as warfarin prevent conversion of vitamin K, thereby decreasing its production in liver
   d. With vitamin K production reduced, several clotting factors (II, VII, IX, and X) are also reduced, thereby prolonging the clotting cascade
   e. Warfarin is bound to plasma proteins, most notably albumin, and is metabolized in liver
   f. Oral anticoagulants are used to manage clients with actual, potential, and recurrent health problems such as deep vein thrombosis (DVT), pulmonary embolism (PE), acute myocardial infarction (AMI), heart valve replacement (bioprosthetic and mechanical), atrial fibrillation, and antiphospholipid syndrome
   g. Selective factor Xa inhibitors inhibit thrombosis through specific action on just factor Xa in the clotting cascade

2. Common medications
   a. Coumarin derivative warfarin sodium is probably the most frequently used oral anticoagulant in the United States
   b. Warfarin is given orally at a usual dose of 1–15 mg daily, with dose titrated to keep INR 2–3
   c. Dabigatran is a direct thrombin inhibitor indicated for stroke prevention in clients with atrial fibrillation and other uses
   d. Fondaparinux, apixaban, edoxaban, and rivaroxaban are factor-Xa inhibitors approved for stroke prevention in clients with atrial fibrillation

3. Administration considerations
   a. Warfarin requires close monitoring (because of a narrow therapeutic range) and frequent dose adjustments (because of individual dose response); there is a high potential for development of food and drug interactions that can lead to ineffective therapy or toxicity
   b. Warfarin's onset of action is slow, and its full anticoagulant effect is not seen until after approximately 1 week; thus, the drug may be started while a client is still on heparin therapy and overlap as heparin is tapered once desirable anticoagulation has been reached
   c. **Prothrombin time (PT)**, a blood test used to measure extrinsic clotting response, and **International Normalized Ratio (INR)**, a standard reference range used to establish consistency in reporting PT levels, may be used to monitor client's response to therapy
   d. Warfarin is usually given in the evening after reviewing pertinent laboratory test results drawn earlier in day
   e. Depending on indication for therapy, desired range of PT or INR will vary; PT levels are usually felt to be effective when they are maintained at 1.5–2.5 times the control value; INR levels range from a usual 2.0–3.0 to a higher range of 3.0–4.5 if client has a mechanical cardiac valve replacement
   f. Duration of therapy can range from several months to lifelong depending on client's specific health problem

  g. Refer to agency protocol and provider's prescription for dose adjustments and monitoring of client's PT and INR levels

  h. Vitamin K is the antidote that reverses the action of warfarin

4. Contraindications

  a. Oral anticoagulants are contraindicated in clients who are pregnant

  b. Lactating women can take warfarin as it will cross through in breast milk but there is little effect on an infant's PT; however, if infant were to require surgery, it would be advisable to obtain infant's PT as a baseline

  c. Oral anticoagulants should not be given to clients who are hemorrhaging or have bleeding tendencies, have malignant hypertension, or have a past history of allergic reaction to coumarin derivatives

  d. Clients with comorbid conditions such as liver failure and heart failure (HF) may have problems with metabolism and utilization of the drug

  e. Dosage reduction for rivaroxaban and dabigatran are indicated in renal impairment

  f. A black box warning for rivaroxaban recommends use of another anticoagulant when rivaroxaban is stopped, since clients have an increased risk for stroke

5. Significant drug interactions

  a. Because warfarin competes for binding sites in liver, there is a high potential for drug interactions relative to enzyme inhibitors and enzyme inducers; these chemical reactions will affect the serum concentration level of warfarin

  b. Warfarin is considered to be a primary example of a medication that has complex interactions with a vast number of medications; it is 99% protein bound, contributing to these interactions

  c. Refer to Table 7-1 for a partial listing of medications that can potentiate and diminish the effect of warfarin

  d. The use of herbal medications is discussed in the next section because the Food and Drug Administration (FDA) considers these to be dietary supplements

6. Significant food interactions

  a. Increased effects are seen with chondroitin and garlic

  b. There is an increased bleeding risk seen with cayenne, feverfew, garlic, ginger, and Gingko biloba

  c. Decreased drug effectiveness is seen with use of green tea, ginseng, and goldenseal

  d. The action of oral anticoagulants can be dramatically diminished by an increase in dietary sources of vitamin K

  e. Foods high in vitamin K such as liver, cheese, egg yolk, leafy vegetables (broccoli, cabbage, spinach, and kale), and oils (peanut, corn, olive, or soybean) should be limited and sources should be taken regularly during therapy to help maintain steady blood levels

Table 7-1   **Partial Listing of Warfarin Drug Interactions**

Drugs That Potentiate Action	Drugs That Decrease Action
Acetaminophen and acetylsalicylic acid (ASA)	Alcohol
Antibiotics	Barbiturates
H_2-histamine-receptor antagonists	Estrogens/oral contraceptives
Loop diuretics	Spironolactone
Nonsteroidal anti-inflammatory drugs (NSAIDs)	Thiazide diuretics
Sulfonamides	Thyroid drugs
Vitamin E	Vitamin K

      f. Dietary supplements of vitamin K should be avoided

      g. Alcohol use should be restricted (if not avoided) to maintain effective drug therapy

      h. Increased effects due to prolonged excretion of warfarin may occur when taken with cranberry juice, fruit, or supplements

      i. Referral to a dietitian is always indicated for clients receiving warfarin therapy because of the many potential dietary interactions and possibility of prolonged treatment with this type of medication

7. Significant laboratory studies

      a. Discoloration of urine (red-orange) can be seen with use of coumarin derivatives and may be of concern to client

      b. A hematologist should evaluate clients who are resistant to anticoagulation treatment with these types of medications for other specific underlying disorders of coagulation that might affect therapy

8. Side effects

      a. Ecchymosis of skin or bleeding from any tissue or organ

      b. Gastrointestinal (GI) and dermatologic problems

      c. Hypotension

      d. Thrombocytopenia

9. Adverse effects/toxicity

      a. Bleeding is the major adverse effect and is usually seen at higher dosage levels

      b. GI: nausea, diarrhea, intestinal obstruction, anorexia, abdominal cramping

      c. Dermatologic manifestations: rash, urticaria, and **purple toe syndrome** (discoloration caused by decreased perfusion from release of microemboli)

      d. Increased serum transaminase levels, hepatitis, jaundice

      e. Burning sensation of feet

      f. Transient hair loss

10. Client-centered nursing care

      a. Monitor client's PT and INR with initiation and continuation of therapy

      b. Review client's medications and dietary history with regard to potential drug and food interactions; be sure to include nutritional and herbal supplements

      c. Notify prescriber of current PT and/or INR results, making note of client's current dose

      d. Communicate with dietitian regarding client's status and anticipate discharge planning needs as therapy continues

      e. Assess client's skin for bleeding tendencies and monitor for GI side effects

      f. Client teaching is critically important because of many potential interactions, length of therapy, and close follow-up monitoring required

      g. Vitamin K may be prescribed to reverse effects of warfarin depending on PT or INR; can be prescribed as a single-dose therapy if high PT and INR values persist; additional doses of vitamin K may be given, and the warfarin dose may be withheld

      h. If the client experiences adverse effects or toxicity, withhold dose of warfarin; depending on INR or client manifestations, administration of phytonadione (vitamin K) may be indicated

      i. If there is significant bleeding, prescriber may order transfusion of fresh frozen plasma (FFP) or prothrombin concentrate

11. Client education

      a. Establish individualized teaching goals that increase client's knowledge of disease process and improve compliance with long-term therapy

      b. Alert client to bleeding problems and how to respond

c. Frequent follow-up blood tests will be required to make sure safe therapeutic therapy is maintained

d. Point-of-care (POC) testing is available for self-monitoring of PT and INR; prescriber may establish a home protocol to help manage care and necessary dosage adjustments

e. Dose must be taken on a daily basis; it cannot be stopped unless prescriber orders a dose to be withheld (pending PT or INR results) or client experiences a bleeding episode

f. Communication between client and all healthcare team members is an essential part of therapeutic management

g. Use a soft-bristle toothbrush and electric razor to minimize even mild trauma that could lead to bleeding

h. Observe for bleeding gums, bruises, nosebleeds, tarry stools, hematuria, hematemesis, and petechiae; report these findings to prescriber

i. Teach client to avoid excessive intake of foods high in vitamin K (see previous section)

j. Teach clients importance of taking dabigatran and rivaroxaban on a daily basis and avoid skipping doses; these drugs have short half-lives and daily intake is important

B. **Heparin and other related medications**

1. Action and use

   a. Heparin is a heterogeneous group of substances that exert anticoagulant effects; they have different molecular weights and other chemical properties that influence vascular system

   b. Heparin plays an active role in **intrinsic pathway** (where fibrin formation occurs and takes several minutes) in clotting cascade

   c. Heparin combines with a plasma heparin cofactor named **antithrombin III (ATIII)**, and this complex causes inactivation of specific clotting factors (II_a, X_a, XII_a, XI_a, and IX_a) in clotting cascade

   d. Heparin/ATIII complex has a very strong anticoagulant effect that inhibits conversion of fibrinogen to fibrin, prevents formation of a fibrin clot, and inhibits thrombin

   e. Molecular weight of the heparin molecule can range from 3,000 to 30,000 daltons (d), with average weight near 15,000 d; the standard measurement used is unfractionated heparin (UFH); **low-molecular-weight heparin (LMWH)** is also available with a molecular weight range of 4,000–6,500 d

   f. Because of its immediate effect, heparin is treatment of choice for clients who have venous thromboembolism, pulmonary emboli, and embolism resulting from atrial fibrillation

   g. Used as prophylaxis in clients at risk for developing thrombi as a result of surgical intervention

   h. Used in a weak concentration as a flush solution to maintain patency and prevent thrombus formation in vascular access devices

   i. Direct thrombin inhibitors inhibit action of thrombin without the intermediate step of antithrombin III inhibition; they are administered intravenously using a 15- to 20-second bolus or by continuous infusion; they are indicated in treatment of heparin-induced thrombocytopenia (HIT) and to prevent associated thromboembolic events

2. Common medications

   a. LMWH is a newer class of heparin molecule consisting of heparin fragments, with enoxaparin being most commonly used

    b. Heparin sodium is the most commonly used anticoagulant for treatment and prevention of recurrent thromboembolic episodes

    c. Argatroban, bivalirudin, and desirudin are direct thrombin inhibitors used in the treatment of HIT

    d. Refer to Table 7-2 for a listing of heparin anticoagulants

3. Administration considerations

    a. Heparin can be administered intravenously (IV) or by subcutaneous (subcut) injection

    b. Heparin bioavailability is influenced by its mode of administration and its chemical formulation; LMWH has a higher bioavailability when compared to standard UFH

Table 7-2   Heparin and Related Medications

Generic Name	Route	Uses
Heparin		
Heparin sodium	IV, subcutaneous	Diagnosis and treatment of deep intravascular clotting, prevention of clotting during dialysis, prevention of clot extension, deep vein thrombosis, pulmonary embolism, post-stroke, post–myocardial infarction, prophylactic in clients with a risk of thrombus formation, atrial fibrillation
Low-Molecular-Weight Heparins		
Dalteparin	Subcutaneous	Unstable angina, non-Q-wave myocardial infarction, prevention of deep vein thrombosis that may lead to pulmonary embolism, status post–abdominal surgery or hip replacement, adjunct to antineoplastic chemotherapy
Enoxaparin	Subcutaneous	Prevention of deep vein thrombosis, prevention of development of thromboembolism following hip replacement, status post–abdominal surgery, treatment of deep vein thrombosis, prevention of ischemic complications of unstable angina, non-Q-wave myocardial infarction
Direct Thrombin Inhibitors		
Argatroban	IV	Used with ASA as an anticoagulant in clients undergoing percutaneous transluminal coronary angioplasty (PTCA) or clients at risk for HIT undergoing percutaneous coronary interventions
Bivalirudin	IV	Prevention of deep vein thrombosis in clients undergoing joint replacement surgery, prevention of stroke in clients with nonvalvular atrial fibrillation
Dabigatran	IV	DVT prophylaxis in clients undergoing hip replacement surgery; off-label uses for prevention of thromboembolic events in clients with unstable angina or undergoing percutaneous coronary interventions
Desirudin	IV	Prevention of deep vein thrombosis in clients undergoing joint replacement surgery, prevention of stroke in clients with nonvalvular atrial fibrillation
Selective Factor Xa Inhibitors		
Rivaroxaban	PO	Prevention of deep vein thrombosis in clients undergoing joint replacement surgery and prevention of stroke in clients with nonvalvular atrial fibrillation
Fondaparinux	Subcutaneous	Prevention of deep vein thrombosis in clients undergoing surgery, treatment of deep vein thrombosis and pulmonary emboli
Apixaban	PO	Reduction of risk of stroke and systemic embolism in atrial fibrillation, prophylaxis of deep vein thromboembolism following surgery, treatment of deep vein thrombosis and pulmonary emboli
Edoxaban	PO	Reduction of risk of stroke and systemic embolism in atrial fibrillation, treatment of deep vein thrombosis and pulmonary emboli

    c. Activated partial thromboplastin time (APTT) is a blood test that determines intrinsic clotting response and is measured in seconds; it is used to monitor a client who is receiving heparin therapy; results are trended over time to determine client response and therapeutic effect

    d. Low-dose UFH therapy is used as a prophylactic treatment for DVT; dosage ranges from 5,000 units subcutaneously every 8–12 hours or three doses in immediate postoperative period per provider protocol; enoxaparin (a LMWH) is used clinically for this purpose and comes in prefilled syringes ready for individual use

    e. High-dose UFH therapy is done to achieve a therapeutic aPTT; aPTT levels should be stabilized at 1.5–2 times the control value

    f. An infusion pump is required for intravenous administration; it should be infused through a dedicated intravenous line because of its incompatibility profile

    g. Heparin weight-based therapy protocol is a standard format used by prescribers in the clinical setting to effectively anticoagulate a client needing immediate intervention (refer to Box 7-1 for specific information relevant to protocol management)

    h. Be sure to carefully identify strength on product label; several concentrations of intravenous heparin are available; some are used only as flushes for intravenous lines

    i. Protamine sulfate is the antidote to reverse heparin's action; dosage depends on dose of heparin given and time period elapsed following its administration; not more than 50 mg should be given in a 10-minute period; protamine sulfate is administered by IV push route

    j. Hypersensitivity or allergic reactions can be seen in clients receiving heparin, so epinephrine 1:1,000 should be readily available if a reaction develops

    k. Thrombin inhibitors should not be administered to clients with active bleeding or those with an aPTT ratio of above 2.5

    l. There is not a specific antidote for thrombin inhibitors, but since they have a very short half-life, discontinuation of an infusion leads to improved coagulation within a few hours

4. Contraindications

    a. Uncontrolled bleeding, known hypersensitivity, and thrombocytopenia

    b. Indirect (heparin) and direct inhibitors should not be given with aspirin (ASA) and nonsteroidal anti-inflammatory drugs (NSAIDS), as this will increase risk of bleeding

    c. LMWH are contraindicated in clients with active bleeding, thrombocytopenia, and/or heparin or pork allergy

---

Box 7-1	• Client weight should be obtained as a baseline for initiation of therapy.
Heparin Weight-Based Therapy Protocol Management Concerns	• Monitor daily weight and pertinent labs (aPTT).
	• Hemoccult all stools to assess for possible adverse effect of bleeding.
	• Titrate heparin dosage as needed based on results of aPTT.
	• aPTT labs are usually ordered q6 hours until two consecutive therapeutic levels are obtained. At that time, aPTT can be ordered q24 hours.
	• Once the client is stabilized, an oral anticoagulant such as warfarin is usually added if client requires long-term therapy.
	• Further monitoring of aPTT, PT, and INR is required as heparin is being discontinued and warfarin is being maintained as the method of anticoagulation.

5. Significant drug interactions: ASA, NSAIDS, and antiplatelet agents can potentiate anticoagulation effect and increase bleeding; herbal supplements such as ginger, garlic, feverfew, green tea, or gingko may increase risk of bleeding

6. Significant food interactions: allergy to pork products may indicate a potential hypersensitivity to LMWH; green leafy vegetables (particularly those high in vitamin K, such as spinach) may be limited if adding warfarin therapy

7. Significant laboratory studies
   a. Heparin prolongs aPPT level that is used to monitor oral anticoagulants
   b. Elevations of serum transaminase levels have been seen

8. Side effects
   a. Hemorrhage, hematuria, epistaxis, bleeding gums
   b. Thrombocytopenia

9. Adverse effects/toxicity
   a. A serious form of thrombocytopenia called **heparin-induced platelet aggregation** (heparin-induced thrombocytopenia and thrombosis [HITT]), also called *white clot syndrome*, can be fatal if not treated aggressively; thrombocytopenia is more pronounced (less than 100,000/mm^3) and begins 3–12 days after starting heparin therapy
   b. Clients on long-term heparin therapy (longer than 6 months' duration) are prone to develop osteoporosis

10. Client-centered nursing care
    a. Monitor client's baseline labs with regard to heparin protocol (specifically aPTT); trend results and titrate medication according to protocol; with continuous intravenous heparin infusion, aPTT is commonly measured every 6 hours; when level is critically high, infusion may be stopped for 1 or more hours and aPTT measured in 2–3 hours
    b. Obtain daily weight for client on weight-based heparin protocol
    c. Monitor client for signs of bleeding, perform a thorough skin assessment, hemoccult all stools to test for blood, and evaluate pertinent labs
    d. Verify with pharmacy or another RN the correct dosage of heparin before administering dose or adjusting heparin infusion
    e. Evaluate dosage for safety and therapeutic range based on normal adult dosage range of 20,000–40,000 units/24 hr; heparin is usually infused in units/hr
    f. Have antidote available (protamine sulfate) for heparin therapy
    g. Subcutaneous administration of heparin requires site rotation; do not aspirate or rub injection site
    h. When administering heparin subcutaneously, inject into abdomen using a small ($5/_8$-inch, 25- to 27-gauge) needle at a 90-degree angle
    i. The preferred administration site for low-molecular-weight heparins, such as enoxaparin, is in antero- and posterolateral sides of the abdomen; do not administer enoxaparin in deltoid area, as hematoma formation may result

11. Client education
    a. Establish specific goals to increase client's knowledge related to heparin administration
    b. Inform client that frequent bloodwork monitoring is required to ensure effective anticoagulation
    c. Teach client to be alert for bleeding problems and how to respond and to prevent injury
    d. Instruct client to observe for hematuria, nosebleeds, blood in stool, and petechiae
    e. Teach to decrease or maintain steady intake of green leafy vegetables if adding warfarin

Practice to Pass

What discharge instructions would you provide to a client who has been placed on anticoagulation therapy?

II. ANTIPLATELET AGENTS

A. Action and use

1. Antiplatelet drugs are substances that inhibit the body's natural clotting mechanism; they prevent or disrupt **aggregation** (accumulation of substances in blood to form a group or cluster) of platelets needed to form a clot
2. Act at specific points in clotting cascade to prevent blood clot formation
3. Used to treat thrombi and are often used as adjunctive therapy to other anticoagulant medications such as warfarin
4. Used as both preventative and treatment measures for clients with history of myocardial infarction, stroke, and cardiac surgery
5. Inhibit or block certain enzyme pathways to prevent clot formation

B. Common medications

1. Aspirin (or acetylsalicylic acid [ASA]) is the most commonly used type of antiplatelet medication
2. Ticlopidine can be used as an antiplatelet medication in clients who cannot take aspirin therapy
3. In addition to its utility as an antiplatelet agent, dipyridamole is also used in cardiac stress testing
4. ASA has many other therapeutic properties such as analgesic, anti-inflammatory, and antipyretic action
5. Clopidogrel bisulfate is used as a form of secondary prevention for clients who have had MI, stroke, and peripheral arterial disease
6. Abciximab is a fab fragment of a specific monoclonal antibody
7. Refer to Table 7-3 for a listing of common antiplatelet medications and their uses

C. Administration considerations

1. ASA is administered in dosages ranging from 81 to 325 mg/day (baby ASA to adult strength); can also be given as an enteric-coated preparation to minimize GI upset
2. Dipyridamole has a better profile when used with clients who have prosthetic mechanical heart valves
3. Ticlopidine has been used effectively as a preventative measure in clients who are at risk for MI
4. Abciximab is administered parenterally and client can receive a bolus dose as well as a constant infusion

D. Contraindications

1. ASA is contraindicated with known hypersensitivity to salicylates, bleeding disorders, asthma, or when gastrointestinal (GI) bleeding is present; ASA should not be given to children because it can be associated with development of Reye syndrome
2. Dipyridamole is contraindicated during pregnancy or lactation
3. Abciximab is contraindicated in clients with evidence of current or recent bleeding, cerebrovascular accident (CVA) or stroke within past 2 years with deficit, and thrombocytopenia
4. Ticlopidine is contraindicated during pregnancy, with a known hypersensitivity, liver disease, or evidence of blood dyscrasias
5. Clopidogrel bisulfate is contraindicated with known hypersensitivity or active bleeding as a result of intracranial hemorrhage or peptic ulcer disease

E. Significant drug interactions

1. With ASA, increased effects are seen with use of ETOH, anticoagulants, methotrexate, and sulfonylureas; decreased effects are seen with use of angiotensin-converting enzyme (ACE) inhibitors, beta-blockers, and diuretics
2. Dipyridamole/ASA can lead to additive effects and to an increased risk for bleeding

Table 7-3	Antiplatelet Agents	
Generic Name	**Route**	**Uses**
ASA		
Aspirin	PO	Reduce incidence of transient ischemic attacks, reduce the risk of nonfatal myocardial infarction in clients with a history of myocardial infarctions
Adenosine ADP Inhibitors		
Dipyridamole	PO	Prevention of thromboembolism in client with heart valves, combination therapy with warfarin sodium, coronary artery disease, angina pectoris
Glycoproteins		
Abciximab	IV	Used in combination with heparin and aspirin in prevention of cardiac ischemic events during transluminal coronary angioplasty
Clopidogrel bisulfate	PO	Treat clients who are at risk for ischemic events, history of myocardial infarction, ischemic stroke, or peripheral arterial disease
Eptifibatide	IV	Acute coronary syndrome, prevention of ischemic events during percutaneous coronary interventions
Tirofiban	IV	In conjunction with heparin to treat acute coronary syndrome, prevent cardiac ischemic events during percutaneous coronary care
Miscellaneous		
Ticagrelor	PO	Prevention of thrombotic events in clients with acute coronary syndrome or myocardial infarction with ST elevation
Anagrelide	PO	Essential thrombocytopenia to decrease platelet count and reduce risk of thrombosis
Cilostazol	PO	Reduce symptoms related to intermittent claudication
Prasugrel	PO	Treatment of unstable angina, non-ST elevation myocardial infarction, reduction of thrombosis in clients with acute coronary syndrome (ACS) or undergoing percutaneous coronary interventions
Cangrelor	IV	Used during percutaneous coronary interventions to reduce the risk of myocardial infarction or stroke
Ticlopidine	PO	Reduce thrombotic stroke in transient ischemic attack clients who cannot tolerate aspirin therapy, sickle cell disease, primary glomerulonephritis, arterial peripheral vascular occlusive disease

      3. Ticlopidine can increase levels of theophylline and phenytoin; cimetidine can lead to increased levels of Ticlid

      4. Clopidogrel bisulfate/NSAIDs may increase risk of bleeding episodes

F. Significant food interactions

      1. Ticlopidine is best taken on a full stomach to help maximize absorption and not in the presence of antacids

      2. ASA is usually taken on a full stomach to minimize GI upset

      3. Avoid these herbal treatments, which can increase risk of bleeding: angelica, cat's claw, chamomile, chondroitin, feverfew, garlic, gingko, golden seal, grape seed extract, green leaf tea, horse chestnut seed, psyllium, or turmeric

G. Significant laboratory studies

      1. ASA can cause false-negative or false-positive results for urine glucose and increase uric acid levels

      2. Ticlopidine has a potential to cause blood dyscrasias and a rise in serum cholesterol levels

H. Side effects

1. ASA: blood dyscrasias, hemorrhage, GI symptoms, as well as central nervous system (CNS) alterations, increased bleeding tendencies, hemorrhage, nausea and vomiting, dizziness, and confusion
2. Dipyridamole: GI complaints, nausea and vomiting, CNS alterations, headache, and dizziness
3. Ticlopidine: serious blood dyscrasias such as agranulocytosis and neutropenia; GI symptoms such as nausea and vomiting; and jaundice
4. Clopidogrel: flulike symptoms, chest pain, edema, and hypertension
5. In general: bruising, hematuria, tarry stools

I. Adverse effects/toxicity

1. ASA toxicity: tinnitus and ototoxicity
2. Abciximab: allergic reaction
3. Ticlopidine: potentially life-threatening decrease in platelets, leading to thrombotic thrombocytopenic purpura (TTP)

J. Client-centered nursing care

1. A baseline level of pertinent hematologic labs should be included at time of client admission
2. Monitor vital signs
3. Monitor bleeding time
4. Monitor client for side effects related to bleeding
5. Use of antiplatelet medications should be stopped for at least 7 days prior to a planned surgery
6. Older adult clients may require closer monitoring with antiplatelet therapy to avoid toxicity because it may be harder to assess for tinnitus and ototoxicity if a client's baseline hearing is already diminished
7. Lifespan concerns: children, pregnant women, and lactating women should not take antiplatelet medications; used in pregnancy only when benefit to mother outweighs risk to fetus; lactating women should be informed of risks to infant if this therapy is considered

K. Client education

1. Instruct client to carry a medical alert bracelet
2. Establish specific individualized goals to increase client's knowledge of therapy and need for continued compliance
3. Instruct client to monitor for side effects related to bleeding and report them
4. Inform client that communication between client and healthcare team members is critical
5. Inform client that adults should not use aspirin for self-medication of pain longer than 5 days without consulting a healthcare provider
6. Instruct to maintain adequate fluid intake to prevent salicylate crystalluria
7. Inform female clients that prolonged use of ASA can lead to iron-deficiency anemia
8. Instruct client and family of measures to prevent bleeding and actions to take if bleeding occurs
9. Instruct clients taking ticlopidine hydrochloride to report fever, chills, sore throat, or other signs of infection immediately

> **Practice to Pass**
>
> A client has been told by his provider to "take an aspirin a day to thin the blood" but is unsure as to the type and dosage. What information would you provide to the client?

III. THROMBOLYTICS

A. Action and use

1. **Thrombolytics**: substances that dissolve or break down a thrombus or blood clot
2. After a thrombus is broken down, blood flow is reestablished to area (increased perfusion) to maintain vascular integrity and prevent ischemia

3. Thrombolytics help activate the **fibrinolytic system** that breaks down a thrombus or blood clot
4. Conversion of plasminogen to plasmin aids clot breakdown by digesting fibrin and degrading fibrinogen and other procoagulant proteins into soluble fragments; plasminogen must be present for thrombolytics to work
5. Process of **fibrinolysis** is activated naturally in the body to prevent excessive clotting or vascular compromise
6. Thrombolytic therapy is indicated for clients at risk for developing thrombus with resultant ischemia such as acute MI, arterial thrombosis, DVT, pulmonary embolism, and occlusion of catheters or shunts
7. Thrombolytic medications are mostly given in emergency and critical care areas

B. **Common medications**
   1. Streptokinase is isolated from group-A beta-hemolytic streptococci (bacteria) and is considered to be antigenic; action is systemic in nature
   2. Alteplase is a natural substance secreted by vascular endothelial cells in body and therefore does not cause an antigenic response; action is specific in nature
   3. Refer to Table 7-4 for a listing of common thrombolytics

C. **Administration considerations**
   1. Thrombolytics are usually given to clients who are acutely ill in emergency and critical care settings where stabilization is the primary goal of intervention
   2. Alteplase has a very short half-life (5 minutes), which may require repeat administration and/or administration with heparin to prevent reocclusion of blood vessels
   3. Baseline vital signs and pertinent coagulation studies are necessary
   4. IV administration is carried out using specific protocols and guidelines to maintain safe and therapeutic effects; monitor IV sites for signs and symptoms of infiltration and/or phlebitis
   5. If intravenous site is not patent or if symptoms suggesting infiltration or phlebitis develop, site should be changed to opposite extremity
   6. Continuous monitoring of blood pressure (BP), mental status, neurologic signs, and response to therapy should be documented; report any signs of chest pain, dizziness, headache, or evidence of bleeding to the healthcare provider
   7. Place client on a cardiac monitor during administration of thrombolytics

D. **Contraindications**
   1. Pregnancy
   2. Not for use in clients who are actively bleeding, have a recent history of stroke, severe uncontrolled hypertension, recent trauma, or neoplasm
   3. Intramuscular route for medication administration is contraindicated when using thrombolytics

Table 7-4	Thrombolytics	
Generic Name	**Route**	**Uses**
Alteplase	IV	Myocardial infarction (MI), acute pulmonary embolism, acute ischemic stroke
Anistreplase	IV	Immediately after onset of acute MI
Reteplase	IV	Coronary artery thrombosis associated with MI
Tenecteplase	IV	Reduces mortality associated with acute MI
Streptokinase	IV	Dissolves blood clots associated with acute MI and pulmonary embolism

E. Significant drug interactions: increased risk of bleeding with anticoagulant and antiplatelet drugs

F. Significant food interactions: none reported

G. Significant laboratory studies

1. Reductions in plasminogen and fibrinogen levels are seen with use of thrombolytic agents
2. Monitoring coagulation profile such as bleeding time, aPTT, and PT is required to ensure safe and therapeutic treatment

H. Side effects

1. Hemorrhage
2. Hypersensitivity reactions; allergic reactions with vascular collapse occur more frequently with streptokinase
3. Nausea and vomiting and hypotension; streptokinase may cause first-dose hypotension
4. Cardiac dysrhythmias

I. Adverse effects/toxicity

1. Side effects of thrombolytic agents are dose-related
2. Dysrhythmias as a consequence of therapy may pose further problems for the client who is already in an acute situation, such as when administered via an intracoronary catheter

J. Client-centered nursing care

1. Monitor pertinent baseline labs and continue to assess client during therapy
2. Monitor client for vital sign changes, as there may be variations in pulse, blood pressure, and temperature caused by thrombolytic administration; watch for signs of impending shock; neurologic checks should be done frequently
3. Maintain adequate intravenous site for medication administration; observe closely for signs and symptoms of infiltration
4. Limit invasive procedures when a client is on thrombolytic therapy to reduce risk of bleeding
5. Assess frequently for signs of bleeding, both obvious and occult
6. If client is found to be bleeding, the medication should be stopped; fresh frozen plasma (FFP) and packed red blood cells (PRBCs) may be prescribed
7. Monitor client closely for development of dysrhythmias
8. Maintain aseptic technique to prevent infection
9. Antidote: aminocaproic acid should be readily available on clinical unit
10. Provide adequate nutrition and rest in order to support client during treatment
11. Support client and family members during acute care management period
12. Maintain effective, open, and therapeutic communication among client, family, and all healthcare team members

K. Client education

1. Treatment methods and medication administration
2. Use methods to reduce risk of bleeding
    a. Use electric razor to reduce risk of bleeding
    b. Brush teeth gently using a soft-bristle toothbrush to reduce risk of bleeding
    c. Avoid trauma to skin and other areas of body to reduce risk of bleeding
3. Lifestyle changes may be instituted in order to prevent further occurrences of abnormal clotting
4. Measurable signs of clinical response may not occur for 6–8 hours after therapy is started
5. Avoid taking aspirin or NSAIDs during therapy because risk of bleeding is enhanced
6. Discontinue medication if bleeding occurs and notify healthcare provider

Practice to Pass

A client in the emergency department is receiving thrombolytic therapy. What nursing interventions should you employ to reduce the risk of bleeding?

IV. HEMOSTATICS

A. Systemic hemostatics

1. Action and use

   a. Systemic **hemostatics** are substances that inhibit bleeding after an injury to maintain hematologic balance

   b. Used to stop/or prevent bleeding in clients who are at risk due to injury

   c. Vitamin K is also used as mandatory treatment to prevent hemorrhagic disease of newborn

   d. Vitamin K works in liver to formulate specific clotting factors (II, VII, IX, and X) that are necessary in coagulation cascade

2. Common medications

   a. Aminocaproic acid and tranexamic acid both impede fibrinolysis

   b. Aminocaproic acid is used to treat postoperative hyperfibrinolysis-induced hemorrhage and for hematologic disorders such as aplastic anemia, hepatic cirrhosis, and some neoplastic disease states; also an antidote to thrombolytic drugs

   c. Tranexamic acid is used 1 day before and 2–8 days after dental or other surgery in clients with hemophilia

   d. Phytonadione, vitamin K_1 is the antidote to warfarin and is fat soluble; reverses excess effects of oral anticoagulants

   e. Menadiol sodium diphosphate, vitamin K_4 is a water-soluble compound

   f. Refer to Table 7-5 for a listing of common systemic hemostatics

3. Administration considerations

   a. Aminocaproic acid and tranexamic acid are administered via oral or intravenous route; close continuous monitoring of the client is required

   b. Phytonadione is usually given intramuscularly to newborns in the delivery room for treatment and prophylaxis of hemorrhagic disease of the newborn

   c. Vitamin K preparations can be given by mouth, intramuscularly, subcutaneously, or intravenously

   d. Monitoring of PT levels will provide information relative to dosing and therapeutic management of client

   e. Desmopressin may be used to treat spontaneous bleeding and trauma-induced hemorrhage

Table 7-5 **Systemic Hemostatics**

Generic Name	Route	Uses
Aminocaproic acid	PO, IV	Excessive bleeding from cardiac surgery, trauma, abruptio placentae, thrombolytic agent antidote
Desmopressin	IV, intranasal	Spontaneous bleeding and trauma-induced hemorrhage
Phytonadine Vitamin K_1	PO, subcutaneous, IM	Promotes liver synthesis of clotting factors; antidote for coumarin overdosage; reverses hypoprothrombinemia secondary to oral antibiotic, quinidine, quinine, salicylate, sulfonamide, and vitamin A; prophylaxis therapy for neonatal hemorrhagic disease
Menadiol sodium diphosphate, Vitamin K_4	PO, subcutaneous, IM, IV	Vitamin K deficiency, promotes blood clotting
Tranexamic acid	PO, IV	Prevents gum hemorrhage during and after tooth extraction in hemophiliac clients

4. Contraindications
   a. Aminocaproic acid is contraindicated in clients who have disseminated intravascular coagulopathy (DIC), postpartum bleeding, upper urinary tract bleeding, or new burns
   b. Contraindicated in any client with a known hypersensitivity
   c. Vitamin K is contraindicated during last few weeks of pregnancy and in clients with liver disease
   d. Tranexamic acid is contraindicated in subarachnoid bleed
   e. Megadoses of iron are contraindicated in first trimester of pregnancy because of risk of fetal teratogenic effects

5. Significant drug interactions
   a. Concurrent use of aminocaproic acid and tranexamic acid with estrogen and oral contraceptives can lead to increased coagulation
   b. Use of aminocaproic acid and certain antibiotics can lead to ototoxicity and nephrotoxicity; check individual antibiotic product literature
   c. Use of antibiotic therapy may lead to a decrease in vitamin K synthesis due to destruction of intestinal bacteria; supplementation may be required
   d. Mineral oil can decrease absorption of vitamin K

6. Significant food interactions
   a. Dietary sources of vitamin K are found in green leafy vegetables, milk, and meats
   b. Vitamin K is a fat-soluble vitamin and can be synthesized by intestinal flora; deficiency states are usually not identified solely with diet, but are more likely caused by malabsorption problems linked to liver disease or alcohol abuse
   c. The addition of yogurt in diet helps to provide a medium for bacterial growth that can lead to maintenance of intestinal flora

7. Significant laboratory studies
   a. PT level is an indicator of response to vitamin K administration
   b. Aminocaproic acid can cause a decrease in potassium levels when used in clients with decreased renal function

8. Side effects
   a. Gastrointestinal: nausea and vomiting, diarrhea, and abdominal cramps
   b. Headache, dizziness, and flushing
   c. Localized reaction at injection site with vitamin K administration
   d. Allergic response with vitamin K products

9. Adverse effects/toxicity
   a. Most drug effects are mild and are usually dose related
   b. Overdose with vitamin K can lead to a serious problem if client is a newborn because of its effect on coagulation cascade

10. Client-centered nursing care
    a. Monitor client for baseline labs related to renal and liver function
    b. Monitor PT levels and response to therapy for vitamin K administration
    c. Monitor client's coagulation profile as antifibrinolytics can cause a **hypercoagulation** or rapid coagulation of blood
    d. Rotate injection sites for administration of vitamin K; assess client for signs of local irritation
    e. Monitor client closely for signs of hypersensitivity and allergic reactions
    f. Monitor client closely during administration via parenteral infusion as there is risk for volume overload and adverse reactions
    g. Use of an infusion pump for intravenous administration is required

11. Client education
    a. Dietary sources of vitamin K previously discussed
    b. Periodic PT levels will be drawn to monitor response to therapy

c. Monitor for signs and symptoms of bleeding

d. Use of dietary yogurt and buttermilk products can help restore normal intestinal flora that will aid in vitamin K synthesis; clients who are on antibiotic therapy or who have intestinal problems may benefit from this supportive therapy

e. Report difficulty urinating or reddish-brown urine (caused by myoglobinuria) while taking aminocaproic acid

f. Report chest pain, arm or leg pain, or difficulty breathing

B. **Local absorbable hemostatic agents**

1. Action and use

a. Localized hemostatics are utilized to stop or inhibit bleeding at a specific site

b. The use of topical local hemostatics leads to absorption of blood in a controlled manner

c. Thrombin can be used following dental extraction procedures to stop bleeding

2. Common hemostatic medications

a. Gelatin products, oxidized cellulose, thrombin, and epinephrine are all examples of topical hemostatic agents

b. Refer to Box 7-2 for a listing of common local hemostatics

3. Administration considerations

a. Topical hemostatics are available in pads, powder, sponge, film, and liquid forms

b. Application involves adherence of the form to a local bleeding site and the material is allowed to remain in place to establish hemostasis

c. Depending on type of local hemostatic used, removal may be done as early as 24–48 hours

d. Irrigation with normal saline may be necessary to prevent further tissue destruction as the topical is removed

e. If product is a sponge or film, it may be completely reabsorbed into body

4. Contraindications

a. Contraindicated if client has a previous allergy to animal protein products or gelatin, since they are composed of animal protein

b. Contraindicated in the presence of infection

5. Significant drug interactions: none reported

6. Significant food interactions: none reported

7. Significant laboratory studies: none reported

8. Side effects: hypersensitivity reactions at site of application, erythema, pruritus, and localized irritations

---

Box 7-2	• Absorbable gelatin sponge: a sterile gelatin that absorbs blood when placed in surgical wound and is absorbed within 4–6 weeks
Local Hemostatics	• Absorbable gelatin film: a sterile absorbable gelatin film often used in neurosurgery, thoracic surgery, or ocular surgery to absorb blood in tissues, act as dural substitute (neurosurgery), or repair pleural defect (thoracic surgery)
	• Epinephrine: a medication that reduces bleeding by causing vasoconstriction
	• Oxidized cellulose: a specially treated form of surgical gauze or cotton that is hemostatic and is usually absorbable in 2–7 days; controls bleeding during surgery involving liver, pancreas, spleen, kidney, thyroid, and prostate
	• Oxidized regenerated cellulose: see oxidized cellulose noted previously
	• Microfibrillar collagen hemostat: an absorbable topical hemostatic substance that attracts platelets and causes platelet aggregation on a bleeding surface
	• Thrombin: a sterile powder treated with thromboplastin in the presence of calcium; catalyzes conversion of fibrinogen to fibrin and may cause platelet aggregation; used topically for capillary bleeding or in combination with absorbable gelatins (previously listed) during surgery

9. Adverse effects/toxicity: same as previously noted

! 10. Client-centered nursing care

   a. Application of topical hemostatics must be done according to prescriber protocol and within guidelines of product information

   b. Assess local site for signs of hypersensitivity and document findings

   c. Remove topical hemostatics as indicated by product guidelines; irrigation of site with normal saline may be required to prevent further tissue destruction; document site appearance in medical record

   d. If client develops an allergic reaction to product or if a reaction is anticipated, an antihistamine such as diphenhydramine may be given

   e. Switching from one material to another may facilitate a better response

! 11. Client education

   a. Removal of topical hemostatics: It is important not to pull off dry materials as this could cause further skin damage and pain

   b. Treatment with local hemostatics may occur over a number of days and weeks

   c. Compliance with treatment regimen is necessary to achieve a good outcome

   d. Monitor site for signs of potential infection

C. Clotting factor replacement therapy

1. Action and use

   a. Refers to specific restoration of blood components necessary for body to regain hemostasis and maintain hematologic integrity

   b. Congenital deficiencies of specific clotting factors can lead to serious (if not fatal) consequences unless there is adequate replacement therapy

   c. Functional platelet and plasma abnormalities can lead to coagulation problems that include specific syndromes, such as hemophilia and von Willebrand disease

   d. Used to stop and prevent hemorrhage in clients who have specific identified factor deficiencies

   e. Used to support clients with specific factor deficiencies who are undergoing a surgical procedure

2. Common medications or blood products

   a. Cryoprecipitate provides a concentrated form of fibrinogen and is a blood product obtained from fresh frozen plasma (FFP)

   b. Antithrombin III works with heparin to provide an anticoagulant effect

   c. Desmopressin acetate is classified as an antidiuretic hormone, but it has adjunctive effects on increasing factor VIII in body

   d. Refer to Box 7-3 for a listing of replacement therapy medications

3. Administration considerations

   a. Antihemophilic factor (AHF) medications are administered via IV route; dosage is individualized based on client's weight, bleeding status, factor deficiency, presence of factor inhibitor, and results of pertinent coagulation lab studies

Practice to Pass

A topical hemostatic agent used on the client now has to be removed. What nursing interventions would you employ to perform this action?

Box 7-3	Antihemophilic factor
	Cryoprecipitated antihemophilic factor–human
Clotting Factor	Antihemophilic factor–porcine
Replacement Therapy	Antihemophilic factor–recombinant
	Antithrombin III
	Desmopressin
	Factor IX complex, human
	Coagulation Factor IX, recombinant

      b. Desmopressin can be administered intranasally; alternate nares when administering drug and document appropriately on medication record

      c. AHF medications are usually refrigerated

      d. Administration of AHF should be done according to protocol; premedicate with antihistamines if ordered; document vital signs during the first 15 minutes of therapy to determine that they stay within client's baseline

4. Contraindications

      a. Clients with a hypersensitivity to bovine, hamster, or mouse protein

      b. Antithrombin III may cause possible infection and hepatitis in pediatric clients and therefore should be used cautiously

      c. Desmopressin is contraindicated in pregnant or lactating clients or clients with known hypersensitivity to drug; it should be used with caution in pediatric or older adult clients due to its antidiuretic effect and potential to develop hyponatremia

5. Significant drug interactions

      a. Concurrent use of antithrombin III and heparin leads to an increased anticoagulant effect

      b. The effects of desmopressin can be potentiated with use of chlorpropamide and carbamazepine

6. Significant food interactions: none reported

7. Significant laboratory studies: sodium levels may need to be monitored with desmopressin therapy because of its effect on this electrolyte

8. Side effects

      a. AHF: hypersensitivity, lethargy, fatigue, nausea, and hypotension

      b. Antithrombin III: none reported

      c. Desmopressin: headaches, nausea, nasal congestion, facial flushing, and chills

9. Adverse effects/toxicity

      a. AHF: developing AIDS and hepatitis, as certain AHF products are derived from human plasma

      b. Desmopressin overdose: increased symptoms noted previously and dyspnea

10. Client-centered nursing care

      a. Proper reconstitution and administration of dose is required according to protocol

      b. Monitoring of pertinent baseline hematologic labs is required

      c. Document baseline vital signs during first 15 minutes of therapy and then according to protocol to monitor client's continued response

      d. Observe client closely for signs of hypersensitivity

      e. Infusion may have to be slowed down or discontinued if client develops increased allergic symptoms

      f. Review client's medication profile for use of concurrent medications that could interfere with clotting

      g. Clients with defined factor deficiencies and their families will need anticipatory support and guidance during a lifetime of therapy

      h. A collaborative healthcare team approach should be instituted to provide continued care to client and family

      i. Clients who have hereditary factor antithrombin III deficiency and become pregnant or require surgery are at risk of developing thrombosis; monitor closely during obstetric and postsurgical time periods

11. Client education

      a. Medication storage and administration if therapy is to be given at home

      b. Disease process and genetic transmission issues; referral to a genetic counselor may be indicated in clients of childbearing age

    c. Refer client to support groups for assistance and strengthening of coping mechanisms

    d. Since client is at risk for bleeding because of factor deficiencies, review concepts of safety as related to lifestyle and job/employment

V. MEDICATIONS TO TREAT ANEMIA

    A. Iron salts

        1. Action and use

            a. Iron is an essential trace element that participates in oxygen transport, tissue respiration, and enzyme reactions

            b. Iron is stored as ferritin in body; ferritin levels reflect visceral stores of iron that are available to body; transferrin levels reflect how iron is transported in body

            c. Iron-deficiency anemia (IDA) is one of the most common nutritional deficiencies in United States

            d. IDA is classified as a microcytic anemia; iron preparations are indicated for treatment of this type of anemia

            e. The use of ferrous salts is indicated for treatment of iron deficiency

            f. Iron medications are available through prescription and over the counter (OTC)

        2. Common medications

            a. Ferrous iron salts provide the largest amount of elemental iron and are available as oral medications

            b. Ferrous fumarate, ferrous gluconate, and ferrous sulfate are three oral iron preparations available; they all are equally effective but require different doses to provide an equivalent amount of iron

            c. Iron dextran is available as an injection when a client cannot tolerate oral administration or if oral therapy is ineffective

            d. Refer to Table 7-6 for a listing of common iron preparations

        3. Administration considerations

            a. Oral iron is given with meals in order to decrease gastric upset

            b. Z-track administration of iron dextran is required to minimize client discomfort, prevent tissue discoloration, and ensure absorption

            c. There is a risk of anaphylactic reaction following iron dextran administration; therefore, a test dose may be ordered over 5 minutes to monitor client response; have epinephrine ready to use if hypersensitivity occurs

            d. Iron can be found in vitamins and nutritional supplements; monitor client for alternate sources of iron so as to avoid potential overdosing and toxicity

            e. Be aware of potential drug interactions that may limit or increase oral iron medications

            f. Liquid (elixir) iron is administered by straw to avoid discoloration of tooth enamel

Table 7-6   **Iron Salts**

Generic Name	Route	Uses
Ferrous fumarate	PO	Correct simple iron deficiency (microcytic, hypochromic anemia) Periods of increased iron needs such as infancy, childhood, and pregnancy
Ferrous gluconate	PO	Correct simple iron deficiency (microcytic, hypochromic anemia) Periods of increased iron needs such as infancy, childhood, and pregnancy
Ferrous sulfate	PO	Correct simple iron deficiency (microcytic, hypochromic anemia) Periods of increased iron needs such as infancy, childhood, and pregnancy
Iron dextran injection	IV, IM	Iron-deficiency anemia when oral administration of iron is unsatisfactory or impossible

4. Contraindications
    a. Contraindicated in clients with ulcerative colitis, peptic ulcer disease, cirrhosis, and hemolytic anemia
    b. Contraindicated in clients with iron overload syndromes (hemosiderosis and hemochromatosis)
    c. Prior history of reaction could lead to a contraindication for use of iron dextran injection (hypersensitivity including anaphylaxis can occur)
    d. Megadoses of iron are contraindicated during first trimester of pregnancy because of risk for teratogenic effects

5. Significant drug interactions
    a. Antacids, antibiotics (quinolones and tetracycline), and thyroid drugs decrease absorption of iron; therefore, oral iron medication should not be administered at same time
    b. Decreased effect of tetracycline and penicillamine
    c. Vitamin C can increase absorption of oral iron medications

6. Significant food interactions
    a. Iron is composed of both heme (animal) and nonheme (plant) sources in the diet; heme sources have a higher bioavailability and are more beneficial in maintaining iron levels
    b. Clients on a strict vegetarian diet may require supplementation to ensure adequate iron levels
    c. Taking iron with vitamin C can lead to increased absorption
    d. Foods that are high in phytates (grains and cereals) can cause a decreased absorption of dietary iron
    e. Iron should not be taken with milk, as decreased absorption will occur

7. Significant laboratory studies
    a. Monitor client's reticulocyte count, which will increase if bone marrow is responding and RBC production is increasing
    b. If hemoglobin and hematocrit levels do not rise following iron therapy, additional testing may be required to determine exact type of anemia

8. Side effects
    a. Gastrointestinal: upset stomach, nausea and vomiting, diarrhea, and constipation
    b. Dark and tarry stools
    c. Dermatologic: discoloration of skin and pain upon injection

9. Adverse effects/toxicity
    a. **Pica** (ingestion of nonfood items in diet) can interfere with iron levels in body, causing individuals to become anemic; pregnant women are the client group most likely to be involved with pica
    b. Iron can accumulate in body, leading to potentially toxic levels
    c. Symptoms of iron overdose can lead a client to progress to shock, seizures, or coma; serum iron levels evaluated greater than 300 mcg/dL is serious and should be treated aggressively
    d. Removal of iron from body during iron overdose is necessary; poison control should be notified if iron overdose is suspected
    e. Chelation therapy should be instituted to remove iron from body in addition to supportive measures such as airway maintenance, correction of acidosis, and administration of intravenous fluids

10. Client-centered nursing care
    a. Monitor client for expected side effects related to iron administration, such as tarry stools
    b. Give oral medication on a full stomach to minimize GI upset

       c. Since anemia is often a symptom of a disease, assess for underlying cause; monitor client lab findings to confirm a diagnosis of IDA

       d. If client does not show a clinical response to iron therapy, notify prescriber

       e. Referral to a dietitian may be indicated to support client's food choices in maintaining adequate iron levels

       f. Evaluate client for pica if there is a high index of suspicion

11. Client education

       a. Proper administration of oral iron medications

       b. Importance of adequate food sources to maintain iron levels; these include foods such as lean meats, liver, egg yolks, dried beans, green vegetables (e.g., spinach)

       c. Expected changes in the characteristics of stool (black, tarry)

B. Vitamin B_{12} (Cyanocobalamin)

1. Action and use

       a. Vitamin B_{12} is a water-soluble vitamin that is utilized as part of many coenzyme reactions during metabolism of carbohydrate, protein, and fat; also essential for DNA synthesis

       b. Vitamin B_{12} is found primarily in foods of animal origin (liver, meat, shellfish, and dairy food items)

       c. Deficiency of vitamin B_{12} affects neurologic, hematologic, and GI systems

       d. Vitamin B_{12} is considered to be the extrinsic factor whereas the intrinsic factor is released by parietal cells in stomach

       e. Clients with GI surgeries that result in partial or complete removal and/or anastomosis of stomach and end the release of intrinsic factor will require injections of vitamin B_{12} on a lifelong basis

       f. **Pernicious anemia** is the anemia that results from vitamin B_{12} deficiency

       g. Vitamin B_{12} deficiency is classified as a megaloblastic macrocytic anemia

       h. Atrophic gastritis is associated with vitamin B_{12} deficiency

       i. Because B-complex vitamins work together, there is likelihood that there is more than one deficiency existing at the same time

2. Common medications

       a. Cyanocobalamin is available as both prescription and OTC

       b. Cyanocobalamin is contained in many multivitamin preparations in addition to being sold as a separate vitamin unit

       c. Vitamin B_{12} is available in oral and injectable forms

       d. Refer to Table 7-7 for a listing of common Vitamin B_{12} preparations

3. Administration considerations

       a. Vitamin B_{12} must be administered parenterally in clients who cannot manufacture intrinsic factor

       b. Therapeutic level for vitamin B_{12} is Schilling test result greater than 30%

       c. Rotation sites with injection of this medication; use Z-track method to minimize burning and local irritation

Table 7-7   Vitamin B_{12} Preparations

Generic Name	Route	Uses
Vitamin B_{12A} (hydroxocobalamin)	IM	Vitamin B_{12} malabsorption, thyrotoxicosis, hemolytic anemia, gluten enteropathy, small-bowel bacterial overgrowth, folic acid deficiency
Vitamin B_{12} (cyanocobalamin)	IM, deep subcutaneous	Pernicious anemia, inadequate secretion of intrinsic factor, dietary deficiency, vitamin B_{12} malabsorption

    d. Cyanocobalamin injection should be protected from light, as light will inactivate drug; it should not be mixed with other medications but given as a separate injection

  4. Contraindications: known prior hypersensitivity

  5. Significant drug interactions

    a. Medications such as anti-epileptics, aminoglycosides, cholestyramine, colchicine, neomycin, and potassium timed-release products will cause decreased absorption of vitamin B_{12}

    b. Monitor potassium levels as use of cyanocobalamin can cause hypokalemia

    c. Chloramphenicol antagonizes the hematologic action of this vitamin

    d. Decreased effectiveness with methotrexate and excessive alcohol use

  6. Significant food interactions

    a. Clients with malabsorption problems may be prone to develop vitamin B_{12} deficiency

    b. Clients with alcoholism are more likely to have malabsorption problems and therefore are likely to have many vitamin deficiencies

    c. A strict vegetarian diet without adequate supplementation may increase a client's risk for developing this vitamin deficiency

  7. Significant laboratory studies

    a. Monitor pertinent hematologic labs to confirm diagnosis of pernicious anemia

    b. Monitor client for potential hypokalemia

  8. Side effects

    a. Flushing

    b. Gastrointestinal: diarrhea with resultant hypokalemia

    c. Dermatologic: itching and pain at the injection site

  9. Adverse effects/toxicity

    a. Vitamin B_{12} is a water-soluble vitamin and as such should not reach toxic levels in body

    b. Some clients can have more serious cardiac effects such as development of heart failure and pulmonary edema

  10. Client-centered nursing care

    a. Review client's medications, both prescription and over the counter, for potential drug interactions

    b. Rotate injection site and document appropriately on medication record

    c. Establish baseline pertinent labs and monitor as needed to document response to treatment

    d. Assess client's pulses and vascular status to determine baseline

    e. Clients with pernicious anemia cannot take oral vitamin therapy alone to correct the problem; medication must be administered via parenteral route

    f. If client's lab values do not indicate a positive response to treatment, notify prescriber and further investigate to determine underlying cause

    g. Refer to dietitian for supportive diet management; foods high in vitamin B_{12} (for those who can absorb it) include liver, kidney, fish, and milk

  11. Client education

    a. Lifelong nature of therapy if diagnosed with pernicious anemia

    b. Food sources of vitamin B_{12} for inclusion in diet (see previous section)

    c. Effects of alcohol on the absorption of vitamin B_{12}

    d. Monitor for signs and symptoms of B_{12} deficiency (numbness and tingling in lower extremities, weakness, fatigue, anorexia, loss of taste, diarrhea, memory loss, and mood changes)

    e. If diarrhea is significant, a change in drug dosage may be required

C. Folic acid
1. Action and use
   a. Folic acid (vitamin B_9) is a water-soluble vitamin needed for DNA synthesis and cellular division
   b. Folic acid may be used either to treat deficiency states or as prophylaxis against a deficiency state, such as in pregnancy
   c. Deficiency states have been associated with neural tube defects in developing fetus and with hematologic manifestations such as megaloblastic macrocytic anemia
   d. Folic acid helps to break down homocysteine (an amino acid) in body; if there is a folic acid deficiency state, then levels of homocysteine can elevate; high homocysteine levels are associated with heart disease
   e. Dietary sources of folic acid are found in fresh green vegetables, yellow fruits and vegetables, liver, yeast, and meats
   f. Folic acid supplements in addition to dietary sources are used to treat deficiency states; supplementation is recommended during pregnancy and lactation
2. Common medications
   a. Folic acid can be obtained as an over the counter medication; therapeutic oral dose is less than 1 mg per day and maintenance dose is less than 0.4 mg per day
   b. Nutritional supplements and/or multivitamin preparations can contain folic acid
   c. Leucovorin calcium may be given intramuscular or intravenously at a usual adult dose of not more than 1 mg per day; this form of folic acid is reserved for use as an adjunct to cancer chemotherapy, not folic acid deficiency
3. Administration considerations
   a. Route of administration can be oral, subcutaneous, intramuscular, or intravenous depending on formulation; folic acid can be given as an intravenous push or added to an infusion; infusion rate should not exceed 5 mcg/minute
   b. Folic acid (0.4 mg) is recommended daily for all pregnant women in the United States to prevent folate deficiency; suggested that therapy start 1 month prior to conception and continue throughout first trimester
   c. Regardless of client's age, daily dose should not be less than 0.1 mg/day
   d. Folic acid should not be mixed with any other medication and should be given as a separate injection
   e. Clients may experience a rash or hypersensitivity at site of injection; rotate injection sites
   f. If client has neurologic deficits, use of folic acid will not correct the problem; attention must be directed to other B vitamins; appropriate therapy must be instituted to correct neurologic compromise
4. Contraindications
   a. Contraindicated for treatment of other anemias not caused by folic-acid deficiency
   b. Folic-acid injections may contain benzyl alcohol and therefore should not be given to neonates; the use of this preservative is contraindicated in neonates
   c. Use cautiously during lactation
5. Significant drug interactions
   a. ASA, phenytoin, and sulfonamides cause decreased folic acid levels
   b. Increased likelihood of seizure activity when used concurrently with phenytoin
   c. Oral contraceptives can increase the risk of folic-acid deficiency
   d. Steroid use increases the need for folic acid in body
   e. Methotrexate, pyrimethamine, triamterene, and trimethoprim act as folic-acid antagonists

    f. Alcohol use can lead to folic-acid deficiency because it increases folic-acid requirements

    g. Continued use of folic acid may interfere with findings associated with vitamin B_{12} deficiency states

6. Significant food interactions

    a. Dietary sources of folic acid should be identified for client

    b. Prolonged cooking of vegetables may destroy the folic acid present

    c. Heating can destroy the vitamin, leading to decreased bioavailability

7. Significant laboratory studies: none specific

8. Side effects: yellow discoloration of urine, nausea, altered sleep, depression, rash, and bronchospasm

9. Adverse effects/toxicity

    a. No toxic effects are reported with oral folic acid

    b. Toxicity can occur if client is on anti-epileptic therapy concurrently with vitamin B_{12} because of competition for binding sites

    c. Hemolytic anemia can occur as a result of increased utilization

10. Client-centered nursing care

    a. Clients who are pregnant should take 0.4 mg of folic acid on a daily basis as neural tube defect prophylaxis

    b. Review client medications for potential drug interactions

    c. Assess and monitor pertinent hematologic labs related to folic acid

    d. Referral to dietitian for dietary support and maintenance of folic acid levels

    e. Counsel client as to the effect that alcohol can have on folic acid levels

    f. Monitor client for potential allergic reactions to medication

    g. Therapeutic effects include improvement in lab studies and reversal of symptoms of folic acid deficiency (diarrhea, constipation, restless legs, fatigue, diffuse muscular pain, forgetfulness, and mental depression)

11. Client education

    a. Importance of neural tube prophylaxis during pregnancy

    b. Potential for increased drug interactions exist with this vitamin

    c. Repeated lab tests are necessary to monitor response to therapy

    d. Remain under close medical supervision while taking folic acid

    e. Food sources high in folic acid include such foods as green leafy vegetables, yellow fruits and vegetables, yeast, and meats

D. Epoetin alfa

1. Action and use

    a. Epoetin alfa is a recombinant form of erythropoietin that stimulates RBC production; chemically identical to erythropoietin produced in kidneys and serves same function, to promote RBC growth

    b. Used to treat clients with anemia from various causes such as renal failure, human immunodeficiency virus infection, and nonmyeloid malignancies with associated chemotherapy-induced anemia

    c. Used as a treatment measure to reduce need for blood transfusions because of its growth potential effect in clients who are undergoing surgery

    d. Ferritin and transferrin saturation levels must be adequate in order to support red blood cell formation

    e. Darbepoetin alfa is closely related to epoetin alfa and is indicated in treatment of anemia associated with cancer chemotherapy or chronic renal failure

2. Common medications

    a. Epoetin alfa dosage varies with client's situation and is calculated in units/kg; dose may range from 3 to 500 units/kg/dose three times/wk and is given subcutaneously or intravenously

      b. Darbepoetin has an extended duration of action, allowing it to be administered once weekly

3. Administration considerations

    a. Medication is refrigerated; let warm to room temperature before administration

    b. Do not use medication that is discolored or contains particulate matter

    c. Do not administer with any other solutions; medication can be administered subcutaneously or intravenously; vial contains no preservative, so unused portion must be discarded

    d. Do not shake medication as this will lead to inactivation

    e. Administration of epoetin alfa must adhere to provider protocol to avoid overdose

    f. Dosages are individualized depending on clinical condition and whether or not dialysis has been instituted

    g. Hemoglobin (Hgb) indicates client response; prescriber identifies target levels (10–12 grams/dL) and therapy is titrated to achieve target; if Hgb level rises too quickly or passes target goal, client may be at risk for developing hypertension and seizures; if Hgb does not rise in response to therapy, dose will be increased depending on adequacy of iron stores; initial effects are usually seen in 1–2 weeks, while achievement of target goal usually takes 2–3 months

    h. Hemoglobin levels should be maintained below 12 grams/dL in clients with renal failure and less than 10 grams/dL in clients with cancer to reduce risk of serious cardiovascular adverse events

    i. Therapy should be discontinued when Hgb levels are greater than 12 grams/dL in renal failure clients and when at 10 grams/dL in clients with cancer

4. Contraindications

    a. Uncontrolled hypertension or known hypersensitivity to human albumin

    b. Complicated anemia from multiple etiologies

    c. Epoetin alfa should not be used in pregnant clients unless benefits outweigh potential risks

5. Significant drug interactions

    a. The use of myelosuppressive agents can interfere with ability of epoetin alfa to work because they have an antagonistic effect; epoetin alfa is usually given following chemotherapy to avoid this effect

    b. The use of epoetin alfa is limited in that it cannot correct underlying problem associated with specific type of anemia; continued use of epoetin alfa leads to potential long-term ineffectiveness as body tries to compensate

6. Significant food interactions: use of iron supplementation is recommended with this medication and can include dietary sources and oral medications

7. Significant laboratory studies

    a. Expected to have an effect on the RBC lineage and raise the serum level, as well as the hematocrit and hemoglobin concentrations

    b. Adjustment of dosage is related to pertinent lab values such as hematocrit, and adequate iron stores; dose is usually adjusted when hematocrit is between 30 and 36%

8. Side effects

    a. Hypertension and edema

    b. Diarrhea, constipation, and nausea and vomiting

    c. Fever, joint pain, and pain at injection site

    d. Thrombocytosis, iron deficiency, sweating, and arthralgias

9. Adverse effects/toxicity

    a. Overcorrection can result in toxic levels, leading to development of polycythemia

    b. Clients can develop hypertension and seizures with toxic levels or a too rapid therapeutic response

10. Client-centered nursing care
   a. Closely monitor client's baseline hematologic labs to provide information relative to treatment response
   b. Monitor BP before initiating therapy and monitor closely during therapy
   c. Rotate injection sites to minimize discomfort
   d. Monitor client for the risk of thrombotic events, such as myocardial infarction, stroke, and transient ischemic accident (TIA), especially for clients with chronic renal failure (CRF)
   e. Follow administration protocols and monitor ongoing pertinent labs
   f. Clients who are on dialysis may require adjusted dosages caused by stress of the hemodynamic process
   g. Monitor client's iron stores (ferritin) and transferrin levels; use of additional supplementation and/or medication may be required to support effects on RBC maturation
   h. Refer to dietitian for nutritional support
   i. Monitor client's baseline vital signs and continue to monitor BP following drug administration
11. Client education
   a. Need for continued lab follow-up and possible dosage adjustment
   b. Possible side effects
   c. Premedicate if necessary with analgesics if bone pain is present or client becomes febrile
   d. Medication can be given in home setting; client can be taught to self-administer dose
   e. Importance of keeping follow-up appointments
   f. Do not drive or be involved in other hazardous activity during the first 90 days of therapy because of possible seizure activity
   g. Importance of compliance with dietary and drug therapy

Practice to Pass

A client asks if medication alone can restore adequate blood cell levels to correct anemia. What would be your best response to this client?

VI. MEDICATIONS TO LOWER SERUM CHOLESTEROL

A. HMG-coenzyme A (HMG-CoA) reductase inhibitors
1. Action and use
   a. Belong to the class of "statins" that work in liver to inhibit cholesterol synthesis
   b. Competitively inhibit this rate-limiting enzyme of mevalonate pathway in liver, which leads to a decrease in cholesterol level
   c. Used to lower LDL cholesterol levels in clients with significant cholesterol elevations and for whom diet therapy has not been effective
   d. Also have an effect on HDL cholesterol that is somewhat dose dependent; lipoprotein levels are not affected by use of statins
2. Common medications
   a. Lovastatin, simvastatin, pravastatin, and rosuvastatin are similar in nature and are isolated from fungal cultures
   b. Fluvastatin and atorvastatin are produced synthetically
   c. Refer to Table 7-8 for a listing and dosage recommendations for common medications
3. Administration considerations
   a. Administration is usually done at night
   b. This dosing schedule increases drug's effectiveness, as cholesterol synthesis normally occurs during evening hours
   c. An FDA advisory was released in 2011 recommending simvastatin 80 mg should only be used in clients who have been taking this dose for 12 or more months

Table 7-8	HMG-CoA Reductase Inhibitors	
Generic Name	**Route**	**Uses**
Atorvastatin	PO	Adjunctive therapy to reduce cholesterol, low-density lipoprotein, and triglycerides
Fluvastatin	PO	Adjunctive therapy to reduce cholesterol, low-density lipoprotein, and triglycerides; slow the progression of coronary artery disease
Lovastatin	PO	Adjunctive therapy to reduce cholesterol, low-density lipoprotein, and triglycerides
Pitavastatin	PO	Adjunctive therapy to reduce cholesterol, low-density lipoprotein, and triglycerides
Pravastatin	PO	Prevention of myocardial infarction in clients who have no increase in cholesterol, slow progression of coronary artery disease; adjunctive therapy to reduce cholesterol, low-density lipoprotein, and triglycerides
Rosuvastatin	PO	Adjunctive therapy to reduce cholesterol, low-density lipoprotein, and triglycerides
Simvastatin	PO	Prevention of myocardial infarction in clients who have no increase in cholesterol, slow progression of coronary artery disease; adjunctive therapy to reduce cholesterol, low-density lipoprotein, and triglycerides

without evidence of myopathy; clients being started on this drug should be started on lower doses

4. Contraindications
    a. Clients with active liver disease and abnormal serum transaminase levels
    b. Pregnant and nursing mothers
5. Significant drug interactions
    a. Increased risk of myositis when used concurrently with immunosuppressives, antifungal agents, fibric acid derivatives, nicotinic acid, and erythromycin
    b. Additive effects are seen when used with cholestyramine
    c. Spironolactone and cimetidine can cause decreased levels of HMG-CoA reductase inhibitors
    d. Rosuvastatin increases serum levels and toxic risk when administered with cyclosporine or gemfibrozil; increased risk of bleeding with sodium warfarin
    e. Simvastatin at any dose is contraindicated with these drugs: itraconazole, ketoconazole, posaconazole, erythromycin, clarithromycin, telithromycin, HIV protease inhibitors, nefazodone, gemfibrozil, cyclosporine, and danazol
    f. Do not exceed 10 mg of simvastatin daily with concurrent use of amiodarone, verapamil, or diltiazem; do not exceed 20 mg with concurrent use of amlodipine or ranolazine
6. Significant food interactions: none reported
7. Significant laboratory studies
    a. Baseline liver function tests (LFTs) should be obtained before starting therapy
    b. LFTs should continue to be monitored at predetermined intervals (12 weeks and with dose adjustment) to confirm response to treatment and prevent possible adverse/toxic reactions
    c. Creatinine phosphokinase (CPK) levels may be monitored to evaluate possible development of myositis
    d. Digoxin level should be monitored if taking concurrently
8. Side effects
    a. Gastrointestinal upset, dyspepsia, flatulence
    b. Pain and myalgias
    c. Headache, rash, dizziness
    d. Sinusitis

9. Adverse effects/toxicity
   a. Altered liver function tests (elevated serum transaminase levels)
   b. Clients with uncontrolled hypothyroidism are at increased risk for muscle-related statin side effects
10. Client-centered nursing care
    a. Drug selection depends on prescriber preference and client tolerance
    b. Not recommended for use in clients younger than age 20
    c. Administer dose with evening meal to coincide with body's timing of cholesterol production
    d. Monitor results of baseline and periodically drawn LFTs
    e. Monitor lipid levels within 2–4 weeks after initiation of therapy
    f. Arrange for consult, if needed, with a dietitian or nutritionist about need for a low-fat diet
11. Client education
    a. Proper self-administration (at evening meal) in order to promote biochemical activity
    b. Lab monitoring is required to maintain compliance and assess client response
    c. Report immediately to prescriber any unexplained muscle pain, tenderness, yellowing of skin or eyes, or loss of appetite
    d. Alcohol intake should be minimized or avoided
    e. Women of childbearing age should use contraceptives while taking a "statin"

B. **Bile acid sequestrants**
   1. Action and use
      a. Bile acid sequestrants are a group of nonabsorbable amine compounds that work in GI tract to bind with bile acids
      b. This binding leads liver cells to respond by sending cholesterol to maintain bile acid synthesis, thereby causing plasma levels of LDL cholesterol to decrease
      c. Indications for use include elevated cholesterol levels with or without high triglyceride levels
      d. Also used as an adjunctive therapy to dietary management of cholesterol elevations
   2. Common medications
      a. Cholestyramine and colestipol are similar in their ability to lower LDL levels
      b. Colestipol is available as a tablet or powder, 5–30 grams/day in two to four doses before meals and at bedtime
      c. Cholestyramine is available as a powder, 4 grams bid to qid before mealtimes and at bedtime; a client may need up to 24 grams/day
      d. Colesevelan hydrochloride binds with bile acids to allow excretion in feces, which lowers cholesterol; dose is up to six 625 mg tablets daily
   3. Administration considerations
      a. Colestipol tablets should not be crushed, chewed, or cut; they should be taken with adequate fluids
      b. Powdered drug forms should be mixed at bedside to prevent overthickening and esophageal obstruction; may be unflavored or orange flavored; because cholestyramine powder contains phenylalanine, it should not be used in clients who have phenylketonuria (PKU)
      c. Bile acid sequestrants should be administered alone due to potential for increased binding effects with other medications; give other drugs 1–2 hours before or 4–6 hours after bile acid administration
      d. Contents of one packet should be mixed with at least 120–180 mL of water or other preferred liquid; undissolved medication is irritating to mucous membranes

4. Contraindications
   a. Colestipol is not recommended for use in pediatric clients
   b. Contraindicated in clients with complete biliary obstruction
5. Significant drug interactions
   a. Bile acid sequestrants can bind to many other medications such as thyroxine, digoxin, diuretics, antibiotics, and warfarin; because of this, they should not be given concurrently with other medications
   b. Additive effects are seen with use of bile acids and HMG-CoA reductase inhibitors and nicotinic acid
   c. Colesevelam is contraindicated with fat-soluble vitamins
6. Significant food interactions: powdered forms must be mixed in appropriate food or fluid to maximize absorption and prevent obstruction
7. Significant laboratory studies
   a. Monitor baseline labs relative to cholesterol and triglyceride levels before starting therapy; continue to trend results to determine client response
   b. Decreased levels of LDL cholesterol should be seen within 1 month of therapy
8. Side effects
   a. Abdominal pain, bloating, reflux, constipation, steatorrhea, and hemorrhoids
   b. Associated vitamin deficiencies (A, D, K)
   c. Rash irritations of skin, tongue, and perianal areas
9. Adverse effects/toxicity
   a. Hypoprothrombinemia
   b. Decreased erythrocyte folate levels
10. Client-centered nursing care
    a. Properly mix and administer medication according to schedule to maximize biochemical activity (see also previous comments on mixing)
    b. Assess and monitor client for side effects of medication
    c. Bile acid sequestrants are not usually used as a first-line therapy to treat elevated cholesterol levels because of poor client tolerance
    d. Vitamin deficiencies may require supplementation, if not discontinuation of bile acid sequestrants, to restore normal levels
    e. Problems related to hemorrhoids and/or constipation may require intervention to provide client comfort
    f. If the client develops GI complaints, a lower dosage may be necessary in order to maintain client compliance with this drug regimen
    g. Serum cholesterol levels are reduced within 24–48 hours after initiation of therapy
    h. Long-term use of cholestyramine can increase bleeding tendency
11. Client education
    a. Properly administer and schedule medication to maximize effect
    b. Be alert for signs and symptoms indicating side effects of these agents
    c. Follow-up bloodwork will be done to monitor cholesterol levels
    d. Increase high-bulk diet with adequate fluid intake
    e. Do not omit doses
    f. Report constipation immediately
    g. Eat frequent, small meals when experiencing heartburn, nausea, or loss of appetite with colesevelam

C. Fibric acid derivatives
1. Action and use
   a. A group of compounds that affect lipoproteins
   b. Act on very low-density lipoprotein (VLDL) and chylomicrons, leading to a reduction of triglyceride levels

      c. HDL cholesterol levels are increased but not the primary effect; also a variable effect on LDL levels

      d. Indicated for treatment of elevated triglyceride levels and elevated cholesterol level that is resistant to dietary management

2. Common medications

      a. Decrease triglyceride and LDL levels and increase HDL levels

      b. Gemfibrozil is also indicated when there is an increased risk for a client to develop pancreatitis

      c. Refer to Table 7-9 for a listing of fibric acid derivatives

3. Administration considerations: dose is usually given in divided doses, 30 minutes prior to morning and evening meals

4. Contraindications

      a. Gallbladder disease, renal problems, liver or biliary cirrhosis

      b. Pregnant or nursing women

5. Significant drug interactions

      a. Drug interactions can be seen with use of anticoagulants; monitor PT or INR levels

      b. Do not use fibric-acid derivatives with statins (HMG-CoA reductase inhibitors) as rhabdomyolysis can occur

6. Significant food interactions: can cause altered taste perception

7. Significant laboratory studies

      a. Obtain baseline lipid levels prior to starting therapy; monitor ongoing labs periodically to document response to treatment

      b. If LFTs are persistently abnormal after 3 months, then therapy should be discontinued

      c. Hypokalemia may be seen in response to therapy

      d. Decreased hemoglobin, hematocrit, and white blood cell (WBC) count may be seen with the use of gemfibrozil

8. Side effects

      a. Abdominal or epigastric pain

      b. Jaundice, blurred vision, headache, and depression

      c. Rash, dermatitis, pruritus with gemfibrozil

      d. Back pain, muscle cramps, myalgia, and swollen joints

9. Adverse effects/toxicity

      a. Client may develop gallbladder disease and acute appendicitis

      b. Eosinophilia

      c. Hypokalemia

10. Client-centered nursing care

      a. Monitor baseline labs and perform ongoing assessments according to protocol

      b. If there is no response to therapy after 3 months, notify prescriber because the medication should be discontinued

      c. Monitor client for potential side effects and adverse effects

      d. Monitor closely for right upper quadrant (RUQ) abdominal pain or vomiting

11. Client education

      a. Labwork will be ongoing in nature to determine client response and evaluate for potential side effects

Table 7-9   **Fibric Acid Derivatives**

Generic Name	Route	Uses
Fenofibrate	PO	Type IV and V hyperlipidemia and hypertriglyceridemia
Gemfibrozil	PO	Reduce VLDL and triglycerides

     b. Report immediately unexplained bleeding

     c. Restrict carbohydrate and alcohol intake

     d. Notify prescriber immediately if any serious side effects, such as acute appendicitis or gallbladder disease, should occur

D. Nicotinic acid (niacin, vitamin B$_{12}$)

  1. Action and use

     a. The active form of vitamin B$_3$ (niacin) in body; water soluble

     b. Works to lower most lipoprotein levels (total cholesterol, LDL, triglyceride, and lipoproteins) and increase HDL levels

     c. Indicated for clients with high cholesterol levels and as adjunctive therapy for clients where diet management is ineffective; dosage is usually started at 1 gram tid in adults

     d. Causes peripheral vasodilation and can be used to treat clients with peripheral vascular disease

     e. Pellagra (dermatitis, diarrhea, and dementia) is the clinical deficiency state associated with niacin deficiency; the required dosage of niacin to treat pellagra is 300–500 mg/day orally in divided doses

  2. Common medications

     a. Vitamin B$_3$ is available both as a prescription and OTC medication

     b. The dosage for lowering cholesterol is higher (more than 3 grams/day) than the normal vitamin dose (500 mg/day in adults)

     c. Nicotinic acid is available in an immediate-release form as well as a sustained-release preparation

  3. Administration considerations

     a. Tablets should be taken whole; do not crush or divide the pill

     b. Medication can be taken with meals to prevent GI upset

     c. Flushing is a common side effect of niacin caused by its vasodilator properties

     d. Oral nicotinic acid should be taken with cold water

  4. Contraindications

     a. Liver disease and/or unexplained levels of elevated serum transaminases and with active peptic ulcer disease

     b. Severe hypotension

  5. Significant drug interactions

     a. Nicotinic acid should not be taken concurrently with statins, as there can be an increase in the occurrence of rhabdomyolysis

     b. Nicotinic acid may potentiate action of other drugs, such as antihypertensive and vasoactive drugs

     c. Nicotinic acid should be used cautiously with clients who are on anticoagulant therapy

     d. Clients with diabetes may need adjustment of their antidiabetic agents when taking nicotinic acid

     e. Niacin can decrease uricosuric effect of probenecid and sulfinpyrazone, leading to increased uric acid levels

     f. Niacin is often used in conjunction with bile resins to enhance effects

  6. Significant food interactions

     a. Since niacin is available in OTC preparations, there is an increased likelihood of higher dosing

     b. 60 mg of dietary tryptophan (amino acid) is necessary to convert to 1 mg of niacin in body

     c. Corn in the diet interferes with conversion of tryptophan to niacin in body

  7. Significant laboratory studies: nicotinic acid leads to increases in blood glucose, uric acid, and serum transaminase levels

   8. Side effects
   a. Flushing
   b. Postural hypotension, vasovagal attacks
   c. Pruritus, increased sebaceous gland activity
   d. Dyspepsia, epigastric pain, and nausea
   9. Adverse effects/toxicity
   a. Clients who report GI symptoms should be monitored closely for possibility of adverse reactions
   b. Shortness of breath or edema
   c. Megadose therapy has been associated with liver damage, hyperglycemia, hyperuricemia, and cardiac dysrhythmias
   10. Client-centered nursing care
   a. Administer dose as prescribed to maximize absorption and minimize potential side effects
   b. Dose is variable depending on whether it is prescribed to reduce cholesterol levels or as a vitamin supplement; be aware of specific dosing levels
   c. Expect side effect of flushing when administering medication
   d. Evaluate client for food sources that are high in niacin (dairy, meats, tuna, and egg) and assess dietary intake
   e. Review list of medications with client and determine if there are any possible drug interactions
   11. Client education
   a. Change position slowly to avoid sudden BP drop
   b. Avoid direct exposure to sunlight
   c. Flushing in face, neck, and ears may occur within 2 hours after oral ingestion and immediately after IV dose and may last several hours
   d. Follow-up labwork will be ongoing to determine response to therapy
   e. Alcohol and niacin cause increased flushing
   f. Do not self-medicate with additional sources of niacin as this can lead to overdose
   g. Premedication with aspirin or ibuprofen can reduce the adverse effect of flushing

E. Cholesterol absorption inhibitors
   1. Action and uses
   a. Ezetimibe blocks absorption of cholesterol in intestinal lumen, thereby decreasing serum cholesterol
   b. Since the liver may compensate by increasing production of cholesterol, a statin is often administered concurrently
   c. Results in decrease of total cholesterol, LDL cholesterol, and triglycerides; these effects are enhanced when taken with a statin
   d. Indicated in treatment of hypercholesterolemia
   2. Common medications
   a. The only drug in this class is ezetimibe, given once daily orally
   b. The drug Vytorin is a fixed combination of ezetimibe and simvastatin
   3. Administration considerations: avoid administering at same time as a bile acid sequestrant; administer ezetimibe 2 hours before or 4 hours following
   4. Contraindications
   a. Extensively metabolized in liver and so contraindicated in clients with severe liver impairment or elevated serum transaminases
   b. Hypersensitivity to ezetimibe
   c. Children younger than 10 years of age
   5. Significant drug interactions
   a. Bile acid sequestrants will interfere with absorption of ezetimibe
   b. Fibric acid derivatives and cyclosporine can increase ezitimibe drug levels

Practice to Pass

Why should cholesterol-lowering medications be taken at bedtime?

6. Significant food interactions; none reported
7. Significant laboratory studies
   a. Monitor baseline and periodic lipid profile, Hgb and Hct, and platelet count
   b. Monitor baseline and periodic liver function tests when used in conjunction with a statin
8. Side effects
   a. Abdominal pain, back pain, diarrhea, and arthralgia
   b. Fatigue, angioedema, myopathy, dizziness, and headache
9. Adverse effects/toxicity: increased risk for myopathy when given with statins
10. Client-centered nursing care
    a. Administer no sooner than 2 hours before or 4 hours after a bile acid sequestrant
    b. Assess for and report unexplained muscle pain
11. Client education
    a. Teach clients to store the drug at 15–30°C (59–86°F)
    b. Report unexplained muscle pain, weakness, or tenderness
    c. Females need to prevent pregnancy while taking the medication
F. **Combination agents:** some drugs contain fixed combinations of lipid-lowering agents
   1. Vytorin contains simvastatin and ezetimibe
   2. Advicor contains lovastatin and niacin
   3. Simcore contains various combinations of simvastatin and niacin

Case Study

C. W., a 48-year-old male client, is being admitted for deep vein thrombosis (DVT) of the left lower extremity and is to be placed on a weight-based heparin protocol. You are the nurse who has been assigned to take care of him.

1. Why is the weight-based heparin protocol being used for this client?

2. What pertinent lab values and diagnostic tests would help to establish therapeutic care of this client?

3. C. W. does not understand why blood tests are done so frequently, and he is becoming quite anxious. What measures can you employ to decrease C. W.'s anxiety?

4. Warfarin is now being added to the treatment regimen and within a few days, C. W. is being discharged. C. W. is concerned about "all the possible risks" associated with warfarin. What collaborative measures could you include in developing a plan of care with regard to warfarin therapy?

For suggested responses, see pages 540–541.

POSTTEST

POSTTEST

① The nurse checks the laboratory values of a client receiving chemotherapy who is scheduled to receive epoetin alfa subcutaneously. Upon finding the hemoglobin is 12.2 grams/dL, the nurse should take which actions? Select all that apply.

1. Administer the medication as prescribed.
2. Withhold the medication dose.
3. Check the client's platelet count before administering the epoetin alfa.
4. Notify the primary care provider of the client's laboratory value.
5. Assess the client for signs of internal bleeding.

2 When the client with pernicious anemia asked why vitamin B$_{12}$ injections are necessary, the nurse should provide which of the following responses?

1. "They contribute to the increased production of red blood cells (RBCs) after a significant blood loss."
2. "Vitamin B$_{12}$ is needed to prevent the red blood cells from sickling."
3. "Your stomach does not produce a substance needed for intestinal absorption of vitamin B$_{12}$."
4. "Vitamin B$_{12}$ is needed to prevent excessive production of red blood cells (RBCs)."

3 When managing the care of a client receiving intravenous (IV) anistreplase, the nurse should take which of the following actions? Select all that apply.

1. Instruct client to avoid activities that could lead to bruising or bleeding.
2. Handle client gently when turning and positioning in bed.
3. Post sign at bedside that states, "No intramuscular injections."
4. Anticipate medicating the client with ibuprofen for joint pain prn.
5. Monitor laboratory results for 50% decrease in bleeding time.

4 A client is prescribed enoxaparin 0.5 mg/kg subcutaneously. The client weighs 50 kg (110 lb) and the enoxaparin comes in a prefilled syringe containing 40 mg/mL. The nurse should prepare a dose of how many mL? Round answer to two decimal places.

_____ mL

5 The home health nurse is scheduling appointments for several clients who are taking folic acid for treatment of folic-acid anemia. Which client should have the *first* appointment?

1. Client taking vitamin B$_{12}$ (hydroxycobalamin) 100 mcg daily by subcutaneous injection for pernicious anemia
2. Client taking tetracycline 500 mg by mouth four times daily for gonorrhea
3. Client taking allopurinol 100 mg by mouth daily for hyperuricemia
4. Client taking an oral contraceptive daily

6 A client treated with heparin sodium exhibits signs and symptoms of a heparin overdose. The nurse should place priority on initiating which action?

1. Administer standard dose of 50 mg of protamine sulfate over a 10-minute period.
2. Draw client's activated partial thromboplastin time (aPTT) level during injection of protamine sulfate.
3. Determine amount of heparin infused along with time frame associated with the infusion.
4. Administer protamine sulfate concurrently with vitamin K to increase its therapeutic effect.

7 A surgical client has suddenly begun to bleed excessively while in the operating room. The nurse should prepare which medication for possible injection?

1. Alteplase
2. Aminocaproic acid
3. Dipyridamole
4. Heparin

8 The nurse anticipates a prescription to administer which drug to a client with aplastic anemia?

1. Dipyridamole
2. Allopurinol
3. Acetylsalicylic acid
4. Cyclosporine

9 The nurse should teach which item of information to a client being discharged on long-term warfarin therapy following cardiac valve replacement surgery?

1. Eat lettuce and tomatoes for lunch only a few times per week.
2. Limit dietary intake of yellow wax beans to twice weekly.
3. Use aspirin for minor aches and pains.
4. Wear shoes that completely enclose the feet.

10 The nurse is monitoring the activated partial thromboplastin time (aPTT) for a client receiving heparin therapy. When the latest aPTT is 2.0 times the normal aPTT, the nurse should perform which action based on this result?

1. Assess for bleeding gums after toothbrushing is complete.
2. Perform a test for occult blood on stool.
3. Assess client for abnormal bruising.
4. Report the value during intershift report.

➤ *See pages 243–244 for Answers and Rationales.*

ANSWERS & RATIONALES

Pretest

1 **Answer: 4** **Rationale:** Oranges and lemons are high in vitamin C, which will enhance absorption of the iron supplement. Green leafy vegetables, whole-grain breads, and raisins are high in iron, but would not enhance the absorption of the medication. **Cognitive Level:** Applying **Client Need:** Pharmacological and Parenteral Therapies **Integrated Process:** Nursing Process: Planning **Content Area:** Pharmacology **Strategy:** Note the critical words in the question are *enhance absorption*. Differentiate the foods that may be sources of iron from the one that is most likely to promote absorption of the iron supplements. **Reference:** Adams, M., Holland, L., & Urban, C. (2017). *Pharmacology for nurses: A pathophysiologic approach* (5th ed.). New York, NY: Pearson, p. 493.

2 **Answer: 4** **Rationale:** A change in clotting is a side effect of antiplatelet drugs. Clients may bruise from minor injuries more readily while receiving antiplatelet therapy. It is important to know how the client previously responded to injury and how he or she does now in order to determine whether the risk for bleeding is increased. Adherence is important but not as relevant as the client's response to therapy. Self-monitoring is an important general safety measure, but data indicating whether bruising has changed helps the nurse determine if the client is at risk. **Cognitive Level:** Applying **Client Need:** Pharmacological and Parenteral Therapies **Integrated Process:** Nursing Process: Assessment **Content Area:** Pharmacology **Strategy:** To choose correctly, you need to determine if the bruise is related to the drug. **Reference:** Adams, M., Holland, L., & Urban, C. (2017). *Pharmacology for nurses: A pathophysiologic approach* (5th ed.). New York, NY: Pearson, pp. 464–466.

3 **Answer: 1** **Rationale:** Ferritin levels reflect the visceral stores of iron in the body. Transferrin levels reflect how iron is transported in the body. Hemoglobin and hematocrit refer to concentration and proportion of red blood cells. The CBC will provide information about blood concentration of all three cell lines (red blood cells, white blood cells, and platelets). **Cognitive Level:** Applying **Client Need:** Pharmacological and Parenteral Therapies **Integrated Process:** Nursing Process: Assessment **Content Area:** Pharmacology **Strategy:** Recall concepts related to physiology and associated drug therapy to choose correctly. **Reference:** Adams, M., Holland, L., & Urban, C. (2017). *Pharmacology for nurses: A pathophysiologic approach* (5th ed.). New York, NY: Pearson, p. 493.

4 **Answers: 1, 2, 5** **Rationale:** Alteplase is a thrombolytic drug that can cause internal bleeding, and vital signs should be monitored closely in the first hour following administration. After dissolution of clots, the heart may respond to reperfusion by developing dysrhythmias, so the client should be placed on a cardiac monitor. Alteplase interferes with clot formation and would produce an increase in the partial thromboplastin time, which should be reported to monitor effects on coagulation. Hourly urinary outputs are not necessary when administering alteplase. **Cognitive Level:** Applying **Client Need:** Pharmacological and Parenteral Therapies **Integrated Process:** Nursing Process: Planning **Content Area:** Pharmacology **Strategy:** Recall first that this drug dissolves clots and evaluate each option to determine the likelihood of each as a consequence of the drug's action. Choose options that relate to bleeding as a primary adverse effect, pertinent effects on cardiac rhythm, and laboratory test results. **Reference:** Wilson, B., Shannon, M., & Shields, K. (2017). *Pearson nurse's drug guide 2017*. New York, NY: Pearson, pp. 55–56.

5 **Answer: 3** **Rationale:** The target goal with epoetin alfa therapy is a hemoglobin level of 10–12 grams/dL and reflects effectiveness of therapy. Bone pain is an adverse effect to epoetin alfa therapy, but the absence of bone pain does not guarantee drug efficacy. A rapid rise in hemoglobin and hematocrit (H&H) is undesirable as it can lead to hypertension and seizures, and it would not reflect an effective therapeutic response. Fever is an adverse response to epoetin alfa, but being afebrile does not guarantee the drug is effective at raising the client's H&H. **Cognitive Level:** Analyzing **Client Need:** Pharmacological and Parenteral Therapies **Integrated Process:** Nursing Process: Evaluation **Content Area:** Pharmacology **Strategy:** Since erythropoietin is produced by the kidneys, *poetin* is an important suffix that should help guide your thinking toward altered hematology. **Reference:** Wilson, B., Shannon, M., & Shields, K. (2017). *Pearson nurse's drug guide 2017*. New York, NY: Pearson, pp. 432–435.

6 **Answers: 2, 5 Rationale:** Facial flushing is a common side effect of niacin, and it occurs shortly after ingesting the drug. Administering aspirin 30 minutes prior to taking niacin can help to reduce this effect. Over time, the flushing will be reduced, but taking the aspirin can help to reduce this very bothersome side effect. Dosages may be adjusted if the client develops side effects; they are not based on lab values. It is not necessary to eat a diet high in niacin in order for the medication to be effective. The medication is given to improve lipid levels, but taking niacin with lovastatin can increase the risk for myopathy and should be avoided. **Cognitive Level:** Applying **Client Need:** Pharmacological and Parenteral Therapies **Integrated Process:** Teaching and Learning **Content Area:** Pharmacology **Strategy:** The wording of the question indicates that the correct response provides true information related to niacin use. Recall the drug's action and side effects to choose correctly. **Reference:** Wilson, B., Shannon, M., & Shields, K. (2017). *Pearson nurse's drug guide 2017*. New York, NY: Pearson, pp. 1097–1098.

7 **Answers: 1, 2, 3, 4 Rationale:** In the treatment of von Willebrand disease, desmopressin stimulates an increase in clotting factors vW and VIII. Desmopressin is the hormone vasopressin, or antidiuretic hormone (ADH), which promotes water reabsorption in the renal tubules. If an excessive amount of drug is used, the client may retain water, and urine output will decrease while the blood pressure could increase. Cryoprecipitate is not used to treat von Willebrand disease since it cannot be filtered safely for HIV. **Cognitive Level:** Analyzing **Client Need:** Pharmacological and Parenteral Therapies **Integrated Process:** Communication and Documentation **Content Area:** Pharmacology **Strategy:** The wording of the question indicates the correct options are true statements. Specific drug knowledge is needed to answer this question, so review it now if needed. **Reference:** Wilson, B., Shannon, M., & Shields, K. (2017). *Pearson nurse's drug guide 2017*. New York, NY: Pearson, pp. 455–456.

8 **Answer: 4 Rationale:** Ibuprofen has an antiplatelet effect and can lead to bleeding as an adverse effect; this would further decrease the platelet count and increase risk of bleeding. Ibuprofen does not affect ferritin levels, although low ferritin levels reflect iron stores, which could indirectly affect bleeding risk. Ibuprofen may be taken when triglyceride levels are low. Low neutrophil counts will affect immune response, but does not necessitate a need to avoid using ibuprofen. **Cognitive Level:** Analyzing **Client Need:** Pharmacological and Parenteral Therapies **Integrated Process:** Teaching and Learning **Content Area:** Pharmacology **Strategy:** Correlate the adverse effect (bleeding) of ibuprofen with the function of platelets to make the correct selection. **Reference:** Wilson, B., Shannon, M., & Shields, K. (2017). *Pearson nurse's drug guide 2017*. New York, NY: Pearson, pp. 790–791.

9 **Answers: 2, 5 Rationale:** After cardiac valve replacement surgery, safe management requires life-long anticoagulation therapy. Clients must be instructed regarding bleeding risks as well as how to modify their environment and activities of daily living accordingly. Follow-up lab testing is required but initially would be weekly or every other week, rather than every 3 months. Warfarin should be taken at the same time of day. Clients are instructed not to double-up doses and to take the medication as specifically ordered to ensure safe and therapeutic effects. Clients should eat a consistent amount of foods containing vitamin K daily. Large amounts of foods high in vitamin K can interfere with the action of warfarin and reduce effectiveness. **Cognitive Level:** Applying **Client Need:** Pharmacological and Parenteral Therapies **Integrated Process:** Teaching and Learning **Content Area:** Pharmacology **Strategy:** Recall that the major adverse effect of anticoagulants is bleeding. With this in mind, select the option that minimizes the risk of bleeding, which is also directly related to the critical term *protection* in the question. **Reference:** Wilson, B., Shannon, M., & Shields, K. (2017). *Pearson nurse's drug guide 2017*. New York, NY: Pearson, pp. 1661–1662.

10 **Answer: 3 Rationale:** The rate of administration must be closely monitored since heparin affects blood clotting. The client could receive a subtherapeutic dose or be at increased risk for bleeding if the infusion was infused too slowly or too quickly, respectively. Vitamin K is the antidote for warfarin therapy, not heparin, and it is not standard policy in most institutions to leave medications at the bedside. Heparin does not require the client to be NPO during IV infusion. Heparin infusion therapies are weight based, and daily weights provide more accurate dosing. **Cognitive Level:** Applying **Client Need:** Pharmacological and Parenteral Therapies **Integrated Process:** Nursing Process: Planning **Content Area:** Pharmacology **Strategy:** Identify the drug action and the risk to the client, and then determine the nursing action that would best protect the client. The core underlying issue is safety during administration of this medication. **Reference:** Wilson, B., Shannon, M., & Shields, K. (2017). *Pearson nurse's drug guide 2017*. New York, NY: Pearson, pp. 760–761.

Posttest

1 **Answers: 2, 4 Rationale:** The dose should not be administered as the hemoglobin has surpassed the target level. When hemoglobin levels are above 12 grams/dL in clients with renal failure and above 10 grams/dL in clients receiving chemotherapy and epoetin alfa is continued, the client is at greater risk to experience serious adverse events, such as heart attack, stroke, and death. The primary care provider should be notified. There is no need to assess for bleeding. Epoetin alfa does not affect platelet levels. **Cognitive Level:** Analyzing **Client Need:** Pharmacological and Parenteral Therapies **Integrated Process:** Nursing Process: Assessment **Content Area:** Pharmacology **Strategy:** First recall the target hemoglobin levels for a client on chemotherapy who is receiving epoetin alfa. Then determine if it is safe to administer the medication to this client. **Reference:** Wilson, B., Shannon, M., & Shields, K. (2017). *Pearson nurse's drug guide 2017*. New York, NY: Pearson, pp. 432–435.

2 **Answer: 3 Rationale:** Intrinsic factor, produced in the stomach, is needed for absorption of vitamin B_{12} Because vitamin B_{12} activates an enzyme that moves folic acid into the cells to contribute to the production of red blood cells, deficiencies of the intrinsic factor results in anemia. Pernicious anemia is due to this absence of intrinsic factor. Significant blood losses are usually replaced with blood transfusions and iron supplements. Sickle cell anemia is treated with hydroxyurea rather than vitamin B_{12}. vitamin B_{12} does not prevent excessive production of red blood cells. **Cognitive Level:** Applying **Client Need:** Pharmacological and Parenteral Therapies **Integrated Process:** Teaching and Learning **Content Area:** Pharmacology **Strategy:** Select the option that remedies the interruption caused by the disease. **Reference:** LeMone, P., Burke, K., Bauldoff, G., & Gubrud, P. (2015). *Medical surgical nursing: Clinical reasoning in patient care* (6th ed.). New York, NY: Pearson, p. 1016.

3 **Answers: 1, 2, 3 Rationale:** Because of the risk of bleeding with infusion of thrombolytic drugs such as anistreplase, vigorous activities or activities that could cause bleeding are discouraged. The client should be moved gently to reduce risk of bleeding. Because of the risk of bleeding, IM injections should be avoided. The client needs to avoid drugs that would prolong bleeding time, such as ibuprofen and aspirin. The client's bleeding time would be increased rather than decreased following administration of a thrombolytic medication. **Cognitive Level:** Applying **Client Need:** Pharmacological and Parenteral Therapies **Integrated Process:** Teaching and Learning **Content Area:** Pharmacology **Strategy:** Associate the drug's action with the greatest risks to the client. **Reference:** Adams, M., Holland, L., & Urban, C. (2017). *Pharmacology for nurses: A pathophysiologic approach* (5th ed.). New York, NY: Pearson, pp. 473–477.

4 **Answer: 0.63 Rationale:** The dose is ordered in mg/kg, so the weight of 110 lb is divided by 2.2 kg/lb, to yield a weight of 50 kg. The ordered dose is 0.5 mg/kg, so 50 multiplied by $0.5\ mg\ =\ 25\ mg$. Use the equation

$$\frac{Desired}{Have} \times 1\ mL$$

$$\frac{25\ mg}{40\ mg} \times 1 = \frac{20}{45}$$

$$= 25x = 40$$

$$x = .625$$

Round appropriately to two decimal places to obtain 0.63 mL. **Cognitive Level:** Applying **Client Need:** Pharmacological and Parenteral Therapies **Integrated Process:** Nursing Process: Implementation **Content Area:** Pharmacology **Strategy:** First recognize the need to convert the client's weight in pounds to kilograms. Then use the "desired over have times quantity" equation to calculate the correct dose. **Reference:** Adams, M., Holland, L., & Urban, C. (2017). *Pharmacology for nurses: A pathophysiologic approach* (5th ed.). New York, NY: Pearson, p. 883.

5 **Answer: 4 Rationale:** Oral contraceptives taken concurrently with folic acid will diminish the effectiveness of the folic acid. Therefore, this client needs the first appointment to determine that drug therapy is effective. Vitamin B_{12} enhances the effects of folic acid, so this client is likely to have a more optimal outcome initially. There are no known negative drug interactions between tetracycline and folic acid or allopurinol and folic acid. **Cognitive Level:** Applying **Client Need:** Pharmacological and Parenteral Therapies **Integrated Process:** Nursing Process: Planning **Content Area:** Pharmacology **Strategy:** The client who should be seen first is the one who is less likely to have a good outcome of therapy or is more at risk for drug interactions. Select the client who correlates best with negative outcomes associated with the drug. **Reference:** Wilson, B., Shannon, M., & Shields, K. (2017). *Pearson nurse's drug guide 2017*. New York, NY: Pearson, pp. 704–705.

6 **Answer: 3 Rationale:** Because protamine has a longer half-life than heparin (protamine 2 hr and heparin 90 minutes) and also has some anticoagulant qualities, the dose of protamine needs to be titrated according to the amount and length of time the heparin was administered. This intervention *precedes* relevant assessment parameters. Monitoring aPTT levels *after* injection of protamine sulfate is the appropriate method for determining effectiveness. Protamine sulfate is the antidote for heparin and vitamin K is the antidote for warfarin; both medications would not be given together. **Cognitive Level:** Analyzing **Client Need:** Pharmacological and Parenteral Therapies **Integrated Process:** Nursing Process: Implementation **Content Area:** Pharmacology **Strategy:** The critical issue of the question is the need to know the antidote specifically associated with heparin,

ANSWERS & RATIONALES

which is protamine sulfate, and data needed for proper dosing. **Reference:** Wilson, B., Shannon, M., & Shields, K. (2017). *Pearson nurse's drug guide 2017.* New York, NY: Pearson, pp. 1335–1336.

7 **Answer: 2** **Rationale:** Hemostatics such as aminocaproic acid are used to control excessive bleeding. They may be applied topically to stop a local hemorrhage or they can be administered parenterally to stop a systemic hemorrhage. Alteplase is a thrombolytic agent and would cause further bleeding. Dipyridamole is an antiplatelet agent used to prevent platelet aggregation and could increase the risk of bleeding. Heparin is an anticoagulant given to prolong the time it takes for blood to clot; it would be contraindicated in a client who is actively bleeding. **Cognitive Level:** Applying **Client Need:** Pharmacological and Parenteral Therapies **Integrated Process:** Nursing Process: Planning **Content Area:** Pharmacology **Strategy:** Differentiate between drugs that cause bleeding and drugs that would reduce bleeding. The correct answer is the drug that reduces bleeding. **Reference:** Wilson, B., Shannon, M., & Shields, K. (2017). *Pearson nurse's drug guide 2017.* New York, NY: Pearson, pp. 69–70.

8 **Answer: 4** **Rationale:** Cyclosporine is used in the treatment of aplastic anemia. It works by preventing destruction of the stem cells by lymphocytes. Dipyridamole is prescribed for clients with polycythemia vera to prevent the increased viscosity resulting from the excessively high numbers of red blood cells. Allopurinol is administered to treat the signs and symptoms of gout associated with polycythemia vera. Acetylsalicylic acid would be contraindicated in the treatment of anemia since it interferes with platelets and can cause gastric bleeding. **Cognitive Level:** Applying **Client Need:** Pharmacological and Parenteral Therapies **Integrated Process:** Nursing Process: Planning **Content Area:** Pharmacology **Strategy:** Correlate the drug with the nature of the disease. **Reference:** Wilson, B.,

Shannon, M., & Shields, K. (2017). *Pearson nurse's drug guide 2017.* New York, NY: Pearson, pp. 405–406.

9 **Answer: 4** **Rationale:** Clients on oral anticoagulant therapy are at increased risk of bleeding and should wear shoes to protect them from possible injury. Lettuce, tomatoes, and yellow wax beans do not contain enough vitamin K to interact negatively with warfarin, so they do not need to be limited. Aspirin increases the risk of bleeding and therefore should not be used while taking an anticoagulant such as warfarin. **Cognitive Level:** Analyzing **Client Need:** Pharmacological and Parenteral Therapies **Integrated Process:** Teaching and Learning **Content Area:** Pharmacology **Strategy:** Recall that warfarin is an anticoagulant that carries an increased risk of bleeding. Select the option that provides the client with the greatest amount of protection against this risk. **Reference:** Wilson, B., Shannon, M., & Shields, K. (2017). *Pearson nurse's drug guide 2017.* New York, NY: Pearson, pp. 1661–1662.

10 **Answer: 4** **Rationale:** Since the therapeutic range for APTT level should be 1.5–2.5 times the control value, no action is necessary and the nurse would provide routine care, including reporting the expected value to the oncoming shift. Monitoring for bleeding gums and excessive or abnormal bruising should be done without regard to the aPTT. Testing for occult blood is a preventative mechanism that would not be related to the therapeutic aPTT range. **Cognitive Level:** Applying **Client Need:** Pharmacological and Parenteral Therapies **Integrated Process:** Nursing Process: Implementation **Content Area:** Pharmacology **Strategy:** The core issue of the question is the appropriate range for activated partial thromboplastin time (aPTT) during anticoagulant therapy. Recall the normal range and use the process of elimination to select the option that reflects ordinary care. **Reference:** Wilson, B., Shannon, M., & Shields, K. (2017). *Pearson nurse's drug guide 2017.* New York, NY: Pearson, p. 762.

References

Adams, M., Holland, L., & Urban, C. (2017). *Pharmacology for nurses: A pathophysiologic approach* (5th ed.). New York, NY: Pearson.

Adams, M. P., & Urban, C. (2016). *Pharmacology: Connections to nursing practice* (3rd ed.). New York, NY: Pearson.

Burchum, J., & Rosenthal, L. (2016). *Lehne's pharmacology for nursing care* (9th ed.). St. Louis, MO: Mosby.

Drug Facts & Comparisons (updated monthly). St. Louis, MO: A. Wolters Kluwer.

Frandsen, G., & Pennington, S. (2017). *Abram's clinical drug therapy: Rationales for nursing practice* (10th ed.). Philadelphia, PA: Lippincott Williams & Wilkins.

Karch, A. M. (2016). *Focus on nursing pharmacology* (7th ed.). Philadelphia, PA: Lippincott Williams & Wilkins.

Kee, J. (2017). *Pearson's laboratory and diagnostic tests with nursing implications* (8th ed.). New York, NY: Pearson.

LeMone, P., Burke, K., Bauldoff, G., & Gubrud, P. (2015). *Medical surgical*

nursing: Clinical reasoning in patient care (6th ed.). New York, NY: Pearson.

Lilley, L. L., Rainforth Collins, S., & Snyder, K. M. (2017). *Pharmacology and the nursing process* (8th ed.). St. Louis, MO: Mosby.

Vallerand, A. H., Sanoski, C. A., & Deglin, J. H. (2017). *Davis's drug guide for nurses* (8th ed.). Philadelphia, PA: F.A. Davis.

Wilson, B., Shannon, M., & Shields, K. (2017). *Pearson nurse's drug guide 2017.* New York, NY: Pearson.

Renal System Medications

8

Chapter Outline

Diuretics
Potassium Supplements
Urinary Anti-infectives and
    Antispasmodics

Medications to Treat Benign
    Prostatic Hyperplasia (BPH)
Medication to Increase Renal
    Perfusion

Hematopoietic Growth Factor
    in Renal Failure

Objectives

➤ Describe general goals of therapy when administering renal
    system medications.
➤ Describe actions, side effects, and adverse effects of commonly
    used diuretics.
➤ Discriminate between potassium-losing and potassium-sparing
    diuretics.
➤ Identify significant laboratory values to monitor in the client taking
    a diuretic.
➤ Explore client adherence concerns related to self-administration of
    diuretic and other urinary medications.
➤ Describe actions, side effects, and adverse effects of commonly
    used urinary anti-infectives, antispasmodics, and analgesics.
➤ Identify client teaching points related to medications prescribed for
    benign prostatic hyperplasia.
➤ Describe rationale for medications prescribed to treat acute and
    chronic renal failure.
➤ Identify significant client education points related to renal system
    medications.

> ### NCLEX-RN® Test Prep
>
> Access the NEW Web-based app
> that provides students with additional
> practice questions in preparation
> for the NCLEX experience.

Review at a Glance

anuria absence of urination and urine
production (less than 400 mL/day)
**benign prostatic hyperplasia
(BPH)** a symptom complex defined as
benign adenomatous hyperplasia of peri-
urethral prostate gland
bactericidal destroying or killing
bacteria

bacteriostatic causing inhibition of
bacterial growth without their destruction
diuretic an agent that increases
amount of urine excreted
orthostatic hypotension a blood
pressure fall of more than 10–15 mmHg
systolic pressure or a fall of more than

10 mmHg diastole pressure and a 10–20%
increase in heart rate
vasodilation widening of blood vessels in response to an internal stimulus
(such as nervous system) or an external
stimulus (such as heat)

PRETEST

1 A client who is starting medication therapy with furosemide 20 mg PO daily asks the nurse what would be the best time of day to take the pill. What time should the nurse recommend?

1. 8:00 a.m.
2. 12 noon
3. 6:00 p.m.
4. At bedtime

2 A client with hypertension and diabetes mellitus is taking hydrochlorothiazide. The client reports onset of an enlarged, red, painful right great toe soon after beginning therapy with this medication. The home health nurse should request a prescription from the healthcare provider for which serum laboratory test?

1. Uric acid level
2. Alanine aminotransferase
3. Serum glucose
4. Serum sodium

3 A client who is taking hydralazine has also been started on drug therapy with amiloride. Which change in client data should the nurse attribute to the interactive effects of these medications?

1. Urine output increase from 40 to 75 mL/hr
2. Pulse rate decrease from 100/min to 85/min
3. Blood pressure decrease from 140 to 120 mmHg when standing
4. Oxygen saturation increase from 90% to 95% on room air

4 The nurse should anticipate that mannitol may be prescribed to reduce symptoms in clients recently admitted to the unit with which conditions? Select all that apply.

1. Pancreatitis
2. Increased intracranial pressure
3. Diarrhea
4. Increased intraocular pressure
5. Congestive heart failure

5 A client is admitted with muscle cramps and frequent premature ventricular contractions associated with hypokalemia. When the client is prescribed a continuous IV infusion containing potassium chloride, the nurse should verify that the infusion rate does not exceed how many milliequivalents (mEq) of potassium per hour? Provide a numerical answer.

Answer: _____

6 A client has been started on medication therapy with nitrofurantoin as chronic suppressive therapy for urinary tract infection. What statements should the nurse include when teaching the client about this medication? Select all that apply.

1. "This medication causes a harmless brown color to the urine."
2. "You should greatly increase your daily fluid intake to about 3 liters/day."
3. "Monitor your urine for cloudiness or foul smell."
4. "Promptly report muscle weakness, tingling, or numbness to the prescriber."
5. "Nausea can be a common side effect of this medication."

7 A client is prescribed trimethoprim. The nurse should assess for changes in which laboratory test to determine possible adverse effects of the drug?

1. Potassium level
2. White blood cell count
3. Uric acid level
4. Serum osmolality

8 The healthcare provider prescribed oxybutynin for a 65-year-old female with urinary frequency and urgency. The nurse should include which instruction to manage a primary side effect when providing medication instruction?

1. "Wear protective underwear."
2. "Avoid activities that may cause injury or bleeding."
3. "Carry an over-the-counter antidiarrheal agent when traveling."
4. "Rinse your mouth or use sugarless hard candy frequently."

9 Because finasteride was prescribed for a 45-year-old man, the nurse should include which priority instruction during a teaching session about the medication?

1. "Use a contraceptive barrier during sexual intercourse."
2. "Sexual performance level may decrease."
3. "Increase daily fluid intake."
4. "Take the drug for 1 month."

10 A client with chronic renal failure is beginning drug therapy with epoetin alfa. The nurse should monitor the trend of which vital sign to detect an adverse effect of this medication?

1. Temperature
2. Pulse
3. Blood pressure
4. Oxygen saturation

➤ *See pages 266–268 for Answers and Rationales.*

I. DIURETICS

A. Loop diuretics

1. Action and use
   a. **Diuretics** (agents that increase amount of urine excreted) inhibit electrolyte reabsorption in thick ascending loop of Henle (Figure 8-1), thereby promoting excretion of sodium, water, chloride, and potassium
   b. Antihypertensive action involves renal **vasodilation** (dilation or widening of vessels), to provide a temporary increase in glomerular filtration rate (GFR) and a decrease in peripheral vascular resistance
   c. Loop diuretics are more potent than thiazide diuretics, causing rapid diuresis; this leads to a reduction in vascular fluid volume, cardiac output, and blood pressure (BP)
   d. Loop diuretics are considered to be "high-ceiling" diuretics, which means dosage can be raised to a greater extent to cause diuresis
   e. They are used in clients with low GFR and hypertensive emergencies
   f. They are also used in clients with edema, pulmonary edema, heart failure (HF), chronic renal failure (CRF), and hepatic cirrhosis
   g. They may be used as treatment in drug overdose to increase renal elimination
2. Common loop diuretic medications (Table 8-1)
3. Administration considerations
   a. Take early in day to avoid nocturia
   b. Give intravenous (IV) doses at recommended rates; rapid injection may cause hypotension
   c. For IV infusion, dilute in 5% dextrose in water, 0.9% sodium chloride (NaCl), or lactated Ringers; use infusion fluids within 24 hours
   d. Administer IV furosemide slowly, as hearing loss can occur if injected rapidly
4. Contraindications: anuria, electrolyte depletion

Figure 8-1

Site of action of diuretics.

Source: Blamb/Shutterstock

Nephron sites of action of diuretics

Table 8-1	**Loop Diuretics**			
Generic Name	**Route**	**Uses**		**Adverse Effects**
Bumetanide	PO, IV	Hypertension, heart failure, hepatic failure, renal failure, postoperative edema		Dizziness, orthostatic hypotension, hypokalemia, hyponatremia, dehydration, ototoxicity (tinnitus, hearing loss)
Furosemide	PO, IV	Acute pulmonary edema, edema, heart failure, chronic renal impairment, hypertension, hypercalcemia		
Torsemide	PO, IV	Heart failure, chronic renal impairment, hepatic cirrhosis, hypertension		

5. Significant drug interactions
   a. Interact with aminoglycosides causing ototoxicity
   b. Interact with digoxin (increase digoxin-induced dysrhythmias), indomethacin, lithium, salicylates, and nonsteroidal anti-inflammatory drugs (NSAIDs), which may decrease efficacy of loop diuretic, tubocurarine, succinylcholine, or antihypertensives
   c. An additive effect with thiazide diuretics and thiazidelike diuretics
   d. Interact with anticoagulants (increase anticoagulant activity), propranolol (increase plasma levels of propranolol), sulfonylureas (hyperglycemia), cisplatin (ototoxicity), and probenecid
   e. Increase risk for lithium toxicity
6. Significant food interactions: licorice may lead to added loss of potassium

7. Significant laboratory studies
   a. Monitor for electrolyte imbalance, especially sodium and potassium
   b. Monitor hemoglobin and hematocrit for increase due to hemoconcentration; monitor platelet count
   c. Monitor for blood dyscrasias, liver, or kidney damage
   d. Monitor blood glucose levels and lipids for possible drug interaction
   e. Monitor lithium levels, if taking lithium for elevation

8. Side effects
   a. CNS: dizziness, headache, orthostatic hypotension, weakness
   b. GI: nausea and vomiting, abdominal pain, elevated lipids with decreased high-density lipoprotein (HDL), pancreatitis, anorexia, constipation
   c. GU: excessive urination, nocturia, urinary bladder spasms
   d. Photosensitivity, sulfonamide allergy, and ototoxicity (tinnitus, hearing impairment, deafness, vertigo, and sense of fullness in ears)
   e. Skin: dermatitis, urticaria, pruritis, and muscle spasm

9. Adverse effects/toxicity
   a. Electrolyte imbalances: hyponatremia, hypochloremia, hypokalemia, hypomagnesemia, hypocalcemia, and hyperuricemia
   b. Thrombocytopenia, systemic vasculitis, interstitial nephritis, thrombophlebitis, agranulocytosis, and aplastic anemia

10. Client-centered nursing care
   a. Monitor vital signs for hypotension and tachycardia
   b. Monitor serum electrolytes, calcium, and uric acid levels
   c. Monitor and record body weight at regular intervals at same time of day and same scale
   d. Monitor intake and output (I&O)
   e. Assess indicators of dehydration: thirst, poor skin turgor, coated tongue
   f. Assess for inadequate tissue perfusion and weakness, decreased muscle strength, restlessness, anxiety, and agitation

11. Client education
   a. Eat foods high in potassium (such as bananas, cantaloupe) to prevent hypokalemia
   b. Restrict sodium intake; do not use salt substitutes if taking potassium supplement
   c. Avoid dehydration by avoiding alcohol and caffeine beverages and replacing fluids during exercise or hot weather
   d. Avoid exposure to intense heat as with baths, showers, and electric blankets
   e. Take small, frequent amounts of ice chips or clear liquids if vomiting
   f. Replace fluids with fruit juice or bouillon if experiencing diarrhea
   g. Diuretics increase amount and frequency of urination, so take medication in morning and afternoon (if twice daily dosing) to avoid nighttime urination
   h. Photosensitivity can occur while taking a loop diuretic
   i. Change position slowly to avoid dizziness and **orthostatic hypotension** (a BP fall of more than 10–15 mmHg systolic or more than 10 mmHg diastolic and a 10–20% increase in heart rate)
   j. Weigh self daily and report sudden weight gains or losses
   k. Report ringing in ears immediately, as this could be a sign of ototoxicity
   l. Do not use loop diuretics while breastfeeding
   m. Eliminate licorice from diet to decrease risk of hypokalemia

B. Thiazide and thiazidelike diuretics
   1. Action and uses
      a. Increased urinary excretion of sodium and water by inhibiting sodium reabsorption in distal convoluted tubule of kidney

---

Practice to Pass

The home healthcare nurse is visiting an older adult client who has been prescribed furosemide. Knowing that ototoxicity is an adverse effect of loop diuretics, what symptoms should the nurse teach the client to report?

      b. Its hypotensive effect may be due to direct arteriolar vasodilation and decreased total peripheral resistance

      c. Used for edema and hypertension (persistent elevation of systolic BP above 140 mmHg and diastolic BP above 90 mmHg)

      d. Not effective for immediate diuresis

  2. Common thiazide and thiazidelike diuretic medications (Table 8-2)

  3. Administration considerations

      a. Administer medication early in day to avoid nocturia

      b. Administer with food or milk to prevent GI upset

      c. Thiazide diuretics are ineffective if creatinine clearance level is less than 30 mL/min

      d. Allow 2–4 weeks for maximum antihypertensive effect

      e. Metolazone is not recommended in children because safety has not been established

Table 8-2   **Common Thiazide and Thiazidelike Diuretics**

Generic Name	Route	Uses	Adverse Effects
Bendroflumethiazide	PO	Edema, congestive heart failure (CHF), calcium nephrolithiasis	Dizziness, vertigo, paresthesia, orthostatic hypotension, headache, blurred vision, photosensitivity, hyperglycemia, hyperuricemia, pancreatitis, gout, impotence, loss of libido
Chlorothiazide	PO, IV	CHF, cirrhosis, corticosteroid and estrogen therapy, hypertension, diabetes insipidus, reduction of osteoporosis	Dizziness, vertigo, paresthesia, orthostatic hypotension, photosensitivity, rash, purpura, nausea, hyperglycemia, hyperuricemia, pancreatitis, gout, impotence, loss of libido
Chlorthalidone	PO	CHF, cirrhosis, corticosteroid and estrogen therapy, hypertension, renal insufficiency	Dizziness, vertigo, paresthesia, fatigue, drowsiness, volume depletion, cardiac dysrhythmia, polyuria, nocturia, nausea, anorexia, diarrhea, constipation, leucopenia, agranulocytosis, pancreatitis, gouty attacks, fluid and electrolyte imbalance
Hydrochlorothiazide	PO	CHF, cirrhosis, corticosteroid and estrogen therapy, hypertension, renal insufficiency	Dizziness, vertigo, paresthesia, orthostatic hypotension, photosensitivity, rash, purpura, nausea, hyperglycemia, hyperuricemia, pancreatitis, gout, impotence, loss of libido
Indapamide	PO	Edema associated with CHF, hypertension, diabetes insipidus	Dizziness, vertigo, paresthesia, weakness, headache, fatigue, volume depletion, dysrhythmia, photosensitivity, nausea, constipation, pancreatitis, polyuria, leukopenia, hypokalemia, gout, muscle cramps
Methyclothiazide	PO	Edema associated with CHF, hypertension, diabetes insipidus	Dizziness, vertigo, paresthesia, weakness, headache, fatigue, volume depletion, dysrhythmia, photosensitivity, nausea, constipation, pancreatitis, polyuria, leukopenia, hypokalemia, gout, muscle cramps
Metolazone	PO	Edema, CHF, hypertension, calcium nephrolithiasis	Dizziness, vertigo, paresthesia, weakness, headache, fatigue, volume depletion, dysrhythmia, photosensitivity, nausea, constipation, pancreatitis, polyuria, leukopenia, hypokalemia, gout, muscle cramps

    4. Contraindications

        a. Hypersensitivity to thiazide diuretics or sulfonamide derivatives

        b. Clients with anuria

        c. Use cautiously in client with severely impaired renal or hepatic function

        d. Contraindicated in pregnancy; women who breastfeed should not use thiazide diuretics

    5. Significant drug interactions

        a. Concomitant use with lithium will increase serum lithium levels

        b. Thiazide diuretics decrease effectiveness of hyperuricemic agents, sulfonylureas, and insulin

        c. There is an additive effect if used with loop diuretics

        d. NSAIDs cause a decreased thiazide diuretic effect

        e. Bile acid resins decrease absorption of thiazide diuretics

        f. Thiazide diuretics may increase hypersensitivity to allopurinol

    6. Significant food interactions: none reported

    7. Significant laboratory studies

        a. May alter serum electrolytes, especially lowering potassium

        b. May increase serum urate, glucose, cholesterol, triglycerides, blood urea nitrogen (BUN), and creatinine

        c. May interfere with tests for parathyroid function

        d. Decreased protein-bound iodine levels without thyroid dysfunction

    8. Side effects

        a. Dizziness, vertigo, headache, and weakness

        b. Dehydration, orthostatic hypotension, nausea and vomiting, abdominal pain, diarrhea, constipation, and frequent urination

        c. Dermatitis and rash

        d. Electrolyte imbalance, impaired glucose tolerance, jaundice, muscle cramps, photosensitivity, impotence, and hyperuricemia

    9. Adverse effects/toxicity: renal failure, aplastic anemia, agranulocytosis, thrombocytopenia, and anaphylactic reaction

  10. Client-centered nursing care

        a. Monitor vital signs for hypotension and tachycardia

        b. Monitor serum electrolytes, calcium, and uric acid levels

        c. Monitor and record body weight at regular intervals at same time of day and same scale

        d. Monitor I&O

        e. Assess indicators of dehydration: thirst, poor skin turgor, coated tongue

        f. Assess for inadequate tissue perfusion and weakness, decreased muscle strength, restlessness, anxiety, and agitation

  11. Client education

        a. Eat foods high in potassium to prevent hypokalemia

        b. Restrict sodium intake; do not use salt substitutes if taking potassium supplement

        c. Avoid dehydration by avoiding alcohol and caffeinated beverages and replacing fluids during exercise or hot weather

        d. Avoid exposure to intense heat as with baths, showers, and electric blankets

        e. Take frequent, small amounts of ice chips or clear liquids if vomiting

        f. Replace fluids with fruit juice or bouillon if diarrhea occurs

        g. Diuretics increase amount and frequency of urination, so take doses in morning and early afternoon to avoid nighttime urination and interruption of sleep

        h. Change position slowly to avoid dizziness and orthostatic hypotension

        i. Weigh self daily and report sudden weight gains or losses

        j. If diabetic, check blood glucose periodically

C. Potassium-sparing diuretics

   1. Action and use

      a. Act directly on distal convoluted tubule to increase sodium excretion and decrease potassium secretion

      b. Used for hypertension and edema associated with HF

      c. Spironolactone is also used for detection of primary hyperaldosteronism, hirsutism, and premenstrual syndrome

   2. Common potassium-sparing diuretic medications (Table 8-3)

   3. Administration considerations

      a. Take with food or milk

      b. Avoid salt substitutes

      c. Avoid excessive ingestion of foods high in potassium

      d. When administering spironolactone to children, crush tablet and mix in flavored syrup as oral suspension

   4. Contraindications

      a. Serum potassium levels greater than 5.5 mEq/mL

      b. Concomitant use with other potassium-sparing diuretics

      c. Fluid and electrolyte imbalances

      d. Anuria, acute and chronic renal insufficiency, diabetic nephropathy, hypersensitivity, and impaired hepatic function

      e. Caution in client with diabetes mellitus

   5. Significant drug interactions

      a. May potentiate hypotensive effects of antihypertensive medications

      b. Increased risk of hyperkalemia with other potassium-sparing diuretics

      c. May increase serum blood levels of lithium due to decreased renal clearance

      d. Reduced effect of digoxin if administered with amiloride

      e. Aspirin may slightly decrease response of spironolactone

      f. Antidiabetic drugs may need adjustment as triamterene may increase blood glucose levels

      g. Corticosteroids may increase electrolyte depletion

   6. Significant food interactions: administering spironolactone with food increases its absorption

   7. Significant laboratory studies

      a. Monitor electrolytes (especially potassium), creatinine, and BUN

      b. Digoxin level

      c. Triamterene may interfere with enzyme assays

Table 8-3	**Common Potassium-Sparing Diuretics**		
Generic Name	**Route**	**Uses**	**Adverse Effects**
Amiloride	PO	Adjunctive therapy with thiazide and loop diuretics to treat edema and congestive heart failure (CHF), hypertension, prevention of hypokalemia	Headache, dizziness, drowsiness, fatigue, paresthesia, tremors, confusion, rash, alopecia, cough, dyspnea, hyperkalemia, decreased libido, impotence, jaundice, gastrointestinal bleeding, muscle cramps
Spironolactone	PO	Diagnosis and treatment of hyperaldosteronism; edema related to CHF, nephrotic syndrome, cirrhosis; prevention and treatment of hypokalemia; essential hypertension	Dizziness, headache, drowsiness, fatigue, rash, cramping, diarrhea, impotence, hyperkalemia, agranulocytosis, hirsutism, gynecomastia, deepened voice
Triamterene	PO	Edema related to CHF, cirrhosis, steroid-related edema, secondary hyperaldosteronism	Headache, rash, hyperkalemia, photosensitivity, nausea and vomiting, dry mouth, renal stones, interstitial nephritis

8. Side effects
    a. CNS: headache, weakness, dizziness, and orthostatic hypotension
    b. GI: nausea and vomiting, diarrhea, and constipation
    c. Impotence, muscle cramps, urticaria, gynecomastia, and breast soreness
    d. Dry mouth, photosensitivity, transient elevated BUN and creatinine
9. Adverse effects/toxicity
    a. Aplastic anemia and thrombocytopenia
    b. Hyperkalemia
10. Client-centered nursing care
    a. Monitor vital signs and urine output
    b. Administer with meals to prevent GI upset
    c. Discontinue potassium supplements
    d. Observe closely older adult and debilitated clients for drug-induced diuresis and hyperkalemia
    e. Monitor for dehydration and electrolyte imbalance
    f. Monitor periodic serum electrolytes and BUN and creatinine
11. Client education
    a. Take medication with food to avoid GI upset with all medications except triamterene
    b. Avoid consumption of large quantities of foods high in potassium
    c. Report any mental confusion or lethargy immediately
    d. Monitor for signs and symptoms of hyperkalemia such as nausea, diarrhea, abdominal cramps, and tachycardia followed by bradycardia
    e. Side effects usually disappear after drug is discontinued except gynecomastia may persist
    f. With spironolactone, maximal diuresis may not occur until day 3 of therapy and diuresis may continue 2–3 days after drug is stopped
    g. Triamterene may turn urine blue
    h. Avoid salt substitutes because they contain potassium
    i. Avoid exposure to direct sunlight

D. **Carbonic anhydrase inhibitors**
    1. Action and use
        a. Noncompetitive reversible inhibition of enzyme carbonic anhydrase, which promotes excretion of bicarbonate, sodium, potassium, and water
        b. Results in slightly acidic urine
        c. Used for open-angle glaucoma to decrease intraocular pressure
        d. Used for treatment of epilepsy
        e. Used to treat metabolic alkalosis
    2. Common carbonic anhydrase inhibitor medications (Table 8-4)
    3. Administration considerations
        a. Increasing dose does not appear to increase diuresis
        b. Do not administer with high-dose aspirin

Practice to Pass

A client was prescribed spironolactone 1 month ago. What key assessments should the nurse make at the client's follow-up visit to the healthcare provider?

Table 8-4		Common Carbonic Anhydrase Inhibitors	
Generic Name	**Route**	**Uses**	**Adverse Effects**
Acetazolamide	PO, IV	Decrease intraocular pressure in clients with open-angle glaucoma, chronic open-angle glaucoma, prevention of acute mountain sickness, adjunctive therapy for seizures, paralysis, drug-induced edema	Confusion, drowsiness, paresthesias, hearing abnormalities, transient myopia, renal calculus, photosensitivity, rash, electrolyte imbalance, aplastic anemia, leukopenia, hyperchloremic acidosis, hypokalemia, hyperuricemia
Methazolamide	PO	Decrease intraocular pressure in clients with open-angle glaucoma	

    4. Contraindications

        a. Pregnancy

        b. Narrow angle or acute glaucoma

        c. Any situation with decreased sodium and/or potassium levels

        d. Marked kidney or liver dysfunction

        e. Cautionary use in clients with chronic obstructive pulmonary disease (COPD), receiving digoxin, or during lactation

    5. Significant drug interactions

        a. Aspirin may cause accumulation and toxicity of acetazolamide

        b. May increase levels of cyclosporine and decreased levels of primidone

        c. Increased excretion of lithium

        d. Decreased renal clearance of amphetamines, anticholinergics, procainamide, quinidine, and tricyclic antidepressants (TCAs)

    6. Significant food interactions: none reported

    7. Significant laboratory studies

        a. Obtain platelet and complete blood cell counts (CBC) prior to and periodically during therapy; may decrease hemoglobin and hematocrit

        b. Monitor serum electrolytes

        c. May cause false-positive proteinuria

        d. May decrease thyroid iodine uptake

        e. May increase uric acid level

    8. Side effects

        a. Confusion, drowsiness, and paresthesias

        b. Hearing dysfunction, GI upset, polyuria, and transient myopia

        c. Electrolyte imbalance, fever, rash, renal calculus, and photosensitivity

    9. Adverse effects/toxicity

        a. Metabolic acidosis

        b. Anaphylaxis

        c. Bone marrow depression

        d. Thrombocytopenia purpura, hemolytic anemia, leukopenia, pancytopenia, and agranulocytosis

        e. Severe reactions to sulfonamides including Stevens–Johnson syndrome, toxic epidermal necrolysis, fulminant hepatic necrosis, coma, and death have occurred

  10. Client-centered nursing care

        a. Monitor for signs and symptoms of dehydration; I&O

        b. Assess for alterations in skin integrity

        c. Assess for edema

        d. Assess vital signs and daily weight

        e. Assess cardiovascular and respiratory status

        f. Assess changes in level of consciousness and activity level

        g. Dietary assessment of high salt-containing foods

        h. Fluid restriction as prescribed

  11. Client education

        a. Do not take aspirin or aspirin-containing medications

        b. Report symptoms of anorexia, lethargy, or tachypnea

        c. Use caution while driving or performing tasks that require alertness, coordination, or physical dexterity because of risk of drowsiness

        d. Monitor for signs of renal calculi

        e. Follow-up scheduled lab tests are important

        f. Weigh self daily at same time of day; report acute weight gain or loss

        g. Be aware of and avoid high-sodium foods and beverages; eat foods high in potassium instead

E. Osmotic diuretics
   1. Action and use
      a. Increase osmotic pressure of glomerular filtrate in proximal tubule and loop of Henle inhibiting reabsorption of water and electrolytes, thus promoting diuresis
      b. Used to prevent and manage acute kidney injury (AKI) and oliguria
      c. Used to decrease intracranial or intraocular pressure
      d. Mannitol is used with chemotherapy to induce diuresis
   2. Common osmotic diuretic medications (Table 8-5)
   3. Administration considerations
      a. Medications are administered IV by slow infusion
      b. Urea turns to ammonia if left standing
      c. Do not infuse with blood or blood products
      d. Mannitol crystallizes at low temperatures
      e. For maximum reduction of intraocular pressure, mannitol should be given 1–1.5 hours before surgery
   4. Contraindications
      a. Severely impaired renal function, marked dehydration, breastfeeding, hepatic failure, active intracranial bleed, and anuria
      b. Severe pulmonary congestion and severe heart failure
   5. Significant drug interactions
      a. Decrease serum lithium levels
      b. Use with cardiac glycosides may cause an increased possibility of digitalis toxicity
      c. Increased effects of other diuretics
   6. Significant food interactions: none reported
   7. Significant laboratory studies: monitor BUN and electrolytes frequently
   8. Side effects
      a. Headache, syncope, and hypotension
      b. Dry mouth, nausea and vomiting, urine retention, electrolyte imbalance, and urticaria
   9. Adverse effects/toxicity
      a. Seizures
      b. Thrombophlebitis
      c. Congestive heart failure
      d. Cardiovascular collapse
   10. Client-centered nursing care
      a. Maintain adequate hydration
      b. Monitor fluid and electrolyte balance
      c. Monitor BUN

Table 8-5 **Common Osmotic Diuretics**

Generic Name	Route	Uses	Adverse Effects
Mannitol	IV	Oliguria, acute renal impairment, edema, ascites, renal failure, hepatic failure, cardiac failure, increased intraocular pressure, increased intracranial pressure, diuresis in drug intoxication, transurethral resection of prostate	Headaches, confusion, seizures, circulatory overload, tachycardia, chest pain, blurred vision, hypotension, hypertension, edema, thrombophlebitis, urticaria, diuresis, fluid and electrolyte imbalance, hyponatremia, pulmonary congestion, rhinitis, water intoxication
Urea	IV	Increased intracranial pressure, cerebral edema, increased intraocular pressure	Syncope, dizziness, headache, disorientation, nausea and vomiting, tissue necrosis at IV site with extravasation, hyponatremia, hypokalemia, thrombophlebitis, febrile episode, hypovolemia

               d. Indwelling catheter should be used in comatose clients for accurate I&O

               e. Monitor I&O and vital signs hourly while on mannitol

               f. Measure daily weight

               g. Monitor renal function, fluid balance, serum, and urinary sodium and potassium levels

               h. Assess for signs of decreasing intracranial pressure if appropriate

               i. Monitor lung and heart sounds for signs of pulmonary edema

         11. Client education

               a. Monitor daily weight and report sudden weight gain or loss

               b. Report immediately pain in chest or legs, shortness of breath, or apnea

               c. Change position slowly to prevent dizziness or orthostatic hypotension

               d. Drink only fluids prescribed even if thirsty and/or experiencing dry mouth

               e. Have family monitor change in neuro status such as decreased level of consciousness (LOC)

II. POTASSIUM SUPPLEMENTS

    A. Action and use

        1. Potassium is main cation in body cells

        2. Acts to maintain intracellular tonicity, maintain balance with sodium across cell membranes, transmit nerve impulses, and maintain cellular metabolism

        3. Help contracting cardiac and skeletal muscle, maintaining acid–base balance, and maintaining normal renal function

        4. Potassium is well absorbed from GI tract and excreted largely by kidneys

        5. Used to prevent and treat hypokalemia

    B. Common potassium supplement (Table 8-6)

    C. Administration considerations

        1. Tablet form should be taken with a full glass of water

        2. Tablets are not to be crushed, chewed, or sucked; if difficulty swallowing, tablet may be broken and dissolved in water

        3. Powder preparations should be mixed with 4 ounces of water or other liquid

        4. Potassium supplements should be taken with meals to decrease GI irritation

        5. Tablets in wax matrix sometimes lodge in esophagus and cause ulceration; in cardiac clients who have esophageal compression due to enlarged left atrium, use liquid form

        6. Enteric-coated tablets are not recommended because of potential for GI bleeding and small bowel ulcerations

        7. Parenteral potassium should be given slowly and in diluted form (often 40 mEg/L or less via peripheral vein) and infused no faster than 10 mEq/hr, even via central line

    D. Contraindications

        1. Severe renal impairment with oliguria, **anuria** (absence of urine), or azotemia

        2. Untreated Addison disease

Table 8-6	Potassium Supplement		
Generic Name	**Route**	**Therapeutic Indications**	**Adverse Effects**
Potassium chloride	PO, IV	Prevention and correction of potassium depletion, IV treatment of cardiac dysrhythmias associated with cardiac glycosides	Hyperkalemia, nausea and vomiting, diarrhea, abdominal pain, rash, GI obstruction, ECG changes with peaked T waves, loss of P waves, ST segment depression, prolongation of QT interval

3. Acute dehydration and heat cramps
4. Hyperkalemia and form of familial periodic paralysis, as well as conditions associated with extensive tissue breakdown
5. Use cautiously with cardiac and renal disease

E. **Significant drug interactions**
   1. Anticholinergics may increase risk of GI irritation and ulceration
   2. Potassium-containing agents increase risk for hyperkalemia
   3. Potassium is not recommended in clients with severe or complete heart block taking digoxin due to potential for dysrhythmias
   4. Use with potassium-sparing diuretics, angiotensin-converting enzyme (ACE) inhibitors, or salt substitutes containing potassium salts can cause severe hyperkalemia
   5. May decrease absorption of vitamin B_{12} in GI tract

F. **Significant food interactions**
   1. Foods high in potassium
   2. Examples include bananas, dates, figs, melons, oranges, peaches, pears, raisins, avocado, green or wax beans, peas, tomatoes, spinach, sweet potatoes, winter squash, chicken, liver, turkey, salmon, beef, yogurt, milk, and chocolate

G. **Significant laboratory studies**: none reported

H. **Side effects**
   1. Paresthesia of extremities, restlessness, confusion, weakness, or heaviness of legs
   2. Hypotension and electrocardiogram (ECG) changes
   3. Abdominal pain, nausea and vomiting, and diarrhea
   4. Hyperkalemia

I. **Adverse effects/toxicity**
   1. Dysrhythmias or cardiac arrest
   2. Respiratory paralysis

J. **Client-centered nursing care**
   1. Monitor serum potassium, BUN, and creatinine
   2. Monitor I&O
   3. Monitor ECG for dysrhythmias
   4. Monitor for side effects such as weakness, feeling of heaviness in legs, confusion, hypotension (signs of hyperkalemia)
   5. Potassium should not be given immediately postoperatively until urine flow is established
   6. Attempt to identify cause of hypokalemia
   7. Assess parenteral infusion site frequently for signs of pain and inflammation

K. **Client education**
   1. Foods high in potassium
   2. Avoid salt substitutes while taking potassium supplements
   3. Sit up while swallowing potassium and contact prescriber if swallowing problems occur
   4. Monitor stools for evidence of GI bleed
   5. Notify prescriber of any other prescription or over-the-counter (OTC) medications
   6. Report immediately confusion; irregular heartbeat; numbness of feet, fingers, or lips; shortness of breath; anxiety; excessive tiredness; or weakness of legs
   7. Take potassium supplement with meals to decrease GI irritation
   8. Take only prescribed amount of potassium to avoid toxicity
   9. Dissolve powder, soluble tablets, or granules completely in at least 4 ounces of water or juice before drinking; take whole tablets with a full glass of liquid if allowed
   10. Do not crush or chew sustained-release capsules but contents can be opened and sprinkled onto soft foods
   11. Expelling a whole sustained-release tablet in stool is normal as body eliminates shell after absorbing potassium

Practice to Pass

A client has been prescribed to take a potassium supplement. What information should the nurse provide during client teaching about this medication?

III. URINARY ANTI-INFECTIVES AND ANTISPASMODICS

A. Anti-infectives

1. Action and use
   a. Has **bacteriostatic** (inhibits growth of bacteria without destruction) and **bactericidal** (destroying bacteria) actions
   b. Act as disinfectants within urinary tract
   c. Used to treat urinary tract infections
2. Common urinary tract anti-infective medications (Table 8-7)
3. Administration considerations
   a. May take with food or milk to decrease GI upset
   b. Check renal and hepatic function before administering
   c. Oral suspension may stain teeth
   d. Complete full course of therapy
4. Contraindications
   a. Hypersensitivity
   b. Megaloblastic anemia and folate deficiency, renal insufficiency, and severe hepatic insufficiency
   c. Severe dehydration, anuria, oliguria, and seizure disorder
5. Significant drug interactions
   a. Methenamine/sulfonamides: may cause formation of an insoluble precipitate in urine
   b. Nalidixic acid/warfarin: increase effect of warfarin
   c. Sulfonamides may increase effects of methotrexate, phenytoin, sulfonylureas, and warfarin
   d. Trimethoprim increases effects of phenytoin
   e. Decreased absorption of nitrofurantoin with magnesium trisilicate
6. Significant food interactions: none reported
7. Significant laboratory studies
   a. May increase liver enzymes and renal function tests
   b. May cause false-positive urinary glucose test
   c. May cause false increase in 17 hydroxycorticosteroids, catecholamines

Table 8-7		Common Urinary Tract Anti-infectives	
Generic Name	**Route**	**Uses**	**Adverse Effects**
Methenamine	PO	Urinary tract infection (UTI), pyelonephritis, cystitis, residual urine, anatomical abnormalities of urinary tract	Bladder irritation, dysuria, urgency, frequency, hematuria, nausea, headache, dyspnea, rash, elevated serum transaminase
Nalidixic acid	PO	UTIs caused by Gram-negative bacteria, *Proteus, Klebsiella, Enterobacter, Escherichia coli*	Rash, pruritis, angioedema, photosensitivity, drowsiness, weakness, headache, vertigo, dizziness, nausea and vomiting, diarrhea
Nitrofurantoin	PO	UTIs caused by *Escherichia coli, Staphylococcus aureus, Klebsiella, Enterobacter, Proteus*	Stevens-Johnson syndrome, exfoliative dermatitis, urticaria, angioedema, nausea, abdominal cramps, hepatotoxicity, pulmonary hypersensitivity, superinfections
Trimethoprim	PO	UTIs caused by *Escherichia coli, Proteus, Klebsiella, Enterobacter, Staphylococcus,* acute otitis media in children	Thrombocytopenia, leukopenia, methemoglobinemia, megaloblastic anemia, exfoliative dermatitis, epigastric distress, nausea and vomiting, diarrhea, rash, pruritus, fever
Sulfisoxazole and phenazopyridine	PO	UTIs, acute otitis media, conjunctivitis, sexually transmitted infections	Exfoliative dermatitis, urticaria, angioedema, nausea, abdominal cramps, hepatotoxicity, pulmonary hypersensitivity, superinfections

8. Side effects
   a. Drowsiness, weakness, headache, dizziness
   b. Sensitivity to light, blurred vision
   c. GI distress and possible nausea, pruritus, rash, arthralgia
9. Adverse effects/toxicity
   a. Seizures, increased intracranial pressure
   b. Leukopenia, thrombocytopenia, angioedema
10. Client-centered nursing care
   a. Drugs work best if client is well (but not overly) hydrated
   b. Administer with meals to decrease GI distress
   c. Monitor renal and liver function and periodic CBC levels
   d. Check urine pH before administration as some drugs work best in acidic urine
   e. Cranberry supplements or vitamin C may be added to acidify urine
   f. Monitor CNS side effects
   g. If using an oral suspension of nitrofurantoin, instruct client to rinse mouth to avoid staining of teeth
   h. Ingestion of large amount of fluid while taking methenamine will reduce antibacterial effects by diluting medication and raising urinary pH
   i. Assess client taking nitrofurantoin for acute pulmonary sensitivity (moderate to severe flulike syndrome)
11. Client education
   a. Long-term therapy is common even if feeling fine
   b. Drink at least eight glasses of water daily but do not overhydrate
   c. Take medications with meals to decrease GI distress
   d. Avoid alkalizing fluids such as milk, fruit juices, or sodium bicarbonate and do not take with antacids
   e. Notify prescriber of any new medications
   f. Use sunscreen to avoid excessive exposure to sunlight
   g. Notify prescriber of any CNS side effects
   h. Nitrofurantoin may discolor urine (brown color); not harmful and will disappear after drug is discontinued
   i. Take methenamine with food

B. **Urinary analgesic**
   1. Action and use
      a. Has a local anesthetic effect on urinary tract mucosa
      b. Used to relieve pain with urinary tract infections or irritation
   2. Common medication: phenazopyridine: 100–200 mg tid, or used with an antibiotic as a combination drug
   3. Administration considerations
      a. Drug colors urine red or orange and may stain fabrics
      b. May be used with antibiotics and should be discontinued after 2 days of antibiotic use
   4. Contraindications
      a. Hypersensitivity
      b. Renal or hepatic diseases
   5. Significant drug interactions: none reported
   6. Significant food interactions: none reported
   7. Significant laboratory studies: may alter results of urinary dipstick
   8. Side effects
      a. Headache and vertigo
      b. Nausea and GI distress

▶ **Practice to Pass**

A client with a UTI is prescribed phenazopyridine and an antibiotic. What information would you teach the client specific to phenazopyridine?

      9. Adverse effects/toxicity

        a. Anaphylaxis

        b. Methemoglobinemia

        c. Renal and hepatic failure

      10. Client-centered nursing care

        a. Assess urinary function and presence of urinary tract infection (UTI)

        b. Monitor I&O

        c. Monitor sclera for yellow tinge

        d. Ensure renal function before administering

        e. Use only as an analgesic

      11. Client education

        a. Maintain perineal hygiene to prevent UTI

        b. Possible side effects

        c. Drug colors urine red-orange and may stain clothing

        d. Do not double dose if a dose is missed

        e. Take medication with food to decrease GI distress

        f. Increase fluid intake to aid in flushing bacteria from bladder

        g. Drug may not be effective for more than 24–48 hours

        h. Notify prescriber if yellowing of eyes develops

        i. Report symptoms that worsen or do not resolve

C. Antispasmodics

      1. Action and use

        a. Relax smooth muscles of urinary tract

        b. Decrease bladder muscle spasms

        c. Used to manage disorders of lower urinary tract associated with hypermotility: dysuria, urgency, nocturia, suprapubic pain, frequency, and incontinence

      2. Common urinary antispasmodic medications (Table 8-8)

      3. Administration considerations: administer 1 hour before antacids or antidiarrheals; do not consume alcohol within 2 hours of dose

      4. Contraindications

        a. Uncontrolled narrow-angle glaucoma

        b. Urinary retention

        c. Paralytic ileus or decreased GI motility

        d. Hypersensitivity to anticholinergics, unstable cardiovascular (CV) status

Table 8-8   **Common Urinary Antispasmodic Medications**

Generic Name	Routes	Uses	Adverse Effects
Darifenacin	PO	Overactive bladder	Xerostomia, constipation, headache, dizziness, dry eyes
Fesoterodine	PO	Prevent urgency, frequency, incontinence	Xerostomia, constipation, dizziness, drowsiness, dry eyes
Oxybutynin	PO, transdermal patch	Neurogenic bladder, incontinence	Xerostomia, constipation, headache, dizziness, somnolence, dry eyes, vision changes, local site reaction (patch)
Solifenacin	PO	Overactive bladder	Xerostomia, constipation, headache, dizziness, dry eyes
Tolterodine	PO	Overactive bladder with frequency, urgency, and urine leakage	Xerostomia, constipation, headache, dizziness, somnolence, dry eyes, vision changes
Trospium	PO	Overactive bladder	Xerostomia, constipation, headache, dizziness, somnolence, dry eyes, vision changes

5. Significant drug interactions
   a. Amantadine increases adverse anticholinergic effects
   b. Phenothiazines or haloperidol will result in decreased antipsychotic effect
   c. Additive effect with other anticholinergic drugs
6. Significant food interactions: none reported
7. Significant laboratory studies: none reported
8. Side effects: dry mouth (xerostomia), constipation, headache, drowsiness, dizziness, dry eyes
9. Adverse effects/toxicity: angioedema, somnolence
10. Client-centered nursing care
    a. Monitor effect of medication on resolution of urinary symptoms
    b. Monitor for CNS manifestations
    c. Monitor I&O
11. Client education
    a. Drowsiness and blurred vision may occur; use caution when driving or operating machinery
    b. Use hard, sugarless candy for dry mouth
    c. Avoid alcohol, which increases drowsiness
    d. Swallow pill whole and do not chew or crush
    e. Shell of medication may appear in stool
    f. Be aware of side effects and to report them to provider

IV. MEDICATIONS TO TREAT *BENIGN PROSTATIC HYPERPLASIA (BPH)*

A. **Action and use**
   1. Block alpha$_1$-receptors in prostate leading to relaxation of smooth muscles, improving urine flow, and decreasing BPH symptoms
   2. Used to increase urine flow and decrease symptoms of BPH
B. **Common BPH medications** (Table 8-9)
C. **Administration considerations**
   1. Do not handle crushed tablets if pregnant
   2. Not indicated for females or pediatric use
   3. Postural effects may occur 2–6 hours after dose
   4. If treatment is interrupted for several days, restart medication at initial dose
D. **Contraindications**
   1. Hypersensitivity
   2. Caution in clients with impaired hepatic function

Table 8-9 Common Medications to Treat Benign Prostatic Hyperplasia

Generic Names	Route	Uses	Adverse Effects
Alpha$_1$-Adrenergic Blockers Alfuzosin Doxazosin Silodosin Tamsulosin Terazosin	PO	Benign prostatic hyperplasia (BPH)—all drugs Essential hypertension—doxazosin, terazosin	Dizziness, headache, fatigue, angina tachycardia, orthostatic hypotension, first-dose phenomenon (hypotension and syncope)
5-Alpha-Reductase Inhibitors Dutasteride Finasteride	PO	BPH	Decreased libido, erectile dysfunction, ejaculation disorder, gynecomastia

E. **Significant drug interactions**
   1. May increase theophylline clearance (finasteride)
   2. Concomitant use with other antihypertensive agents or diuretics (terazosin)
   3. Do not use with alpha-adrenergic blockers (decreased blood pressure)
   4. Cimetidine may decrease alfuzosin levels
   5. Use cautiously with warfarin
   6. Doxazosin may decrease effects of clonidine
   7. Dutasteride levels increased with cimetidine, diltiazem, verapamil, ketoconazole, macrolides, and protease inhibitors

F. **Significant food interactions**: none reported

G. **Significant laboratory studies**
   1. Decrease WBC and neutrophil counts with doxazosin
   2. Decreased hematocrit, WBC, hemoglobin, total protein, and albumin levels with terazosin
   3. Finasteride may decrease prostate-specific antigen (PSA), even in prostate cancer

H. **Side effects**
   1. Impotence, decreased volume of ejaculate, decreased libido, asthenia
   2. Dizziness, headache, nervousness, palpitations, peripheral edema, postural hypotension, nasal congestion, myalgia
   3. Diarrhea and nausea

I. **Adverse effects/toxicity**: hypotension, shock, and arrhythmias

J. **Client-centered nursing care**
   1. Assess client for severity of symptoms
   2. Provide treatment options
   3. Monitor for decreased BP
   4. Rule out cancer of prostate before initiating therapy
   5. Monitor for concomitant medications for interactions
   6. Monitor urine volume
   7. Take alfuzosin with same meal each day

K. **Client education**
   1. Change position slowly to prevent orthostatic hypotension
   2. Avoid driving and hazardous tasks for first 12–24 hours or after increasing dose due to drowsiness and somnolence
   3. Report side effects to prescriber
   4. Take medication at same time each day
   5. Women who are or may become pregnant should not handle crushed finasteride tablets due to risk of adverse effect to male fetus
   6. A male client whose sexual partner is or may become pregnant should avoid exposing her to his semen or else discontinue finasteride
   7. Volume of ejaculate may be decreased but does not impair fertility

V. MEDICATION TO INCREASE RENAL PERFUSION

A. **Action and use**
   1. Primary focus of pharmacological management of renal failure is to restore and maintain renal perfusion and to eliminate drugs that are directly nephrotoxic
   2. Diuretics to improve urinary outflow have been previously discussed and are not covered in this category
   3. Dopaminergic receptors cause vasodilation in renal, mesenteric, coronary, and intracerebral vascular beds and increase urine flow

B. **Common medication**: dopamine, 2–5 mcg/kg/min to increase renal perfusion; may increase to 50 mcg/kg/min IV to raise blood pressure

Practice to Pass

A client is prescribed finasteride for BPH. What would you say to explain how the drug works?

C. **Administration considerations**
   1. Administered IV using an infusion device to control rate of flow
   2. Administered into a large vein to prevent possibility of extravasation
   3. Hypovolemia should be corrected before initiation of dopamine therapy
   4. Decrease dose as soon as hemodynamic condition is stabilized
   5. Do not mix with other medications
   6. Discard solutions after 24 hours
D. **Contraindications**
   1. Uncorrected tachydysrhythmias, pheochromocytoma, or ventricular fibrillation
   2. Caution in use with occlusive vascular disease, cold injuries, diabetic endarteritis, and arterial embolism
E. **Significant drug interactions**
   1. MAOIs may prolong and intensify effect of dopamine
   2. Beta blockers antagonize cardiac effects
   3. General anesthetics may cause ventricular arrhythmias and hypertension
   4. Diuretics may result in increased diuretic effects
F. **Significant food interactions**: none reported
G. **Significant laboratory studies**: increased catecholamines and increased serum glucose levels
H. **Side effects**
   1. Headache, tachycardia, angina, palpitations, hypotension, bradycardia, vasoconstriction, widening of QRS complex
   2. Nausea and vomiting, piloerection, azotemia
I. **Adverse effects/toxicity**: anaphylaxis, asthmatic episodes, severe hypertension
J. **Client-centered nursing care**
   1. Carefully monitor I&O
   2. Assess infusion site frequently for extravasation; use 5–10 mg phentolamine mesylate in 10–15 mL of normal saline as an antidote
   3. Monitor vital signs, cardiac output, and ECG frequently
   4. Monitor for side effects
K. **Client education**: report side effects and monitor vital signs and I&O

VI. HEMATOPOIETIC GROWTH FACTOR IN RENAL FAILURE

A. **Action and use**
   1. Used to stimulate red blood cell (RBC) production
   2. Reverses anemia associated with chronic renal failure
B. **Common medication**: epoetin alfa, subcutaneous/IV 300–500 units/kg/dose 3 times/wk
C. **Administration considerations**
   1. Initial effects can be seen within 1–2 weeks
   2. Hematocrit (Hct) reaches normal levels (30–33%) in 2–3 months
   3. Do not shake solution
   4. IV administration: epoetin alfa may be given undiluted by direct IV as a bolus dose
D. **Contraindications**
   1. Uncontrolled hypertension
   2. Known hypersensitivity to mammalian cell-derived products and albumin
E. **Significant drug interactions**: none reported
F. **Significant food interactions**: none reported
G. **Significant laboratory studies**
   1. CBC with differential and platelet count
   2. Monitor BUN, creatinine, phosphorus, and potassium
   3. Monitor partial thromboplastin time (APPT)
   4. Evaluate transferrin and serum ferritin prior to initiation of therapy

> **H. Side effects**
>   1. Hypertension
>   2. Headache, seizure
>   3. Iron deficiency, sweating
> **I. Adverse effects/toxicity**
>   1. Thrombocytosis, clotting of AV fistula
>   2. Bone pain, arthralgias
> **J. Client-centered nursing care**
>   1. Blood pressure may rise during early therapy as Hct increases; notify prescriber of a rapid rise in Hct greater than 4 points in 2 weeks
>   2. Do not give with any other drug solution
>   3. Use only one dose per vial, and do not reenter vial
>   4. Inspect solution for particulate matter prior to use
>   5. Monitor for hypertensive encephalopathy in clients with CRF during period of increasing Hct
>   6. Client may require additional heparin during dialysis to prevent clotting of vascular access
> **K. Client education**
>   1. Self-monitor vital signs, especially BP
>   2. Headache is a common adverse effect; it should be reported if it is severe
>   3. Avoid driving or other hazardous activity because of possible seizure activity, especially during first 90 days of therapy
>   4. Important to keep all follow-up appointments

Case Study

A 78-year-old male with a history of heart failure (HF) and hypertension (HTN) is admitted to the hospital for repair of an inguinal hernia. His medications include lisinipril po 40 mg daily, furosemide po 20 mg bid, spironolactone 25 mg po daily, metoprolol 25 mg bid, and aspirin 81 mg po daily. Laboratory values are:

- Potassium – 5.2 mEq/L
- Sodium – 138 mmol/L
- Chloride – 102 mmol/L
- Carbon dioxide – 25 mmol/L

- BUN – 29 mmol/L
- Creatinine – 1.8 mg/dL
- Est glomerular filtration rate (GFR) – 57
- Glucose – 86 mg/Dl

1. Explain the rationale for use of each of the medications.

2. What concerns do you have with his laboratory findings and why?

3. What factors could be contributing to his elevated potassium level, since he is taking a loop diuretic, which is potassium wasting?

4. What action should the nurse take?

5. Although the medication profile will most likely be adjusted, what teaching is indicated regarding potassium-sparing diuretics?

For suggested responses, see page 541.

POSTTEST

1 A client was started on drug therapy with bumetanide 1 month ago. At a follow-up health visit, the nurse should be most concerned with which most recent laboratory test result?

1. Blood urea nitrogen 22 mg/dL
2. Blood glucose 130 mg/dL
3. Potassium 3.1 mEq/L
4. Calcium 9.5 mEq/L

- -

2 A 45-year-old female has been taking indapamide 2.5 mg daily. She reported to the clinic today with leg cramps and a blood pressure of 126/70. The nurse should consult with the prescriber to do which of the following?

1. Stop the indapamide.
2. Evaluate the electrolytes.
3. Change prescription to furosemide.
4. Change prescription to a nonsteroidal anti-inflammatory drug.

- -

3 A client will be starting drug therapy with spironolactone to manage edema associated with cirrhosis of the liver. The nurse should encourage the client to avoid excessive amounts of which foods? Select all that apply.

1. Bananas
2. Cantaloupe
3. Grapes
4. Green beans
5. Spinach

- -

4 The nurse notes that the diuretic acetazolamide is listed on the client's medication reconciliation sheet. The nurse should check the client's health history for which anticipated health problem?

1. Addison disease
2. Open-angle glaucoma
3. Liver cirrhosis
4. Heart failure

- -

5 A client has received a prescription for supplemental potassium chloride. Which client teaching points should the nurse include in a discussion with the client? Select all that apply.

1. "Take supplement with meals to reduce GI upset."
2. "Report irregular pulse, fatigue, or weakness in legs."
3. "Expect diarrhea or vomiting as side effects."
4. "Dissolve soluble tablet in at least 120 mL (4 oz) of water or juice."
5. "Avoid use of salt substitutes while taking potassium."

- -

6 A nurse notes that a client has methenamine on the list of prescribed medications. The nurse should suspect that the client has a diagnosis of which health problem?

1. Urinary tract infection
2. Bladder incontinence
3. Acute kidney injury
4. Chronic renal failure

- -

7 The nurse is providing information to a client who has started drug therapy with sulfisoxazole. Which instruction would be the highest priority of the nurse to provide?

1. "Check the urine pH to prevent crystals from forming in the urine."
2. "Report sudden onset of fever, pruritus, and malaise."
3. "Restrict your oral fluid intake to an amount between 500 and 1,000 mL/day."
4. "Keep your urine at an alkaline level."

- -

8 After phenazopyridine is prescribed for a client, the nurse teaches the client which of the following items of information?

1. "Continue taking drug until infection is resolved."
2. "Long-term use of drug requires no follow-up."
3. "With appropriate hydration, it is safe to breastfeed."
4. "Report sign of yellow-tinged skin or sclera."

- -

9 A client has been started on medication therapy with tolterodine. The home health nurse making a follow-up visit should assess for resolution of which symptoms? Select all that apply.

1. Reduced urine output
2. Urinary urgency
3. Urinary frequency
4. Leakage of urine
5. Hematuria

10 A nurse administering tamsulosin to a client would expect to note which therapeutic outcomes of drug therapy? Select all that apply.

1. Hypotension
2. Syncope
3. Decreased urethral obstruction
4. Increased urine flow
5. Decreased urinary frequency

➤ *See pages 268–269 for Answers and Rationales.*

ANSWERS & RATIONALES

Pretest

1 Answer: 1 Rationale: If the nurse is to advise the client appropriately, knowledge of pharmacokinetics is necessary. For example, onset: 20–60 minutes; peak: 60–70 minutes; duration: 2 hours; elimination: 50% every 24 hours. Since clients may not respond as expected, the client should ingest the drug as early as possible to prevent nocturia that could disrupt the client's sleep. Therefore, 8:00 a.m. is the best answer. While 12 noon is a more appropriate time than 6:00 p.m. or bedtime, it is not the best time. Since 50% will remain in the body for each 24-hour period, a cumulative effect could disrupt the client's sleep–rest pattern. An onset of 20–60 mins would result in a direct interruption of the sleep–rest pattern. Cognitive Level: Applying Client Need: Pharmacological and Parenteral Therapies Integrated Process: Teaching and Learning Content Area: Pharmacology Strategy: Associate the drug actions and pharmacokinetics with the client's lifestyle. Knowing the drug is a diuretic will help to avoid times that would result in nocturia. Reference: Wilson, B. A., Shannon, M., & Shields, K. (2016). *Pearson nurse's drug guide 2016*. New York, NY: Pearson, pp. 689–690.

2 Answer: 1 Rationale: Hyperuricemia is a side effect of thiazide diuretics such as hydrochlorothiazide, and this could lead to symptoms resembling gout (such as an enlarged, painful great toe). An increase in liver enzymes such as alanine aminotransferase (ALT) is not associated with thiazide diuretics. Clients may experience hyperglycemia, but this is more likely related to the comorbidity of diabetes mellitus than

to a drug side effect, and pain from diabetic neuropathy (if present) is not likely to occur in the toe. The drug is more likely to cause hypokalemia than a change in sodium level. Cognitive Level: Applying Client Need: Pharmacological and Parenteral Therapies Integrated Process: Nursing Process: Planning Content Area: Pharmacology Strategy: The core issue of the question is knowledge that symptoms of gout can occur with thiazide diuretics because of an increase in uric acid level. Eliminate the option referring to the liver first, based on location of symptoms and the option related to blood glucose for the same reason. Choose correctly between the remaining two by recalling that potassium is the electrolyte of concern or by associating the client's symptoms with an elevated uric acid level. Reference: Wilson, B. A., Shannon, M., & Shields, K. (2016). *Pearson nurse's drug guide 2016*. New York, NY: Pearson, pp. 749–751.

3 Answer: 3 Rationale: A blood pressure decrease when standing up from a lying or sitting position is called *orthostatic hypotension*. This can occur when a diuretic such as amiloride is added to antihypertensive drug therapy with hydralazine. An increase in urine output is an intended drug effect of a diuretic such as amiloride, but it is not an interactive drug effect. The pulse rate should not decrease with the addition of a diuretic to the client's medication list. A change in oxygen saturation is not expected with the addition of amiloride (a diuretic) to the client's medication list. Cognitive Level: Analyzing Client Need: Pharmacological and Parenteral Therapies Integrated Process: Nursing Process: Assessment Content Area: Pharmacology Strategy: The core issue of the question is knowledge of orthostatic hypotension as a interactive drug effect when a client receives both an antihypertensive drug and a diuretic. **Reference:** Wilson, B. A., Shannon, M., & Shields, K. (2016). *Pearson nurse's drug guide 2016*. New York, NY: Pearson, pp. 68–69.

4 **Answer: 2, 4 Rationale:** Mannitol may be prescribed for clients with increased intracranial pressure or increased intraocular pressure by causing diuresis. It would not be prescribed for clients with pancreatitis, diarrhea, and congestive heart failure. Clients with pancreatitis would not experience a benefit from a drug that promotes diuresis. Mannitol is known to precipitate pulmonary edema and heart failure because of its osmotic action. **Cognitive Level:** Applying **Client Need:** Pharmacological and Parenteral Therapies **Integrated Process:** Nursing Process: Implementation **Content Area:** Pharmacology **Strategy:** Consider first that mannitol is an osmotic diuretic. Then systematically review each option to determine which health problems would benefit from a state of diuresis. **Reference:** Lehne, R. (2015). *Pharmacology for nursing care* (9th ed.). St. Louis, MO: Elsevier, p. 451.

5 **Answer: 10 Rationale:** Because rapid administration of potassium chloride can lead to cardiac dysrhythmias and cardiac arrest, the recommended IV infusion rate should not exceed 10 mEq/hr. **Cognitive Level:** Applying **Client Need:** Pharmacological and Parenteral Therapies **Integrated Process:** Nursing Process: Planning **Content Area:** Pharmacology **Strategy:** The core issue of the question is knowledge of principles of safe administration of potassium chloride. Specific knowledge is needed to answer the question. **Reference:** Wilson, B. A., Shannon, M., & Shields, K. (2016). *Pearson nurse's drug guide 2016*. New York, NY: Pearson, pp. 1264–1265.

6 **Answers: 1, 3, 4, 5 Rationale:** Nitrofurantoin does cause a harmless brown discoloration to the urine. Clients should be made aware of this so it does not cause them concern. The client should continue to monitor for signs and symptoms of urinary tract infection, which can include cloudy or foul-smelling urine, in addition to classic symptoms of frequency, urgency, and dysuria. Muscle weakness, tingling, and numbness can be signs of neuropathy, which can be severe and irreversible. For this reason, these symptoms should be reported immediately to the prescriber. Nausea is a common side effect of this medication, although it can be reduced by using the macrocrystal form of nitrofurantoin. The client should maintain adequate fluid intake, but fluids are not generally "forced" or increased to high levels during chronic therapy. **Cognitive Level:** Applying **Client Need:** Pharmacological and Parenteral Therapies **Integrated Process:** Nursing Process: Planning **Content Area:** Pharmacology **Strategy:** The core issue of the question is knowledge of client teaching points related to nitrofurantoin drug therapy. Consider each

statement as true or false to aid in making correct selections. **Reference:** Wilson, B. A., Shannon, M., & Shields, K. (2016). *Pearson nurse's drug guide 2016*. New York, NY: Pearson, pp. 1094–1095.

7 **Answer: 2 Rationale:** Trimethoprim can cause serious adverse effects on the hematologic system, decreasing the red blood cell count, white blood cell count, and platelet count. These changes can be detected by a complete blood count. A potassium level would most commonly be of concern with drugs such as diuretics or digoxin. A uric acid level would be useful to detect side effects of thiazide diuretics or to detect gout. A serum osmolality would be useful in determining fluid volume status, such as for clients who have increased intracranial pressure. **Cognitive Level:** Applying **Client Need:** Pharmacological and Parenteral Therapies **Integrated Process:** Nursing Process: Evaluation **Content Area:** Pharmacology **Strategy:** The core issue of the question is knowledge of adverse effects of trimethoprim. Consider the hematologic adverse effects to choose correctly. **Reference:** Wilson, B. A., Shannon, M., & Shields, K. (2016). *Pearson nurse's drug guide 2016*. New York, NY: Pearson, pp. 1582–1583.

8 **Answer: 4 Rationale:** Oxybutynin is an antispasmodic used for urinary incontinence and bladder spasms. It causes anticholinergic side effects such as dry mouth, constipation, urinary hesitancy, and decreased gastroenteritis motility. For this reason the client needs to use measures to counteract dry mouth. Wearing protection is an appropriate action for urinary incontinence, but retention and hesitancy is associated with this drug. The drug has no effect on the clotting process so there is no unusual risk of injury. The anticholinergic actions are more likely to cause constipation than diarrhea. **Cognitive Level:** Applying **Client Need:** Pharmacological and Parenteral Therapies **Integrated Process:** Teaching and Learning **Content Area:** Pharmacology **Strategy:** First recall that oxybutynin is an antispasmodic that causes anticholinergic effects. Then evaluate each option to find the recommendation that matches the side effects of this drug. **Reference:** Wilson, B. A., Shannon, M., & Shields, K. (2016). *Pearson nurse's drug guide 2016*. New York, NY: Pearson, pp. 1147–1149.

9 **Answer: 1 Rationale:** Finasteride is an androgen inhibitor that may be used to treat enlarged prostate. It reduces the serum levels of testosterone, resulting in decreased prostate gland size and indirectly improving the flow of urine during voiding. Because of the risk of abnormalities to the fetus, pregnant women or women of childbearing age should not be exposed to semen fluid of a male taking finasteride. The decreased serum level of testosterone may result in decreased libido, but is not as relevant as the risk to the developing fetus. Because of urinary stasis that accompanies enlarged prostate, the client should increase fluid intake to prevent infection. Once again, however, this is not as relevant as the health of a developing fetus. It may take 6–12 months to reach full therapeutic effectiveness so 3 weeks is too short a time frame. **Cognitive Level:** Analyzing **Client Need:** Pharmacological and Parenteral Therapies **Integrated Process:** Teaching and Learning **Content Area:** Pharmacology **Strategy:** Recall first that finasteride (Proscar) is an androgen inhibitor, and then associate fetal deformities with the drug. **Reference:** Wilson, B. A., Shannon, M., & Shields, K. (2016). *Pearson nurse's drug guide 2016.* New York, NY: Pearson, pp. 144–145.

10 **Answer: 3 Rationale:** The client's blood pressure may increase during early therapy as the hematocrit rises. The nurse should monitor the trend in this vital sign and alert the healthcare provider if there is significant increase, which could warrant a dosage reduction. Epoetin alfa does not cause a rise or drop in body temperature. The client's pulse rate is not expected to change significantly during drug therapy with epoetin alfa. A change in oxygen saturation is not an adverse drug effect of epoetin alfa. **Cognitive Level:** Applying **Client Need:** Pharmacological and Parenteral Therapies **Integrated Process:** Nursing Process: Evaluation **Content Area:** Pharmacology **Strategy:** The core issue of the question is knowledge of adverse effects of epoetin alfa. Consider possible consequences of a rapidly rising hematocrit to choose correctly. **Reference:** Wilson, B. A., Shannon, M., & Shields, K. (2016). *Pearson nurse's drug guide 2016.* New York, NY: Pearson, pp. 576–577.

Posttest

1 **Answer: 3 Rationale:** The nurse should be most concerned with the low serum potassium result (normal 3.5–5.1 mEq/L) because bumetanide is a potassium-wasting diuretic. The blood urea nitrogen is within normal limits (8–22 mg/dL) and is not of concern. The blood glucose is only slightly elevated (normal 70–110 mg/dL) so it is not the priority and is not related to therapy with bumetanide. The calcium level is within normal limits (8.5–11 mg/dL). **Cognitive Level:** Analyzing **Client Need:** Pharmacological and Parenteral Therapies **Integrated Process:** Nursing Process: Assessment **Content Area:** Pharmacology **Strategy:** The core issue of the question is knowledge of the effects of drug therapy on laboratory values. Recall concerns with potassium-wasting diuretics to choose correctly. **Reference:** Wilson, B. A., Shannon, M., & Shields, K. (2016). *Pearson nurse's drug guide 2016.* New York, NY: Pearson, pp. 212–213.

2 **Answer: 2 Rationale:** Indapamide is a thiazide diuretic that may cause hypokalemia. Because the function of potassium involves the action potential of smooth muscles such as arteries, hypokalemia can result in irregular muscle contractions. Hence, muscle weakness and leg cramps can occur. Since the cause of the signs and symptoms is manageable and the problems do not significantly impact the client's health, terminating the drug is not necessary. Furosemide is a loop diuretic that can also result in hypokalemia. Since the leg cramps are the result of hypokalemia, a nonsteroidal anti-inflammatory drug (NSAID) is not the appropriate treatment for the symptom. **Cognitive Level:** Analyzing **Client Need:** Pharmacological and Parenteral Therapies **Integrated Process:** Nursing Process: Implementation **Content Area:** Pharmacology **Strategy:** First determine that indapamide is a diuretic. Then correlate the category of the drug with potential side effects that could result in leg cramps. **Reference:** Wilson, B. A., Shannon, M., & Shields, K. (2016). *Pearson nurse's drug guide 2016.* New York, NY: Pearson, pp. 790–791.

3 **Answers: 1, 2, 5 Rationale:** Spironolactone is a potassium-sparing diuretic, so the client should avoid excessive intake of foods high in potassium. Bananas, cantaloupe (and other melons), and spinach are high in potassium and should be avoided or limited while taking spironolactone. Grapes and green or wax beans are lower in potassium and may be eaten regularly while taking spironolactone. **Cognitive Level:** Analyzing **Client Need:** Pharmacological and Parenteral Therapies **Integrated Process:** Nursing Process: Assessment **Content Area:** Pharmacology **Strategy:** The core issue of the question is knowledge of spironolactone as a potassium-sparing diuretic and foods to avoid or limit during therapy. **Reference:** Wilson, B. A., Shannon, M., & Shields, K. (2016). *Pearson nurse's drug guide 2016.* New York, NY: Pearson, pp. 1442–1444.

4 **Answer: 2 Rationale:** Acetazolamide is a carbonic anhydrase inhibitor that has uses as a diuretic and antiglaucoma agent. The nurse should anticipate that the client has open-angle glaucoma as part of the health history. Addison disease or other adrenocortical insufficiency would be a contraindication to the use of acetazolamide. Acetazolamide is contraindicated for use in severe liver disease. Diuretics such as loop diuretics or thiazide diuretics are commonly used to treat heart failure. **Cognitive Level:** Analyzing **Client Need:** Pharmacological and Parenteral Therapies **Integrated Process:** Nursing Process: Assessment **Content Area:** Pharmacology **Strategy:** The core issue of the question is knowledge of the intended uses for acetazolamide, a carbonic anhydrase inhibitor. **Reference:** Wilson, B. A., Shannon, M., & Shields, K. (2016). *Pearson nurse's drug guide 2016.* New York, NY: Pearson, pp. 13–14.

5 **Answer: 1, 2, 4, 5 Rationale:** Potassium can be irritating to the GI tract so the client should take the dose with meals. Because hyperkalemia is a risk if there is excessive potassium supplementation, the client should report signs of hyperkalemia such as irregular pulse, fatigue, or weakness in legs. Soluble tablets should be dissolved in at least 4 ounces of liquid, while whole tablets should be taken with a large glass of liquid (if allowed). The client should avoid the use of salt substitutes while taking potassium chloride because salt substitutes are high in potassium and could lead to hyperkalemia. Diarrhea and vomiting are not expected side effects and should be reported. **Cognitive Level:** Analyzing **Client Need:** Pharmacological and Parenteral Therapies **Integrated Process:** Teaching and Learning **Content Area:** Pharmacology **Strategy:** The core issue of the question is knowledge of principles of safe self-administration of potassium. Because more than one option is correct, evaluate each option as a true–false statement. **Reference:** Wilson, B. A., Shannon, M., & Shields, K. (2016). *Pearson nurse's drug guide 2016*. New York, NY: Pearson, pp. 1265–1266.

6 **Answer: 1 Rationale:** Methenamine is a urinary tract anti-infective that is useful in treating urinary tract infections. Some types of bladder incontinence may be treated with drugs that reduce bladder spasm. Methenamine is not useful in treating acute kidney injury, which would be characterized by a sudden drop in urine output. Methenamine would not counteract the effects of chronic renal failure, which is an irreversible health problem. **Cognitive Level:** Applying **Client Need:** Pharmacological and Parenteral Therapies **Integrated Process:** Nursing Process: Analysis **Content Area:** Pharmacology **Strategy:** The core issue of the question is knowledge of uses for methenamine, a urinary anti-infective. Use this knowledge and the process of elimination to make a selection. **Reference:** Wilson, B. A., Shannon, M., & Shields, K. (2016). *Pearson nurse's drug guide 2016*. New York, NY: Pearson, pp. 981–983.

7 **Answer: 2 Rationale:** Early signs of hypersensitivity require immediate intervention, so the client should report sudden onset of fever, pruritis, or malaise. Checking the urine pH decreases the potential for stone formation, a very painful but not life-threatening problem. Fluid intake should produce 1,500 mL/day, and the client needs to take in at least 2 liters of fluid per day. The medication is more soluble in alkaline urine, but attending to a hypersensitive reaction takes priority. **Cognitive Level:** Analyzing **Client Need:** Pharmacological and Parenteral Therapies **Integrated Process:** Teaching and Learning **Content Area:** Pharmacology **Strategy:** Note the syllable *sulf* in the drug and associate this with a sulfa drug, which has high allergenic potential. Correlate this with the signs and symptoms in the correct option and the immediacy of need. **Reference:** Wilson, B. A., Shannon, M., & Shields, K. (2016). *Pearson nurse's drug guide 2016*. New York, NY: Pearson, p. 1453.

8 **Answer: 4 Rationale:** Phenazopyridine is a urinary tract analgesic that may be prescribed alone or may be combined with an antibiotic appropriate for urinary tract infections. Yellow-tinged skin is a sign of drug accumulation related to renal impairment. This sign should be reported to the prescriber, if noted. Although it may be manufactured in combination with an antibiotic, it could also be discontinued after pain with urination is relieved, often after 1–2 days of antibiotic therapy. Any drug that is used long term would require follow-up, but this drug is used on a short-term basis. The safety of the drug during breastfeeding is unsubstantiated. **Cognitive Level:** Applying **Client Need:** Pharmacological and Parenteral Therapies **Integrated Process:** Teaching and Learning **Content Area:** Pharmacology **Strategy:** Associate the characteristics of the drug with the significant risks to the client. Frequently, medication questions seek to determine knowledge of adverse effects and the action needed if they occur. **Reference:** Wilson, B. A., Shannon, M., & Shields, K. (2016). *Pearson nurse's drug guide 2016*. New York, NY: Pearson, pp. 1211–1212.

9 **Answers: 2, 3, 4 Rationale:** Tolterodine is an antimuscarinic type of anticholinergic agent used to control symptoms of overactive bladder. It helps to control symptoms such as urinary frequency, urgency, and leakage of urine. Tolterodine does not treat conditions leading to decreased urine output. Tolterodine does not treat urinary infection or other conditions associated with hematuria. **Cognitive Level:** Analyzing **Client Need:** Pharmacological and Parenteral Therapies **Integrated Process:** Nursing Process: Evaluation **Content Area:** Pharmacology **Strategy:** The core issue of the question is knowledge of intended effects of tolterodine. Because more than one option is correct, evaluate each option as a true–false statement. **Reference:** Wilson, B. A., Shannon, M., & Shields, K. (2016). *Pearson nurse's drug guide 2016*. New York, NY: Pearson, pp. 1553–1554.

10 **Answers: 3, 4, 5 Rationale:** Therapeutic outcomes of tamsulosin would include decreased urethral obstruction, increased urine flow, and decreased urinary frequency. Hypotension and syncope are adverse effects of tamsulosin. **Cognitive Level:** Analyzing **Client Need:** Pharmacological and Parenteral Therapies **Integrated Process:** Nursing Process: Evaluation **Content Area:** Pharmacology **Strategy:** The critical words in the question are *therapeutic outcomes*. With this in mind, select the options that are intended effects of the drug. **Reference:** Lehne, R. A. (2016). *Pharmacology for nursing care* (9th ed.). St. Louis, MO: Saunders, p. 782.

References

Adams, M., Holland, L., & Bostwick, P. (2017). *Pharmacology for nurses: A patho-physiologic approach* (5th ed.). New York, NY: Pearson.

Adams, M., & Urban, C. (2016). *Pharmacology: Connections to nursing practice* (3rd ed.). New York, NY: Pearson.

Drug Facts & Comparisons (Updated monthly). St. Louis, MO: A. Wolters Kluwer.

Karch, A. M. (2017). *Focus on nursing pharmacology* (7th ed.). Philadelphia, PA: Lippincott Williams & Wilkins.

Kee, J. (2017). *Handbook of laboratory and diagnostic tests and nursing implications* (8th ed.). New York, NY: Pearson.

Lehne, R. (2016). *Pharmacology for nursing care* (9th ed.). St. Louis, MO: Mosby.

LeMone, P. T., Burke, K. M., Bauldoff, G., & Gubrud, P. (2015). *Medical surgical nursing: Clinical reasoning in patient care* (6th ed.). New York, NY: Pearson.

Wilson, B. A., Shannon, M. T., & Shields, K. M. (2016). *Pearson nurse's drug guide 2016*. New York, NY: Pearson.

Gastrointestinal System Medications

9

Chapter Outline

Gastrointestinal (GI) Stimulants
Medications to Decrease
    GI Tone and Motility
    (Anticholinergics and
    Antispasmodics)
Antidiarrheals
Laxatives

Antiemetics
Histamine H_2 Antagonists
Proton Pump Inhibitors
Mucosal Protective Agents
Antacids
Antimicrobials for *Helicobacter
    pylori* Organisms

Medications Used to Dissolve
    Gallstones
Pancreatic Enzyme
    Replacement

Objectives

➤ Describe general goals of therapy when administering gastrointestinal system medications.
➤ Describe the use and side effects of antacids.
➤ Identify the actions of various forms of laxatives.
➤ Explain the effects of H_2-receptor antagonists, proton pump inhibitors, and mucosal protectants on the gastrointestinal tract.
➤ Describe client-centered nursing care related to administration of antiemetics.
➤ Identify specific food and drug interactions associated with various gastrointestinal system medications.
➤ Describe nursing considerations related to administration of pancreatic enzyme replacements.
➤ List significant client education points related to gastrointestinal system medications.

NCLEX-RN® Test Prep

Access the NEW Web-based app that provides students with additional practice questions in preparation for the NCLEX experience.

Review at a Glance

antacid agent that reduces or neutralizes acidity
anticholinergic antagonist to parasympathetic action or other cholinergic receptors
antispasmodic agent that prevents or relieves spasms

cathartic agent with purgative action
H₂ antagonist antagonist agent against histamine that decreases gastrin secretion
Helicobacter pylori bacteria found in gastric mucosa that produces urease

and is associated commonly with gastric and duodenal ulcers
laxative agent used to cause a bowel movement or loosening of the bowels
surfactant a surface-active agent also known as a wetting agent, tension depressant, detergent, and emulsifier

PRETEST

1 A constipated client is given a prescription to use psyllium mucilloid. What information should the nurse provide during client education about the medication?

1. Refrain from physical activity for 2 hours.
2. Follow the initial dose with an additional 8 ounces of water.
3. Take an antiemetic.
4. Sprinkle the powder formulation on food.

2 A client with gastroesophageal reflux disease (GERD) is taking metoclopramide as prescribed. What client statement indicates to the nurse that the medication instruction was effective?

1. "The purpose of this drug is to increase GI motility."
2. "This drug decreases the tone of the lower esophageal sphincter."
3. "This drug will prevent or stop diarrhea from occurring."
4. "This drug kills the *H. pylori* organism that causes peptic ulcer disease."

3 A client is taking dicyclomine for irritable bowel syndrome (IBS). Which nursing assessment is the best indicator that the client is self-administering the medication properly?

1. Presence of mucus in stool
2. Weighs 4.5 kg (10 lb) less than last examination
3. Bowel sounds are hypoactive
4. Nutritional intake within normal ranges

4 A client who is allergic to aspirin has acute diarrhea. Based on the aspirin allergy, which medication should the nurse avoid administering?

1. Attapulgite
2. Bismuth subsalicylate
3. Diphenoxylate with atropine
4. Loperamide

5 The nurse determines that further instructions are needed if a client with diarrhea makes which statement?

1. "I need to avoid intake of dairy products."
2. "I should take bismuth subsalicylate as directed."
3. "I should call my healthcare provider if diarrhea lasts more than 2 days."
4. "If the diarrhea persists, I should start taking psyllium mucilloid."

6 The nurse is selecting candidates for a health screening project regarding the abuse of laxatives. The *best* client group includes which of the following?

1. Older adult clients with congestive heart failure (CHF)
2. Clients with irritable bowel syndrome (IBS)
3. Clients with bulimia nervosa or anorexia nervosa
4. Clients who are obese

7 A healthy adult client has been taking a laxative 3 days per week for 9 months. What primary risk should the nurse address in a teaching plan with this client?

1. Risk of electrolyte imbalance
2. Risk of drug dependence
3. Risk of fluid imbalance
4. Risk for inadequate nutritional status

8 After noting a new prescription for loperamide 4 mg by mouth, every 6 hours as needed for a 71-year-old client, the nurse should provide which instruction to unlicensed assistive personnel (UAP)?

1. Set up seizure precautions.
2. Set up safety precautions.
3. Measure vital signs every 4 hours.
4. Place a commode at the bedside.

9 After being diagnosed with an open-cratered gastric ulcer, a 19-year-old female client starts crying and refuses to take the prescribed medications. The nurse should perform which activities at this time? Select all that apply.

1. Explain in detail the action of ranitidine.
2. Sit with client to allow her to express her feelings.
3. Teach client about ways to prevent future ulcerations.
4. Explain risks associated with not treating the open-crater gastric ulcer.
5. Encourage the client to ingest the dose of misoprostol.

10 Because magnetic resonance imaging (MRI) revealed an open-cratered gastric ulcer, a semi-comatose female client is receiving misoprostol. In what order should the nurse prioritize directions about client care to the unlicensed assistant personnel (UAPs)? Place the activities in order of priority.

1. Maintain head of bed at 35 degrees.
2. Report restlessness.
3. Place bed protector beneath client.
4. Keep a log of client's bowel pattern.
5. Report vaginal spotting.

➤ *See pages 297–298 for Answers and Rationales.*

I. GASTROINTESTINAL (GI) STIMULANTS

A. Action and use
1. Decrease reflux by increasing sphincter tone, enhancing acid clearance, and decreasing gastric emptying
2. Decrease or prevent nausea and vomiting due to chemotherapy, and facilitate small bowel intubations
3. Used for delayed gastric emptying caused by diabetic gastroparesis, gastroesophageal reflux disease (GERD), or postoperative nausea and vomiting
4. Stimulate gastric motility without stimulating gastric, biliary, or pancreatic secretion
5. Sensitize tissues to action of acetylcholine and induce release of prolactin
6. Dexpanthenol minimizes risk of paralytic ileus after major abdominal surgery

B. Common GI stimulant medications: see Table 9-1

C. Administration considerations
1. Metoclopramide PO should be taken 30 minutes before meals and bedtime
2. Metoclopramide IV should be given 30 minutes prior to chemotherapy for anti-emetic effect

D. Contraindications
1. Hypersensitivity, history of seizure disorders, pheochromocytoma, and Parkinson's disease (metoclopramide)

Table 9-1 **Gastrointestinal Stimulants**

Generic Name	Route	Uses
Dexpanthenol [dextro-pantothenyl alcohol]	IM, IV, Topical	Prophylactic use immediately after major abdominal surgery to minimize paralytic ileus development, intestinal atony, postoperative or postpartum flatus, resumption of GI motility following paralytic ileus, eczema, dermatosis, diaper rash, chafing
Metoclopramide	PO, IM, IV	Relief of acute symptoms or recurrent symptoms of diabetic gastroparesis or GERD, prevention of nausea and vomiting, facilitation of small bowel intubation (single dose), stimulation of gastric emptying and movement of barium, improvement of lactation, relief of nausea or vomiting associated with many etiologies including pregnancy

2. Contraindicated in clients where overstimulation may be dangerous, such as with GI hemorrhage, obstruction, or perforation
3. Contraindicated with allergy to dextran, marked hemostatic defects, congestive heart failure (CHF), and renal failure (dexpanthenol)
4. Use with caution in clients with a history of depression, seizure disorder, or hypertension
5. Lactation: excreted in breast milk, so caution should be used in nursing mothers

E. **Significant drug interactions**
1. Metoclopramide is metabolized by P450 liver enzyme system and should not be taken with inhibitors of this enzyme such as macrolides, antifungals, and some protease inhibitors; may decrease absorption of digoxin
2. Concomitant use of metoclopramide, hyoscyamine, and tricyclic antidepressants may antagonize effects of metoclopramide
3. Levodopa has the opposite effect and may antagonize metoclopramide effect
4. Metoclopramide may increase hypertensive effects of monoamine oxidase inhibitors (MAOIs) and decrease absorption of digoxin from GI tract
5. Increased toxic and immunosuppressive effects of cyclosporine

F. **Significant food interactions**: none reported

G. **Significant laboratory studies**: serum electrolyte levels, falsely elevated glucose level

H. **Side effects**
1. Drowsiness, diarrhea, restlessness, fatigue
2. Parkinsonlike symptoms
3. Transient hypertension
4. Constipation

I. **Adverse effects/toxicity**
1. Seizures, extrapyramidal symptoms, neuroleptic malignant syndrome
2. Agranulocytosis
3. Depression with suicide ideations

J. **Client-centered nursing care**
1. Monitor for possible hypernatremia and hypokalemia, particularly if client has CHF or liver cirrhosis
2. Extrapyramidal symptoms may occur in young and older adults and with high-dose treatment of metoclopramide
3. Monitor BP carefully when administering metoclopramide IV

K. **Client education**
1. Report signs and symptoms of side effects
2. Report signs of acute dystonia immediately
3. Do not drive for a few hours after taking metoclopramide
4. Drink adequate amounts of fluids
5. Avoid humid environments with methoscopolamine

II. MEDICATIONS TO DECREASE GI TONE AND MOTILITY (ANTICHOLINERGICS AND ANTISPASMODICS)

A. **Action and use**
1. **Anticholinergics** antagonize the action of acetylcholine at specific cholinergic receptor sites
2. **Antispasmodics** are similar; they are believed to relax smooth muscle
3. Used for treatment of spasms of GI tract such as pylorospasm, ileitis, and irritable bowel syndrome
4. Methoscopalamine blocks effect of acetylcholine, relaxing smooth muscles

B. **Common medications for GI tone and motility**: see Table 9-2

Table 9-2	**Medications to Decrease GI Tone and Motility: Anticholinergics/Antispasmodics**	
Generic Name	**Route**	**Uses**
Dicyclomine hydrochloride	PO	Functional bowel or irritable bowel syndrome
Hyoscyamine sulfate	PO	Irritable bowel syndrome, peptic ulcer disease, spastic or functional disorders, cystitis, neurogenic bladder, parkinsonism, biliary and renal colic, rhinitis, anticholinesterase poisoning, partial heart block associated with vagal activity, and to decrease operative secretions
Methscopolamine bromide	PO	Peptic ulcer disease
Propantheline bromide	PO	Peptic ulcer disease

C. **Administration considerations:** give medication 30–60 minutes before meals and at bedtime for therapeutic effect

D. **Contraindications**
1. Angle-closure glaucoma, obstructive GI disease, paralytic ileus, obstructive uropathy, adhesions between iris and lens, myocardial ischemia, toxic megacolon
2. Excreted in breast milk; may cause infant toxicity and decreased milk production
3. Use with caution with renal dysfunction

E. **Significant drug interactions**
1. Use of another anticholinergic drug may result in increased anticholinergic side effects
2. Atropine may increase the effect of phenothiazines
3. Increased effects of atenolol with anticholinergic drugs
4. Decreased effectiveness of all antipsychotic medications with dicyclomine
5. Decreased effects of haloperidol and phenothiazines with propantheline bromide
6. Antacids decrease absorption of anticholinergics

F. **Significant food interactions:** none reported

G. **Significant laboratory studies:** serum electrolyte levels

H. **Side effects**
1. Hypersensitivity
2. Urticaria, rash, dry mouth, nausea and vomiting, constipation, urinary hesitance and retention
3. Impotence, blurred vision, worsening of glaucoma
4. Palpitations, headache, flushing, drowsiness, dizziness, confusion

I. **Adverse effects/toxicity**
1. May cause dilated, nonreactive pupils, visual changes
2. Tachycardia
3. Dysphagia, decreased or absent bowel sounds
4. Hyperthermia, hypertension, increased respiratory rate

J. **Client-centered nursing care**
1. An understanding of the factors contributing to the diarrhea is essential in effective treatment
2. Clients who lose significant potassium with diarrhea are at risk for the development of paralytic ileus and cardiac dysrhythmias
3. They should also be monitored for metabolic acidosis because of the loss of bicarbonate and impaired renal excretion of acids
4. Document indications and present medications
5. Monitor vital signs, urine output, and visual changes
6. Monitor intake and output (I&O)

K. Client education

1. Avoid exposure to high temperatures because of risk of hyperthermia
2. Report side effects to healthcare provider
3. Dietary and fluid interventions to decrease constipation
4. Report any additional medications prescribed
5. Self-monitor I&O
6. Take drug as prescribed

III. ANTIDIARRHEALS

A. Action and use

1. Slow and/or inhibit GI motility by acting on nerve endings of the intestinal wall, thereby reducing the volume of stools, increasing viscosity, and decreasing fluid and electrolyte loss
2. Used for symptomatic relief of acute nonspecific diarrhea and diarrhea of inflammatory disease

B. Common antidiarrheal medications: see Table 9-3

C. Administration considerations

1. Shake suspensions well; chew tablets thoroughly
2. Stool may appear gray-black (may mask GI bleeding)
3. Do not give concurrently with other medications
4. Seek medical care if diarrhea persists for more than 2 days in an adult
5. Do not use to treat diarrhea in children; seek medical attention
6. Do not give to clients with *C. difficile*

D. Contraindications

1. Presence of bloody diarrhea, diarrhea associated with pathogens such as *E. coli*, salmonella, shigella or pseudomembranous colitis, or other bacterial toxins
2. Avoid use if obstructive bowel disease is suspected
3. Avoid bismuth subsalicylate if allergic to aspirin
4. Difenoxine/atropine sulfate may cause serious side effects in nursing infants; therefore, should not be used for children under 2 years of age

E. Significant drug interactions

1. Allergies to aspirin or other salicylates since bismuth subsalicylate contains salicylate
2. Avoid aspirin use as concomitant use with bismuth subsalicylate, which may cause aspirin toxicity
3. Bismuth may also decrease tetracycline absorption in the GI tract

Table 9-3	Antidiarrheals	
Generic Name	**Route**	**Uses**
Bismuth subsalicylate	PO	Indigestion, nausea, diarrhea, control and prevention of traveler's diarrhea, relieve gas and abdominal cramping, chronic infantile diarrhea
Diphenoxylate	PO	Diarrhea, traveler's diarrhea
Loperamide	PO	Acute nonspecific diarrhea, chronic diarrhea associated with inflammatory bowel disease, reduction of discharge volume from ileostomy, traveler's diarrhea
Octreotide acetate	Subcut, IM, IV	Suppression or inhibition of severe diarrhea associated with metastatic carcinoid tumors, profuse watery diarrhea, reduction of growth hormone in clients with acromegaly
Rifaximin	PO	Clients 12 years and older with traveler's diarrhea caused by noninvasive *E. coli*

      4. Diphenoxylate/atropine sulfate and difenoxin/atropine sulfate may increase the sedative effects of barbiturates, narcotics, and alcohol

      5. Concurrent use with MAOIs may increase risk of hypertensive crisis

  F. Significant food interactions: none reported

  G. Significant laboratory studies: diphenoxylate may increase serum amylase levels

  H. Side effects

      1. Nausea and vomiting

      2. Dry mouth, dizziness, drowsiness, constipation

      3. Temporary darkening of stools and tongue may occur with bismuth salicylate

  I. Adverse effects/toxicity

      1. Clinical signs and symptoms of overdose include drowsiness, decreased blood pressure (BP), seizures, apnea, blurred vision, dry mouth, and psychosis

      2. Risk of aspirin toxicity with concurrent use of aspirin and bismuth subsalicylate

      3. Other adverse effects include central nervous system (CNS) depression, respiratory depression, hypotonic reflexes, angioedema, anaphylaxis, and paralytic ileus

  J. Client-centered nursing care

      1. Note allergies

      2. Document onset, duration, and frequency of symptoms

      3. Document previous therapies used

      4. Note current medications

      5. Identify any causative factors; perform stool analysis if necessary and prescribed

      6. Assess for evidence of dehydration or electrolyte imbalance

      7. Monitor vital signs and I&O

      8. Note presence of comorbid conditions

      9. Check abdomen for tenderness, distention, bowel sounds, or masses

     10. Administer bismuth and tetracycline 1 hour apart

  K. Client education

      1. Withhold solid food for 24 hours with acute diarrhea

      2. Foods that aggravate diarrhea include milk products, fruit and fruit juices, coffee or tea with caffeine, and chocolate

      3. Drink fluids to avoid dehydration and alleviate dry mouth

      4. Follow BRAT diet—bananas, rice, applesauce, tea/toast—to avoid dehydration if recommended by healthcare provider (controversial)

      5. Do not exceed prescribed dose

      6. Consult healthcare provider if diarrhea persists over 2 days

      7. Use caution in activities requiring alertness if dizziness or drowsiness is present (possible side effects)

      8. Report fever, nausea and vomiting, abdominal pain, or distention

      9. Avoid OTC antacids, dairy products, and other foods that aggravate diarrhea

     10. Use good personal hygiene to avoid skin irritation or breakdown because of diarrhea

     11. Avoid alcohol ingestion while taking medication

     12. Notify healthcare provider if pregnant or breastfeeding

     13. Report tinnitus if using bismuth products as it may be a sign of salicysm (salicylate toxicity)

IV. LAXATIVES

  A. Bulk-forming laxatives

      1. Action and use

         a. Include nonabsorbable polysaccharide and cellulose derivatives

         b. Bulk-forming **laxatives** absorb water to increase bulk in fecal mass

---

Practice to Pass

How long should a client take an over-the-counter (OTC) anti-diarrheal medication before consulting a healthcare provider?

      c. Peristalsis is stimulated by increased fecal mass, which decreases bowel transit time

      d. They generally produce a laxative effect within 12 to 14 hours but may require 2–3 days for full effect

      e. Are frequently used to prevent straining with defecation in clients who are post–myocardial infarction or have other conditions in which straining at stool could be harmful

    2. Common laxative medications: see Table 9-4

    3. Administration considerations

      a. Since these agents rely on water to increase their bulk, it is essential that adequate fluids be given for bowel absorption

      b. These agents may also cause intestinal and esophageal obstruction when insufficient liquid is administered with dose

      c. Each dose should be given with a full glass of liquid (240 mL) and followed with a full glass of liquid (240 mL)

      d. Use sugar-free preparations in clients with phenylketonuria

Table 9-4   **Laxatives**

Generic Name	Usual Adult Dosage Range	Route
Bulk-Forming Laxatives		
Methylcellulose	1 tsp (19 grams) in 8 oz of water 1–3 times a day	PO
Calcium polycarbophil	2 tablets 1–4 times a day	PO
Psyllium mucilloid	3–4 grams in 8 oz of liquid 1–3 times a day	PO
Stimulant Laxatives		
Bisacodyl	10–15 mg at HS	PO
Castor oil	15–60 mL	PO
Glycerin	1 suppository	PR
Senna	2 tablets at HS	PO
Hyperosmotic Laxatives		
Lactulose	10–20 grams in 4 oz water	PO
Polyethylene glycol	17 grams in 8 oz water daily	PO
Glycerin	3-gram suppository	Rectal
Stool Softeners (Surfactants)		
Docusate sodium	50–300 mg daily	PO
Docusate potassium	100–300 mg daily	PO
Docusate calcium	240 mg daily	PO
Lubiprostone	8–24 mg daily	PO
Saline Laxatives		
Magnesium hydroxide	30–60 mL at HS	PO
Sodium biphosphate	1.25 oz enema	Rectal
Miscellaneous Laxatives		
Mineral oil	15–30 mL	PO
Nalogexol	25 mg daily	PO
Linaclotide	145–290 mg/day	PO

4. Contraindications
    a. Not recommended for clients with intestinal stenosis, ulceration, or adhesions
    b. Use cautiously in clients with swallowing difficulties to ensure aspiration does not occur
    c. Do not use if fecal impaction is present
5. Significant drug interactions: decreased GI absorption may occur with digitalis, anticoagulants, nitrofurantoin, and salicylates
6. Significant food interactions
    a. Dietary management of constipation can be aided by encouraging intake of fluid and fiber
    b. Fiber increases stool bulk and water retention in bowel
    c. A dietary bulk-forming nutrient such as bran is an appropriate adjunctive therapy for constipation
    d. Bran is only partially fermented by bacteria, resulting in increased stool bulk, accelerated transit time, and promotion of normal defecation
    e. Rapid increases in dietary roughage may cause abdominal bloating and flatulence
    f. Adequate fluid intake is also necessary in order to prevent fecal impaction
    g. Generally 240–360 mL of fluid with each tablespoon of bran is sufficient
    h. Avoid foods that reduce stool, such as bananas, rice, breads, and cheeses
7. Significant laboratory studies: none reported
8. Side effects
    a. Abdominal discomfort and/or bloating, flatulence
    b. Nausea and vomiting, diarrhea
9. Adverse effects/toxicity
    a. Rare reports of allergic reactions to karaya such as urticaria, rhinitis, dermatitis, bronchospasm
    b. Esophageal obstruction, swelling, or blockage may occur when insufficient fluid is used in mixing a bulk-forming laxative
10. Client-centered nursing care
    a. Assess degree of abdominal distention, bowel sounds, and bowel elimination patterns
    b. Assess swallowing ability, adequately mix agents in liquid and encourage additional fluid intake
    c. Monitor for aspiration
    d. If administered via feeding tube, it must be a large-bore tube, and medication must be adequately dissolved in liquid and given rapidly with adequate flushing
    e. Add at least 240 mL (8 oz) of water or juice to drug
    f. Separate psyllium administration from digoxin, salicylates, and anticoagulants by 2 hours
    g. Use sugar-free preparations in diabetic clients
11. Client education
    a. These agents require adequate hydration to be effective
    b. Additional fluids and exercise are helpful in aiding bowel elimination
    c. Mix powder preparation with at least 240 mL (8 oz) fluid and drink immediately and follow with another 240 mL (8 oz) of fluid
    d. Bulk-forming laxatives may decrease appetite if taken before meals
    e. Take bulk-forming laxative 2 hours after meals and any oral medications
    f. Use sodium and sugar-free preparations if they are appropriate to individual diet restrictions
    g. Full effect of medication may not occur for 2–3 days

B. Stimulant cathartics
  1. Action and use
     a. **Cathartics** are agents with purgative actions
     b. Called stimulants because they stimulate peristalsis via mucosal irritation or intramural nerve plexus activity, which results in increased motility
     c. Stimulant laxatives may alter permeability of colonic mucosal cells, which results in intraluminal fluid and electrolyte secretion
     d. Defecation occurs between 6 and 12 hours after oral administration of these agents
     e. Rectal administration of bisacodyl and senna produces catharsis within 15 minutes to 2 hours
  2. Common medications (see Table 9-4 again)
  3. Administration considerations
     a. Bedtime administration of dose promotes a morning bowel movement
     b. Swallow tablet whole; do not crush
     c. Do not take within 1 hour of antacids; do not take with milk
  4. Contraindications
     a. Contraindicated with abdominal pain, nausea and vomiting, symptoms of appendicitis, rectal bleeding, gastroenteritis, intestinal obstruction, fecal impaction
     b. Use senna cautiously with nursing mothers as senna is excreted in breast milk
  5. Significant drug interactions: antacids and drugs that increase gastric pH may result in GI irritation or cramping
  6. Significant food interactions: do not take within 1 hour of milk
  7. Significant laboratory studies: none reported
  8. Side effects
     a. Nausea and vomiting, abdominal cramps, diarrhea, laxative dependence
     b. Muscle weakness, fluid and electrolyte imbalance
     c. Rectal burning or irritation with suppository use
  9. Adverse effects/toxicity
     a. Hypokalemia, hypocalcemia
     b. Metabolic acidosis or alkalosis
  10. Client-centered nursing care
     a. Evaluate for nausea and vomiting, abdominal pain, or diarrhea
     b. Evaluate for medication effectiveness
     c. Monitor for fluid and electrolyte imbalances
     d. Administer medication 1 hour before or after ingestion of milk or an antacid
     e. Encourage increased fluids and diet alterations to include increased amounts of high-fiber foods
     f. Evaluate for laxative dependence and offer counseling
  11. Client education
     a. Discourage client from chronic use of laxatives; use beyond 1 week should be avoided
     b. These agents may produce a cathartic colon if used for several years; colon develops abnormal motor function and on x-ray resembles ulcerative colitis; usually discontinuation of laxative use restores normal bowel function
     c. Increase fluid intake and diet high in fiber
     d. Report signs and symptoms of side effects immediately
     e. Take medications 1 hour before or after ingestion of milk or an antacid

C. Hyperosmotic cathartics
  1. Action and use
     a. Increase osmotic pressure within intestinal lumen, which results in luminal retention of water, softening stool
     b. Lactulose is an unabsorbed disaccharide metabolized by colonic bacteria primarily to lactic acid, formic, and acetic acids

         c. It has been proposed that these organic acids may contribute to osmotic effect

         d. Used for treatment of occasional constipation

         e. Used to reduce ammonia levels (lactulose)

    2. Common medications (see Table 9-4 again)

    3. Administration considerations

         a. Glycerin is available only for rectal administration (suppository or enema) for treatment of acute constipation; its laxative effect occurs within 15 to 30 minutes

         b. Lactulose may require 24–48 hours for effect; it is also more costly and should be reserved for acute constipation

         c. Dissolve 17 grams polyethylene glycol 3350 in 240 mL (8 oz) water and use once daily for up to 2 weeks; it may take 2–4 days for results to occur

    4. Contraindications

         a. Contraindicated in bowel obstruction

         b. Use lactulose cautiously in clients with diabetes mellitus

    5. Significant drug interactions: antibiotics may decrease laxative effect by elimination of bacteria needed to digest active form

    6. Significant food interactions: none reported

    7. Significant laboratory studies: serum electrolyte levels

    8. Side effects

         a. Glycerin: rectal irritation and burning, hyperemia of rectal mucosa

         b. Lactulose and polyethylene glycol 3350: flatulence, abdominal cramps and bloating, diarrhea

    9. Adverse effects/toxicity: fluid and electrolyte imbalances

    10. Client-centered nursing care

         a. Polyethylene glycol 3350 should always be dissolved in 240 mL of water

         b. Dilute lactulose in water or juice to decrease sweet taste

         c. Monitor frequency and consistency of stools

         d. Monitor for electrolyte imbalances, especially in older adults

    11. Client education

         a. Polyethylene glycol 3350 should be dissolved in 240 mL water

         b. Medication may take 2–4 days for effect

         c. Contact prescriber if unusual bloating, cramping, or diarrhea occurs

         d. Prolonged use may result in electrolyte imbalance and laxative dependence

         e. Take medication with juice to improve taste

D. Stool softeners (surfactants)

    1. Action and use

         a. Used on a scheduled basis for clients who are likely to become constipated, such as with hospitalization, bedrest, postsurgical status, and for those receiving opioid analgesic medications

         b. Stool softeners are often referred to as emollient laxatives

         c. They are anionic **surfactants** that lower fecal surface tension in vitro by allowing water and lipid penetration

         d. Softening of feces generally occurs after 1–3 days

         e. Some preparations combine a stool softener such as docusate sodium with a stimulant such as casanthranol to make a single combination product

         f. Used for constipation associated with dry, hard stools and to decrease strain of defecation

         g. Lubiprostone is used to treat irritable bowel syndrome (IBS) with constipation and chronic idiopathic constipation

    2. Common medications (see Table 9-4 again)

    3. Administration considerations

         a. Do not give with mineral oil

         b. Offer fluids after each oral dose

4. Contraindications
   a. Contraindicated with any hypersensitivity to drug
   b. Contraindicated with intestinal obstruction, undiagnosed abdominal pain, vomiting, or other signs of appendicitis, fecal impaction, or acute abdomen
   c. Docusate sodium should not be used by clients with congestive heart failure (CHF) because of sodium content
5. Significant drug interactions: may increase absorption of mineral oil
6. Significant food interactions: none reported
7. Significant laboratory studies: none reported
8. Side effects
   a. Mild abdominal cramping, diarrhea
   b. Dependence with long-term or excessive use
   c. Bitter taste
9. Adverse effects/toxicity (all rare)
   a. Throat irritation has occurred with docusate sodium solution
   b. Docusate potassium has been associated with hyperkalemia when used in clients who have renal insufficiency or renal failure
10. Client-centered nursing care
    a. Monitor frequency and consistency of stools
    b. Monitor for electrolyte imbalances, especially in older adults
11. Client education
    a. Take medication with milk or juice to decrease bitter taste
    b. Increase fluid intake if not contraindicated by another condition such as CHF or renal failure
    c. It may require 1–3 days to soften fecal matter
    d. Consult with dietitian regarding dietary changes to increase fiber foods
    e. Avoid prolonged use

E. **Saline laxatives**
   1. Action and use
      a. Magnesium, sulfate, phosphate, and citrate salts are used when rapid bowel evacuation is required, as in bowel evacuation in preparation for procedures or surgery
      b. Mechanism of action of these poorly absorbed ions is unclear, but it is believed that they produce an osmotic effect that increases intraluminal volume and stimulates peristalsis
      c. Magnesium may cause cholecystokinin release from duodenal mucosa, promoting increased fluid secretion and motility of small intestine and colon
      d. Orally administered magnesium and sodium phosphate salts are effective within 30 minutes to 6 hours
      e. Phosphate-containing rectal enemas evacuate bowel within 2 to 15 minutes
   2. Common medications (see Table 9-4 again)
   3. Administration considerations
      a. Use magnesium salts cautiously for clients with renal impairment because absorption may cause hypermagnesemia
      b. Use sodium phosphate salts cautiously for clients with CHF when sodium restriction is necessary
   4. Contraindications
      a. Saline agents are not recommended for children under 2 years of age because of potential for hypocalcemia in this population
      b. Abdominal pain, nausea and vomiting, or other signs and symptoms of appendicitis or acute abdomen
      c. Intestinal obstruction, edema, CHF, megacolon, or impaired renal function

5. Significant drug interactions: concomitant use with antacids may inactivate both
6. Significant food interactions: none reported
7. Significant laboratory studies: none reported
8. Side effects: cramping and urgency to defecate
9. Adverse effects/toxicity
   a. Safe when administered for short-term management
   b. May cause significant fluid and electrolyte imbalances when used for prolonged periods or in certain clients
10. Client-centered nursing care
    a. Dehydration and electrolyte imbalances may occur from repeated administration without appropriate fluid replacement
    b. Encourage increased fluid intake
    c. Monitor drug effectiveness
11. Client education
    a. Use appropriate dose and avoid frequent or prolonged use due to risk of laxative dependence
    b. Report side effects or lack of effectiveness to healthcare provider
    c. Increase fluid intake as allowed or tolerated

F. Miscellaneous laxatives

1. Mineral oil
   a. Lubricates feces and hinders water reabsorption into colon
   b. Indigestible; may impair absorption of fat-soluble vitamins (A, D, E, K), anti-coagulants, birth control pills, cardiac glycosides, and sulfonamides
   c. Contraindicated with abdominal pain, nausea and vomiting; signs and symptoms of appendicitis or acute abdomen, and fecal impaction or bowel obstruction
   d. Because of possible aspiration and diminished vitamin absorption, do not administer to young children (younger than 6 years of age), pregnant women, older adults, and debilitated clients
   e. Avoid administration of drug to clients lying flat in bed because of risk of aspiration
2. Nalogexol is a newer laxative used to treat opioid-induced constipation
3. Linaclotide is a newer laxative used to treat irritable bowel syndrome (IBS) with constipation

V. ANTIEMETICS

A. Action and use

1. Emesis is a complex reflex brought about by activation of vomiting center (a nucleus of neurons located in medulla oblongata)
2. Certain stimuli activate vomiting center directly (e.g., gastrointestinal irritation) while other stimuli (e.g., drugs, toxins, radiation) act within medulla to stimulate chemoreceptor trigger zone (CTZ); presumably, emetogenic compounds and anti-emetic drugs produce their effects by altering function of these neuroreceptors; once vomiting reflex is triggered, wavelike contractions of stomach propel its contents upward and out of body
3. Receptors involved are influenced by acetylcholine, histamine, serotonin, dopamine, benzodiazepines, and cannabinoids
4. Phenothiazines: suppress emesis by blockade of dopamine receptors in CTZ
5. Butyrophenones: suppress emesis by blocking dopamine receptors in CTZ
6. Metoclopramide: inhibits dopamine receptors in CTZ
7. Cannabinoids are approved to treat nausea and vomiting associated with cancer chemotherapy; mechanism of action is unknown

8. Dronabinol is also approved as an appetite stimulant for clients with acquired immunodeficiency syndrome (AIDS)
9. Glucocorticoids: mechanism for suppression of emesis is unknown; they are effective alone and in combination with other antiemetics in treatment of emesis associated with cancer chemotherapy
10. Antihistamines: anticholinergic effect reducing motion sickness and vomiting
11. Ondansetron: blocks serotonin receptors to reduce nausea
12. Aprepitant: a substance P and neurokinin 1 receptor antagonist that does not affect serotonin

B. **Common antiemetic medications:** see Table 9-5
C. **Administration considerations**
1. Frequently, antiemetic combinations are more beneficial than single-drug treatment, particularly for cancer chemotherapy management of emesis; this may suggest that there is more than one mechanism triggering emesis
2. As a rule, prophylactic drugs are generally given by mouth; however, management of active emesis is usually through parenteral or rectal administration of medications

Table 9-5 **Antiemetics**

Generic Name	Route	Uses
Aprepitant	PO	Combined with other antiemetics to prevent acute or prolonged nausea and vomiting (N/V) associated with emetogenic cancer chemotherapy, particularly high-dose cisplatin
Buclizine	PO	Control N/V and dizziness associated with motion sickness
Chlorpromazine	PO, suppository	Control N/V and intractable hiccups
Cyclizine	PO	Control N/V and dizziness associated with motion sickness
Dexamethasone	IV	Glucocorticoid given before chemotherapy to control N/V
Dimenhydrinate	PO	Antihistamine that also controls N/V associated with motion sickness
Dolasetron	PO, IM, IV	Prevent N/V associated with chemotherapy; prevent and treat postoperative N/V
Doxylamine	PO	Antihistamine combined with pyridoxine (vitamin B6) to treat N/V associated with pregnancy
Dronabinol	PO	N/V associated with cancer chemotherapy in clients who do not respond to other antiemetic medications
Granisetron	IV	Prevent N/V associated with chemotherapy; prevent and treat postoperative N/V
Hydroxyzine	PO, IM	Treat N/V
Meclizine	PO	Prevent N/V and motion sickness
Metoclopramide	PO, IM, IV	Prophylaxis of postoperative nausea
Netupitant and palonosetron	PO	Used with dexamethasone 1 hour before chemotherapy to prevent N/V
Ondansetron	PO, IV	Treat N/V associated with chemotherapy or postoperative N/V
Perphenazine	PO, IM, IV	Severe N/V and intractable hiccups
Prochlorperazine	PO, IM, IV	Severe N/V
Promethazine	PO, IM, IV	N/V and motion sickness
Rolapitant	PO	Used with dexamethasone and serotonin receptor antagonist 1–2 hours before chemotherapy to prevent N/V
Scopolamine	Topical	N/V and motion sickness

3. Anticipatory nausea and vomiting should be treated 1 hour before meals or treatment
4. Parenteral preparations should be given deep IM to avoid leakage of drug into subcutaneous tissues

D. Contraindications
1. Generally contraindicated with CNS depression and coma
2. Use cautiously in clients with glaucoma, seizures, intestinal obstruction, prostatic hyperplasia, asthma, and cardiac, pulmonary, or hepatic disease
3. Aprepitant is contraindicated with hypersensitivity, lactation, or concurrent use of pimozide; use cautiously with warfarin, vinblastine, vincristine, docetaxel, ironotecen, imatinib, and paclitaxel
4. Dolasetron mesylate is contraindicated with prolonged QT interval or second- or third-degree AV block
5. Dronabinol is contraindicated with allergy to sesame oil, or with use of ritonavir, alcohol, sedatives or hypnotics, psychotomimetics, or tricyclic antidepressants

E. Significant drug interactions
1. Epinephrine, including ephedrine, may increase hypotension
2. Avoid use with MAOIs
3. Antihistamines and CNS depressants may increase CNS depression
4. Levodopa may have decreased action
5. Phenytoin may increase toxicity
6. Meclizine may mask signs of ototoxicity with such medications as aminoglycosides, salicylates, and loop diuretics
7. Glucocorticoids cause hyperglycemia
8. Rifampin decreases dolasetron levels

F. Significant food interactions: none reported

G. Significant laboratory studies
1. Monitor BUN and creatinine (kidney function)
2. May mask response of skin testing; discontinue 4 days prior to testing
3. May cause hyperglycemia, false-positive or false-negative pregnancy test; may increase liver enzyme levels
4. Dexamethasone may increase glucose and cholesterol levels, decrease potassium, calcium, and thyroxine levels

H. Side effects
1. Phenothiazines can produce extrapyramidal reactions, anticholinergic effects, hypotension, and sedation; be alert for aspiration
2. Butyrophenones can also produce extrapyramidal reactions, sedation, and hypotension
3. Cannabinoids may cause temporal disintegration, dissociation, depersonalization, and dysphoria

I. Adverse effects/toxicity
1. Cannabinoids are contraindicated for clients with psychiatric disorders
2. Phenothiazines: agranulocytosis, thrombocytopenia

J. Client-centered nursing care
1. Dronabinol has potential for abuse
2. Check vital signs regularly for risk of hypotension or tachycardia
3. Observe for side effects and adverse reactions
4. Monitor I&O for urine retention
5. Obtain baseline electrocardiogram with dolasetron
6. Observe for mood changes or involuntary movements
7. Monitor lab values: liver function tests, electrolytes, and renal function tests (blood urea nitrogen and creatinine)

8. Store dronabinol in refrigerator
9. Ensure client safety

10. Monitor for anticholinergic effects: dry mouth, constipation, or visual changes
11. Ask client to empty bowel/bladder prior to administering antiemetics to reduce risk of falls

K. Client education
1. Avoid activities that require alertness
2. Report adverse effects to healthcare provider
3. Avoid alcohol and CNS depressant drugs
4. Diabetic clients need to monitor blood glucose
5. Take medications as prescribed
6. Avoid excessive sunlight and ultraviolet light because of risk for photosensitivity
7. Use sugarless hard candy or ice chips to avoid dry mouth
8. Increase fluids and dietary fiber to decrease risk of constipation
9. Take medication 30–60 minutes before any activity that causes nausea for best effect

VI. HISTAMINE H₂ ANTAGONISTS

A. Action and use
1. Reduce gastric acid secretion by blocking histamine H_2 in gastric parietal cells
2. Reduce total pepsin output
3. Histamine **H_2 antagonists** (agents against histamine decreasing gastric secretion) are used to treat duodenal ulcer, gastric ulcer, hypersecretory conditions such as Zollinger-Ellison syndrome, reflux esophagitis
4. Used to prevent stress ulcers in critically ill clients and as combination therapy to treat ***Helicobacter pylori*** (bacteria found in gastric mucosa) infection

B. Common histamine H_2 antagonist medications: see Table 9-6

C. Administration considerations
1. Intravenous (IV) administered drugs should not be mixed with other medications
2. Avoid antacid use within 1 hour of administration
3. May be given as single dose, twice daily, or with meals and at bedtime

D. Contraindications
1. Hypersensitivity to drug
2. Use caution in clients with impaired renal or hepatic function

Table 9-6	Histamine H_2 Antagonists	
Generic Name	**Route**	**Uses**
Cimetidine	PO, IM, IV	Short-term treatment for duodenal ulcer or benign gastric ulcer, pathologic hypersecretory condition such as Zollinger-Ellison syndrome, prophylactic of stress-induced ulcers, acute upper GI bleeding in critically ill clients, gastroesophageal reflux disease, heartburn and indigestion
Famotidine	PO, IV	Short-term treatment for duodenal ulcer or benign gastric ulcer, pathologic hypersecretory condition such as Zollinger-Ellison syndrome, prophylactic of stress-induced ulcers, acute upper GI bleeding in critically ill clients, gastroesophageal reflux disease, heartburn and indigestion
Nizatidine	PO	Short-term treatment of duodenal ulcer and benign gastric ulcer, gastroesophageal reflux disease, prevention of heartburn and acid indigestion
Ranitidine	PO, IM, IV	Short-term treatment for duodenal ulcer or benign gastric ulcer, pathologic hypersecretory condition such as Zollinger-Ellison syndrome, prophylactic of stress-induced ulcers, acute upper GI bleeding in critically ill clients, gastroesophageal reflux disease, heartburn and indigestion, erosive esophagitis

E. **Significant drug interactions**
   1. Decreased ketaconazole absorption with famotidine
   2. Cimetidine: decreased metabolism of beta-adrenergic blockers, phenytoin, lidocaine, procainamide, quinidine, benzodiazepines, metronidazole, tricyclic antidepressants, oral contraceptives, and warfarin causing increased risk of toxicity
   3. Cimetidine alters absorption of ketoconazole, ferrous salts, indomethacin, and tetracyclines, and may decrease concentration of digoxin
   4. Nizatidine may increase salicylate levels with high doses of aspirin
   5. Ranitidine may increase diazepam absorption, increase hypoglycemic effects of glipizide, increase procainamide levels, and increase warfarin effect
   6. Antacids should not be given with H2 antagonist because they decrease absorption of iron and vitamin B12, which depend on an acidic environment

F. **Significant food interactions**: none reported

G. **Significant laboratory studies**
   1. Ranitidine: false-positive urine prolactin
   2. Cimetidine: false-negative allergen skin test, increased prolactin, alkaline phosphatase and creatinine levels and may alter gastroccult testing caused by blue dye used in tablets
   3. Famotidine may cause false-negative allergen results and may increase liver enzyme levels
   4. Nizatidine may cause false-positive urobilinogen

H. **Side effects**
   1. Somnolence, diaphoresis, rash, headache, hypotension
   2. Taste disorder, diarrhea, constipation, dry mouth
   3. Cardiac dysrhythmias
   4. Impotence with cimetidine

I. **Adverse effects/toxicity**
   1. Rare but may include agranulocytosis, neutropenia, thrombocytopenia, aplastic anemia, and pancytopenia
   2. Anaphylaxis

J. **Client-centered nursing care**
   1. Reduced dosages usually required for clients with hepatic or renal impairment
   2. Assess medications for possible interactions
   3. Evaluate nutritional status and dietary interventions
   4. Evaluate need for smoking cessation and alcoholic abuse programs
   5. Give cimetidine with meals and at bedtime

K. **Client education**
   1. Avoid smoking, which causes gastric stimulation
   2. Avoid **antacid** (agent reducing acidity) use within 1 hour of dose
   3. Take medications only as directed
   4. Once-a-day dosage should be taken at bedtime; if prescribed more than daily, take before meals
   5. Avoid gastric irritants such as alcohol, aspirin, or nonsteroidal anti-inflammatory drugs (NSAIDs)
   6. Report any side effects to healthcare provider
   7. Cigarette smoking decreases drug effectiveness

VII. PROTON PUMP INHIBITORS

A. **Action and use**
   1. Block acid production by inhibiting H^+, K^+-ATPase at secretory surface of gastric parietal cells, thereby blocking formation of gastric acid

2. Used for treatment of erosive or ulcerative gastroesophageal reflux disease (GERD) or duodenal ulcers, active benign gastric ulcers, and nonsteroidal anti-inflammatory drug (NSAID)–associated gastric ulcers (short term)
3. Used for healing and reduction in relapse rates of heartburn symptoms in erosive or ulcerative GERD (maintenance)
4. Used for treatment of pathologic hypersecretory conditions such as Zollinger-Ellison syndrome (long term)

B. **Common medications:** see Table 9-7
C. **Administration considerations**
   1. May give with antacids
   2. If unable to swallow capsules, lansoprazole and esomeprazole capsules may be opened and sprinkled on applesauce before taking
   3. To give per nasogastric (NG) tube, dilute capsule contents in 40 mL juice
   4. Omeprazole, pantoprazole, and rabeprazole must be swallowed whole
   5. Pantoprazole IV: should be administered over a period of 15 minutes at a rate not greater than 3 mg/min (7 mL/min)
   6. Pantoprazole IV should be administered using in-line filter provided
D. **Contraindications:** not recommended in children or nursing mothers
E. **Significant drug interactions**
   1. Rabeprazole and pantoprazole may alter absorption of gastric pH-dependent drugs such as ketoconazole, digoxin, iron preparations, and ampicillin
   2. Esomeprazole may affect drugs metabolized by CYP2C19
   3. Lansoprazole may alter theophylline levels; give at least 30 minutes before sucralfate
   4. Omeprazole may potentiate diazepam, phenytoin, and warfarin
   5. Omeprazole should be taken 30 minutes before sucralfate; it may alter absorption of pH-dependent medications
   6. Hypoglycemia could occur if rabeprazole is combined with itraconazole or gemfibrozil
   7. Esomeprazole increases serum levels and increases risk of toxicity of benzodiazepines
   8. Esomeprazole interferes with absorption of ketoconazole, iron salts, and digoxin
F. **Significant food interactions:** none reported but administer before meals
G. **Significant laboratory studies**
   1. May increase liver enzymes
   2. Monitor theophylline levels with lansoprazole

Table 9-7	Proton Pump Inhibitors	
Generic Name	**Route**	**Uses**
Esomeprazole	PO	GERD, heartburn, erosive esophagitis, duodenal ulcer, duodenal ulcer with *Helicobacter pylori*, gastric ulcer related to nonsteroidal anti-inflammatory drugs (NSAIDs)
Lansoprazole	PO	Short-term treatment of erosive esophagitis, GERD, duodenal or gastric ulcer, long-term treatment of pathologic hypersecretory conditions, maintenance therapy for healing erosive esophagitis and duodenal ulcers
Omeprazole	PO	Heartburn, *Helicobacter pylori* with amoxicillin, metronidazole, and clarithromycin, treatment of pathologic hypersecretory conditions, benign gastric ulcer, duodenal ulcer, first-line therapy for GERD
Pantoprazole	PO, IV	Short-term and long-term treatment of GERD, erosive esophagitis, pathologic hypersecretory conditions such as Zollinger-Ellison syndrome, neoplastic conditions, peptic ulcer
Rabeprazole	PO	*Helicobacter pylori*, pathologic hypersecretory conditions such as Zollinger-Ellison syndrome, erosive and ulcerative GERD, daytime and nighttime heartburn

3. May need to monitor diazepam and phenytoin levels and prothrombin times more frequently with omeprazole

H. Side effects

1. Headache, diarrhea, constipation, abdominal pain, nausea, flatulence
2. Rash, hyperglycemia, dizziness, pruritis, dry mouth
3. Injection site reaction with pantoprazole

I. Adverse effects/toxicity

1. Pancreatitis, liver necrosis, hepatic failure, toxic epidermal necrolysis
2. Stevens–Johnson syndrome
3. Agranulocytosis, myocardial infarction (MI), shock, cerebral vascular accident (CVA)
4. GI hemorrhage

J. Client-centered nursing care

1. Dosage should be reduced in severe liver disease
2. Document reason for therapy, duration of symptoms, and drug efficacy
3. Monitor for side effects
4. Monitor laboratory test results including liver function tests, CBC, and measures of renal function (BUN, creatinine)
5. Review any diagnostic findings
6. Assess for pregnancy or lactation
7. Increase water intake to 8–10 glasses per day to prevent constipation
8. Administer 30 minutes before first meal of day because food activates proton pump

K. Client education

1. Be aware of side effects; report diarrhea
2. Take medications as prescribed; do not increase dose
3. Follow prescribed diet and activities to decrease symptoms
4. Medication is generally for short-term therapy; keep healthcare appointments for treatment of continued signs and symptoms
5. Esomeprazole and omeprazole should be taken before meals
6. Notify healthcare provider of any difficulty swallowing since omeprazole, pantoprazole, and rabeprazole must be swallowed whole
7. Lansoprazole and esomeprazole capsules may be opened and sprinkled on soft food

VIII. MUCOSAL PROTECTIVE AGENTS

A. Action and use

1. Misoprostol inhibits gastric secretion, protects gastric mucosa by increasing bicarbonate and mucus production, and decreases pepsin levels
2. Sucralfate protects site of ulcer from gastric acid by forming an adherent coating with albumin and fibrinogen; absorbs pepsin, decreasing its activity
3. Misoprostol is used for prevention of gastric ulcers; investigational use with duodenal ulcers
4. Sucralfate is used for short-term treatment of duodenal ulcers with continued maintenance treatment at lower doses; investigational use for gastric ulcers

B. Common mucosal protective medications: see Table 9-8

> **Practice to Pass**
>
> A proton pump inhibitor has been prescribed for a client who recently had a stroke (cerebrovascular accident or CVA). What nursing assessment should be performed?

Table 9-8	Mucosal Protective Agents		
Generic Name	**Route**	**Uses**	
Misoprostol	PO	Prevention of NSAID- or aspirin-induced gastric ulcers, gastric ulcer, duodenal ulcer	
Sucralfate	PO	Short-term care for duodenal ulcer given up to 8 weeks, oral and esophageal ulcers related to radiation or chemotherapy, gastric ulcer, reflux and peptic esophagitis, gastritis related to aspirin or NSAID, stress ulcer	

C. Administration considerations

1. Sucralfate should be taken 1 hour before meals and bedtime or 2 hours after meals
2. Sucralfate should be taken 2 hours after medications and not within 2 hours of antacids
3. Misoprostol should be taken on empty stomach and not within 30 minutes (before or after) food intake

D. Contraindications

1. Misoprostol is contraindicated in clients who are allergic to prostaglandins or who are pregnant or lactating
2. Use cautiously with clients with renal impairment and clients older than 64 years old
3. Safety has not been established for children under 18 years old
4. Misoprostol may cause miscarriage with serious bleeding
5. No known contraindications with sucralfate, but safety in children and during lactation is not fully established

E. Significant drug interactions

1. Sucralfate: decreased absorption of digoxin, fluoroquinolones, ketoconazole, phenytoin, quinidine, ranitidine, tetracycline, and theophylline; dosing medications 2 hours before sucralfate eliminates interactions
2. Antacids may decrease binding of sucralfate
3. Misoprostol decreases availability of aspirin

F. Significant food interactions: none reported

G. Significant laboratory studies

1. Misoprostol may decrease basal pepsin secretion
2. No laboratory interactions with sucralfate

H. Side effects

1. Dizziness, headache, constipation, diarrhea, nausea and vomiting, flatulence, dry mouth, and rash
2. Misoprostol may cause spotting, cramping, dysmenorrhea, menstrual disorders, and postmenopausal bleeding

I. Adverse effects/toxicity

1. Angioedema
2. Respiratory difficulty, laryngospasm
3. Seizures

J. Client-centered nursing care

1. Assess GI symptoms
2. Assess for pregnancy via serum test prior to beginning misoprostol and should be negative within first 2 weeks of therapy
3. Monitor concomitant medications
4. Give medications according to prescription
5. Monitor for side effects
6. Assess respiratory status, swallowing, or change in gag reflex

K. Client education

1. Avoid gastric irritants such as caffeine, alcohol, smoking, and spicy foods
2. Take medication as prescribed and do not share with others
3. Report side effects to healthcare provider for possible dosage change
4. Use contraception while on misoprostol
5. Female clients should report any abnormal vaginal bleeding
6. Do not take misoprostol if pregnant; if client becomes pregnant while taking misoprostol, she should stop taking it
7. Avoid pregnancy at least 1 month or 1 menstrual cycle after stopping medication
8. Increase fluids and fiber to decrease constipation
9. Use antacids properly to decrease interaction
10. Report immediately any difficulty swallowing or breathing

Practice to Pass

What information would you share with a pregnant female client with peptic ulcer disease who asks you about taking misoprostol?

IX. ANTACIDS

A. **Action and use**
   1. Neutralize gastric acid
   2. Used for symptomatic relief of hyperacidity associated with GI disorders
   3. Used as an antiflatulent to alleviate symptoms of gas and bloating

B. **Common antacid medications:** see Table 9-9

C. **Administration considerations**: antacids should be taken at least 2 hours apart from other drugs where a drug interaction may occur

D. **Contraindications**
   1. Safety has not been established for use of antacids by lactating women
   2. Magnesium hydroxide is contraindicated in presence of abdominal pain, nausea and vomiting, diarrhea, severe renal dysfunction, fecal impaction, rectal bleeding, colostomy, and ileostomy
   3. Aluminum carbonate antacids: prolonged use of high doses in presence of low-serum phosphate
   4. Calcium carbonate antacids: hypercalcemia and hypercalciuria, severe renal disease, renal calculi, GI hemorrhage or obstruction, dehydration
   5. Dihydroxyaluminum sodium carbonate: aluminum sensitivity, severe renal disease, dehydration, clients on sodium-restricted diets

E. **Significant drug interactions**
   1. Antacids increase gastric pH, which may decrease absorption of other drugs, such as digoxin, ciprofloxacin, ofloxacin, norfloxacin, phenytoin, iron supplements, isoniazid, ethambutol, and ketoconazole
   2. Antacids may bind with other drugs, therefore decreasing drug's absorption and effectiveness, such as tetracycline

F. **Significant food interactions**: none reported

G. **Significant laboratory studies**: prolonged use of antacids may alter aluminum, calcium, sodium, and phosphate levels

H. **Side effects**
   1. Belching, constipation, flatulence, diarrhea
   2. Gastric distention
   3. Acid rebound if antacids are given frequently

I. **Adverse effects/toxicity**
   1. Hypophosphatemia (anorexia, malaise, tremors, muscle weakness)
   2. Aluminum toxicity (dementia) may occur with repeated dosing
   3. Hypercalcemia and metabolic alkalosis may occur with antacids containing calcium carbonate
   4. May worsen hypertension and heart failure from increased sodium intake with use of those antacids containing sodium carbonate

Table 9-9 Antacids

Generic Name	Route	Uses
Aluminum hydroxide	PO	Relief of gastric acidity, esophageal reflux, hiatal hernia, duodenal ulcer
Calcium carbonate	PO	Hyperacidity, acid indigestion, peptic esophagitis, hiatal hernia, control of hyperphosphatemia in CRF
Calcium carbonate with magnesium hydroxide	PO	Peptic ulcer, hyperacidity, gastritis, peptic esophagitis, hiatal hernia
Magnesium hydroxide, aluminum hydroxide, and simethicone	PO	Peptic ulcer, hyperacidity, gastritis, peptic esophagitis, hiatal hernia
Sodium bicarbonate	PO	Hyperacidity, acid indigestion; can be given IV to treat metabolic acidosis

J. Client-centered nursing care
1. Shake suspension well
2. Flush NG tube with water after administration
3. Observe for signs and symptoms of altered phosphate levels: anorexia, muscle weakness, and malaise

K. Client education
1. Increase fluids, fiber, and exercise to avoid constipation
2. Take as directed; do not exceed maximum dose
3. Keep medication out of reach of children
4. Drink sufficient fluids (8–10 glasses/day)
5. Antacids may interact with certain medications; notify healthcare provider of any prescribed medications; do not take antacids within 45 minutes to 2 hours of other medications or absorption of other drug may be decreased
6. Do not use unless prescribed if diagnosed with kidney disease

X. ANTIMICROBIALS FOR *HELICOBACTER PYLORI* ORGANISMS

A. Action and use
1. Antisecretory and antimicrobial action against most strains of *Helicobacter pylori*
2. Used for eradication of *Helicobacter pylori* infection and reduce risk of duodenal ulcer recurrence
3. Common drugs are amoxicillin, clarithromycin, metronidazole, and tetracycline; often two or more drugs are used together for increased effectiveness; may also be combined with a proton pump inhibitor or bismuth compound

B. Common medications: see Table 9-10

C. Administration considerations
1. Swallow all pills whole except bismuth, which should be chewed and not swallowed whole
2. If dose is missed, continue with normal dosage regimen, do not double-dose

D. Contraindications
1. Allergy to any component of therapy
2. Avoid coadministration with pimozide or terfenadine because of risk of cardiac dysrhythmias
3. Pregnant women should not take regimens containing clarithromycin

Table 9-10 Drug Regimens that Include Antimicrobials for *Helicobacter pylori*

Generic Name	Usual Adult Dosage Range	Route
Lansoprazole, amoxicillin, clarithromycin	Twice daily for 10–14 days	PO
Bismuth subsalicylate, metronidazole, tetracycline	Four times daily for 14 days	PO
Omeprazole, clarithromycin	Omeprazole 40 mg daily and clarithromycin 500 mg three times daily for 2 weeks then omeprazole 20 mg daily for 2 weeks	PO
Ranitidine, bismuth citrate, clarithromycin	Ranitidine bismuth citrate 400 mg twice daily and clarithromycin 500 mg three times daily for 2 weeks then ranitidine bismuth citrate 400 mg twice daily for 2 weeks	PO
Lansoprazole, amoxicillin	Lansoprazole 30 mg and amoxicillin combination (1 gram three times daily for 14 days)	PO

E. **Significant drug interactions**
   1. May alter absorption of drugs dependent on gastric pH: ketoconazole, ampicillin, iron, or digoxin
   2. Safety in children is not established
F. **Significant food interactions**: none reported
G. **Significant laboratory studies**
   1. Abnormal liver function tests
   2. May increase theophylline levels
   3. May interfere with prothrombin times
   4. May alter serum levels of drugs metabolized by P450 enzyme system
H. **Side effects**
   1. Rash, nausea and vomiting, diarrhea, abnormal taste, abdominal pain, dyspepsia
   2. Headache, photosensitivity
   3. Transient CNS reactions such as anxiety, behavior changes, tinnitus, and vertigo
I. **Adverse effects/toxicity**: ventricular dysrhythmias
J. **Client-centered nursing care**
   1. Note signs and symptoms, onset, and duration of symptoms
   2. Document allergy status
   3. Determine pregnancy status
   4. Document previous therapies used
   5. Document confirmation of infection
K. **Client education**
   1. Compliance with drug therapy is important to eliminate infection
   2. Avoid gastric irritants such as smoking, alcohol, and caffeine
   3. Use stress reduction techniques as indicated
   4. Report side effects to prescriber
   5. Report continued symptoms to prescriber
   6. Bismuth-containing preparations may cause darkening of tongue and stool
   7. Review drug packaging as some preparations are prepackaged
   8. Do not double dose if dose is missed
   9. Use additional contraceptive measures as antibiotics can decrease birth control pill effectiveness
   10. Avoid prolonged exposure to sun

XI. MEDICATIONS USED TO DISSOLVE GALLSTONES

A. **Action and use**
   1. Ursodiol is used to dissolve gallbladder stones smaller than 20 mm; absorbed in small bowel, secreted into hepatic bile ducts, and expelled into duodenum in response to eating; a natural-occurring bile acid that inhibits hepatic synthesis and secretion of cholesterol
   2. Chenodiol reduces cholesterol content of gallstones (must have high cholesterol content and not be radiopaque stones)
B. **Common medications**: Ursodiol and chenodiol
C. **Administration considerations**: use beyond 24 months has not been established
D. **Contraindications**
   1. Do not use for clients with calcified cholesterol stones, radiopaque stones, or radiolucent bile pigment stones
   2. Excretion in breast milk is not known; use with caution
   3. Avoid in clients with acute cholecystitis, biliary obstruction, pancreatitis, allergy to bile acids, and chronic liver disease

E. **Significant drug interactions**: antacids and bile acid sequestrants (cholestyramine, colestipol) may interfere with action of ursodiol by decreasing its absorption

F. **Significant food interactions**: none reported

G. **Significant laboratory studies**: none reported

H. **Side effects**
   1. Nausea and vomiting, abdominal pain, constipation, diarrhea, rash
   2. Headache, fatigue, anxiety, sweating
   3. Thinning of hair, arthralgia

I. **Adverse effects/toxicity**: diarrhea

J. **Client-centered nursing care**
   1. If no dissolution of partial stone is observed in 12 months, drug will probably not be effective
   2. Gallbladder ultrasound should be done every 6 months during first year of therapy
   3. Document indications and length of therapy
   4. Determine pregnancy status
   5. If infection present, combine with anti-infective agents

K. **Client education**
   1. Avoid antacid use with drug unless prescribed
   2. Therapy may take up to 24 months
   3. Stones may recur
   4. Limit dietary fat
   5. Report any side effects to prescriber
   6. Discuss contraceptive methods because birth control pills may decrease drug effect
   7. Stress importance of follow-up visits and diagnostic tests

XII. PANCREATIC ENZYME REPLACEMENT

A. **Action and use**
   1. Replacement of pancreatic enzyme in conditions where there is a deficiency of exocrine pancreatic secretions, such as with cystic fibrosis, chronic pancreatitis, postpancreatectomy, steatorrhea, malabsorption syndrome, or postgastrectomy
   2. Helps to digest fat and absorb fat, proteins, and carbohydrates
   3. Dosage is adjusted on an individual basis according to extent of enzyme deficiency, dietary fat content, and enzyme activity of individual drug formulation

B. **Common pancreatic enzyme replacement medication**: pancrelipase

C. **Administration considerations**
   1. Swallow tablets or capsules whole, do not crush or chew
   2. If swallowing is difficult, open capsules and give contents in applesauce or pudding to swallow without chewing
   3. Take medications with meals and snacks

D. **Contraindications**
   1. Hypersensitivity to pork protein or enzymes
   2. Contraindicated in acute pancreatitis

E. **Significant drug interactions**
   1. If given with antacids, rise in gastric pH may cause enteric-coated capsules to dissolve in stomach and inactivate drug
   2. Pancreatic lipase is inactivated at pH less than 4
   3. If antacids allow enteric coating to dissolve too soon, drug will be inactivated by gastric acid
   4. This drug needs to travel into less acidic duodenum before breaking down for therapeutic effect; if given with oral iron supplements, enzymes may decrease effect of iron

F. **Significant food interactions**: none reported

G. **Significant laboratory studies**: elevated serum and urinary uric acid

H. Side effects

!

    1. Nausea

    2. Diarrhea

    3. Abdominal cramps

I. Adverse effects/toxicity: hyperuricemia

J. Client-centered nursing care

!

    1. Monitor for side effects and monitor steatorrhea, as it should diminish with appropriate dose of medication

    2. Assess and monitor to maintain good nutritional status

    3. Document indications for therapy

    4. Document allergies

    5. Assess swallowing ability or difficulty

K. Client education

    1. Take before or with meals with plenty of water

    2. Report any side effects to healthcare provider

    3. Report joint pain and swelling

    4. Review dietary interventions with clients; consult with dietitian for counseling and meal planning

Case Study

A 45-year-old male client comes to the nurse practitioner stating he wakes often at night with coughing and burning he describes as heartburn. He drinks one or two alcoholic beverages per evening, usually with distilled liquor, and then wine with dinner. He eats heavy dinners with dessert. He prefers mint ice cream and coffee for dessert. The nurse practitioner prescribes a regimen with omeprazole every morning and aluminum/magnesium antacid 30 mL qid.

1. How should you instruct the client about gastroesophageal reflux disease and its relationship to symptoms?

2. What information will you provide to the client about his diet, particularly the evening meal?

3. What type of medications are likely to be prescribed if the client is diagnosed with *H. pylori*?

4. What information and instructions should you provide to the client about his medications?

For suggested responses, see page 541.

POSTTEST

❶ When the nurse teaches a client about the side effects of anticholinergic medications, what set of signs or symptoms should be included?

    1. Urinary retention, constipation, or dilated pupils

    2. Pupillary constriction, bronchoconstriction, or bradycardia

    3. Inability to obtain an erection, irregular heart rhythm

    4. Increased salivation, dysphagia, confusion, restlessness

❷ A pregnant client asks the nurse about laxative use during pregnancy. After recommending that the healthcare provider be consulted before using any drug, the nurse should instruct the client to avoid using which laxative during pregnancy?

    1. Bisacodyl

    2. Mineral oil

    3. Castor oil

    4. Sodium biphosphate

POSTTEST

3 After a family member reported altered mental function in a client with end-stage liver disease, the healthcare provider prescribed lactulose 30 mL by mouth, three times daily. The home health nurse reviews the client's chart for which laboratory test(s) to monitor medication effectiveness?

1. Alanine aminotransferase (ALT) and aspartate amino-transferase (AST)
2. Blood urea nitrogen (BUN) and creatinine
3. Bilirubin and urobilinogen
4. Serum ammonia

4 A client asks, "How does diphenoxylate help stop diarrhea?" Which of the following is the *best* response by the nurse?

1. "It slows down the motility of the intestine, thereby increasing fluid absorption."
2. "Because of the increased sodium in the stool, fluid moves into the bloodstream."
3. "It increases the bulk in the intestines, resulting in decreased peristalsis."
4. "It decreases circulation of blood to the bowels, making them less reactive to stimulation."

5 The nurse should consult with the prescriber if oral mineral oil is prescribed for which of the following clients? Select all that apply.

1. Client with dysphagia following a cerebral vascular accident (CVA)
2. Client who has suspected appendicitis
3. Client who has a fecal impaction
4. Client who has infrequent heartburn
5. Client who has steatorrhea

6 The nurse concludes that docusate sodium is appropriate for use in which of the following clients? Select all that apply.

1. A client preparing for a colonoscopy who needs a bowel prep
2. A postoperative client taking opioid analgesics for pain
3. A client who experienced a myocardial infarction 24 hours ago
4. A client trying to reduce the chances of chronic constipation
5. A client with painful hemorrhoids

7 An otherwise healthy client diagnosed with chole-cystitis reports to the emergency department with severe pain. The nurse is most likely to administer which of the following drugs with an appropriate order?

1. Codeine sulfate
2. Bethanecol
3. Dicyclomine
4. Morphine sulfate

8 A client has cholelithiasis, but is a poor surgical candidate because of comorbid conditions. The nurse is most likely to teach the client about which of the following medications?

1. Ursodiol
2. Omeprazole
3. Cimetidine
4. Ibuprofen

9 A client who has a history of a seizure disorder is newly diagnosed with a gastric ulcer. The client has maintained seizure-free status using phenytoin. The nurse would question a new prescription for which of the following drugs to treat symptoms caused by the ulcer?

1. Famotidine
2. Cimetidine
3. Nizatidine
4. Ranitidine

10 A client has a new prescription to take bisacodyl. To enhance a rapid medication effect, the nurse instructs the client to take the medication in which way?

1. On an empty stomach
2. With plenty of fluids
3. With meals
4. At bedtime

➤ *See pages 298–300 for Answers and Rationales.*

ANSWERS & RATIONALES

Pretest

1 **Answer: 2 Rationale:** Psyllium mucilloid should be mixed with 8 ounces of water and an additional 8 ounces of water should be consumed after the initial dose to avoid esophageal obstruction. There is no need to refrain from physical activity while taking psyllium mucilloid. Psyllium mucilloid typically does not cause nausea so there is no need for an antiemetic. Psyllium mucilloid should be mixed in water for consumption, not sprinkled on food. **Cognitive Level:** Analyzing **Client Need:** Pharmacological and Parenteral Therapies **Integrated Process:** Nursing Process: Implementation **Content Area:** Pharmacology **Strategy:** Apply knowledge of drug characteristics to the question. The critical thinking question within the test item is, "What is the risk to the client if proper fluid is not ingested with psyllium mucilloid?" **Reference:** Adams, M. P., Holland, L. N., & Urban, C. Q. (2017). *Pharmacology for nurses: A pathophysiologic approach* (5th ed.). Boston: Pearson, pp. 696–697.

2 **Answer: 1 Rationale:** Metoclopramide is a GI stimulant, increasing motility of the GI tract, shortening gastric emptying time, and thus reducing the risk of the esophagus being exposed to gastric contents. Decreased lower esophageal sphincter (LES) tone will increase the risk of gastric contents being regurgitated upward into the esophagus. Because the drug increases GI motility, it can cause diarrhea rather than combating it. GERD can place clients at increased risk for *H. pylori* bacterial infection; however, anti-infectives would be used to treat this infection. **Cognitive Level:** Applying **Client Need:** Pharmacological and Parenteral Therapies **Integrated Process:** Nursing Process: Evaluation **Content Area:** Pharmacology **Strategy:** First recall the pathophysiology of GERD. Consider that if GERD results in backward flow of gastric contents, it is logical for the drug prescribed to promote forward movement of gastric contents. **Reference:** Wilson, B. A., Shannon, M. T., & Shields, K. M. (2017). *Pearson nurse's drug guide 2017*. New York, NY: Pearson, pp. 998–1000.

3 **Answer: 4 Rationale:** Dicyclomine hydrochloride relieves GI smooth muscle spasm, alleviating the symptoms and leading to a balanced state of nutritional and fluid status. Presence of mucus in the stool is one of the Manning criteria associated with irritable bowel syndrome (IBS). During the recovery phase the weight should be stable with no further weight loss. Bowel sounds should be normal, not hypoactive. **Cognitive Level:** Analyzing **Client Need:** Pharmacological and Parenteral Therapies **Integrated Process:** Nursing Process: Evaluation **Content Area:** Pharmacology **Strategy:** The drug name Antispas is a clue that the drug is an antispasmodic by action. Recall that spasms are a major sign or symptom of IBS and focus on the data that is the most normal as the answer to the question. **Reference:** Wilson, B. A., Shannon, M. T., & Shields, K. M. (2017). *Pearson nurse's drug guide 2017*. New York, NY: Pearson, pp. 464–466.

4 **Answer: 2 Rationale:** Bismuth subsalicylate has a salicylate base and is contraindicated in clients who are allergic to aspirin, also known as acetylsalicylic acid. Attapulgite and loperamide may be given safely to a client allergic to aspirin. Diphenoxylate with atropine contains codeine as well as atropine as ingredients. **Cognitive Level:** Applying **Client Need:** Pharmacological and Parenteral Therapies **Integrated Process:** Nursing Process: Planning **Content Area:** Pharmacology **Strategy:** Associate the word *salicylate* with aspirin and use the process of elimination to pick the medication that contains salicylate in the generic name. **Reference:** Wilson, B. A., Shannon, M. T., & Shields, K. M. (2017). *Pearson nurse's drug guide 2017*. New York, NY: Pearson, pp. 183–184.

5 **Answer: 4 Rationale:** Metamucil is a bulk-forming laxative that could aggravate diarrhea, and this statement indicates that the client has a lack of understanding. The other statements made by the client are true and indicate proper understanding. Dairy products may aggravate diarrhea and it is helpful to avoid these during a bout of diarrhea. Kaopectate is an antidiarrheal agent that is commonly used to manage this health problem, which is usually self-limiting. The client should contact the healthcare provider if diarrhea persists more than 2 days. **Cognitive Level:** Applying **Client Need:** Pharmacological and Parenteral Therapies **Integrated Process:** Nursing Process: Evaluation **Content Area:** Pharmacology **Strategy:** The critical words in the question are *further instructions*, indicating that the correct option is an incorrect client statement. Associate the primary problem (diarrhea) with the action of psyllium fiber (accelerated peristalsis). Since this drug would worsen the client's symptoms, this is the incorrect statement and is therefore the answer to the question. **Reference:** Wilson, B. A., Shannon, M. T., & Shields, K. M. (2017). *Pearson nurse's drug guide 2017.* New York, NY: Pearson, pp. 1313–1314.

6 Answer: 3 Rationale: Clients with eating disorders such as anorexia nervosa or bulimia nervosa are most likely to abuse laxatives. Older adults often believe having a stool every day is healthy and they are also a group that may excessively use laxatives, but they are not as at risk as clients who have eating disorders. Clients with irritable bowel syndrome (IBS) are not likely to disturb the GI tract with drugs that could further irritate the tissue. Clients who are obese are more likely to be inactive and ingest diets high in fat and cholesterol. **Cognitive Level:** Analyzing **Client Need:** Pharmacological and Parenteral Therapies **Integrated Process:** Nursing Process: Assessment **Content Area:** Pharmacology **Strategy:** First eliminate two options because they are least likely to abuse laxatives overall. Next associate the characteristic of laxative abuse with the group most likely to demonstrate compulsive behaviors, which helps you to choose correctly between the clients who are older adults and those with eating disorders. **Reference:** Adams, M. P., & Urban, C. (2016). *Pharmacology: Connections to nursing practice* (3rd ed.). New York, NY: Pearson, pp. 1030–1032.

7 Answer: 2 Rationale: Laxatives are included on the list of drugs in which misuse results in dependence. A healthy client who regularly ingests a laxative needs to be taught about laxatives and physical dependence. A fluid and/or electrolyte imbalance may be present, but the primary focus is to address the cause and not the outcome. Since the client is healthy, one can presume the nutritional status is adequate. **Cognitive Level:** Applying **Client Need:** Pharmacological and Parenteral Therapies **Integrated Process:** Teaching and Learning **Content Area:** Pharmacology **Strategy:** The critical terms are *healthy* and *9 months*. The term *healthy* indicates the laxative is not needed physically, suggesting that there may be a psychosocial concern. Focus on the term *9 months* to consider drug misuse or abuse. **Reference:** Adams, M. P., & Urban, C. (2016). *Pharmacology: Connections to nursing practice* (3rd ed.). New York, NY: Pearson, pp. 1030–1032.

8 Answer: 4 Rationale: Loperamide is indicated for the treatment of diarrhea. If this is a new prescription, then critical thinking suggests that the diarrhea is relatively new in onset. Placing a commode at the bedside would provide for proper management of an older adult client with diarrhea. There is no evidence that ingestion of normal dosages of this drug usually causes seizures. There is also no evidence that ingestion of normal dosages of this drug places the client at significant risk for falls or significant changes in vital signs. **Cognitive Level:** Applying **Client Need:** Management of Care **Integrated Process:** Communication and Documentation **Content Area:** Pharmacology **Strategy:** First recognize that the drug in the question is an antidiarrheal agent, and then select

the option that addresses meeting bowel elimination needs in an older adult client. **Reference:** Wilson, B. A., Shannon, M. T., & Shields, K. M. (2017). *Pearson nurse's drug guide 2017.* New York, NY: Pearson, pp. 910–911.

9 Answer: 2, 4, 5 Rationale: Discussion of feelings with another person helps the client manage emotional reactions. The nurse does not know why the client is crying. Although the client is emotionally upset, the nurse is obligated to inform the client of the risks associated with refusing medication. Although the client does need to know that ranitidine is an H_2-receptor blocker that reduces gastric acid production, resulting in less exposure of the open crater to irritants, the client does not appear to be ready for teaching. Because it seals the open crater and protects it from gastric contents, misoprostol is commonly used in open-crater gastric ulcers. The nurse should encourage the client to take the medication to reduce risk of perforation. **Cognitive Level:** Analyzing **Client Need:** Pharmacological and Parenteral Therapies **Integrated Process:** Communication and Documentation **Content Area:** Pharmacology **Strategy:** Discriminate between risks to the client and client needs. Think about the conditions that would ensure client rights and guarantee quality nursing care. **Reference:** Wilson, B. A., Shannon, M. T., & Shields, K. M. (2017). *Pearson nurse's drug guide 2017.* New York, NY: Pearson, pp. 1024–1025.

10 Answer: 1, 2, 3, 4, 5 Rationale: Misoprostol is administered for open-cratered gastric ulcers. The nurse may want to elevate the head of the bed because of the high risk of aspiration of blood. Maintaining an airway and breathing are high in priority. One side effect is abdominal pain, and increased restlessness could indicate the client is experiencing pain, making this second in priority. Ingestion of misoprostol can result in diarrhea. To prevent skin breakdown, placing a bed protector beneath the buttocks as the third action will help the skin to remain clean and dry. A log would help determine the bowel pattern and would be done fourth as it is a routine care activity. One side effect of the drug is spotting. This problem lacks the immediacy of aspiration, pain, and maintaining skin integrity, and would be done last if it occurs. **Cognitive Level:** Analyzing **Client Need:** Pharmacological and Parenteral Therapies **Integrated Process:** Nursing Process: Planning **Content Area:** Pharmacology **Strategy:** Make decisions about the priorities by determining what will place the client most at risk, followed by routine care activities and then items that may not occur at all. **Reference:** Wilson, B. A., Shannon, M. T., & Shields, K. M. (2017). *Pearson nurse's drug guide 2017.* New York, NY: Pearson, pp. 1024–1025.

Posttest

1 Answer: 1 Rationale: Anticholinergic effects include drying of mucous membranes, dilated pupils, and decreased motility of the GI tract, which may result in constipation. Pupillary constriction, bronchoconstriction, and bradycardia are the opposite of anticholinergic outcomes. The parasympathetic system participates in establishing an erection, hence, blockers would result in erectile dysfunction, and the drugs increase the heart rate. Because dry mouth is an anticholinergic effect, excessive salivation is incorrect. **Cognitive Level:** Applying **Client Need:** Pharmacological and Parenteral Therapies **Integrated Process:** Teaching and Learning **Content Area:** Pharmacology **Strategy:** Recall that when there is more than one part to an option, all parts must be correct for that option to be correct. Next, recall that side effects are exaggerations of parasympathetic function to help you choose correctly. **Reference:** Adams, M. P., & Urban, C. (2016). *Pharmacology: Connections to nursing practice* (3rd ed.). New York, NY: Pearson, pp. 214–217.

2 **Answer: 3 Rationale:** Because it may induce premature labor, castor oil is a Pregnancy Category X preparation. Bisacodyl is Pregnancy Category C. Mineral oil and sodium biphosphate are listed as unknown. It is recommended that the client utilize preventive methods such as adequate dietary fiber and at least 8 glasses of fluid per day. **Cognitive Level:** Applying **Client Need:** Pharmacological and Parenteral Therapies **Integrated Process:** Teaching and Learning **Content Area:** Pharmacology **Strategy:** Correlate the characteristics of the laxative with the risks to the fetus. Specific knowledge is needed to answer this question. **Reference:** Adams, M. P., & Urban, C. (2016). *Pharmacology: Connections to nursing practice* (3rd ed.). New York, NY: Pearson, pp. 1030–1032.

3 **Answer: 4 Rationale:** Elevated serum ammonia levels are commonly associated with hepatic encephalopathy. AST and ALT are liver enzymes indicating liver impairment. The enzyme level does not have a direct relationship to the cause of the impaired mental function. BUN and creatinine levels provide evidence of renal function. Bilirubin is elevated and urobilinogen may be normal or decreased in liver disease. Neither test would provide information regarding the hepatic encephalopathy. **Cognitive Level:** Applying **Client Need:** Pharmacological and Parenteral Therapies **Integrated Process:** Nursing Process: Assessment **Content Area:** Pharmacology **Strategy:** Correlate the altered mental function with the elevated ammonia levels. Next, recall that this medication helps to reduce ammonia levels in clients with severe liver disease. **Reference:** Wilson, B. A., Shannon, M. T., & Shields, K. M. (2017). *Pearson nurse's drug guide 2017.* New York, NY: Pearson, pp. 725–726.

4 **Answer: 1 Rationale:** Diphenoxylate inhibits nerve endings that cause intestinal movement. Decreasing the velocity increases opportunity for absorption of fluid resulting in increased viscosity of the stools. The drug is a narcotic with a structure similar to meperidine and has no effect on the shifts of sodium. Increased bulk would increase peristalsis. The drug primarily affects the nervous system, not the circulatory system. **Cognitive Level:** Analyzing **Client Need:** Pharmacological and Parenteral Therapies

Integrated Process: Teaching and Learning **Content Area:** Pharmacology **Strategy:** The core issue of the question is specific information about the drug action of diphenoxylate (Lomotil). Associate "low" mobility (motil) with Lomotil. **Reference:** Wilson, B. A., Shannon, M. T., & Shields, K. M. (2017). *Pearson nurse's drug guide 2017.* New York, NY: Pearson, pp. 493–494.

5 **Answer: 1, 2, 3, 5 Rationale:** Mineral oil should not be administered to clients with swallowing problems due to increased risk of aspiration leading to lipoid pneumonia. If a drug that may increase peristalsis is introduced, it may intensify the signs or symptoms or blur the clinical picture in a client with appendicitis. The client with fecal impaction needs to be disimpacted and may require enemas. Steatorrhea causes excessive stimulation of peristalsis because of the excessive fat content in the stool. There is no contraindication to giving this medication to a client with occasional heartburn, since this is likely due to food intolerance. **Cognitive Level:** Applying **Client Need:** Pharmacological and Parenteral Therapies **Integrated Process:** Nursing Process: Planning **Content Area:** Pharmacology **Strategy:** Correlate the clinical profile of the diseases or alterations with the actions of the drug. **Reference:** Adams, M. P., & Urban, C. (2016). *Pharmacology: Connections to nursing practice* (3rd ed.). New York, NY: Pearson, pp. 1030–1031.

6 **Answer: 2, 3, 5 Rationale:** Docusate sodium is appropriate for the postoperative client taking opioid analgesics, the client who had a myocardial infarction 24 hours ago, and the client with painful hemorrhoids. The client preparing for a colonoscopy would likely use a stimulant laxative. The client trying to reduce the chances of chronic constipation would likely use a bulk-forming laxative. **Cognitive Level:** Analyzing **Client Need:** Pharmacological and Parenteral Therapies **Integrated Process:** Nursing Process: Assessment **Content Area:** Pharmacology **Strategy:** Recall the specific drug action of a stool softener and match that to the benefit needed in a client with the conditions listed. Note that the wording of the question indicates that more than one option is correct. **Reference:** Adams, M. P., & Urban, C. (2016). *Pharmacology: Connections to nursing practice* (3rd ed.). New York, NY: Pearson, pp. 1030–1032.

7 **Answer: 4 Rationale:** Morphine sulfate is the drug of choice of the options listed because it is an opioid analgesic that is strong enough to relieve the pain, and it does not intensify biliary spasms, although this was a widely held notion in the past. Codeine sulfate is not utilized because it is a weaker opioid analgesic, although morphine sulfate is commonly administered. Bethanechol is a cholinergic drug that results in increased smooth muscle tone and motility. Dicyclomine is an antispasmodic that could decrease the biliary spasms, but is not an analgesic. The pain is also related to the inflammatory process. **Cognitive Level:** Applying **Client Need:** Pharmacological and Parenteral Therapies **Integrated Process:** Nursing Process: Planning **Content Area:** Pharmacology **Strategy:** The core issue of the question is which drug will relieve severe pain in a client with cholecystitis. Eliminate two options because they are not opioid analgesics. Choose between the remaining two options because one is stronger. Correlate the best remedy in relation to the total disease profile. **Reference:** Wilson, B. A., Shannon, M. T., & Shields, K. M. (2017). *Pearson nurse's drug guide 2017.* New York, NY: Pearson, pp. 436–438.

8 **Answer: 1 Rationale:** Ursodiol is a naturally occurring bile acid used to dissolve gallstones. It is believed to suppress hepatic synthesis and secretion of cholesterol as well as intestinal absorption. Omeprazole is a proton pump inhibitor that reduces gastric acid production. Cimetidine is an H_2 antagonist that reduces gastric acid production, but is not designed to treat cholelithiasis. Ibuprofen is a nonsteroidal anti-inflammatory drug (NSAID) and may be needed should the client develop a fever secondary to the process of inflammation. **Cognitive Level:** Applying **Client Need:** Pharmacological and Parenteral Therapies **Integrated Process:** Nursing Process: Planning **Content Area:** Pharmacology **Strategy:** The wording of the question suggests that the correct answer will be a drug that will treat the gallstones since surgery is not an option. Determine the actions of each of the drugs listed and then correlate the disease process with the action of the drug. **Reference:** LeMone, P. T., Burke, K. M., Bauldoff, G., & Gubrud, P. (2015). *Medical surgical nursing: Clinical reasoning in patient care* (6th ed.). New York, NY: Pearson, p. 723.

9 **Answer: 2 Rationale:** All of the drugs listed are histamine 2 (H_2)–receptor blockers that inhibit the secretion of gastric acid. Cimetidine interacts with a large number of drugs. Because it decreases the hepatic metabolism of phenytoin, they should not be administered concurrently. Famotidine has no known drug interactions with phenytoin. Nizatidine does not interfere with phenytoin therapy. Ranitidine reduces the absorption of several antibiotics. **Cognitive Level:** Applying **Client Need:** Pharmacological and Parenteral Therapies **Integrated Process:** Nursing Process: Planning **Content Area:** Pharmacology **Strategy:** Review each of the drugs in the options and determine the one that has the highest risk of negative interaction with the antiepileptic drug. **Reference:** Wilson, B. A., Shannon, M. T., & Shields, K. M. (2017). *Pearson nurse's drug guide 2017.* New York, NY: Pearson, pp. 1463–1465.

10 **Answer: 1 Rationale:** Taking bisacodyl on an empty stomach will result in a more rapid effect. Drinking plenty of fluids is a good general measure to reduce the risk of constipation. Taking the medication with a meal will delay absorption. If taking at bedtime, the client will have a bowel movement in the morning. **Cognitive Level:** Applying **Client Need:** Pharmacological and Parenteral Therapies **Integrated Process:** Nursing Process: Implementation **Content Area:** Pharmacology **Strategy:** Note that two options are opposites, making it more likely that one of them is correct. Consider that food will slow down or delay drug action to help choose the option citing to take the medication on an empty stomach. **Reference:** Wilson, B. A., Shannon, M. T., & Shields, K. M. (2017). *Pearson nurse's drug guide 2017.* New York, NY: Pearson, pp. 179–180.

References

Adams, M. P., Holland, N., & Urban, C. (2017). *Pharmacology for nurses: A pathophysiologic approach* (5th ed.). New York, NY: Pearson.

Adams, M. P., & Urban, C. (2016). *Pharmacology: Connections to nursing practice* (3rd ed.). New York, NY: Pearson.

Burchum, J., & Rosenthal, L. (2016). *Lehne's pharmacology for nursing care* (9th ed.). St. Louis, MO: Mosby.

Drug Facts & Comparisons (2017) (Updated monthly). St. Louis, MO: Wolters Kluwer.

Frandsen, G., & Pennington, S. (2017). *Abram's clinical drug therapy: Rationales for nursing practice* (10th ed.). Philadelphia, PA: Lippincott Williams & Wilkins.

Ignatavicius, D. D., & Workman, M. L. (2016). *Medical-surgical nursing: Patient centered collaborative care* (8th ed.). Philadelphia, PA: Elsevier.

Karch, A. M. (2017). *Focus on nursing pharmacology* (7th ed.). Philadelphia, PA: Lippincott Williams & Wilkins.

Kee, J. (2017). *Pearson's laboratory and diagnostic tests with nursing implications* (8th ed.). New York, NY: Pearson.

LeMone, P. T., Burke, K. M., Bauldoff, G., & Gubrud, P. (2015). *Medical-surgical nursing: Clinical reasoning in patient care* (6th ed.). New York, NY: Pearson.

Lilley, L. L., Rainforth Collins, S., & Snyder, K. M. (2017). *Pharmacology and the nursing process* (8th ed.). St. Louis, MO: Mosby.

Wilson, B. A., Shannon, M. T., & Shields, K. M. (2016). *Pearson nurse's drug guide 2016.* New York, NY: Pearson.

Immune System Medications

10

Chapter Outline

Immunomodulators
Immunizations
Medications to Treat Multiple
   Sclerosis

Medications to Treat
   Myasthenia Gravis
Medications to Treat
   Rheumatoid Arthritis

Medications to Treat Systemic
   Lupus Erythematosus

Objectives

➤ Describe the general goals of therapy when administering immune system medications.
➤ Identify the primary uses, interactions, major side effects, and adverse or toxic effects of commonly prescribed immunostimulant and immunosuppressant medications.
➤ Describe components of the recommended childhood immunization schedule.
➤ Identify side effects and adverse effects associated with the administration of immunizations.
➤ List contraindications associated with the administration of vaccines.
➤ Explain the nursing considerations related to the administration of medications commonly used to treat multiple sclerosis (MS), myasthenia gravis, rheumatoid arthritis, and systemic lupus erythematosus.
➤ List the significant client education points related to immune system medications.

NCLEX-RN® Test Prep

Access the NEW Web-based app that provides students with additional practice questions in preparation for the NCLEX experience.

Review at a Glance

active immunity immunity acquired by having a disease or by injection of infectious organisms
antigen a substance that produces formation of antibodies
cellular immunity host immunity that has been enhanced with increases in white blood cells and both helper and suppressor T-cell function
colony-stimulating factors factors that stimulate glycoproteins to produce

blood cells, thus stimulating immunity and bone marrow development
glycoprotein compounds of carbohydrates and proteins that, when produced, increase blood cell production
immune globulin an injection that provides passive immunity following exposure to certain communicable diseases
immunosuppression ability to suppress body's response to an antigen

neutropenia abnormally low neutrophil count
vaccine injections of living attenuated organisms or dead organisms that assist a human host to develop protection from a communicable disease

PRETEST

1 A client is scheduled to receive filgrastim 5 mcg/kg/day. The nurse considers that the dose should be withheld and the prescriber notified if which assessment data is noted?

1. Hematocrit 37%, hemoglobin 12 grams/dL
2. Mental depression
3. Bone pain
4. White blood cells 11,000/mm^3

2 A client being cared for at home is taking sargramostim. The nurse manager at the home health agency is most concerned when the unlicensed assistive personnel (UAP) reports which finding?

1. Early-morning oral temperature of 37.2°C (99°F)
2. Nausea and occasional diarrhea
3. Dyspnea on exertion and dependent edema
4. Mental depression and fatigue

3 A 61-year-old female client has severe rheumatoid arthritis that is being managed with leflunomide and infliximab. After the client reported having an elevated temperature of 37.7°C (99.8°F), the nurse should consider which possible etiology for this symptom?

1. Development of infection
2. Joint inflammation
3. Probable dehydration
4. Drug interaction

4 After the intramuscular administration of immune globulin, the nurse should provide which instructions to the client? Select all that apply.

1. Apply ice pack to injection site if swelling occurs.
2. Postpone receiving live vaccine for at least 3 months.
3. Use protective measures for the next 2 months until immunity develops.
4. Notify nurse if chills and fever develop.
5. Urinary output is likely to decrease.

5 A client with a seizure disorder is taking an antiepileptic medication along with cyclosporine. Which nursing interventions should the nurse include in the plan of care? Select all that apply.

1. Consult with the prescriber regarding the need to increase the cyclosporine dosage.
2. Evaluate for symptoms of elevated blood pressure.
3. Consult with the prescriber regarding the need to lower the antiepileptic dosage.
4. Routinely monitor blood glucose levels for hyperglycemia.
5. Monitor the client for seizures.

6 A client is scheduled to receive a high-dose regimen of aldesleukin. What should the nurse include when teaching about the drug? Select all that apply.

1. "Flulike symptoms are rare and indicate a potentially serious complication."
2. "This drug has potential interactions with most other drugs."
3. "This drug should help your body fight cancer cells."
4. "If severe fatigue occurs, the drug will need to be discontinued."
5. "This drug can only be given by brief intravenous infusions."

7 The nurse would place highest priority on which nursing concern and associated intervention when working with a client who is receiving cyclosporine?

1. Decreased blood flow to tissues: monitor for high blood pressure.
2. Severe pain: administer analgesic as prescribed.
3. Loss of intravascular fluids: encourage fluids.
4. Tremors: set up safety precautions.

8 Several clients were exposed to hepatitis A. The nurse should question a prescription for immune serum globulin by the intramuscular route with which client situation?

1. Diagnosis of diabetes insipidus
2. Exposure to rubeola
3. Exposure to hepatitis B
4. Platelet count less than 100,000/mm^3

9 A new parent asks the maternal-newborn nurse for information about immunizations for the infant. Which information should be included in client teaching? Select all that apply.

1. "Immunizations to prevent contagious diseases are required by law."
2. "Infants tend to be more susceptible to contagious diseases."
3. "Immunizations are safe without side effects."
4. "The injections are inexpensive or free at the health department."
5. "Immunity to disease develops immediately after the first immunization, so you may consider not having booster vaccines."

10 A client being treated for myasthenia gravis presents to the emergency department with severe ataxia and tremors. The nurse immediately prepares to administer which medication per protocol order?

1. Edrophonium
2. Ambenonium
3. Neostigmine
4. Atropine

➤ *See pages 326–328 for Answers and Rationales.*

I. IMMUNOMODULATORS

A. Description
1. Immunomodulators alter immune system actions in body by either suppressing or enhancing a client's immune response
2. Depending on desired immune response, client is given either an immune stimulant or an **immunosuppressant**, a drug that suppresses the body's response to an **antigen** (a substance that triggers antibody formation)

B. Immunostimulants
1. **Colony-stimulating factors (CSFs)**
   a. Action and use
      1) Colony-stimulating factors are **glycoproteins** that increase production of blood cells that enhance an individual's **cellular immunity** (host immunity characterized by increases in white blood cells and both helper and suppressor T-cell functions) by increasing number of lymphocytes and inhibiting tumor growth
      2) They increase development of leukocytes, which are adversely affected by chemotherapy agents used to treat cancer or after bone marrow transplantation
      3) These medications reduce **neutropenia** (abnormally low neutrophil count) and decrease incidence of infection; they assist in mobilization of stem cells, allowing for stem cell collection

     b. Common immunostimulant medications (Table 10-1)
     c. Administration considerations
       1) Sargramostim (GM-CSF)
        a) Multiple results—including increasing number of neutrophils, eosinophils, and monocytes—and increasing bactericidal activity of other immune cells
        b) Commonly used for clients with neutropenia caused by chemotherapy, acute lymphocytic leukemia, or Hodgkin disease
       2) Filgrastim
        a) Has two actions: increases bone marrow production of neutrophils and enhances function of existing neutrophils
        b) Generally given by subcutaneous route, although it may be given IV
        c) With each further chemotherapy administration, dose of filgrastim may be increased by 5 mcg/kg; with bone marrow transplantation or collection of stem cells, increase dose by 10 mcg/kg/day; dose for severe chronic neutropenia is 5–6 mcg/kg, one to two times per day

     d. Contraindications
       1) Sargramostim: pregnancy or lactation, hypersensitivity to yeast products or *E. coli* products, leukemic myeloblasts in bone marrow; use cautiously with hepatic or renal insufficiency and increased growth of tumor size
       2) Filgrastim and pegfilgrastim: pregnancy (Category C) and hypersensitivity to *E. coli* products (*E. coli* is used to produce this drug)
     e. Significant drug interactions
       1) Lithium and corticosteroids may increase the effectiveness of CSFs, especially sargramostim
       2) Do not administer either 24 hours before or 24 hours after chemotherapy because these drug types produce opposing effects
     f. Significant food interactions: none reported
     g. Significant lab studies

       1) Baseline and twice weekly complete blood count (CBC) with differential and platelet count; report to prescriber a WBC count over 10,000 cells/mm^3 or absolute neutrophil count (ANC) over 8,000/mm^3 (normal 1,500–8,000/mm^3)

Table 10-1   **Common Immunostimulants: Colony-Stimulating Factors**

Generic Name	Route	Uses
Sargramostin (GM-CSF)	IV or subcut	Stimulates granulocyte (neutrophil) and macrophage production
		Treats neutropenia following bone marrow transplant or chemotherapy
		Myeloid reconstitution after autologous bone marrow transplantation
		Accelerates myeloid recovery in non-Hodgkin lymphoma and acute lymphoblastic leukemia
		Mobilizes hematopoietic progenitor cells for collection by leukopheresis
Filgrastim (granulocyte-CSF)	IV or subcut	Stimulates granulocyte (neutrophil) production
		Reduces incidence of infections in client with nonmyeloid malignancies receiving myelosuppressive anticancer drugs
		Reduces time for neutrophil recovery following chemotherapy, severe chronic neutropenia
		Orphan drug use—myelodysplastic syndrome, aplastic anemia
Pegfilgrastim (G-CSF)	Subcut	Stimulates granulocyte (neutrophil) production
		Reduces time for neutrophil recovery following chemotherapy

2) Assess creatinine, blood urea nitrogen (BUN), liver enzymes before and after administration

3) Elevations in leukocyte alkaline phosphatase, serum alkaline phosphatase, lactate dehydrogenase, and uric acid (appear to be related to increased bone marrow activity)

    h. Side effects

        1) Bone pain, especially to bones with large amounts of bone marrow; usually managed with nonopioid analgesics

        2) Splenomegaly occurs in up to 30% of clients with long-term therapy

        3) Supraventricular dysrhythmia, tachycardia, myocardial infarction (MI) (with high leukocyte counts)

        4) Nausea and vomiting, anorexia, constipation, diarrhea

    i. Adverse effects/toxicity

        1) General

            a) MI, gastrointestinal (GI) hemorrhage, thrombus formation, and stroke (generally from high leukocyte counts)

            b) Adult respiratory distress syndrome (ARDS), pleural effusion

        2) Sargramostim

            a) Plan to withhold medication and notify prescriber if ANC rises above 8,000 cells/mm^3; dosage may be reduced or drug discontinued

            b) Respiratory distress occurring during first IV infusion administration, reduce IV rate by 50% if dyspnea occurs: signs include shortness of breath, hypotension, and tachycardia

        3) Filgrastim and pegfilgrastim: report neutrophil count of 8,000/mm^3 or higher to healthcare provider

    j. Client-centered nursing care

        1) Assess CBC and platelet count before administration and two times per week during medication administration

        2) Assess renal and hepatic function

        3) Assess for excessive myeloid blasts in bone marrow

        4) Do not administer during pregnancy and cautiously with lactation

        5) Client is at an increased risk for infection due to low WBC counts; evaluate for symptoms such as fever, chills, rash, or nonhealing areas; teach to avoid exposure to infection

        6) Leukocytosis may occur as a medication effect; evaluate for elevated WBCs during therapy

    k. Client education

        1) Report pain in joints and bones

        2) Maintain good hygiene and avoid exposure to crowds because of susceptibility to infection

        3) Teach to report even mild symptoms of infection such as fever, sore throat, chills, and rash

        4) Teach symptoms of allergic response, though this risk is low for this class of medications

2. Cell-stimulating medications

    a. Action and use

        1) Interferons (IFNs)

            a) Biologic response modifiers with antiviral, anti-inflammatory, and antineoplastic activity; a natural cytokine that has been modified by recombinant DNA technology, interferons warn surrounding cells that a viral infection has occurred; by attaching to uninfected cells, protective antiviral protein production is induced

---

Practice to Pass

What three assessments for hypersensitivity reaction are necessary for a client with hypersensitivity to *E. coli* products?

Practice to Pass

What assessment related to laboratory values should the nurse make when administering colony-stimulating factors?

      b) Reduce spread of viral infections by stimulating activities of leukocytes, phagocytes, and T-cells; interferons also promote cell death of infected cells

      c) "Peg" formulations have the molecule polyethylene glycol (PEG) bonded to INF to extend drug's half-life, which allows for once-weekly dosing

    2) Interleukins

      a) Biologic response modifiers that prevent thrombocytopenia and stimulate platelet production; they also possess an antitumor action and promote inflammation

      b) Cause cytotoxic T-cell replication, which results in lymphokine-activated killer cells that destroy only cancer cells and maintain normal cells; interleukins activate and increase production of natural killer (NK) cells, increase B-cell and plasma cell production, and increase neutrophil chemotaxis (movement in response to a stimulus)

  b. Common cell-stimulating medications (Table 10-2)

  c. Administration considerations

    1) Interferons

      a) Administer per accompanying drug insert

      b) Black box warning (IFN alfa2-b): may cause or aggravate fatal or life-threatening neuropsychiatric (including depression, suicidal ideation), autoimmune, ischemic, or infectious disorders; discontinue if symptoms are persistent or severe

    2) Aldesleukin

      a) Because of drug's ability to cause serious effects in every body system, it is given in a hospital that has an intensive care unit with medical specialists available

      b) High-dose regimen is associated with toxicities and is administered in multiple brief IV infusions because of short half-life; low-dose regimens may be given subcut at home

      c) Withhold if moderate to severe fatigue occurs

      d) Alert healthcare provider of symptoms of capillary leak syndrome or infection

      e) Treatment of overdose: dexamethasone

Table 10-2	**Common Cell-Stimulating Medications**	
Generic Names	**Route**	**Uses**
Interferon (IFN) alfa-2b	Subcut, IM	AIDs-related Kaposi sarcoma, chronic hepatitis B and C, leukemia, non-Hodgkin lymphoma, genital warts (condylomata acuminata)
IFN alfacon-1	Subcut, IM	Relapsing forms of multiple sclerosis
IFN alfa-n3	Intralesion	Warts
IFN beta-1a	IM or subcut	Severe multiple sclerosis
IFN beta-1b	Subcut	Severe multiple sclerosis
Peginterferon alfa-2a	Subcut	Hepatitis C
Peginterferon alfa-2b	Subcut	Hepatitis C
IFN gamma-1b	Subcut	Chronic granulomatous disease and severe osteoporosis
Aldesleukin; interleukin-2 (IL-2)	IV	Metastatic renal cell carcinoma and metastatic malignant melanoma Considered an orphan drug when used for non-Hodgkin lymphoma and acute myelogenous leukemia; used off-label to treat leprosy

    d. Contraindications

      1) Interferons

        a) Autoimmune hepatitis or hepatic decompensation

        b) Neonates and infants: contains benzyl alcohol, which may cause neurologic complications

        c) Use caution in clients with liver impairment, cardiac disease, herpes zoster, or who have recent exposure to chickenpox

        d) Do not use if hypersensitivity to albumin or mannitol

      2) Interleukins: aldesleukin

        a) Multiple contraindications; clients with significant cardiac, nervous system, pulmonary, renal, or hepatic problems should not use this drug

        b) May worsen clients with autoimmune diseases including scleroderma, thyroiditis, diabetes mellitus, and rheumatoid arthritis (RA)

        c) Treat bacterial infections before initiating therapy

        d) May induce coma in patients with developing moderate to severe lethargy

        e) Use cautiously in patients with epilepsy as can cause seizures

    e. Significant drug interactions

      1) Interferons—zidovudine levels may increase to toxic levels

      2) Interleukins

        a) Potential interaction with almost any drug, causing additive effects or organ damage

        b) Because of increased bleeding risk, use caution with aspirin, NSAIDs, and platelet inhibitors

        c) Avoid vaccines during and for 3 months after therapy

    f. Significant food interactions: none specific

    g. Significant laboratory studies

      1) Interferons: monitor platelets and white blood cells (myelosuppression), and liver enzymes (elevation)

      2) Interleukins: baseline CBC, electrolytes, renal, and liver panel (renal and hepatic impairment is likely during therapy)

    h. Side effects

      1) Interferons

        a) Most common effects are flulike symptoms, which include fever, chills, and fatigue, that generally improves over time

        b) Others include headache, myalgia, anorexia, nausea and vomiting, diarrhea, cough, dyspnea, pharyngitis, hair loss, injection site reactions (IFN betas)

      2) Aldesleukin: flulike symptoms, lethargy, rash, anorexia, nausea and vomiting, diarrhea, confusion or agitation, lethargy, dyspnea

    i. Adverse effects/toxicity

      1) Interferons: myelosuppression (anemia, leukopenia, thrombocytopenia), hepatotoxicity, suicidal ideation, myocardial infarction, anaphylaxis, severe depression, seizures (IFN beta), myasthenia gravis (IFN beta)

      2) Interleukins: capillary leak syndrome (which can cause death), tachycardia, hypotension, oliguria or anuria, pulmonary edema, cardiac arrest, sepsis

    j. Client-centered nursing care

      1) Interferons

        a) Monitor body weight due to lack of appetite

        b) Evaluate for symptoms of thrombocytopenia or neutropenia

        c) Monitor cardiac function especially in older adults, who are at increased risk for cardiotoxicity

        d) Monitor hydration status along with ability to consume fluids and food

        2) Interleukins

           a) Assess for renal and hepatic impairment

           b) Perform thorough comprehensive assessment before administering initial dose to assess for presence or history of diseases

           c) Maintain fluid and electrolyte balance particularly to prevent encephalopathy and mental status changes

           d) Assess for neutropenia or thrombocytopenia

        3) Provide optimal hygiene practices

        4) Monitor for weight gain

    k. Client education

        1) Interferons

           a) Avoid exposure to infection such as crowded places or public transportation

           b) Notify healthcare provider immediately for symptoms of infection such as rash, sore throat, or diarrhea

           c) Report signs of depression, lethargy, or excessive sleeping immediately

           d) Teach to rotate injection site, apply ice briefly before and after the injection, and apply a warm, moist compress after injection; antihistamines or topical hydrocortisone may be used to reduce itching and erythema; report worsening symptoms to healthcare provider

        2) Interleukins

           a) Plan for fatigue and flulike symptoms by prevention of overscheduling and taking acetaminophen before and after injections

           b) Report symptoms of bleeding or infection to healthcare provider

           c) Report symptoms of depression, kidney, or liver failure immediately

C. Immunosuppressants

    1. Action and use

        a. Inhibit inflammatory response and block immune response to an antigen

        b. Inhibit T-cell function and also block production of antibodies by B cells

        c. Prevent rejection of transplanted organs and treat autoimmune disorders (i.e., rheumatoid arthritis, systemic lupus erythematosus, myasthenia gravis, Hashimoto thyroiditis, as discussed later in this chapter).

        d. Immunosuppressants may include antibodies, cytotoxic agents and antimetabolites, calcineurin inhibitors, kinase inhibitors, and corticosteroids

           1) Cytotoxic drugs and antimetabolites class: inhibits aspects of lymphocyte replication and includes some drugs that treat cancer

           2) Calcineurin inhibitors: preferred drug class to prevent transplant rejection; block interleukin-2 and disrupt T-cell function by binding to intracellular messenger calcineurin; often used in treatments for psoriasis and rheumatoid arthritis

           3) Antibodies: act against T cells or T-cell receptors (note suffix -*mab* in these medication names); monoclonal antibodies (MAB) are specific to a single type of target cell or receptor and have less adverse effects than polyclonal antibodies; majority used to fight cancer cells but some are approved for treating autoimmune disorders; one is approved to prevent transplant rejection

           4) Kinase inhibitors; used with cyclosporine and corticosteroids to prevent organ rejection

           5) Corticosteroids: potent anti-inflammatory agents; affect almost every part of the immune response; have significant long-term adverse effects but are drug of choice for short-term therapy of severe inflammation

    2. Common immunosuppressant medications (Table 10-3)

Table 10-3	Common Immunosuppressant Medications	
Generic Name	**Route**	**Uses**
Cytotoxic Drugs and Antimetabolites		
Anakinra	Subcut	Severe, acute rheumatoid arthritis in clients over age 17 who have not responded to methotrexate and other drug therapies
Azathioprine	PO	Prevent rejection of kidney transplant; severe refractory rheumatoid arthritis
Betalacept	IV	Prevent rejection of kidney transplant
Cyclophosphamide	PO, IV	Prevent transplant organ rejection
Etanercept	Subcut	Moderate to severe forms of ankylosing spondylitis (AS), juvenile arthritis, plaque psoriasis, and rheumatoid and psoriatic arthritis
Methotrexate	PO	Severe psoriasis or rheumatoid arthritis (note different dosage formulation if used for treatment for cancer)
Mycophenolate	PO, IV	Prevent organ rejection with allogenic renal, hepatic, and heart transplants; moderately severe systemic lupus erythematosus
Thalidomide	PO	Skin conditions related to Hansen's disease (formerly leprosy), multiple myeloma
Monoclonal Antibodies		
Basiliximab	IV	Prophylaxis of acute rejection in kidney transplant; used in combination with cyclosporine and corticosteroids
Belimumab	IV	Suppresses B cells; for use in severe systemic lupus erythematosus
Infliximab	IV	Blocks tumor necrosis factor; useful in severe inflammatory disorders, including Crohn disease
Kinase Inhibitors (Rapamycins)		
Everolimus	PO	Prevention of kidney or liver transplant rejection
Sirolimus	PO	Prophylaxis for kidney transplant rejection; used with corticosteroids and cyclosporine; unlabeled use: psoriasis treatment
Calcineurin Inhibitors		
Cyclosporine	PO, IV	Prevent kidney, liver, and heart transplant rejection; treat chronic rejection in clients who have received immunosuppressive agents; rheumatoid arthritis, recalcitrant plaque psoriasis; often administered concurrently with corticosteroid such as prednisone
Tacrolimus	PO	Prevent liver or kidney organ rejection, moderate to severe atopic dermatitis; unlabeled use: prophylaxis in bone marrow, cardiac, pancreas, pancreatic island cell, small bowel transplants, autoimmune disease, recalcitrant psoriasis

3. Administration considerations
    a. When used to prevent rejection of organ transplant, generally used in conjunction with other medications, such as corticosteroids
    b. Read product directions carefully
    c. Monoclonal antibodies: avoid vaccinations for at least 2 weeks following last dose of drugs
4. Contraindications
    a. Allergy to drug
    b. Pregnancy or lactation

    c. Use cautiously with renal or hepatic impairment and with exposure to viral infections

  5. Significant drug interactions

    a. General

      1) Increased risk of hepatic or renal toxicity in clients taking other renal or hepatotoxic medications

      2) Multiple medication interactions may increase or decrease effectiveness of medications; see product literature

    b. Calcineurin inhibitors

      1) Cyclosporine: antiepileptic medications decrease cyclosporine levels; angiotensin-converting enzyme (ACE) inhibitors, NSAIDs increase cyclosporine levels

      2) Tacrolimus: increased risk of toxicity with metoclopramide, nicardipine, cimetidine, clarithromycin

  6. Significant food interactions: increased serum levels of calcineurin inhibitors (by 50–200%) are associated with administration of cyclosporine and grapefruit juice or grapefruit

  7. Significant laboratory studies: liver enzymes (AST, ALT), BUN and creatinine, CBC with platelet count, blood glucose (hyperglycemia), serum potassium (hyperkalemia)

  8. Side effects

    a. Antimetabolites: nausea and vomiting, bone marrow suppression

    b. Calcineurin inhibitors: hypertension and reduction in renal output

    c. Monoclonal antibodies: local site reactions and influenza-like symptoms

    d. General effects: increased risk for infection

    e. Hypertension

    f. Bone marrow suppression

  9. Adverse effects/toxicity

    a. Antimetabolites: leukopenia, thrombocytopenia, anemia

    b. Azathioprine: drug has high potential for toxicity, causing decreased leukocyte or platelet count

    c. Calcineurin inhibitors: nephrotoxicity and hepatotoxicity

    d. Monoclonal antibodies: anaphylaxis, infections

  10. Client-centered nursing care

    a. Assess for signs and symptoms of infection and opportunistic infections

    b. Provide supportive care for flulike symptoms

    c. Review drug interactions, as there are multiple drug interactions for all of these drug classes that may either increase or decrease drug effectiveness

    d. Assess nutritional status

    e. Encourage well-balanced meals with frequent, small feedings

    f. Avoid use of live vaccines

    g. Maintain blood studies as prescribed such as CBC, platelet count, and renal and hepatic function tests

  11. Client education

    a. Need for lab studies, prevention of infection, and all aspects of medication administration including action, side effects, and nursing implications; also report signs of infection

    b. Birth control methods should be utilized until after discontinuation of drug therapy

    c. Grapefruit can raise cyclosporine levels, increasing the risk of toxicity

Practice to Pass

What learning objectives are appropriate for the nurse to develop for a client who will be receiving immunosuppressant agents?

II. IMMUNIZATIONS

  A. Vaccines

  1. Action and use

  a. Vaccines are injectable or oral suspensions containing live but weakened (attenuated) or inactivated (killed) microorganisms, toxoid, or recombinant technology vaccine, that when injected produce antibodies to fight against a disease

  b. Active immunity results from introduction of a specific protein antigen by way of a vaccine; body responds by developing antibodies to confer a long-lasting immunity to that organism

  c. Vaccines are used to prevent diseases that may have high mortality and morbidity

  d. Some vaccinations are needed only once; others require boosters

  e. Effectiveness assessed by measuring number of antibodies produced after vaccine has been administered (titer)

  2. Common immunization medications (Figure 10-1 and Table 10-4)

Figure 10-1A

Recommended immunizations from birth to 6 years.

Source: Department of Health and Human Services. Retrieved from https://www.cdc.gov/vaccines/schedules/easy-to-read/child.html.

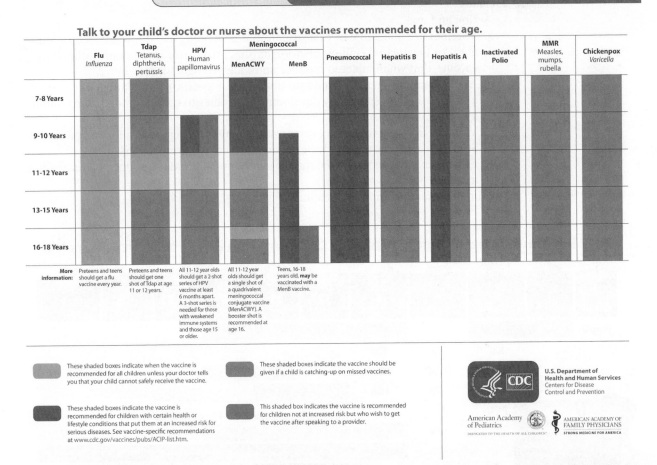

Figure 10-1B

Immunizations from 7 to 18 years.

Source: Department of Health and Human Services. Retrieved from https://www.cdc.gov/vaccines/schedules/easy-to-read/preteen-teen.html.

3. Administration considerations
   a. Live vaccines should be administered at least 1 month apart
   b. Hepatitis A is a two-dose series for clients at risk
   c. Hepatitis B: initial dose followed by second dose 1 month later, and a third dose 6 months after initial dose
   d. Measles, mumps, and rubella; total amount of reconstituted vial is administered subcut
   e. Immunization schedules are established by the Centers for Disease Control and Prevention (CDC); see Figure 10-1

4. Contraindications
   a. Vaccines should not be administered during a moderate to severe febrile illness, pregnancy, cancer, leukemia, and while on immunosuppressive drug therapy; use caution if administering to any immunocompromised individuals as their immune system may not be able to develop effective immunity
   b. Do not administer for 3 months after blood products have been administered

(*text continues on page 315*)

Figure 10-1C

Immunizations for adults.

Source: Department of Health and Human Services. Retrieved from https://www.cdc.gov/vaccines/schedules/downloads/adult/adult-schedule-easy-read-bw.pdf.

Table 10-4   Immunizations

Generic Name	Route	Actions	Uses
BCG (TICE BCG) haemophilus B conjugate vaccine and hepatitis B surface antigen	Percutaneously	Prevention of tuberculosis with high-risk exposure Active immunity against haemophilus B and hepatitis B	Prevention of tuberculosis, haemophilus B, and hepatitis B
Diphtheria and tetanus toxoids, combined (Dt, Td) diphtheria and tetanus toxoids and acellular pertussis vaccine absorbed (DTaP)	IM	Stimulates active immunity against diphtheria, tetanus, and pertussis	Prevention of diphtheria, tetanus, and pertussis
Diphtheria and tetanus toxoids and whole cell pertussis vaccine with haemophilus B conjugate vaccine DTwp-HIB	IM	Stimulates active immunity against diphtheria, tetanus, pertussis, and haemophilus B	Prevention of diphtheria, tetanus, pertussis, and haemophilus B Administered to children 2 months to 5 years

(*continued*)

Table 10-4	Immunizations (*continued*)			
Generic Name	**Route**	**Actions**		**Uses**
Diphtheria and tetanus toxoid	IM	Stimulates active immunity against diphtheria and tetanus		Prevention of diphtheria and tetanus
Hepatitis A vaccine	IM	Simulates immunity against hepatitis A		Prevention of hepatitis A infection
Hepatitis B vaccine	IM	Stimulates immunity against hepatitis B		Prevention of hepatitis B infection
Human papillomavirus (HPV) vaccine	IM	Stimulates immunity against HPV		Prevention of HPV-associated cancers and genital warts
Influenza virus vaccine, trivalent inactivated (TiIV)	IM	Stimulates active immunity to influenza virus antigens		Prevention of influenza virus
Influenza virus vaccine; live attenuated intranasal vaccine (LAIV)	Intranasal 2 mL	Stimulates active immunity to influenza virus antigens		Prevention of influenza virus
Measles	Subcut	Stimulates active immunity to measles		Immunization of persons older than age 1 year who reside or travel to endemic regions
Measles, mumps, and rubella (MMR-II)	Subcut	Stimulates active immunity to measles, mumps, and rubella		Immunization of persons greater than 15 months of age
Measles and rubella, live (MR vax II)	Subcut	Stimulates active immunity to measles and rubella		Immunization of children age 1 year and older
Meningococcal polysaccharide vaccine (MPSV-4) or meningococcal conjugate vaccine (MCV)	Subcut (MPSV-4), IM (MCV)	Stimulates immunity to meningococcal infections caused by *Neisseria meningitidis*; not effective against meningococcus serogroup B		Immunization against meningococcal infections in endemic regions; MPSV-4 for patients age 2–10 or over 55, MCV for those age 11–55
Mumps virus vaccine live	Subcut	Stimulates active immunity to mumps		Immunization against mumps in persons age 1 year and older
Pneumococcal vaccine polyvalent	Subcut or IM	Stimulates active immunity to pneumococcal infection; developed from 23 strains of *S. pneumoniae*		Immunization against pneumococcal infections; not recommended for children under age 2
Pneumococcal 7-valent conjugate vaccine	IM	Stimulates active immunity to pneumococcal infection		Assists prevention of invasive pneumococcal disease in infants and children
Poliovirus vaccine: inactivated (IPOL)	IM	Stimulates active immunity to polio		Immunization against polio in children and adults; oral polio vaccine still used in other parts of the world but has a rare risk of vaccine-associated polio
Rotavirus vaccine	PO	Stimulates active immunity against rotavirus		Immunization for infants 6–32 weeks of age to prevent gastroenteritis
Rubella virus vaccine live	Subcut	Stimulates active immunity to rubella virus		Immunization for children older than age 1 year and adults. Do not administer to clients who are pregnant or hypersensitive to neomycin
Rubella and mumps vaccine live	Subcut	Stimulates immunity to rubella and mumps		Immunization of children older than age 1 year and adults
Typhoid vaccine	Subcut	Stimulates active immunity to typhoid fever		Immunization against typhoid fever
Varicella virus vaccine	Subcut	Stimulates active immunity against chickenpox		Initial vaccination in childhood, repeat vaccination after age 60 months

      c. Do not administer influenza vaccine to clients who are hypersensitive to chicken or egg products; do not administer hepatitis B vaccine if known hypersensitivity to yeast

      d. Use during pregnancy – consider potential benefits of disease prevention versus risk to the mother and fetus

      e. Smallpox is believed to have been eradicated through vaccinations and the vaccine is no longer administered

  5. Significant drug interactions: immunosuppressive drug therapy

  6. Significant food interactions: none reported

  7. Significant laboratory studies: monitor antibody titer levels

  8. Side effects

      a. Pain, swelling, or redness at injection site

      b. Flulike symptoms

      c. Hypersensitivity (rarely noted)

  9. Adverse effects/toxicity: rarely clients may experience a hypersensitivity reaction, most often a response to preservatives; must be reported to the Vaccine Adverse Event Reporting System (VAERS)

  10. Client-centered nursing care

      a. Determine administration guidelines and timing of immunization administration

      b. Adhere to individual vaccine storage recommendations to ensure vaccine potency

      c. Assess client for acute infection prior to administration

      d. Maintain documentation of immunization administration and client reaction to administration; provide client or caretaker with a record of immunizations administered

      e. Administer all vaccines for which client is eligible at different sites, using different syringes

      f. Observe client for manifestations of adverse reactions and have epinephrine available in case of hypersensitivity reactions

      g. Provide acetaminophen after administration as needed

      h. Apply heat to injection site as needed for comfort

  11. Client education

      a. Discuss with client and family risk of contracting vaccine-preventable illnesses as well as signs and symptoms

      b. Instruct on treatment of flulike symptoms using acetaminophen or NSAIDs such as ibuprofen

      c. Instruct on importance of keeping a record of immunizations and being up to date in immunization administration

      d. Provide a copy of the Current Vaccine Information Statement for each vaccine administered; available from the Centers for Disease Control and Prevention

      e. Adults should be immunized against tetanus every 10 years

      f. Women of childbearing age should not become pregnant for 3 months after receiving a rubella immunization

B. Immune globulins

  1. Action and use

      a. **Immune globulins** provide passive immunity to a disease; immune system is not activated so does not provide long-term protection

      b. Can be used prophylactically to prevent disease following exposure

  2. Common immune globulin medications (Table 10-5)

  3. Administration considerations: if given IM, monitor for injection site reactions; IVIG contains antibodies to live viruses so active vaccinations should not be given until 3–5 months after IVIG administered

Practice to Pass

What client education should be implemented during a hepatitis A outbreak?

Table 10-5 Common Immune Globulin Medications

Immune Globulin	Route	Use
Cytomegalovirus (CMV) immune globulin	IV	Prevent CMV after organ transplant
Hepatitis B immune globulin	IM	Prevent hepatitis B after exposure
Immune globulin intravenous (IVIG)	IV	Treat primary immunodeficiency, reduce infection risk in immunocompromised individuals, increase platelets in individuals with idiopathic thrombocytopenic purpura, prevent aneurysm associated with Kawasaki syndrome
Rabies immune globulin	IM	Postexposure prevention of rabies; follow with five doses of rabies vaccine over a 28-day period
Respiratory syncytial virus (RSV) immune globulin	IV	Prevent RSV in high-risk individuals
Rh_0(d) immune globulin	IM, IV	Prevent mother's immune system from developing antibodies against Rh-positive fetus
Tetanus immune globulin	IM	Prevent tetanus after injury
Varicella zoster immune globulin	IM	Prevent varicella after exposure

4. Contraindications: hypersensitivity to immune globulin; use cautiously with thrombocytopenia and disorders affecting coagulation
5. Significant drug interactions: none reported
6. Significant food interactions: none reported
7. Significant laboratory studies: none reported
8. Side effects
   a. Allergic reaction
   b. Flulike symptoms
   c. Irritation at injection site
9. Adverse effects/toxicity: anaphylaxis
10. Client-centered nursing care
   a. Monitor for signs and symptoms of hypersensitivity reaction following administration
   b. Provide comfort for flulike symptoms
   c. Apply heat to irritated injection site
   d. Do not administer to clients with a history of coagulation disorders
   e. Document the medication administered, dosage, date, and response to medication
11. Client education
   a. Treatment of flulike symptoms (client and family)
   b. Signs and symptoms of anaphylaxis and to seek emergency care if noted (client and family)
   c. There is no evidence to support linkage of immunization such as MMR to autism
   d. Provide documentation to the client and family on the medication administered

C. Antitoxins
   1. Action and use: antibodies provided in immune sera for specific toxins that are released from invading pathogens; provides passive immunity
   2. Common antitoxin medications (see Table 10-6)
   3. Administration considerations: antirabies serum can be applied to animal bite wound
   4. Contraindications: hypersensitivity to antitoxin or horse serum, malignancy, and use cautiously with pregnancy
   5. Significant drug interactions: immunosuppressive drug therapy

Table 10-6	Common Antitoxin Medications	
Generic/Trade Names	**Route**	**Uses**
Antirabies serum, equine	IM or to bite wound	Horse serum used if human rabies immune globulin is unavailable
Botulism antitoxin	See drug insert	Obtained from horses immunized against *Clostridium botulinum*; used to treat botulism

6. Significant food interactions: none reported
7. Significant laboratory studies: none reported

8. Side effects: irritation and pain at injection site
9. Adverse effects/toxicity: hypersensitivity to medication and severe pain at injection site
10. Client-centered nursing care
    a. Monitor client response to medication
    b. Assess vital signs before and after administration
    c. Cleanse wound in case of animal bite
    d. Document client's response to medication
    e. Test sensitivity to horse serum and have epinephrine available

    f. Assess for neurologic response to botulism antitoxin
11. Client education
    a. Intended effects of medication
    b. Adverse effects of medication
    c. Wound care of client's animal bite

III. MEDICATIONS TO TREAT MULTIPLE SCLEROSIS (MS)

A. Action and use
1. The goal of medication therapy for multiple sclerosis (MS) is to decrease inflammation, suppress immune system to prevent nerve tissue destruction, and to reduce fatigue and ataxia
2. A wide variety of disease-modifying drugs are used to treat MS, including corticosteroids, anti-inflammatory agents, immunomodulators, and immunosuppressants
3. Medications are aimed at slowing disease progression and decreasing severity of attacks
4. Immunomodulators and immunosuppressants are given to slow progression of disease
5. Adrenocorticosteroid agents are used to relieve symptoms associated with myelin swelling: prednisone and methylprednisolone
6. Muscle relaxants are given to relieve spasticity associated with MS: baclofen, dantrolene, and diazepam
7. Miscellaneous drugs are also used for specific symptoms
    a. Amantadine (a dopaminergic drug) and modafinil (a central adrenergic drug) may help relieve fatigue, weakness, and memory loss
    b. Gabapentin (antiseizure drug) may relieve anxiety, insomnia, and neuropathic pain

B. Common medications for multiple sclerosis (Table 10-7)

C. Administration considerations
1. Typically, medications are started as soon as a diagnosis of MS is made and should be continued indefinitely unless toxicity occurs or no benefit is noted
2. Beta-1b should be discontinued in 6 months if disease does not enter remission

Table 10-7	Common Medications to Treat Multiple Sclerosis			
Generic Name	**Route**	**Actions**		**Uses**
Alemtuzumab	IV	Immunosuppressant		For progressive forms of MS
Dalfampridine	PO	Potassium channel blocker; treats difficulty with walking		For relapsing forms of MS
Dimethyl fumarate	PO	Myelin oxidative stress reducer		For relapsing forms of MS
Fingolimod	PO	Immunomodulator		For relapsing forms of MS
Glatiramer acetate	Subcut	Immunomodulator; protects myelin sheath		For relapsing forms of MS
Interferon beta-1a	IM, subcut	Immunomodulator		For relapsing forms of MS
Interferon beta-1b	Subcut	Immunomodulator		For relapsing and remitting form of MS
Mitoxantrone	IV	Antineoplastic and immunosuppressant		For progressive forms of MS
Natalizumab	IV	Immunomodulator; prevents WBCs from migrating to CNS		For relapsing forms of MS
Peginterferon beta-1a	Subcut	Immunomodulator		For relapsing forms of MS
Teriflunomide	PO	Immunomodulator; suppresses division of B and T cells		For relapsing forms of MS

　　D. **Contraindications**
　　　　1. These medications should be administered cautiously in presence of hepatic or renal insufficiency and when client has been diagnosed with a neoplasm
　　　　2. Contraindicated in pregnancy, lactation, and hypersensitivity to drug
　　E. **Significant drug interactions:** do not administer these medications with hepatotoxic or nephrotoxic medications; see individual product literature for others
　　F. **Significant food interactions:** do not administer these medications with grapefruit juice or grapefruit; effectiveness of medication will be reduced if this occurs
　　G. **Significant laboratory studies**
　　　　1. Liver enzymes (AST/ALT)
　　　　2. Blood glucose
　　　　3. BUN and creatinine
　　　　4. Calcium, phosphorus, uric acid
　　　　5. CBC and platelet count
　　H. **Side effects**
　　　　1. See earlier section for general side effects of immunomodulators and immunosuppressants
　　　　2. Glatiramer acetate: anxiety, diarrhea, flulike symptoms, hypertonia, and pain at injection site; may cause a reaction resembling myocardial ischemia
　　I. **Adverse effects/toxicity**
　　　　1. See earlier section for general adverse effects of immunomodulators and immunosuppressants
　　　　2. Depending on specific drug, severe adverse effects may include anaphylaxis, hepatotoxicity, dysrhythmias, cardiotoxicity, shortness of breath
　　J. **Client-centered nursing care**
　　　　1. Assess client for signs and symptoms of pulmonary edema, chest pain, shortness of breath, GI symptoms, or other side/adverse effects
　　　　2. Assess laboratory tests as prescribed by prescriber
　　　　3. Monitor blood pressure (BP), pulse, and cardiac output

Practice to Pass

What nursing interventions should be implemented to relieve the flulike symptoms that are side effects during administration of medications to treat multiple sclerosis?

4. Provide comfort measures when client experiences flulike symptoms
5. Assess injection sites for inflammation and pain

K. Client education

1. Side effects of medication and need for periodic laboratory studies; report side and adverse effects to prescriber
2. Need for supportive care of flulike symptoms, including adequate fluid intake, rest, and use of acetaminophen for relief of pain and fever
3. How to recognize signs and symptoms of pulmonary edema and hepatotoxicity and to report them

IV. MEDICATIONS TO TREAT MYASTHENIA GRAVIS

A. Action and use

1. The goal of anticholinesterase (acetylcholinesterase inhibitor) medications is to treat symptoms of myasthenia gravis (MG)
2. MG causes formation of antibodies to anti-acetylcholine receptors; anticholinesterase medications increase concentration of acetylcholine at neuromuscular junction
3. Used to increase conduction of nerve impulses and their strength

B. Common medications for myasthenia gravis (Table 10-8)

C. Administration considerations

1. Edrophonium: for diagnostic purposes only; discontinue all cholinesterase inhibitors (anticholinesterases) at least 8 hours before test; administer IV slowly while observing client response; response will often be immediate
   a. Myasthenic (positive) response is brief improvement in muscle strength without lingual or skeletal muscle fasciculations; indicates need for therapy with cholinesterase inhibitor

Table 10-8	**Common Medications to Treat Myasthenia Gravis**		
Generic Name	**Route**	**Actions**	**Uses**
Ambenonium	PO	Cholinesterase inhibitor: increases acetylcholine (Ach) concentration at sites of cholinergic transmission; prolongs and inhibits enzyme acetylcholinesterase, causing parasympathomimetic effects, facilitating transmission at skeletal neuromuscular junction	Symptom control of myasthenia gravis
Edrophonium	IV, IM	Cholinesterase inhibitor and muscle stimulant: increases concentration of Ach at sites of cholinergic transmission by inhibiting the destruction of Ach by cholinesterase; facilitates transmission of impulses at skeletal neuromuscular junction	Diagnosis of myasthenia gravis; differentiation between myasthenic crisis (insufficient neostigmine, indicated by improvement of symptoms) and cholinergic crisis (excess neostigmine, indicated by worsening of symptoms)
Neostigmine	IM, subcut, IV	Cholinesterase inhibitor: increases concentration of Ach at cholinergic transmission sites and prolongs effect of Ach at skeletal neuromuscular junction	Symptom control of myasthenia gravis
Pyridostigmine	PO	Cholinesterase inhibitor: increases Ach concentration at sites of cholinergic transmission and prolongs effects of Ach by inhibiting acetylcholinesterase, facilitating transmission at skeletal neuromuscular junction	Symptom control of myasthenia gravis

          b. Cholinergic response is lacrimation, diaphoresis, salivation, abdominal cramps, diarrhea, nausea and vomiting, decreased muscle strength; indicates overtreatment with cholinesterase inhibitor

          c. Adequate response is no change in muscle strength; minimal cholinergic adverse effects; indicates at or near optimal dosage level of cholinesterase inhibitor

    2. Neostigmine: can be administered subcut during an acute exacerbation of MG

    3. Pyridostigmine: a timed-release preparation can be administered PO at bedtime; can also be administered IM/IV during acute exacerbation

    4. Corticosteroids or immunosuppressants may be added to plan of care during exacerbation or over time if medications become ineffective

D. Contraindications

    1. Pregnancy and lactation

    2. Bradycardia, intestinal or urinary obstruction, peritonitis, aplastic anemia, lactation

    3. Hypersensitivity to drug

    4. Use cautiously in clients with asthma, heart disease, Parkinson disease, and seizure disorders

E. Significant drug interactions

    1. Combination of MG medications and NSAIDs poses a threat of GI bleeding because of increase in GI secretions

    2. Decreased effects of neostigmine occur with ambenonium and corticosteroids

F. Significant food interactions: none reported

G. Significant laboratory studies: monitor ALT/AST, BUN, and creatinine

H. Side effects

    1. Bradycardia, hypotension, or cardiac arrest

    2. Increased gastric secretions or diarrhea

    3. Increased urinary urgency

    4. Involuntary incontinence of stool

    5. Nausea and vomiting

I. Adverse effects/toxicity

    1. Severe cholinergic reaction includes excessive salivation, sphincter relaxation, diarrhea, and vomiting

    2. During administration of edrophonium, observe for cholinergic reaction and have atropine available as an antidote

J. Client-centered nursing care

    1. Assess respiratory and general muscle strength including swallowing and heart rate prior to administration

    2. Administer oral doses with meals to enhance absorption and decrease GI irritation; sustained release, so do not chew or crush

    3. Administer doses on time to prevent difficulty with respirations and swallowing caused by undermedication or late medication administration

    4. Administer IV preparations slowly to prevent cholinergic reaction; IM administrations should be deep into a large muscle

    5. Have atropine available to counteract cholinergic reaction but also be aware that atropine may mask parasympathetic effects of anticholinesterase overdose

    6. Assess client's response to the medication and ability to perform activities of daily living (ADLs)

K. Client education

    1. All aspects of medication administration

    2. How to coordinate medication administration with ADLs

    3. Overmedication will result in cholinergic reaction

    4. Assessment of apical pulse

    5. Side effects of medications

    6. Take medications with food to decrease GI irritation

    7. Report muscle weakness promptly to prescriber

V. MEDICATIONS TO TREAT RHEUMATOID ARTHRITIS

A. Action and use

1. Management of rheumatoid arthritis (RA) in early stages is accomplished with use of NSAIDs and disease-modifying antirheumatic drugs (DMARDs)
2. DMARDs reduce inflammation stiffness, swelling, and pain; anti-inflammatory effect is noted by decrease in erythrocyte sedimentation rate (ESR)
3. In severe cases of RA, or if clients have not responded to anti-inflammatories and DMARDs (nonbiologic therapies), biologic response modifiers (mainly monoclonal antibodies) may be added to treatment regimen

B. Common medications for rheumatoid arthritis (Table 10-9)

Table 10-9   Common Medications to Treat Rheumatoid Arthritis (RA)

Generic Name	Route	Actions	Uses
Nonbiologic Drugs			
Azathioprine	PO	Antimetabolite cytotoxic drug with immunosuppressant properties	RA and kidney transplant; high risk of malignancy (black box warning) limits its use
Hydroxychloroquine	PO	Unclear action; may interfere with communication between cells in immune system	RA, juvenile idiopathic arthritis, other autoimmune diseases; relieves some symptoms of systemic lupus erythematosus
Leflunomide	PO	Pyrimidine synthesis inhibitor: inhibits enzyme dihydro-orotate dehydrogenase (DHODH) (active in RA); inhibits B-cell and T-cell function	Relieves symptoms and slow progression of RA
Methotrexate	PO	Folic acid inhibitor: inhibits folic acid reductase, which inhibits DNA synthesis and cellular replication; selectively affects most rapidly dividing cells	Management of severe RA
Sulfasalazine	PO	Anti-inflammatory drug	RA, ulcerative colitis
Biologic Therapies			
Abatacept	IV	Selective T-cell costimulation blocker	Moderate to severe RA in adults, juvenile idiopathic RA; do not administer concurrently with TNF blockers
Adalimumab	Subcut	Monoclonal antibody, tumor necrosis factor (TNF) blocker	RA, other immune diseases
Anakinra	Subcut	Interleukin-1 receptor blocker	Moderate to severe active RA
Certolizumab pegol	Subcut	Monoclonal antibody; TNF blocker	RA, Crohn disease, psoriatic arthritis, ankylosing spondylitis
Etanercept	Subcut	Immunosuppressant, TNF blocker	Moderate to severe RA
Golimumab	Subcut	Manmade protein; binds to and blocks TNF-alpha when injected	RA, psoriatic arthritis, ankylosing spondylitis
Infliximab	IV	Monoclonal antibody, blocks TNF-alpha	RA, severe plaque psoriasis, psoriatic arthritis, ankylosing spondylitis, and inflammatory bowel disease (Crohn disease, ulcerative colitis)
Rituximab	IV	Monoclonal antibody, binds CD20 on B lymphocytes, thus reducing inflammation	Treat moderate to severe RA that is nonresponsive to treatment with TNF blockers
Tocilizumab	IV	Monoclonal antibody, interleukin-6 receptor blocker	RA in adults, polyarticular juvenile rheumatoid arthritis (PJIA), systemic form of juvenile idiopathic arthritis (SJIA)
Tofacitinib	PO	Inhibits janus kinase (JAK) enzyme that is responsible for inflammation in RA	Moderate to severe RA; used alone or in combination with other drugs such as methotrexate

   C. **Administration considerations:**
   1. DMARDs: may take several months to achieve therapeutic effects
   2. Therapy is administered in a step-wise progression
      a. When DMARD therapy is started, a single nonbiologic drug is prescribed (often hydroxychloroquine, methotrexate, leflunomide, or sulfasalazine)
      b. If symptoms worsen or do not improve after 3 months, a second DMARD is added, and later a third if needed
      c. Biologic therapies are prescribed for severe RA or for clients who have not responded to nonbiologic DMARDs

   D. **Contraindications**
   1. Never administer medications to clients who have a known allergy to animal products
   2. Contraindicated with pregnancy, lactation, liver disease, or renal disease
   3. Use cautiously in clients with immunosuppression or malignancy

   E. **Significant drug interactions**
   1. Do not administer these drugs with any agents known to be hepatotoxic
   2. Use caution when administering anakinra with etanercept (tumor necrosis factor blocker) because of increased risk for neutropenia and resulting risk for severe infection
   3. Methotrexate: multiple solution incompatibilities
   4. Do not administer biologic response modifiers with vaccinations
   5. Biologic response modifiers may be used with other DMARDs, but are generally contraindicated with each other due to similar mechanism of action

   F. **Significant food interactions**
   1. Methotrexate results may be decreased with increased caffeine intake
   2. Echinacea increases liver toxicity

   G. **Significant laboratory studies:** liver function tests, BUN and creatinine, CBC and platelet count

   H. **Side effects**
   1. Vary depending on drug and are numerous; read individual product literature
   2. May include GI symptoms such as anorexia, nausea and vomiting, or diarrhea
   3. Many increase risk of infection because of neutropenia secondary to myelosuppression
   4. Hydroxychloroquine: can cause unusual pigmentation of skin (to a blue-black color)

   I. **Adverse effects/toxicity**
   1. Vary depending on drug and are numerous; read individual product literature
   2. Hepatotoxicity, pericarditis
   3. Pulmonary edema
   4. Thrombosis, Stevens–Johnson syndrome, and death
   5. Increased eosinophil count or decreased neutrophils, total WBC count, or platelet count

   J. **Client-centered nursing care**
   1. Avoid use of antacids for at least 2 hours after dose administration
   2. Assess for bone marrow suppression, pulmonary fibrosis, and GI ulceration or bleeding with methotrexate
   3. Protect from exposure to sunlight
   4. Assess for side effects to medication
   5. Assess for signs of infection with all DMARDs
   6. Stop medications if signs of severe infection develop

   K. **Client education**
   1. Use measures to protect self from infection
   2. Use good oral hygiene to protect from stomatitis
   3. Monitor for and report bruising, petechiae, bleeding gums, or blood in stool

4. Monitor blood glucose if indicated and report elevations
5. Take medications as directed and be aware of side effects, action, use, and contraindications
6. Use contraceptive measures to protect against pregnancy with cytotoxic drugs such as methotrexate

VI. MEDICATIONS TO TREAT SYSTEMIC LUPUS ERYTHEMATOSUS

A. **Action and use**
1. Cytotoxic and antimetabolite drugs (also called *purine analogs*) are used along with NSAIDs and corticosteroids to treat symptoms of systemic lupus erythematosus (SLE)
2. They provide immunosuppressive action to treat autoimmune diseases
3. Cytotoxic and antineoplastic drugs are used as immunosuppressive agents to decrease cell proliferation in immune system; administered concurrently with corticosteroid therapy

B. **Common medications for systemic lupus erythematosus** (Table 10-10)

C. **Administration considerations**: see individual product literature or information discussed earlier in chapter

D. **Contraindications**
1. Do not administer with agents that are known to be hepatotoxic
2. Do not administer during pregnancy or lactation

E. **Significant drug interactions**: if azathioprine is administered with allopurinol, the azathioprine dose should be reduced

F. **Significant food interactions**: do not administer azathioprine with grapefruit juice

G. **Significant laboratory studies**
1. Liver and renal function tests
2. Blood glucose
3. CBC and platelet count
4. Calcium, phosphorus, and uric acid

H. **Side effects**
1. Alopecia
2. Stomatitis, diarrhea, and colitis
3. Dizziness
4. Itching or rash
5. Leukopenia or thrombocytopenia

Table 10-10	Common Medications to Treat Systemic Lupus Erythematosus (SLE)		
Generic Name	**Route**	**Actions**	**Uses**
Azathioprine	PO	Cytotoxic agent: suppresses cell-mediated hypersensitivity and alters antibody production	Administered for autoimmune component of disease; blocks inflammation pathways and helps to lower steroid dosage
Cyclophosphamide	PO, IV	Cytotoxic agent: lymphocytes are sensitive to drug effects in immunosuppression	Treatment of SLE
Cyclosporine	PO	Calcineurin inhibitor: inhibits T-helper and T-suppressor cells, lymphokine production, and release of interleukin-2 and T-cell growth factor	Prophylaxis against kidney, liver, and heart transplantation; treatment of chronic rejection in clients who have received immunosuppressants; RA, recalcitrant plaque psoriasis, and SLE
Methotrexate	PO	Folic acid inhibitor: inhibits folic acid reductase, which inhibits DNA synthesis and cellular replication in rapidly dividing cells	Management of SLE; especially effective in treating skin lesions, arthritis, and pleuritis

I. Adverse effects/toxicity
1. Black furry tongue
2. Hepatotoxicity
3. Pericarditis
4. Pulmonary edema
5. Stevens–Johnson syndrome
6. Death

J. Client-centered nursing care
1. Assess for side effects of medications
2. Assess for pulmonary edema and shortness of breath
3. Assess laboratory tests as prescribed by provider

K. Client education
1. How to protect self from infection
2. Need for proper oral hygiene to protect from stomatitis
3. How to self-monitor blood glucose level and report elevations
4. Be aware of all aspects of medication therapy, including side effects, actions, use, and contraindications
5. How to recognize pulmonary edema and to report to provider

Case Study

A 15-year-old girl is diagnosed with untreatable liver failure and esophageal varices with hemorrhage, and her name is placed on the national transplant list. Two weeks later, she received a liver transplant. Both before and after surgery she stated she was anxious and depressed. Three weeks after surgery she was discharged on these medications:

- Tacrolimus 3 mg PO bid
- Magnesium oxide 1 tablet PO bid
- Azathioprine 50 mg 2½ tablets PO every other day
- Esomeprazole 1 tablet PO bid
- Milk of magnesia 30 mL PO every other day

One week after discharge, she experienced extreme abdominal pain and was readmitted with signs of liver transplant rejection. A liver biopsy was performed and surgery was done to repair a closing portal vein. A prescription for methylprednisolone 125 mg IVP every 8 hours was added to her medication list. Laboratory studies obtained included AST/ALT, CBC with platelets, chemistry profile, arterial blood gases, and serum bilirubin.

1. What are the priority nursing concerns for this client both preoperatively and postoperatively?
2. Prior to the administration of the previously listed medications, what diagnostic studies and assessments should the nurse make?
3. What should be included in a teaching plan for this client and her family?
4. What nursing interventions should be implemented prior to discharge following the portal vein repair?
5. What is the rationale for the administration of methylprednisolone following the portal vein repair?

For suggested responses, see pages 541–542.

POSTTEST

1 The client asks how filgrastim will help with the management of cancer. The nurse should provide which response?

1. "Filgrastim will reduce your fatigue level."
2. "Filgrastim will increase your ability to resist infection."
3. "Filgrastim reduces the nausea and vomiting that accompanies chemotherapy."
4. "Filgrastim will protect your heart during chemotherapy administration."

2 Following an autologous bone marrow transplant, a client is receiving sargramostim. The nurse should give *priority* to assessing for which drug side effects?

1. Bone pain, myalgia, or arthralgia
2. Hypotension, tachycardia, or cardiac rhythm changes
3. Nausea and vomiting and diarrhea
4. Myalgia, weight gain, and increased uric acid levels

3 The nurse should anticipate that clients receiving which medications will have acetaminophen prescribed to prevent or treat flulike symptoms? Select all that apply.

1. Interferon alfa-2b
2. Aldesleukin
3. Cyclosporine
4. Azathioprine
5. Basiliximab

4 A client is receiving cortisone after receiving a liver transplant. Several months later, what assessment data is of greatest concern to the home health nurse?

1. Ability to perform activities of daily living (ADLs)
2. Psychological response to receiving another person's body part
3. Eye examination results of intraocular pressure (IOP) and lens density
4. Presence of fine tremors and gingival hyperplasia

5 A client has neutropenia from chemotherapy. The nurse anticipates that which medications are likely to be prescribed? Select all that apply.

1. Epoetin alfa
2. Pegfilgrastim
3. Oprelvekin
4. Filgrastim
5. Sargramostim

6 A client with a renal transplant is receiving tacrolimus. The nurse reviews the results of which set of laboratory tests prior to drug administration?

1. Lactic dehydrogenase (LDH) and creatinine phosphokinase (CPK)
2. Serum uric acid and serum protein
3. Serum calcium level and serum albumin level
4. Aspartate aminotransferase (AST) and alanine aminotransferase (ALT)

7 A client with multiple sclerosis (MS) has been prescribed interferon alfa-2b. Which intervention should the nurse include in the plan of care?

1. Request a prescription to treat clinical depression.
2. Instruct the client to change body positions slowly.
3. Encourage the client to seek grief counseling.
4. Encourage routine hydration with water.

POSTTEST

8 An infant girl with a tympanic membrane temperature of 38.3°C (101°F) is scheduled to receive the second diphtheria, pertussis, and tetanus (DPT) vaccine along with the inactivated poliovirus vaccine (IPV). The nurse should take which action?

1. Withhold vaccines and reschedule her visit when she is not febrile.
2. Administer injection and instruct mother to administer an antipyretic when she gets home.
3. Administer acetaminophen orally and give immunizations.
4. Obtain titers on needed immunizations and withhold them until results are obtained.

9 A client with multiple sclerosis who receives cyclophosphamide and digoxin reports nausea to the outpatient clinic nurse. The nurse should place highest priority on taking which action?

1. Evaluate the cyclophosphamide level.
2. Administer an oral antiemetic daily.
3. Provide six frequent, small meals.
4. Evaluate the digoxin level.

10 When a nurse discovers that a renal transplant recipient eats grapefruit for breakfast and is taking cyclosporine as an immunosuppressant drug, the nurse should provide which instructions? Select all that apply.

1. "This combination is likely to cause epigastric burning."
2. "Grapefruit and cyclosporine have interactions that affect the drug dosage."
3. "Take loperamide for diarrhea if it occurs."
4. "Be sure to watch for signs and symptoms of organ rejection."
5. "This combination could cause confusion or kidney failure."

➤ *See pages 328–329 for Answers and Rationales.*

ANSWERS & RATIONALES

Pretest

1 **Answer: 4 Rationale:** Filgrastim is a colony-stimulating factor. The goal of the therapy is to increase the neutrophil count to a normal level. The WBC range is 5,000–10,000/mm³. Thus, if the count is above normal level, the nurse should withhold the dose and confirm future prescriptions. Although the drug can cause anemia, the hemoglobin and hematocrit are within normal limits. There is no evidence that mental depression is caused by this drug. Because of the nature of the drug, the depression would probably be treated and the medication continued. Because of the risks to the client, the drug would be continued and the bone pain would be managed with opioid analgesics. **Cognitive Level:** Applying **Client Need:** Pharmacological and Parenteral Therapies **Integrated Process:** Nursing Process: Planning **Content Area:** Pharmacology **Strategy:** The critical words are *withholding the dose*. Consider the action of the drug to reason that the correct answer must either identify the intended outcome or a severe adverse effect. With this in mind, recall that the drug is intended to stimulate white blood cell production and note the normal value to choose it as the correct option. **Reference:** Adams, M. P., &

Urban, C. (2015). *Pharmacology: Connections to nursing practice* (3rd ed.). New York, NY: Pearson, p. 646.

2 **Answer: 3 Rationale:** Pericarditis, a side effect of this drug, can result in heart failure. Signs and symptoms include dyspnea on exertion and dependent edema. Unlicensed assistive personnel (UAP) are capable of noting this data while performing or assisting with activities of daily living. A slight temperature elevation accompanies pericarditis but is not representative of impaired cardiac function. Nausea and diarrhea are common, but dyspnea and edema take priority. Mental depression and fatigue need to be addressed but the dyspnea and the edema take priority over these elements. **Cognitive Level:** Analyzing **Client Need:** Pharmacological and Parenteral Therapies **Integrated Process:** Communication and Documentation **Content Area:** Pharmacology **Strategy:** Use the syllable *gram* in the word *sargramostim* to recall the increase in heart size associated with congestive heart failure. Next, recall the scope of practice of unlicensed assistive personnel (UAP) to select the most important abnormal data that is within their scope to collect. **References:** Wilson, B. A., Shannon, M. T., & Shields, K. M. (2017). *Pearson nurse's drug guide 2017.* New York, NY: Pearson, pp. 1424–1426; Adams, M. P., & Urban, C.

(2015). *Pharmacology: Connections to nursing practice* (3rd ed.). New York, NY: Pearson, p. 649.

3 **Answer: 1 Rationale:** A client taking medication that interferes with the immune response may be at risk for infection. The nurse should assess for other signs and symptoms of infection. Joint inflammation would produce more localized symptoms and is not likely to cause the temperature to rise to that degree. There is no indication that the client is dehydrated. The elevated temperature is not caused by drug interaction. **Cognitive Level:** Analyzing **Client Need:** Pharmacological and Parenteral Therapies **Integrated Process:** Nursing Process: Assessment **Content Area:** Pharmacology **Strategy:** Remember that drugs that interrupt the immune response may also put the client at risk for infection. **References:** Wilson, B. A., Shannon, M. T., & Shields, K. M. (2017). *Pearson nurse's drug guide 2017.* New York, NY: Pearson, pp. 146, 405, 836, 896, 1431; Adams, M. P., & Urban, C. (2015). *Pharmacology: Connections to nursing practice* (3rd ed.). New York, NY: Pearson, pp. 691–703.

4 **Answers: 1, 2, 4 Rationale:** Significant pain and tenderness is likely to occur at the injection site and a cold compress may be used. The drug may interfere with the development of antibodies following administration of live viruses so vaccinations should be postponed for at least 3 months. Immune globulin provides passive immunity, which is immediately active but only lasts for a few weeks or months. Fever and chills are indicative of hypersensitivity. Because of the diuretic effect of maltose (a preservative), urinary output may increase rather than decrease. A decrease in urine output would indicate a complication that should be reported. **Cognitive Level:** Analyzing **Client Need:** Pharmacological and Parenteral Therapies **Integrated Process:** Teaching and Learning **Content Area:** Pharmacology **Strategy:** Correlate drug characteristics with the purpose of the prescription. **References:** Wilson, B. A., Shannon, M. T., & Shields, K. M. (2017). *Pearson nurse's drug guide 2017.* New York, NY: Pearson, pp. 808–811; Adams, M., Holland, L., & Urban, C. (2017). *Pharmacology for nurses: A pathophysiologic approach* (5th ed.). New York, NY: Pearson, p. 520.

5 **Answer: 1, 2, 4, 5 Rationale:** Because concurrent administration of antiepileptic medications and cyclosporine will cause decreased therapeutic levels of the cyclosporine, an increase in the cyclosporine dosage needs to be made to ensure the appropriate therapeutic effect. Hypertension is seen in over half of the patients who take cyclosporine. The antiepileptic medication will need to be administered at the proper dosage level that controls the seizures. Cyclosporine can elevate the blood glucose and so this should be monitored. Monitoring for seizures should continue in the plan of care. **Cognitive Level:** Analyzing **Client Need:** Pharmacological and Parenteral Therapies **Integrated Process:** Nursing Process: Implementation **Content Area:** Pharmacology **Strategy:** Use knowledge of cyclosporine and the relationship between

antiepileptics and cyclosporine to make the correct selections. **References:** Wilson, B. A., Shannon, M. T., & Shields, K. M. (2017). *Pearson nurse's drug guide 2017.* New York, NY: Pearson, pp. 405–408; Adams, M. P., & Urban, C. (2015). *Pharmacology: Connections to nursing practice* (3rd ed.). New York, NY: Pearson, p. 699.

6 **Answers: 2, 3, 4, 5 Rationale:** Aldesleukin is an interleukin-2 agent that stimulates production of B cells, T cells, macrophages, and natural killer (NK) cells. The drug has potential interactions with almost any other drug, so the healthcare provider should be consulted before adding or stopping medications. Aldesleukin increases the body's ability to fight cancer cells. If moderate to severe fatigue develops, the drug should be withheld and the provider notified. The high-dose regimen can only be given IV. A low-dose regimen is less common and can be given subcutaneously. Flulike symptoms are common and can be managed with premedication. **Cognitive Level:** Analyzing **Client Need:** Pharmacological and Parenteral Therapies **Integrated Process:** Communication and Documentation **Content Area:** Pharmacology **Strategy:** Apply knowledge of drug side effects with client's clinical profile. Note that the wording of the question indicates more than one answer is correct. **Reference:** Adams, M. P., & Urban, C. (2015). *Pharmacology: Connections to nursing practice* (3rd ed.). New York, NY: Pearson, p. 694.

7 **Answer: 1 Rationale:** A side effect of cyclosporine is hypertension that places the client at risk for ineffective tissue perfusion to the kidneys, brain, and heart. Chest pain and leg cramps, but not severe pain, are occasionally associated with cyclosporine. Nephrotoxicity is associated with the drug, but hypervolemia is more likely than hypovolemia. Tremors are a side effect of the drug, but this does not override the significance of uncontrolled hypertension. **Cognitive Level:** Applying **Client Need:** Pharmacological and Parenteral Therapies **Integrated Process:** Nursing Process: Implementation **Content Area:** Pharmacology **Strategy:** Specific drug knowledge is needed to answer the question. If needed, use the ABCs—airway, breathing, and circulation—to choose correctly. **Reference:** Adams, M. P., & Urban, C. (2015). *Pharmacology: Connections to nursing practice* (3rd ed.). New York, NY: Pearson, p. 698.

8 **Answer: 4 Rationale:** Intramuscular immune serum globulin should not be administered to clients with a history of coagulation disorders (platelet count of less than $100,000/mm^3$). It can be administered to clients with diabetes insipidus, but should be avoided in clients with diabetes mellitus. It is administered to clients exposed to rubeola and hepatitis B to provide passive immunity. **Cognitive Level:** Applying **Client Need:** Pharmacological and Parenteral Therapies **Integrated Process:** Nursing Process: Planning **Content Area:** Pharmacology **Strategy:** Think of immunoglobulin therapy and hypocoagulation as repelling each other. Choose the option that represents this connection in thinking. **Reference:** Wilson, B. A.,

ANSWERS & RATIONALES

Shannon, M. T., & Shields, K. M. (2017). *Pearson nurse's drug guide 2017*. New York, NY: Pearson, p. 808.

9 Answers: 1, 2, 4 Rationale: The client does need to understand that immunizations are required by law; without immunizations, it would be difficult to control contagious diseases, leading to a high rate of mortality and morbidity in children. Because of reduced immunity, infants are more prone to many contagious diseases. All immunizations commonly have minor side effects. Information about cost may allay fears that the parent cannot afford the immunization, thus increasing compliance. Immunity begins with the first vaccine, but the child does not have full immunity until all doses are given. **Cognitive Level:** Applying **Client Need:** Pharmacological and Parenteral Therapies **Integrated Process:** Communication and Documentation **Content Area:** Pharmacology **Strategy:** When determining the appropriate responses, consider the client and intended recipient along with facts about immunizations. **Reference:** Adams, M. P., Holland, N., Urban, C. (2017). *Pharmacology for nurses: A pathophysiologic approach* (5th ed.). New York, NY: Pearson, p. 712.

10 Answer: 4 Rationale: Side effects of cholinesterase inhibitors used to treat myasthenia gravis include dysrhythmic muscular contractions. Atropine (an anticholinergic medication) counteracts the cholinergic effect of a cholinesterase inhibitor drug. Edrophonium is a cholinesterase inhibitor that is used to diagnose myasthenia gravis. Its use would worsen the client's symptoms. Ambenonium and neostigmine are also cholinesterase inhibitors, which would worsen the side effects that the client is experiencing. **Cognitive Level:** Applying **Client Need:** Pharmacological and Parenteral Therapies **Integrated Process:** Nursing Process: Planning **Content Area:** Pharmacology **Strategy:** Consider from the symptoms described that the client may be experiencing excessive drug effects, after recalling that the symptoms of the disease include muscle weakness. From there, choose the medication that is the antidote to the prescribed medication. **Reference:** Adams, M. P., Holland, N., Urban, C. (2017). *Pharmacology for nurses: A pathophysiologic approach* (5th ed.). New York, NY: Pearson, p. 153.

Posttest

1 Answer: 2 Rationale: Filgrastim increases the number of neutrophils whose function is to act against invading microorganisms. The drug may cause anemia, which may compound the feelings of fatigue rather than reduce them. The drug may cause nausea and vomiting rather than reduce it. It may cause changes in the electrocardiogram and is not cardioprotective. **Cognitive Level:** Applying **Client Need:** Pharmacological and Parenteral Therapies **Integrated Process:** Teaching and Learning **Content Area:** Pharmacology **Strategy:** Associate the syllable *fil* in *filgrastim* with filling the gap in the neutrophil count caused by chemotherapy. Recall the function of neutrophils to then choose the correct option.

Reference: Wilson, B. A., Shannon, M. T., & Shields, K. M. (2017). *Pearson nurse's drug guide 2017*. New York, NY: Pearson, pp. 674–676.

2 Answer: 2 Rationale: Hypotension, tachycardia, and thrombocytopenia are major side effects of sargramostim. They take priority because they affect circulation. The other options indicate signs or symptoms that are side effects of the drug but they do not have priority over those that affect circulatory status. Bone pain, myalgia, and arthralgia are common side effects. Nausea and vomiting and diarrhea are side effects that should be managed, but would *not* receive priority over cardiovascular changes. Myalgia, weight gain, and increased uric acid levels are side effects of the drug that would also be secondary priorities. **Cognitive Level:** Applying **Client Need:** Pharmacological and Parenteral Therapies **Integrated Process:** Nursing Process: Assessment **Content Area:** Pharmacology **Strategy:** Associate the drug with musculoskeletal and cardiac complications. Then prioritize using the ABCs (airway, breathing, and circulation). **References:** Adams, M. P., Holland, N., Urban, C. (2017). *Pharmacology for nurses: A pathophysiologic approach* (5th ed.). New York, NY: Pearson, p. 649 Wilson, B. A., Shannon, M. T., & Shields, K. M. (2017). *Pearson nurse's drug guide 2017*. New York, NY: Pearson, pp. 1424–1426.

3 Answers: 1, 2, 5 Rationale: Immunomodulators, including interferon, aldesleukin, and basiliximab, are associated with the common side effect of flulike symptoms. Acetaminophen is commonly used to treat these symptoms. Cyclosporine and azathioprine have several side effects, but are not likely to cause flulike symptoms. **Cognitive Level:** Analyzing **Client Need:** Pharmacological and Parenteral Therapies **Integrated Process:** Nursing Process: Assessment **Content Area:** Pharmacology **Strategy:** Specific drug knowledge is needed to answer the question. Consider the class of each drug to help make a selection. **Reference:** Adams, M. P., & Urban, C. (2015). *Pharmacology: Connections to nursing practice* (3rd ed.). New York, NY: Pearson, p. 1155.

4 Answer: 3 Rationale: Long-term use of corticosteroids to prevent organ rejection can result in the development of cataracts and glaucoma. While fatigue and weakness prevented normal activities before the transplant, the client's ability to manage personal needs increases after the transplant. Clients often experience mental depression following the transplant. While psychosocial needs are important as well, the nurse should give the potential loss of sight priority. Overgrowth of gums and fine tremors are minor side effects of the drug. **Cognitive Level:** Applying **Client Need:** Pharmacological and Parenteral Therapies **Integrated Process:** Nursing Process: Assessment **Content Area:** Pharmacology **Strategy:** The time line in the question refers to long-term intended and adverse effects associated with the use of cortisone. Use specific knowledge about the drug to make a selection. **Reference:** Adams, M. P., & Urban, C. (2015). *Pharmacology: Connections to nursing practice* (3rd ed.). New York, NY: Pearson, pp. 691–696.

ANSWERS & RATIONALES

5 **Answers: 2, 4, 5 Rationale:** Colony-stimulating factors that stimulate the production of white blood cells include pegfilgrastim, filgrastim, and sargramostim. Epoetin stimulates the production of red blood cells. Oprelvekin stimulates the production of platelets. **Cognitive Level:** Applying **Client Need:** Pharmacological and Parenteral Therapies **Integrated Process:** Nursing Process: Planning **Content Area:** Pharmacology **Strategy:** Note that the drugs that stimulate the white blood cells all have the suffix *-stim.* **Reference:** Adams, M. P., & Urban, C. (2015). *Pharmacology: Connections to nursing practice* (3rd ed.). New York, NY: Pearson, pp. 645–649.

6 **Answer: 4 Rationale:** AST (aspartate aminotransferase) and ALT (alanine aminotransferase), which are liver enzymes, are relevant since tacrolimus and other immunosuppressant drugs are hepatotoxic. LDH (lactic dehydrogenase) is found in many tissues and is not specifically used for determining liver damage. CPK (creatinine phosphokinase) is used in the diagnosis of cardiac, neurologic, and muscle damage. The drug does not significantly affect these tissues. Changes in uric acid levels are related to gout. Serum protein is used more commonly for the diagnosis of lymphoma or myeloma. Serum calcium levels are more likely to be elevated with decreased parathyroid function or with decreased bone resorption. Because of the long half-life (12–18 days) of albumin, it is not an effective test for determining whether or not the drug should be administered. **Cognitive Level:** Applying **Client Need:** Pharmacological and Parenteral Therapies **Integrated Process:** Nursing Process: Assessment **Content Area:** Pharmacology **Strategy:** The core issue of the question is knowledge that this medication is hepatotoxic. With this in mind, select the laboratory tests that best reflect liver function. **Reference:** Wilson, B. A., Shannon, M. T., & Shields, K. M. (2017). *Pearson nurse's drug guide 2017.* New York, NY: Pearson, pp. 1492–1495.

7 **Answer: 4 Rationale:** Interferon alfa-2a is a biologic response modifier used in treatment of multiple illnesses, including multiple sclerosis (MS). A history of depression or suicidal tendencies may prevent the use of the drug; however, an antidepressant would not generally need to be requested from the healthcare provider. Dizziness, hypotension, and tachycardia are not common side effects of interferon. The need for grief counseling would not be related to administration of this drug. Hydration status should be monitored by the nurse, particularly in the initial stage of treatment, due to renal excretion of the drug, in order to prevent toxicity. **Cognitive Level:** Applying **Client Need:** Pharmacological and Parenteral Therapies **Integrated Process:** Nursing Process: Implementation **Content Area:** Pharmacology **Strategy:** Specific drug knowledge is needed to answer this question. Associate need for hydration with this medication. **Reference:** Wilson, B. A., Shannon, M. T., & Shields, K. M. (2017). *Pearson nurse's drug guide 2017.* New York, NY: Pearson, pp. 834–836.

8 **Answer: 1 Rationale:** Since fever is a side effect of the vaccine, the immunization should be withheld. It would be difficult to separate a response to the immunization from a febrile disease. Diagnosis of the problem should be made before treatment is initiated. Administering an antipyretic is more appropriate for prevention of a fever after the vaccine is administered. The fever remains of unknown origin and further diagnosis is needed. Titers should be performed after immunization or actually having the disease. **Cognitive Level:** Applying **Client Need:** Pharmacological and Parenteral Therapies **Integrated Process:** Nursing Process: Implementation **Content Area:** Pharmacology **Strategy:** Recall that immunization stimulates the immune process, which could make it difficult to interpret the significance of fever. Use general nursing knowledge of vaccines and the immune response to make a selection. **Reference:** Adams, M. P., & Urban, C. (2015). *Pharmacology: Connections to nursing practice* (3rd ed.). New York, NY: Pearson, pp. 723–725.

9 **Answer: 4 Rationale:** Cyclophosphamide combined with digoxin may result in digoxin toxicity, so the healthcare team must continually assess for signs and symptoms of toxicity. Nausea is an early sign of digoxin toxicity. Nausea and vomiting are also side effects of cyclophosphamide, but because cyclophosphamide may increase the risk of digoxin toxicity, the best response is to explore the digoxin level first. The nurse should administer an antiemetic but not orally. Nausea needs to be relieved before eating. **Cognitive Level:** Applying **Client Need:** Pharmacological and Parenteral Therapies **Integrated Process:** Nursing Process: Assessment **Content Area:** Pharmacology **Strategy:** As an early strategy for many questions, consider the possibility of drug toxicity when symptoms are reported. Next, associate the symptom of nausea with digoxin toxicity to answer this particular question. **Reference:** Adams, M. P., & Urban, C. (2015). *Pharmacology: Connections to nursing practice* (3rd ed.). New York, NY: Pearson, p. 964.

10 **Answers: 2, 5 Rationale:** The combination of grapefruit and cyclosporine will result in an increased serum cyclosporine level. The most common adverse effects include nephrotoxicity and neurotoxicity. Epigastric burning may be related to the ingestion of the fruit, but is not related to the combination with the drug. Diarrhea is not a consequence of this combination. Since the combination is more likely to increase the cyclosporine levels, organ rejection is not likely. **Cognitive Level:** Applying **Client Need:** Pharmacological and Parenteral Therapies **Integrated Process:** Communication and Documentation **Content Area:** Pharmacology **Strategy:** Consider that a question that focuses on a food and a drug or on two or more drugs usually aims at testing knowledge of the interactions between them. With this in mind, eliminate two options first and then use drug knowledge to choose between the remaining two. **References:** Wilson, B. A., Shannon, M. T., & Shields, K. M. (2017). *Pearson nurse's drug guide 2017.* New York, NY: Pearson, pp. 405–408; Adams, M. P., & Urban, C. (2015). *Pharmacology: Connections to nursing practice* (3rd ed.). New York, NY: Pearson, p. 462.

ANSWERS & RATIONALES

References

Adams, M., Holland, L., & Urban, C. (2017). *Pharmacology for nurses: A pathophysiologic approach* (5th ed.). New York, NY: Pearson.

Adams, M. P., & Urban, C. (2015). *Pharmacology: Connections to nursing practice* (3rd ed.). New York, NY: Pearson.

Drug Facts & Comparisons (Updated monthly). St. Louis, MO: A. Wolters Kluwer.

Holland, L., Adams, M., & Brice, J. (2018). *Core concepts in pharmacology* (5th ed.). New York, NY: Pearson.

Karch, A. M. (2016). *Focus on nursing pharmacology* (7th ed.). Philadelphia, PA: Lippincott Williams & Wilkins.

Kee, J. L. (2017). *Pearson handbook of laboratory and diagnostic tests with nursing implications* (8th ed.). New York, NY: Pearson.

Lehne, R. (2016). *Pharmacology for nursing care* (9th ed.). St. Louis, MO: Mosby.

LeMone, P., Burke, K., Bauldoff, G., & Gubrud, P. (2015). *Medical surgical nursing: Clinical reasoning in patient care* (6th ed.). New York, NY: Pearson.

Wilson, B. A., Shannon, M. T., & Shields, K. M. (2017). *Pearson nurse's drug guide 2017.* New York, NY: Pearson.

Anti-Infective Medications

11

Chapter Outline

Antibiotics
Antimycobacterials

Antivirals
Antifungals

Antiprotozoals
Antihelminthics

Objectives

➤ Describe general goals of therapy when administering anti-infective medications.

➤ Explain why antibiotics should not be discontinued until the prescribed therapy is complete.

➤ Identify actions and common side effects of various anti-infective medications.

➤ Describe most common adverse reactions to anti-infective medications.

➤ Explain nursing considerations related to anti-infective medications prescribed to treat human immunodeficiency virus and acquired immunodeficiency syndrome.

➤ Describe why medication combinations are commonly used to treat tuberculosis and leprosy.

➤ Identify significant client education points related to the use of anti-infective medications.

NCLEX-RN® Test Prep

Access the NEW Web-based app that provides students with additional practice questions in preparation for the NCLEX experience.

Review at a Glance

amebiasis infection of large intestine by a protozoan parasite called *Entamoeba histolytica*; transmitted via fecal to oral route from contaminated food or water or from person-to-person contact; found worldwide

bactericidal term for an agent that *destroys* a bacterial microorganism

bacteriostatic agent that *inhibits* growth of bacteria and depends on host's immune system to destroy bacteria

candidiasis a fungal infection caused by *Candida albicans* transmitted by direct contact or as a superinfection; occurs in mucous membranes in warm, dark, moist areas such as oral cavity (thrush), vagina, intestine, and cutaneously beneath breasts and in diaper areas of infants

cross-sensitivity a condition in which one class of drugs is chemically very similar to another; allergy to one class may suggest allergy to another class of drugs; cross-sensitivity occurrence between penicillins and cephalosporins has been reported to be 1–18%

cytomegalovirus (CMV) a common virus that resides in salivary glands; may cause CMV pneumonia (potentially fatal) and CMV retinitis (with potential blindness) in immunosuppressed clients; newborns are also at higher risk if mother is infected; requires use of standard precautions

disulfiram-like reaction also called antabuse effect; a reaction when certain medications are taken with even small amounts of alcohol; causes abdominal cramping, facial and upper body flushing, pulsating headache, weakness, uneasiness, vertigo, hypotension, palpitations, shortness of breath, sweating, pruritic macular rash, tachycardia, nausea and vomiting; may occur within 10–30 minutes of alcohol ingestion and last 30 minutes to several hours

empiric therapy drug therapy initiated based on clinical manifestations of a pathologic or infectious process rather than diagnosis by culture and sensitivity (C&S); selection of agent is based on most common known cause of infection and may be adjusted if needed after C&S results are known

giardiasis most common protozoan intestinal (usually duodenal) infection transmitted by contaminated food or water or stool of infected clients; causes diarrhea, abdominal distention, and malodorous stools

helminths disease-producing parasites such as *Nematoda* (roundworms) and *Platyhelminthes* (flatworms) that include *Cestodes* (tapeworms) and *Trematodes* (flukes), which may be isolated in stool, urine, blood, sputum, or host tissues

herpes simplex a viral infection classified as Type 1 (of facial areas including cold sore or fever blister) or Type 2 (genital herpes)

herpes varicella virus that causes chickenpox

herpes zoster virus of chickenpox that has lain dormant in nerves; eruptions of infection occur along nerve routes, especially of trunk; may be activated by immunosuppressed states or stress of disease

peak drug level serum blood level of antibiotic drawn 15–30 minutes after IV infusion is complete to determine that peak level is not at a toxic level

***Pneumocystis jiroveci* pneumonia** very serious protozoan infection of lungs occurring only in immunosuppressed clients

pseudomembranous colitis a type of superinfection that occurs when an antibiotic decreases or completely eliminates normal flora needed to maintain normal function in GI tract; permits overgrowth of other bacteria or fungi or yeasts (not susceptible to antibiotic) that cause infection

Stevens–Johnson syndrome an adverse skin reaction that resembles appearance of partial-thickness burns with erythema multiforme, fever, and bullae (blister) lesions of mucous membranes of oropharynx, conjunctiva, vagina, and anus

superinfection a condition in which an antibiotic decreases or eliminates

normal bacterial flora that consists of certain bacteria and fungi or yeasts needed to maintain normal function in various organs; permits overgrowth of other bacteria or fungi or yeasts (not susceptible to antibiotic) that cause infection (e.g., vaginal yeast infection, pseudomembranous colitis, candidiasis)

tinea fungal infections, called ringworm, caused by dermatophytes on foot (tinea pedis or "athlete's foot"), on scalp (tinea capitis), on body (tinea corporis), and in groin (tinea cruris or "jock itch")

toxoplasmosis protozoan systemic infection transmitted by contact with oocysts in feces of domesticated animals, primarily in feline species

trough drug level blood specimen drawn just prior to next scheduled IV dose of antibiotic to determine that therapeutic level has been maintained between drug doses and that adequate renal clearance of drug has occurred to avoid toxicity

PRETEST

1 When overseeing drug therapy for a client taking isoniazid, the nurse should assess for which of the following? Select all that apply.

1. Elevated aspartate aminotransferase (AST)
2. Clinical manifestations of hypercalcemia
3. Concurrent self-administration of aluminum antacids
4. Compliance with ingestion of pyridoxine vitamin Vitamin B_6 supplements
5. Excessive bruising on the skin

2 A client receiving an intravenous infusion of a cephalosporin medication reports pain and irritation at the infusion site. After noting thrombophlebitis at the site, in what order should the nurse complete these actions?

1. Elevate extremity.
2. Remove the peripheral catheter.
3. Apply a warm compress to the site per agency policy.
4. Stop the infusion.
5. Apply a sterile dressing.

3 A client is receiving oseltamivir for *influenza A*. The nurse should monitor for which common side effect?

1. Stevens–Johnson syndrome
2. Diarrhea
3. Excessive urination
4. Nephrotoxicity

4 Which intervention is of highest priority for the nurse working with a client who has *herpes zoster* (shingles) and who recently began drug therapy with acyclovir?

1. Monitor for jaundice and elevated liver enzymes.
2. Teach client to avoid sexual intercourse during therapy.
3. Administer the dose early in the day, as it may cause insomnia.
4. Encourage fluid intake of 2,500–3,000 mL daily if not contraindicated.

5 The nurse should conclude that a client with bacterial pneumonia understands self-administration of a prescribed oral antibiotic after the client makes which statement?

1. "I will continue to take the antibiotic as it is prescribed, even though I no longer have a cough with yellow sputum."
2. "When I missed a dose of my antibiotic this morning, I made up by taking two doses at the time of the next dose."
3. "I am careful to take the antibiotic every day at breakfast, lunch, and dinner."
4. "Even though my provider prescribed a chewable tablet, I have no problem swallowing it whole."

6 After taking amoxicillin for 10 days, the client has developed diarrhea, with approximately eight watery stools per day. The nurse should anticipate the need for which priority interventions? Select all that apply.

1. Monitor for clinical manifestations of metabolic acidosis.
2. Administer an antiperistaltic agent such as dicyclomine hydrochloride.
3. Administer an antidiarrheal agent such as kaolin and pectin.
4. Collect stool specimen for a cytotoxin assay to detect *Clostridium difficile.*
5. Instruct client to increase intake of fruit juices.

7 When assessing a client for toxicities associated with tobramycin therapy, the nurse should include evaluation of which client data? Select all that apply.

1. Hand strength
2. Creatinine levels
3. Alanine aminotransferase (ALT) levels
4. Amylase levels
5. Ringing in the ears

8 Which client statement indicates an understanding of the use of erythromycin? Select all that apply.

1. "I will always take this medication with fruit juices."
2. "If I experience abdominal fullness I will contact my provider."
3. "I know I should not crush the pills."
4. "I understand it is common to have some hearing loss while taking this medication."
5. "I will let my provider know if I begin to have a lot of diarrhea."

9 The prescriber has just ordered cefdinir, a third-generation cephalosporin, for a client with a staphylococcal infection. The nurse collaborates with the prescriber about which data related to the client?

1. Blood urea nitrogen (BUN) 14 mg/dL
2. Elevated granulocyte count
3. Culture and sensitivity (C&S) results not yet available
4. History of Type I hypersensitivity to penicillin

10 A client's sputum specimen is sent to the laboratory for gram stain testing. The nurse should assess the client for signs of what type of infection?

1. Bacterial
2. Acute viral
3. Parasitic
4. Fungal

➤ *See pages 384–386 for Answers and Rationales.*

I. ANTIBIOTICS

A. Aminoglycosides

1. Action and use
   a. **Bactericidal**: aminoglycosides kill bacteria cells by interfering with protein synthesis
   b. Effective against aerobic gram-negative infections; used in combination with another antibiotic to treat gram-positive infections
   c. Because of minimal absorption from GI tract, can be used to remove enterococcal bacteria (sterilize bowel) prior to bowel surgery
   d. Used to destroy urease-producing bacteria in bowel to prevent absorption of ammonia in hepatic encephalopathy
   e. Toxicity limits drug's use to serious gram-negative infections and specific conditions involving gram-positive cocci
2. Common aminoglycoside medications (Table 11-1)
3. Administration considerations
   a. Intravenous (IV) route preferred for optimal distribution to tissues
   b. May be used intramuscularly (IM) as well
   c. Oral route: poorly absorbed so effective orally only to cleanse bowel prior to abdominal surgery or to prevent absorption of ammonia in hepatic encephalopathy
   d. Intrathecal or intraventricular injection: may be used because of poor penetration of cerebrospinal fluid (CSF) by other routes
   e. Periocular instillations: because of poor penetration of eye fluids, direct instillations may be used
   f. Topical route: neomycin combined with other antibiotics provides broad-spectrum coverage in a cream or ointment
4. Contraindications/cautions
   a. Allergy to aminoglycosides
   b. Should be used cautiously if preexisting renal disease or hearing loss, myasthenia gravis, neuromuscular disease, or in neonates and preterm infants (immaturity of renal system)
   c. Concurrent order for renal toxic agents such as amphotericin B, vancomycin, or loop diuretics such as furosemide
   d. Contraindicated in pregnancy and lactation
5. Significant drug interactions
   a. Aminoglycosides may be microbiologically inactivated with concurrently high concentration of penicillins greater than 200 mcg/mL
   b. Do not mix other medications in same IV fluid

Table 11-1 Aminoglycosides

Generic Name	Route
Amikacin	IM, IV
Gentamicin	IM, IV, topical
Kanamycin	PO, IM, IV, irrigation, intraperitoneal, inhalation
Neomycin	PO, IM
Paromomycin	PO
Streptomycin	IM
Tobramycin	IM, IV, topical

       c. With oral anticoagulant therapy, bleeding may increase because aminoglycosides decrease vitamin K synthesis in intestinal tract

       d. Concurrent administration of dimenhydrinate may mask signs of toxicity

6. Significant food interactions: none reported

7. Significant laboratory studies

       a. Peak drug level: blood specimen drawn 30–60 minutes after IM administration and 30 minutes after completion of IV infusion of aminoglycoside to determine that toxic level does not occur; dose may need to be decreased if peak too high; peak levels may not be drawn with once-daily dosing since dose is short-lived

       b. Trough drug level: blood specimen drawn immediately prior to administering next IV dose of aminoglycoside to ensure that therapeutic levels of drug are maintained between doses and also adequate renal clearance of drug has occurred; if a therapeutic level is not sustained, an increase in dose and/or dosing frequency may be needed; if trough levels are too high, dosage will need to be decreased

       c. White blood count (WBC) to monitor effectiveness of drug therapy

          1) Neutrophils and immature neutrophils, called stabs or bands, are increased in acute bacterial infections

          2) Neutrophils and lymphocytes make up 75–90% of leukocytes; a "shift to the left" signifies an increase in neutrophil production and, therefore, an acute bacterial infection

       d. Serum creatinine and blood urea nitrogen (BUN) before first dose and to monitor renal function; expected BUN-to-creatinine ratio is 20:1 or 15:1 depending on criteria of laboratory; if creatinine level rises 3–4 days into treatment, it indicates renal damage has occurred

       e. Culture and sensitivity prior to first dose to ensure microorganisim is susceptible to antibiotic

8. Side effects: headache, paresthesia, skin rash, fever, nausea and vomiting, and fatigue

9. Adverse effects/toxicity

       a. Nephrotoxicity and ototoxicity are two common toxicities associated with therapy with aminoglycosides

       b. Occur when trough levels are elevated

       c. Nephrotoxicity: risk factors include infancy or advanced age (with associated immature or declining renal function), hypotension, dehydration, preexisting renal disease, and coadministration of other nephrotoxic drugs

       d. Ototoxicity: may be irreversible

          1) Auditory impairment and vestibular damage with possible damage to 8th cranial nerve

          2) Risk increased with nephrotoxic drugs, prolonged treatment with aminoglycosides, impaired renal function, and other ototoxic drugs, such as furosemide, vancomycin, amphotericin B, and certain antineoplastic agents

       e. Neuromuscular blockade and respiratory paralysis: secondary to inhibition of acetylcholine release; may be seen in clients with myasthenia gravis or those receiving neuromuscular blocking agents such as pancuronium or succinylcholine; use calcium salts to reverse blockade

       f. Hypersensitivity reactions include purpura, rash, urticaria, and exfoliative dermatitis

       g. Superinfection: a secondary infection caused by eradication of normal flora

          1) Candidiasis: secondary infection usually of skin and mucous membranes caused by *Candida albicans*; often associated with immunosuppression

            a) Occurs on mucous membranes of oropharynx (thrush), bronchi, vagina, and anus

             b) Appears as discrete white plaques; red, scaly, papular skin rash can occur in warm, moist, dark areas, such as in breast folds, axilla, and/or groin

        2) Pseudomembranous colitis: secondary infection of bowel usually caused by *Clostridium difficile*

             a) Manifested by four to six watery stools/day with blood and/or mucus, abdominal pain, and fever

             b) Antibiotic is discontinued and vancomycin orally (PO) or metronidazole IV or PO is prescribed

10. Client-centered nursing care

    a. Collect appropriate specimen for culture and sensitivity (C&S) prior to initiating anti-infective therapy to ensure appropriate drug is prescribed; **empiric therapy** (based on probable offending organism) is usually begun before test results become available because of seriousness of infection

    b. Assess for other current medications that could cause drug–drug interaction (e.g., other nephrotoxic drugs)

    c. Ensure client takes complete course of antibiotic for full beneficial effects, even if clinical manifestations of infection resolved; premature discontinuation can result in regrowth of microorganisms as well as development of drug resistance

    d. Encourage increased fluid intake to 2-3L/day (to reduce risk of nephrotoxicity) unless contraindicated by another condition and calculate intake and output (I&O)

    e. Monitor peak and trough aminoglycoside levels

    f. Monitor for nephrotoxicity: serum creatinine (normal 0.8–1.6 mg/dL), BUN (normal 8–22 mg/dL), urine creatinine clearance, and urinalysis results (urinary casts and proteinuria)

    g. Monitor for ototoxicity

        1) Assess baseline hearing and existing hearing impairments (may be noted by presence of hearing aids) and monitor for hearing loss once therapy begins; may include audiometry testing

        2) Clinical signs of ototoxicity include dizziness, light-headedness, tinnitus, fullness in ears, and hearing loss

        3) Monitor vestibular integrity: perform Romberg test, if possible; have client stand alone with hands at sides and eyes open, then have client close eyes; minimum swaying of body is expected, but if unable to maintain standing position or balance, Romberg test is positive indicating problem with balance

    h. Consult with prescriber about dosage adjustment or medication change if indicated by results of above tests or assessments

    i. Observe for evidence that infection is resolving within 48–72 hours of therapy (fever and local manifestations)

    j. Provide small, frequent, nutritious meals with high-quality proteins; drugs that may be taken with food may be associated with decreased gastrointestinal (GI) upset

    k. See Box 11-1 for other general principles of nursing care for client receiving anti-infective therapy

11. Client education

    a. See universal teaching points for anti-infectives (Box 11-2)

    b. Keep premixed drug refrigerated as recommended

    c. Take safety precautions according to side effects that occur

    d. Take oral aminoglycoside on an empty stomach, 1–2 hours before any meal or other drugs

    e. Eat frequent, small meals with at least six to eight glasses of fluid daily

Box 11-1	*Before drug therapy is initiated:*
General Principles of Nursing Care During Anti-Infective Therapy	• Obtain health history, including allergies, current medication profile (for possible drug interactions), history of illness (noting especially GI, liver, kidney, and neurologic disorders). • Gather physical examination data, including vital signs, height and weight, and specific signs and symptoms of infection. • Assess results of baseline laboratory tests, such as BUN and creatinine (kidney), liver enzymes, electrolytes, complete blood count (note WBC particularly), possible lipid panel, and others as indicated to provide a baseline if adverse drug effects or toxicity occur. • Ensure that specimen for culture and sensitivity (C&S) is obtained before administering first dose of anti-infective therapy. *During anti-infective drug therapy:* • Administer medication correctly using six "rights" of medication administration. • Monitor for hypersensitivity reaction with first dose, especially within first 2–30 minutes, after second dose (if sensitization occurred with first dose), and be aware that delayed reactions may occur even after 72 hours. • If drug is being administered IV, assess for signs of phlebitis or infiltration and instruct client to report pain or other site symptoms during administration of dose. • Ensure adequate fluid intake and if indicated by specific drug, increased fluid intake to 2–3 L/day. • Monitor client's fever (if present) and local symptoms of infection to see if they are resolving; report unchanged or worsening symptoms to provider after 48–72 hours (depending on infection and antiinfective being used). • Monitor for adverse drug effects that are specific to anti-infective drug class, signs of superinfection (occurs during antibiotic therapy because of reduction of normal flora), photosensitivity and skin sensitivity (increased risk of sunburn) depending on drug in use. • Review results of periodic labwork: WBC should decrease and adverse changes should not occur in labs (commonly CBC, liver, and renal studies). • Ensure client takes full course of prescribed therapy to prevent infection from returning and to reduce risk of client developing resistance to drug (antibiotics).

Box 11-2	

Universal Client Teaching Points for Anti-Infective Therapy	• Know drug name, dose, route, administration schedule, what adverse effects to observe for and when to report, and whether to take with or without food
	  • Avoid or eliminate alcohol
	  • Increase overall fluid intake and take oral doses with a full glass of water
	• Take at evenly spaced intervals around the clock as much as possible (but without interrupting sleep) in order to maintain therapeutic levels between doses
	• Take full course of therapy as prescribed to prevent repeat infection or development of drug resistance
	• Do not double the next dose if a dose is skipped or missed
	• Discard any outdated or unused drug; self-administration or use of drugs with decreased potency could adversely affect future treatment and increase risk of development of drug resistance
	• Do not use drug if expiration date has passed
	• Before taking any over-the-counter (OTC) drugs, check efficacy and possible adverse reactions with healthcare provider
	• Report symptoms of infection that do not improve after 48 hours of therapy or worsening symptoms to healthcare provider
	• Monitor for and report signs of superinfection (candidiasis or pseudomembranous colitis)

        f. Report sore throat, watery stools greater than four to six per day and severe nausea and/or vomiting, which indicate possible superinfection

        g. Instruct on signs and symptoms of ototoxicity: headache, nausea, unsteady balance or gait, tinnitus, vertigo, high-frequency hearing loss, and dizziness

B. Carbapenems

  1. Action and use

    a. Inhibit cell wall synthesis and are bactericidal; effective against many gram-positive organisms and most gram-negative cocci and bacilli and anaerobic bacteria

    b. Imipenem is always combined with cilastatin, which increases serum levels of imipenem

    c. May be used in serious infections of urinary tract, lower respiratory tract, skin, and abdominopelvic area

    d. Meropenem used for peritonitis and bacterial meningitis (because of its ability to enter CSF)

  2. Common carbapenem medications (Table 11-2)

  3. Administration considerations

    a. Carbapenems have been associated with drug-induced seizure activity in a small percentage of clients; they are contraindicated in anyone with a history of hypersensitivity to any of their ingredients

    b. Reduced doses are indicated in presence of renal insufficiency

    c. If administering IM, inject deep into gluteal muscle

  4. Contraindications

    a. A small risk (about 1%) of allergenicity exists in clients with penicillin allergies; clients with anaphylactic-type reactions to penicillin should not receive carbapenem

    b. Use caution in clients with central nervous system (CNS) disorders, renal dysfunction, asthma, or in pregnancy or lactation

  5. Significant drug interactions

    a. CNS effects may be additive when given with cyclosporine, ganciclovir, and theophylline

    b. Meropenem may interact with valproic acid; monitor levels of valproic acid to ensure they are therapeutic

    c. Concurrent use of imipenem-cilastatin with cyclosporine, tramadol, theophylline, or ganciclovir may increase risk of seizures and other CNS effects

    d. Concurrent administration with penicillin, cephalosporins may antagonize antimicrobial effects with imipenem-cilastatin or aztreonam

  6. Significant food interactions: none specific

  7. Significant laboratory studies

    a. Monitor renal function; reduced doses of imipenem-cilastatin may be needed in renal insufficiency since this drug is substantially excreted by kidneys

    b. Monitor liver function tests (LFTs), electrolytes, BUN, creatinine, and complete blood count (CBC) with differential

Table 11-2   **Carbapenems**

Generic Name	Route
Imipenem-cilastatin	IV
Doripenem	IV
Ertapenem	IV, IM
Meropenem	IV

8. Side effects
   a. Nausea and vomiting, anorexia, dizziness, diarrhea, rash, pruritus, headache, and thrombophlebitis at IV injection site
   b. Drug fever
   c. Hyperkalemia, hyponatremia, polyuria, oliguria, weakness, arthralgias
9. Adverse effects/toxicity
   a. Superinfections such as pseudomembranous colitis and blood dyscrasias may occur
   b. CNS effects such as seizures, especially in older adults with compromised renal function, or when concurrently taking ganciclovir
   c. Hypersensitivity reactions with fever, chills, dyspnea, chest discomfort, hyperventilation, pruritus
10. Client-centered nursing care (see Box 11-1 again)
    a. Clients allergic to other beta-lactam antibiotics may be cross-allergic to imipenem
    b. Monitor for neurotoxicity, nephrotoxicity, hepatotoxicity, transient hearing loss
    c. Provide measures for seizures and other CNS alterations when appropriate; call prescriber to discontinue drug if seizures occur
    d. Do not interchange IM and IV solutions
11. Client education
    a. See Box 11-2 for universal teaching points for anti-infective therapy
    b. Determine whether or not client is pregnant before starting imipenem-cilastatin
    c. Instruct client to inform nurse if IV site is burning or painful
    d. Instruct client to report severe or persistent diarrhea, other secondary infection (sore throat, vaginal irritation), intense itching, difficulty breathing, confusion, or seizures
    e. Teach not to breastfeed or become pregnant while taking imipenem-cilastatin

C. Cephalosporins
1. Action and use
   a. Structurally and chemically related to penicillins; like penicillins, they also contain a beta-lactam ring; **cross-sensitivity** may occur between penicillins and cephalosporins, meaning that allergy to one class may indicate hypersensitivity to the other in some clients
   b. Five generations of cephalosporins; differences between generations include activity against gram-negative bacteria, resistance to beta-lactam drugs, and distribution in CSF; usually bactericidal in action
   c. Used to treat sexually transmitted infections (STIs), respiratory infections such as bronchitis, pharyngitis, otitis media, sinusitis, and pneumonia, urinary tract infections (UTIs), skin and tissue infections, and Lyme disease
   d. Used prophylactically and therapeutically in orthopedic disorders
   e. Used for endocarditis prophylaxis prior to surgery for clients with history of rheumatic heart disease
   f. Important to reserve use for appropriate clinical infections because bacterial resistance increasing
   g. Most cephalosporins are excreted through urine except cefoperazone and ceftriaxone, which are excreted in bile
2. Common cephalosporin medications (Table 11-3)
3. Administration considerations
   a. Well absorbed from GI tract, absorption is delayed with food but amount absorbed is not affected; exceptions are cefadroxil and cefprozil, whose absorption is not delayed with food
   b. Check renal function before and during therapy to allow for appropriate dosage adjustment; renal impairment significantly extends drug half-life

Practice to Pass

The client taking an antibiotic develops diarrhea. What assessments and interventions would you perform?

Table 11-3	Cephalosporins
Generic Name	**Route**
First Generation	
Cefadroxil	PO
Cefazolin	IM, IV
Cephalexin	PO
Cephapirin (no longer produced in U.S.)	PO, IM, IV
Cephradine	PO, IM, IV
Second Generation	
Cefaclor	PO
Cefotetan	IM, IV
Cefoxitin	IM, IV
Cefprozil	PO
Cefuroxime	PO, IM, IV
Third Generation	
Cefdinir	PO
Cefditoren	PO
Cefixime	PO
Cefotaxime	IM, IV
Cefpodoxime	PO
Ceftazidime	IM, IV
Ceftibuten	PO
Ceftizoxime	IM, IV
Ceftriaxone	IM, IV
Fourth and Fifth Generations	
Cefepime	IM, IV
Ceftraroline	IV

    c. Separate oral administration of antacids, histamine H2-receptor blockers, iron supplements, and foods fortified with iron by 2 hours before and after oral administration of cephalosporins

    d. Separate oral administration of cefdinir from iron supplements and foods fortified with iron by 2 hours

    e. Intramuscular administration is painful and irritating; administer deep IM into large muscle; avoid repeated IM injections; IV is preferred parenteral route; addition of prescribed 1% xylocaine solution can help to reduce pain with IM injections

    f. Shake suspensions to disperse or dissolve particles of drug immediately before measurement

4. Contraindications

    a. Cross-sensitivity with penicillins; not recommended for those who have had a Type I (anaphylactic) reaction to penicillin

    b. Use extreme caution if creatinine clearance is less than 50 mL/minute

     c. Hepatotoxicity with cefoperazone and ceftriaxone

     d. Should be used cautiously in pregnancy (crosses placenta) and lactation

5. Significant drug interactions

     a. Probenecid: increases and prolongs half-life of cephalosporins

     b. Loop diuretics and aminoglycosides increase risk of nephrotoxicity

     c. Anticoagulants increase risk of bleeding

     d. Use of ethanol with some cephalosporins such as cefoperazone and cefotetan can cause **disulfiram-like reaction** (weakness, pulsating headache, and abdominal cramps) during therapy and up to 72 hours after drug discontinued; can occur within 30 minutes of alcohol ingestion

     e. Antacids: concurrent use interferes with absorption of cefaclor, cefdinir, cefpodoxime

     f. Histamine H2-receptor antagonists: decrease plasma concentration of cephalosporins

6. Significant food interactions

     a. Iron supplements and iron-fortified foods decrease absorption of cefdinir

     b. May take with food or milk if drug causes gastric irritation except ceftibuten, which is taken 1 hour before and 2 hours after meals

     c. Drug absorption enhanced with food with cefuroxime and cefpodoxime

7. Significant laboratory studies

     a. With parenteral use and/or prolonged therapy, check urinalysis, BUN, and serum creatinine to monitor renal function

     b. Monitor liver function tests when giving cefoperazone and ceftriaxone

     c. Monitor baseline and periodic INR if taking oral anticoagulants and long-term parenteral cefamandole, cefoperazone, cefotetan, or moxalactam; also assess for increased bleeding, such as bleeding gums and easy bruising

8. Side effects

     a. Central nervous system (CNS): lethargy, hallucinations, anxiety, depression, twitching, seizures, coma

     b. GI: nausea and vomiting, mild diarrhea, abdominal cramps or distress, increased LFTs such as aspartate aminotransferase (AST) and alanine aminotransferase (ALT), abdominal pain, colitis

     c. Hematologic: anemia, increased bleeding time, bone marrow depression, granulocytopenia

     d. Rash, pruritus, pain at injection site

     e. Other: taste alteration, sore mouth; dark, discolored, or sore tongue; oral or vaginal candidiasis

9. Adverse effects/toxicity

     a. Anaphylaxis; some form of hypersensitivity occurs in 5–16% of clients

     b. Serum sickness–like illness

          1) Erythema multiforme and other skin rashes, arthralgia, and fever

          2) Usually follows second course of treatment and may be delayed at least 10 days after initiation of drug

          3) Treated with antihistamines and corticosteroids

     c. Seizure activity (especially with renal impairment or intraventricular administration); discontinue cephalosporin to resolve activity

     d. In renal impairment, cancer, impaired vitamin K synthesis, malnutrition, or low vitamin K stores, there is increased risk for the following:

          1) Coagulation disturbances with parenteral use or concurrent anticoagulant use

          2) Disulfiram-like reaction in those who consume or, less frequently, inhale or absorb alcohol as in perfume, aftershave, alcohol swabs

    e. Pseudomembranous colitis: treated by stopping cephalosporin and giving oral vancomycin or metronidazole

    f. Accumulation of biliary sludge or pseudolithiasis with ceftriaxone; clears after drug is discontinued

10. Client-centered nursing care (see again Box 11-1)

    a. Monitor clinical therapeutic response; client may have repeat culture if improvement is not observed in 48 hours

    b. Monitor IM injection sites for induration and tenderness; provide warm compresses and gentle massage to injection sites if painful or swollen; if phlebitis or redness at IV site develops, remove IV device and restart IV

    c. Monitor for nephrotoxicity: check serum creatinine, BUN, and urine creatinine clearance and keep accurate I&O

    d. Monitor for unusual lethargy beginning after drug started; provide safety measures, including adequate lighting, partial side-rails, and assistance with ambulation

    e. Monitor blood glucose in client with diabetes mellitus; although urine glucose testing is generally outdated, false-positive urine glucose can occur with copper sulfate technique

    f. Offer frequent, small meals with quality protein as tolerated

    g. Provide frequent oral care; offer ice chips or sugarless candy if stomatitis and sore mouth occur

    h. Monitor for superinfections

        1) Often subtle and nonspecific with clinical manifestations of oral or pharyngeal discomfort with oral candidiasis or perineal itching or discharge with vaginal candidiasis

        2) Differentiate antibiotic diarrhea from pseudomembranous colitis; the latter is characterized by fever, abdominal cramping, at least four to six watery stools/day, stools with blood and/or mucus; send stool specimen culture for *Clostridium difficile*

    i. Monitor for easy bruising or bleeding if taking anticoagulants; administer vitamin K as prescribed for prlonged INR

11. Client education

    a. See again Box 11-2 for universal teaching points for anti-infectives

    b. Take safety precautions including changing position slowly and avoiding driving and hazardous tasks if CNS effects occur

    c. Drink fluids and maintain nutrition, especially protein, to ensure adequate protein for drug binding and efficacy of action

    d. Shake suspensions well to dispense or dissolve particles of drug immediately before measurement: to ensure dosage accuracy, use a measuring device for suspension or other liquid and not a kitchen teaspoon (may vary from 2 to 10 mL/teaspoon)

    e. Report manifestations of hypersensitivity or superinfection to healthcare provider

        1) Hypersensitivity: difficulty breathing, severe rash, hives, severe headache, dizziness or weakness, aching joints

        2) Severe diarrhea: call healthcare provider; do not take antiperistaltic agent that would promote retention of toxins, such as *C. difficile* in pseudomembranous colitis; mild diarrhea: may take absorbent antidiarrheal agent

        3) Vaginal itching or discharge, sore mouth or throat, white patches on oral mucous membranes

    f. Report side effects to healthcare provider: anorexia, epigastric pain, or nausea and vomiting indicating biliary sludge or pseudolithiasis if on ceftriaxone; discontinue drug and manifestations will resolve

    g. Refrain from alcohol use during therapy and for 72 hours after drug discontinued to avoid disulfiram-like reaction

D. Fluoroquinolones

1. Action and use
   a. Broad-spectrum bactericidal antibiotics that interfere with enzyme DNA gyrase
   b. More effective against gram-negative and selected gram-positive organisms (especially later generations of fluoroquinolones); used in various bacterial infections depending on bacteria and site: lower respiratory tract infections, sinusitis, bone and joint infections, infectious diarrhea, skin and soft tissue infections, intra-abdominal infections, STIs, and UTIs
   c. Postexposure prophylaxis to anthrax
   d. Moxifloxacin effective against anaerobes
2. Common fluoroquinolone medications (Table 11-4)
3. Administration considerations
   a. Administer evenly spaced around the clock and do not interrupt sleep, if possible, to maintain therapeutic blood level
   b. Oral drug is tolerated better with food
4. Contraindications
   a. Known hypersensitivity to fluoroquinolones
   b. Use cautiously in clients with renal dysfunction including those with advanced age, children, pregnant or lactating women, those with history of seizures
   c. Contraindicated in clients with myasthenia gravis
5. Significant drug interactions
   a. Oral antacids, iron, zinc preparations, and sucralfate reduce absorption; separate fluoroquinolones from these drugs by 2 hours
   b. Probenecid prolongs half-life of fluoroquinolones
   c. Beta-agonist effects of theophylline may be increased; monitor clients with hypertension, ischemic heart disease, coronary insufficiency, heart failure (HF), or history of cerebrovascular accident (CVA or stroke)
   d. Class IA or Class III antidysrhythmics may enhance adverse cardiovascular (CV) effects
   e. Cimetidine may prolong half-life
   f. Cyclosporine increases risk of nephrotoxicity
   g. Glucocorticosteroids may increase risk for rupture of tendon, especially in older adults
   h. Use of ciprofloxacin with phenytoin may lower levels of phenytoin
   i. Nitrofurantoin may reduce efficacy of norfloxacin
   j. Use of nonsteroidal anti-inflammatory drugs (NSAIDs) with levofloxacin increases CNS stimulation including seizures; levofloxacin may also increase or decrease blood glucose in clients taking oral antidiabetic agents

Table 11-4 Fluoroquinolones

Generic Name	Route
Ciprofloxacin	PO, IV, ophthalmic
Gatifloxacin	PO, IV
Levofloxacin	PO, IV
Norfloxacin	PO, ophthalmic
Ofloxacin	PO, IV, otic, ophthalmic
Besifloxacin	Ophthalmic
Finafloxacin	Eardrops
Gemifloxacin	PO
Moxifloxacin	PO, IV, ophthalmic

      k. Risk of significant CV side effects may occur with use of certain CV agents and sparfloxacin or moxifloxacin

      l. Increased bleeding risk may occur with oral anticoagulants because antibiotic alters intestinal flora and interferes with vitamin K synthesis

  6. Significant food interactions

      a. Limit alkaline foods such as dairy products, vegetables, and legumes that can alter pH of stomach and absorption

      b. Ciprofloxacin and norfloxacin can increase serum levels of caffeine

  7. Significant laboratory studies: monitor ALT (SGPT), AST (SGOT), alkaline phosphatase, and bilirubin for elevation in liver toxicity; monitor PT or INR if on warfarin

  8. Side effects

      a. Headache, dizziness, fatigue, lethargy, restlessness

      b. Nausea and vomiting, diarrhea, epigastric distress, oral candidiasis, dysphagia, elevated liver enzymes, bilirubin, and alkaline phosphatase

      c. Rash, pruritus, urticaria, photosensitivity, flushing

  9. Adverse effects/toxicity

      a. Superinfections: more common in prolonged therapy

      b. Anaphylaxis

      c. Peripheral neuropathy

      d. Tendonitis and tendon rupture (FDA black box warning), which occurs more often in older adults and clients with renal failure or receiving a glucocorticoid; not approved for use under age 18

  10. Client-centered nursing care (see Box 11-1 again)

      a. Monitor PT, INR, and manifestations of increased bleeding or bruising if also on oral anticoagulants

      b. Provide more frequent meals with complete or complementary proteins to better ensure adequate albumin levels for drug efficacy

      c. Monitor for increased CNS irritability if client has history of epilepsy, ethanol abuse, or is concurrently taking theophylline

      d. Maintain hydration with 3 liters of fluid/day, if not contraindicated, to prevent crystalluria, and monitor renal function

  11. Client education

      a. Refer to Box 11-2 again for universal teaching points for anti-infective therapy

      b. Take safety precautions including changing position slowly and avoiding driving and hazardous tasks if CNS effects occur

      c. Drink fluids and maintain nutrition, especially protein, to provide adequate protein for drug binding and drug efficacy

      d. Report difficulty breathing, severe headache, dizziness, or weakness to healthcare provider

      e. May obtain baseline electrocardiogram with sparfloxacin or moxifloxacin

      f. Teach to wear sunglasses, long-sleeved and long-legged garments, and hat to protect from direct sunlight; sunscreen or sunblock may not prevent photosensitivity reaction; avoid ultraviolet lights, tanning beds, and direct sunlight

      g. Report unexplained joint or muscle pain

E. Macrolides and lincosamides

  1. Action and use

      a. **Bacteriostatic** (inhibiting growth of bacteria) but can be bactericidal in high doses with some bacteria

      b. Highly protein-bound

      c. Inhibit bacterial protein synthesis by binding to 50S ribosomal subunit; do not bind to human ribosome, thus providing selective toxicity

      d. Used in upper and lower respiratory tract infections, skin and soft tissue infections caused by *Streptococcus* or *Haemophilus* organisms, syphilis, gonorrhea, chlamydia, Lyme disease, and *Mycoplasma*, *Listeria*, and *Corynebacterium* infections

      e. Clarithromycin is used with omeprazole to treat *Helicobacter pylori* associated with peptic ulcers

      f. Lincosamides may be bactericidal and bacteriostatic; used to treat chronic bone infections, genitourinary (GU) infections, intra-abdominal infections, pneumonia, and streptococcal or staphylococcal septicemia

      g. Fidaxomicin approved for infections caused by *C. difficile*; not absorbed orally so remains in digestive tract

2. Common macrolide and lincosamide medications (Table 11-5)

3. Administration considerations

      a. If erythromycin form has bitter taste, give with juice or applesauce

      b. Give clindamycin and lincomycin with at least 8 ounces of fluid or on an empty stomach

      c. If clindamycin is given IV, give by infusion, not by intravenous push (IVP) method

      d. Azithromycin has longer half-life with less frequent dosing, shorter term of therapy, and fewer or less intense GI side effects than others (may contribute to better compliance)

      e. Give azithromycin suspension on an empty stomach, as food can significantly inhibit absorption

4. Contraindications

      a. Hypersensitivity

      b. Use caution with liver or renal dysfunction, GI disorders, in older adults and pregnant or lactating women

      c. Lincosamides are also contraindicated in ulcerative colitis or enteritis and children less than 1 year of age

5. Significant drug interactions

      a. Many drug interactions can occur; read individual product literature

      b. Erythromycin may increase risk of bleeding with warfarin

      c. Erythromycin and clarithromycin increase risk of myopathy and rhabdomyolysis with lovastatin or simvastatin

6. Significant food interactions: grapefruit juice may increase bioavailability of erythromycin

7. Significant laboratory studies: monitor for hepatotoxicity (e.g., ALT, AST, alkaline phosphatase, bilirubin elevations) and nephrotoxicity (e.g., serum creatinine, BUN, creatinine clearance, urinalysis)

Table 11-5   **Macrolides and Lincosamides**

Generic Name	Drug Type	Route
Azithromycin	Macrolide	PO, IV, ophthalmic
Clarithromycin	Macrolide	PO
Erythromycin	Macrolide	PO, topical
Clindamycin	Lincosamide	PO, IM, IV, topical
Lincomycin	Lincosamide	PO, IM, IV
Fidaxomicin	Macrolide	PO

8. Side effects
   a. Nausea and vomiting, diarrhea, abdominal cramping, abnormal taste (clarithromycin)
   b. Dry skin or burning if topical route; thrombophlebitis at peripheral IV site
9. Adverse effects/toxicity
   a. Ototoxicity (erythromycin) with tinnitus often preceding hearing loss, hepatotoxicity (jaundice, pruritis, and elevated liver enzymes), and nephrotoxicity
   b. Superinfections (e.g., pseudomembranous colitis, candidiasis)
   c. High doses of erythromycin may be cardiotoxic, increasing risk for a *torsades de pointes* dysrhythmia; client may experience palpitations and chest pain
10. Client-centered nursing care (see Box 11-1 again)
    a. Assess GI function and elimination pattern
    b. Observe for bleeding if taking oral anticoagulants
    c. Monitor for development of superinfections
    d. Monitor liver enzymes, serum creatinine, BUN, creatinine clearance
    e. Assess baseline hearing and monitor for hearing loss; arrange for discontinuation of drug if occurs
    f. Hydrate with at least 2,000–2,400 mL/day if not contraindicated
11. Client education
    a. See again Box 11-2 for universal teaching points for anti-infective therapy
    b. Include protein in diet since these drugs are highly protein-bound and need protein for therapeutic efficacy
    c. Report signs of ototoxicity including dizziness, vertigo, nausea, tinnitus, roaring noises, or hearing impairment

F. Penicillins

1. Action and use
   a. Beta-lactams are chemical structure of penicillins; derived from fungus or mold evidenced on bread or fruit
   b. One of oldest antibiotic drug classes and is therefore most likely to cause hypersensitivity
   c. There is similarity among penicillins, cephalosporins, monobactams, carbapenems, and beta-lactamase inhibitors; they share many of the same actions and uses; cross-sensitivity is possible
   d. Penicillin is least toxic beta-lactam; is usually antibiotic of choice because of low toxicity potential in nonallergic client
   e. Bactericidal; bacteriostatic effect with adequate dosing or blood levels
   f. Only cross blood–brain barrier if meningeal inflammation present
   g. Penicillins are classified as natural penicillins, penicillinase-resistant penicillins (antistaphylococcal), broad-spectrum penicillins (aminopenicillins), and extended-spectrum penicillins (antipseudomonal)
   h. Used to treat a broad range of infections, such as upper respiratory infections (e.g., strep throat), pneumonia, STIs such as syphilis but not gonorrhea, wound infections, and UTIs
   i. Used prophylactically against endocarditis for oral, GI, pulmonary procedures when bacteria may enter circulation; usually amoxicillin or ampicillin is used
   j. Because of history of possible overuse by prescribers, increasing resistance is developing, especially in facility-acquired infections
2. Common penicillin medications (Table 11-6)
3. Administration considerations
   a. Oral dosing needs to be three to four times the parenteral dose because of hepatic first-pass effect and instability of penicillin in acidic environment of stomach
   b. For serious systemic infections, parenteral route is recommended

Table 11-6	Penicillins	
Generic Name	**Type of Drug**	**Route**
Penicillin G (benzathine, potassium, or procaine)	Natural penicillin	IM (benzathene, procaine), IM or IV (potassium)
Penicillin V	Natural penicillin	PO
Dicloxacillin	Penicillinase-resistant	PO
Nafcillin	Penicillinase-resistant	IV, IM
Oxacillin	Penicillinase-resistant	IV
Amoxicillin	Broad-spectrum	PO
Amoxicillin-clavulanate	Broad-spectrum	PO
Ampicillin	Broad-spectrum	PO, IM, IV
Ampicillin and subactam	Broad-spectrum	IM, IV
Piperacillin	Extended-spectrum	IM, IV
Piperacillin-tazobactam	Extended-spectrum	IV
Ticarcillin-clavulanate	Extended-spectrum	IV

    c. Absorption erratic from IM route; limit due to irritability of tissue; IM injection should be slow and steady over 12–15 seconds to minimize discomfort and prevent obstruction of needle, especially with thick preparations

4. Contraindications

    a. Hypersensitivity reaction and anaphylaxis, serum sickness, exfoliative dermatitis, blood dyscrasias

    b. Penicillin G procaine or benzathine not to be given IV: lethal

    c. Use caution in anemia, thrombocytopenia, bone marrow depression, and concurrently with anticoagulants because some penicillins cause increased bleeding

5. Significant drug interactions

    a. Loop and thiazide diuretics may exacerbate hypokalemia and rash

    b. Potassium-sparing diuretics may contribute to hyperkalemia

    c. Leads to decreased efficacy of oral contraceptives

    d. Probenecid delays excretion and increases serum level of penicillins

    e. Avoid coadministration with tetracycline because it may interfere with effectiveness of penicillins and increases risks of adverse effects

    f. Atenolol levels may be decreased when given with ampicillin; increased risk for anaphylaxis

    g. Allopurinol increases risk for rash

    h. Piperacillin may alter elimination of lithium

    i. Aspirin, phenylbutazone (ibuprofen-like), sulfonamides, furosemide, thiazide diuretics, and indomethacin prolong half-life of penicillin-G

    j. When penicillin is administered concurrently with aminoglycosides and both are given parenterally, the aminoglycoside may be inactivated

6. Significant food interactions: take on empty stomach although amoxicillin is not affected by food

7. Significant laboratory studies

    a. CBC with WBC and differential

    b. PT or INR if on oral anticoagulants; activated partial thromboplastin time (aPPT) if receiving heparin

    c. Liver function studies: ALT, AST, bilirubin, alkaline phosphatase

    d. Electrolytes, especially potassium and sodium

8. Side effects

   a. Most common allergic responses are skin rash, urticaria, pruritis, angioedema; a maculopapular, pruritic rash that is like measles with ampicillin or amoxicillin is not a true allergic reaction, but develops after 7–10 days of therapy and may last a few days after drug discontinuation; not a contraindication to give drug in future

   b. Most common side effects are GI, such as nausea and vomiting, diarrhea, epigastric distress, abdominal pain, colitis, elevated liver enzymes; also taste alteration, sore mouth, or dark, discolored, sore tongue

   c. Hypokalemia or hyperkalemia, metabolic alkalosis

9. Adverse effects/toxicity

   a. Type I hypersensitivity often fatal immediately if untreated within 2–30 minutes; signs include urticaria, pruritis, severe dyspnea, stridor, tachycardia, diaphoresis, hypotension, dizziness, loss of consciousness and circulatory collapse

   b. Serum sickness–like reaction: skin rash, arthralgia, fever

   c. Exfoliative dermatitis: red, scaly skin

   d. Blood dyscrasias: hemolytic anemia, neutropenia, leukopenia

   e. Superinfections with broader-spectrum penicillins, especially with prolonged therapy; pseudomembranous colitis possible up to several weeks after drug discontinued; treated with anti-infectives such as metronidazole PO or IV or vancomycin PO

10. Client-centered nursing care (see Box 11-1 again)

   a. Assess for allergies and hypersensitivity history

   b. Do not administer with fruit juices, milk, or carbonated beverages because of poor absorption

   c. Monitor renal studies, liver enzymes, and electrolytes; many penicillins contain sodium salts that can result in hypokalemia

   d. Consult with prescriber about dose or drug adjustment if indicated by lab results

   e. Monitor for adverse effects; may not be necessary to discontinue drug if mild diarrhea develops; give yogurt or buttermilk to restore normal flora; use absorbent antidiarrheal agents (kaolin and pectin); avoid antiperistaltic agents that delay or prevent elimination of intestinal toxins

   f. Provide nutritious diet and adequate hydration

   g. Some penicillins cause false-positive results on urine glucose testing; blood glucose monitoring is standard

11. Client education

   a. See Box 11-2 for universal teaching points for anti-infectives

   b. Take oral drug on empty stomach; take 1 hour before meals or 2 hours after meals, except amoxicillin (which is not affected by food); take dose with a full glass of water

   c. Chewable tablets must be crushed or chewed in order for penicillin to be effectively absorbed

   d. Shake suspensions to disperse particles prior to measurement; use a calibrated device to measure liquid since kitchen teaspoons may vary by 2–10 mL; most suspensions maintain potency for 14 days if refrigerated

   e. Ensure antibiotic drops used for correct route (i.e., oral, eye, ear)

   f. Report rash, urticaria, pruritis, difficulty breathing

   g. Report sore throat, watery stools equal to or greater than four to six stools/day or stools with blood/mucus, severe nausea and vomiting, unusual bleeding or bruising

   h. Take frequent, small meals with high-quality protein and drink equal to or greater than six to eight glasses of water per day, if not contraindicated by other conditions

G. Sulfonamides

1. Action and use

   a. First effective group of antibiotics (1935)

   b. Bacteriostatic; inhibit folic acid synthesis to prevent cell growth

   c. Used to treat UTIs (most commonly caused by *Escherichia coli*), *Chlamydia trachomatis* causing blindness, pneumonia, brain abscesses, mild to moderate ulcerative colitis, active Crohn disease, and rheumatoid arthritis; with pyrimethamine as only effective drug treatment for toxoplasmosis; drugs of choice for treatment of nocardiosis

   d. Sulfacetamide to prevent bacterial growth in burns and wounds

   e. Cross-sensitivity possible with penicillins and cephalosporins

2. Common sulfonamide medications (Table 11-7)

3. Administration considerations

   a. Fluid intake should be 3,000–4,000 mL/day if tolerated to promote urinary output at least 1,500 mL/day to prevent crystalluria/stone formation; an alkaline ash diet may be helpful, which includes fruit (except plums, prunes, and cranberries), vegetables, and milk

   b. Store in light-resistant, tightly closed container at room temperature

4. Contraindications

   a. History of hypersensitivity to sulfonamides, salicylates, penicillins, or cephalosporins

   b. During pregnancy because of risk of birth defects or kernicterus; use cautiously

   c. During lactation and in children younger than 2 months unless used to treat congenital toxoplasmosis

   d. In porphyria, advanced or severe renal or hepatic dysfunction, or intestinal and urinary blockage; use cautiously with impaired renal or hepatic function, asthma, blood dyscrasias, or glucose-6-phosphate dehydrogenase (G6PD) deficiency

5. Significant drug interactions

   a. Increased risk for bleeding with oral anticoagulants

   b. More significant drop in blood glucose with oral antidiabetic agents (such as tolbutamide, tolazamide, glyburide, glipizide, or chlorpropamide)

   c. Increased risk for phenytoin toxicity with phenytoin

   d. Trimethoprim and sulfamethoxazole: combines sulfonamide with folic acid antagonist; increases synergistic effect

6. Significant food interactions: some drugs, such as sulfamethoxazole, may be crushed and taken with liquids of choice

7. Significant laboratory studies

   a. Creatinine, BUN, creatinine clearance, urinalysis to monitor renal function

   b. ALT, AST, bilirubin, alkaline phosphatase to monitor hepatic function

   c. CBC to monitor for blood dyscrasias and response to therapy

8. Side effects: commonly include anorexia, nausea and vomiting, rash (maculopapular with urticaria), photosensitivity, and crystalluria

Table 11-7 Sulfonamides

Generic Name	Route
Sulfisoxazole	PO
Sulfadiazine	PO, topical
Trimethoprim-sulfamethoxazole	PO, IV
Sulfadoxine-pyrimethamine	PO

9. Adverse effects/toxicity
   a. Peripheral neuritis and neuropathy
   b. Tinnitus, hearing loss, vertigo, ataxia, seizures
   c. Hepatitis, pancreatitis
   d. Blood dyscrasias: anemia, agranulocytosis, thrombocytopenia, leukopenia, eosinophilia, hypothrombinemia
   e. Exfoliative dermatitis, **Stevens–Johnson syndrome** (an adverse reaction of skin that resembles appearance of partial-thickness burns)
   f. Serum sickness, drug fever

10. Client-centered nursing care (see Box 11-1 again)
    a. Assess baseline laboratory findings for liver function and renal function (creatinine) and monitor during therapy; a baseline skin assessment will provide a basis for detecting hypersensitivity reaction later if it occurs
    b. Provide hydration to ensure daily urinary output of equal or greater than 1,500 mL to prevent stone and crystal formations; alkalinize urine as indicated; keep accurate I&O record
    c. Consult prescriber for dose adjustment or discontinuation of drug if toxicities develop
    d. Provide for safety if neurotoxicities develop, such as ataxia or seizures
    e. Provide frequent, small nutritious meals with high-quality proteins; drugs that may be taken with food may decrease GI upset
    f. Assess for clinical improvement, adverse effects, and effectiveness of client education

11. Client education
    a. See Box 11-2 for universal teaching points for anti-infectives
    b. Take safety precautions if client experiences vertigo, ataxia, seizures
    c. Avoid driving or performing hazardous tasks if drowsiness occurs
    d. Take with food, if not contraindicated, to minimize GI upset
    e. Eat frequent, small meals with at least 2,500–3,000 mL fluid intake a day
    f. Empty bladder frequently, at least every 2 hours while awake
    g. Report flank or suprapubic pain, increased dysuria, disruption of skin integrity to healthcare provider

H. Urinary tract antiseptics

1. Action and use
   a. These drugs act against bacteria in urine but have little or no systemic antibacterial effects
   b. Used for UTIs only; destruction of bacteria based on acidification of urine
2. Common urinary tract antiseptic medications (Table 11-8)
3. Administration considerations: shake suspensions well just prior to measuring with a calibrated device (household teaspoons may vary by 2–10 mL); because methenamine suspension contains a vegetable oil base, use caution to prevent lipid aspiration pneumonia; nitrofurantoin suspension should be diluted and mouth rinsed thoroughly after taking
4. Contraindications
   a. Methenamine hippurate: avoid concurrent use of drugs that could alkalinize urine and interfere with effectiveness (e.g., antacids, carbonic anhydrase inhibitors, citrates, sodium bicarbonate, thiazide diuretics)
   b. Sulfamethizole: increased risk for crystalluria
   c. Caution with nitrofurantoin: can increase neurotoxicity in clients with neurologic disorders such as peripheral neuropathy and seizures and can cause pulmonary reaction in clients with pulmonary conditions

Table 11-8	**Urinary Tract Antiseptics**
Generic Name	**Route**
Fosfomycin	PO
Methenamine	PO
Nalidixic acid	PO
Nitrofurantoin	PO

    d. Use caution in clients with impaired renal and/or hepatic function
    e. Use caution during lactation and pregnancy
5. Significant drug interactions
    a. See contraindications listed earlier
    b. Probenecid: may increase risk for toxicity with sulfinpyrazone; decreased urinary tract effectiveness may occur with nitrofurantoin
6. Significant food interactions
    a. Controversial if pH of urine has any effect on UTI (acidity may inhibit adherence of bacteria to bladder wall)
    b. Acid ash foods that may increase urine acidity include meat, cheese, eggs, and whole grains, as well as cranberries, prunes, and plums
    c. Fluids that may acidify urine and potentially facilitate drug action include cranberry or prune juice; cranberry supplements may also help
7. Significant laboratory studies
    a. Urinalysis and urine C&S: baseline and repeated regularly
    b. CBC with WBC and differential
    c. Baseline ALT, AST, alkaline phosphatase, and bilirubin; repeat as necessary
    d. Baseline creatinine, BUN, creatinine clearance; repeat as needed
    e. Pulmonary function tests with nitrofurantoin
8. Side effects vary among drugs but may include:
    a. Nausea and vomiting, anorexia, diarrhea, epigastric distress
    b. Rash, pruritus, headache, dizziness, drowsiness, blurred vision
    c. Low back pain
    d. Nitrofurantoin: urine may become brown
9. Adverse effects/toxicity: anaphylaxis, superinfections, hemolytic anemia (nalidixic acid), crystalluria (methenamine), interstitial pneumonitis (nitrofurantoin), and Stevens-Johnson syndrome (nitrofurantoin)
10. Client-centered nursing care (see also Box 11-1)
    a. Monitor for resolution of signs of upper or lower urinary infection
    b. Monitor for clinical manifestations of adverse effects
    c. Encourage at least 3,000 mL/day fluids, including cranberry juice if not contraindicated by fluid restriction, diabetes mellitus, or other conditions
    d. Give medication with or after food to limit GI adverse effects
11. Client education
    a. See Box 11-2 for universal teaching points for anti-infectives
    b. Take with or after food to minimize GI distress
    c. Drink at least 3 liters of fluid a day including cranberry and prune juice unless contraindicated by other conditions
    d. Include acid ash foods in diet, such as cranberries or cranberry juice, prunes, plums, cheese, eggs, meat, whole grains; limit or avoid alkaline ash foods, such as citrus fruits and juices, vegetables

   e. Do not take other medications unless approved by prescriber; avoid drugs that may alkalinize urine, such as antacids, sodium bicarbonate (baking soda); consult with prescriber regarding use of ascorbic acid (vitamin C) or cranberry supplements, which acidify urine

   f. Nalidixic acid can cause photophobia; avoid bright sunlight, wear sunglasses, and report any visual disturbances; photosensitivity can also occur several weeks after drug is discontinued so client should avoid direct sunlight or ultraviolet light

   g. Nitrofurantoin may cause urine to be brown

   h. Do not drive or perform hazardous tasks if drowsiness or dizziness occurs

   i. Instruct client on urinary hygiene measures and perineal care, including a cotton liner in underwear, avoiding hot tubs and bubble baths, wiping from front to back, and voiding after intercourse

I. Tetracyclines

   1. Action and use

   a. Broad spectrum; bacteriostatic (by inhibiting protein synthesis); can be bactericidal in high concentrations

   b. Effective against many microorganisms, including mycoplasmas, rickettsiae, cholera, certain protozoa, and organisms causing many sexually-transmitted infections (chlamydia; syphilis, or gonorrhea if penicillin allergy)

   c. Suppress *Proprionibacteriium acnes* in treating acne, and *Helicobacter pylori* in peptic ulcer disease

   d. Drug of choice for Rocky Mountain spotted fever, **amebiasis** (a protozoan infection), brucellosis, shigellosis, cholera, tetanus, chronic bronchitis, Lyme disease

   e. Used as a sclerosing agent for pleural and pericardial effusion, such as in metastasis of cancer; causes inflammation resulting in fibrosis, leaving scar tissue that does not allow fluid to accumulate

   f. Used to treat traveler's diarrhea and is used with quinine for treatment of malaria

   g. Used to treat syndrome of inappropriate antidiuretic hormone (SIADH) with demeclocycline by inhibiting antidiuretic hormone (ADH)

   2. Common tetracycline medications (generic name ends in -*cycline*; Table 11-9)

   3. Administration considerations

   a. Avoid administering outdated drug: Fanconi-like syndrome (polyuria, polydipsia, nausea and vomiting, glycosuria, proteinuria), acidosis, renal tubular dysfunction and lupus erythematosus–like syndrome have occurred and are attributed to preparations used beyond expiration date

   b. Oral: give with full glass of water on empty stomach at least 1 hour before or 2 hours after meals; food, milk, and milk products decrease absorption by half

   c. Shake oral suspension well to distribute particles

   d. Use calibrated measuring device (kitchen teaspoon can vary by 2–10 mL)

   e. If topical, clean area with soap and water, rinse and dry well prior to application

   4. Contraindications

   a. Hypersensitivity to tetracyclines

   b. Severe renal or hepatic dysfunction

   c. Contraindicated during last half of pregnancy when tooth development occurs, from birth to 8 years of age, and in lactating women; tetracyclines bind to calcium, preventing normal bone growth and causing tooth hypoplasia in developing fetus or child younger than 8 years old; this produces discoloration of teeth

   d. Use caution with history of renal or liver dysfunction, allergy, asthma, hay fever, urticaria, or in myasthenia gravis

   e. Use caution with concurrent use of oral anticoagulants

   f. Tetracyclines may antagonize other antibiotics; see product literature

   g. Doxycycline, tigecycline, and minocycline hydrochloride are Pregnancy Category D drugs

Table 11-9	Tetracyclines
Generic Name	**Route**
Demeclocycline	PO
Tetracycline	PO
Doxycycline	PO, IV
Minocycline	PO, IV
Tigecycline	IV

5. Significant drug interactions
   a. Antacids and antidiarrheal agents with kaolin and pectin decrease absorption
   b. Oral anticoagulants potentiate hypoprothrombinemia
   c. Decreased effectiveness of oral contraceptives
   d. Increased effect against brain abscess with sulfonamide
   e. Decreased effect of penicillin
   f. Increased or decreased level of digoxin depending on specific tetracycline
   g. Can cause fatal nephrotoxicity with methoxyflurane, an anesthetic
6. Significant food interactions
   a. Milk and dairy products and iron supplements interfere with absorption
   b. Take on empty stomach; an exception is doxycycline, which should be taken with food or a full glass of milk
7. Significant laboratory studies
   a. After initial culture prior to initiating drug therapy; obtain follow-up culture from gonoccocal infection site 3–7 days post-treatment to ensure elimination of infection, or culture from other sites if improvement not observed
   b. Baseline and periodic renal and liver function tests
   c. CBC including WBC with differential to monitor response to therapy (decreased WBC), to check for thrombocytopenia, and for hemolytic anemia
8. Side effects
   a. Nausea and vomiting, diarrhea, epigastric distress, abdominal discomfort, flatulence, dry mouth, dysphagia, bulky or loose stools, steatorrhea
   b. Headache, photosensitivity, increased intracranial pressure (rare)
   c. Maculopapular rash, urticaria, exfoliative dermatitis, angioedema
   d. Stinging or burning with topical application
   e. Discoloration of developing teeth
   f. Pigmentation of conjunctiva related to drug deposits
   g. Discoloration and loosening of nails
   h. Retrosternal pain
9. Adverse effects/toxicity
   a. Elevated liver function tests and decreased cholesterol level
   b. Drug fever, serum sickness, and anaphylaxis
   c. Hepatotoxicity, pancreatitis, nephrotoxicity
   d. Blood dyscrasias such as thrombocytopenia, hemolytic anemia
   e. Superinfections: increased risk for candidiasis in clients taking oral contraceptives, with diabetes mellitus, leukemia, systemic lupus erythematosus (SLE); possible stomatitis, glossitis, black, hairy tongue (lingua nigra), and pseudomembranous colitis
   f. Fatty degeneration of liver results in jaundice, azotemia, increased nitrogen retention, hyperphosphatemia, and metabolic acidosis
   g. Tetracycline topical application can cause itching, wheezing, and anaphylaxis in client with asthma allergies

10. Client-centered nursing care (see Box 11-1 again)
    a. Assess history of immunosuppression
    b. Check CBC including WBC with differential, RBC indices, and platelet count
    c. Collaborate with prescriber regarding dosage or drug change if indicated by adverse effects
    d. Monitor I&O
11. Client education
    a. See Box 11-2 for universal teaching points for anti-infectives
    b. Unstable with age and light exposure; store in tightly covered container in dry area, protected from light at room temperature
    c. Report side effects, particularly severe diarrhea
    d. Practice good oral care and hygiene
    e. Avoid exposure to direct sunlight or ultraviolet light or tanning beds; wear hat, long sleeves, long-legged pants, and sunglasses outside during and for a few days after treatment; sunscreen or sunblock may not prevent erythema
    f. If on long-term treatment, report onset of severe headache or visual disturbances that may indicate increased intracranial pressure (rare); requires discontinuation of tetracycline to prevent irreversible vision loss
    g. Take oral doses with full glass of water on empty stomach (1 hour before or 2 hours after meal or dairy product) to promote absorption and decrease risk of esophagitis; report sudden dysphagia to healthcare provider
    h. Topical form may stain clothing
    i. Topical application can cause affected skin to reflect yellow or green fluorescence under an ultraviolet or "black" light

J. **Miscellaneous antibiotics** (Table 11-10)
    1. Aztreonam
        a. Action and use: bactericidal against gram-negative rods; has similar activity as beta-lactam antibiotic (penicillins) and cephalosporins; used for infections with gram-negative aerobes, such as *pseudomonas aeruginosa*
        b. Administration considerations: given inhalation, IV/IM; cautious use if history of hypersensitivity to penicillins or cephalosporins
        c. Contraindications: known hypersensitivity to aztreonam, viral infections
        d. Significant drug interactions: cefoxitin, imipenem; incompatible with nafcillin sodium, cephradine, vancomycin, or metronidazole; yields false-positive results with cupric sulfate-type urine glucose testing products
        e. Significant food interactions: none significant
        f. Significant laboratory studies
            1) Monitor for hepatotoxicity (ALT, AST, bilirubin, alkaline phosphatase) and nephrotoxicity for hepatotoxicity (creatinine, creatinine clearance, and BUN)

Practice to Pass

Tetracycline capsules have been prescribed for an 18-year-old female client to treat acne. What specific teaching would you include on the client education plan?

Table 11-10 Miscellaneous Antibiotics

Classification	Generic Name	Route
Monobactam	Aztreonam	IM, IV, inhalation
Streptogramins	Quinupristin/dalfopristin	IV
None (unique cell wall inhibitor)	Vancomycin	IV, off-label PO use
Ketolide (similar to macrolide)	Telithromycin	PO
Oxazolidinones	Linezolid	PO, IV
Cyclic lipopeptide	Daptomycin	IV
None (antibacterial and antiparasitic)	Metronidazole	PO, IV

       2) Monitor WBC with differential to monitor therapeutic effectiveness; note linezolid may decrease WBC count, neutrophils, and platelet count

   g. Side effects: nausea and vomiting diarrhea, candidiasis, local pain at injection site

   h. Adverse effects/toxicity (rare): anaphylaxis, pseudomembranous colitis

   i. Client-centered nursing care (see Box 11-1)

   j. Client education: same as for penicillins and cephalosporins; see also Box 11-2

2. Quinupristin and dalfopristin

   a. Action and use

       1) Two streptogramin antibacterials work synergistically; in a new class of antibiotics called *streptogramins* that work by binding 50S ribosome, similar to action of macrolides

       2) Used to treat bacteremia and life-threatening infections caused by *Vancomycin-resistant Enterococcus faecium* (VREF) and complicated skin and skin structure infections

   b. Administration considerations

       1) For IV use only, preferably via central line

       2) Incompatible with normal saline or heparin; flush line with D_5W before and after each dose and to reconstitute drug

       3) Infuse using an infusion pump

   c. Contraindications: known hypersensitivity to quinupristin and dalfopristin

   d. Significant drug interactions: do not mix with other drugs; use cautiously with cephalosporins; inhibits metabolism of tacrolimus, cisapride, and cyclosporine (close monitor cyclosporine levels for increase)

   e. Significant food interactions: none reported

   f. Significant laboratory studies: baseline and periodic liver and renal function tests

   g. Side effects: hepatotoxicity, arthralgias, myalgias (possibly severe), pruritus, vomiting, and diarrhea

   h. Adverse effects/toxicity: with peripheral IV administration, frequently pain, inflammation, edema, and thrombophlebitis

   i. Client-centered nursing care: see Box 11-1; avoid infusion into peripheral sites (associated with high incidence of phlebitis)

   j. Client education: same as with other antibiotics; see Box 11-2 again

3. Vancomycin

   a. Action and use

       1) Bactericidal; antibiotic of choice for methicillin-resistant *Staphylococcus aureus* (MRSA) and other gram-positive bacteria, yeast, fungi

       2) Oral: for antibiotic-induced pseudomembranous colitis caused by *Clostridium difficile* and for staphylococcal enterocolitis

       3) IV: for bone and joint infections or septicemia caused by staphylococcal organisms

   b. Administration considerations

       1) Poorly absorbed from GI tract so oral therapy for treatment of local, surface-infected areas of GI tract

       2) IV administration should be through a central venous access device because of high risk for phlebitis; can cause necrosis if it extravasates

       3) Increasing reports of resistance to enterococcus strains; concern about MRSA resistance developing; quinupristin and dalfopristin used in place of vancomycin sometimes to limit evolution of resistance to vancomycin

       4) Incidence of "red neck syndrome" (see under side effects) minimized by infusing over at least 60 minutes, preferably 90 minutes

   c. Contraindications: known hypersensitivity; use cautiously in renal dysfunction, prior hearing loss, pregnancy and lactation, and older adults and neonates

    d. Significant drug interactions

       1) Do not mix intravenously with other drugs

       2) Increased risk of ototoxicity and nephrotoxicity when used with other drugs having potential for these toxicities

    e. Significant food interactions: none reported

    f. Significant laboratory studies

       1) Serum creatinine, BUN, creatinine clearance, urinalysis (for casts in urine)

       2) Peak and trough drug levels

       3) ALT, AST, bilirubin, alkaline phosphatase

       4) CBC with WBC and differential

       5) Audiometry testing

    g. Side effects

       1) Nausea, hypotension, flushing

       2) Pain and thrombophlebitis at injection site

       3) "Red neck syndrome": too-rapid IV infusion (less than 60 minutes) results in profound hypotension, erythematous rash on face, neck, upper chest, and arms

       4) Too-rapid infusion can cause increased sense of warmth, nausea, and generalized tingling and paresthesia

    h. Adverse reactions/toxicity

       1) Ototoxicity of auditory branch of 8th cranial nerve; possible irreversible hearing loss

       2) Nephrotoxicity with possible uremia

       3) Hypersensitivity: anaphylaxis

       4) Superinfections

       5) Leukopenia and eosinophilia: temporary

    i. Client-centered nursing care (see Box 11-1)

       1) Monitor baseline and regular lab results for early detection of toxicities

       2) Ensure central venous access available

       3) Assess baseline hearing; assess regularly for early detection of hearing loss, tinnitus, and loss of hearing high-pitched tones that may precede deafness

       4) Record accurate I&O

       5) Assess for improvement in clinical manifestations of infection

       6) Give over 60–90 minutes to avoid too-rapid administration

       7) Monitor for hypotension and tachycardia during infusion; if red neck syndrome occurs, stop infusion and report to healthcare provider

       8) Consult with prescriber for dose adjustment or drug discontinuation if toxicities develop

       9) Ensure adequate nutrition and hydration

    j. Client education (see Box 11-2 again)

       1) Keep appointments for laboratory testing and follow-up visits with healthcare provider

       2) If to receive IV therapy in home, ensure appropriate person's knowledge and ability to perform procedures correctly, including monitoring blood pressure (BP) and heart rate

       3) Report ringing in ears or change in hearing

       4) Report sore throat, watery stools more than four to six per day or if blood or mucus in stools, severe nausea and vomiting, change in color or consistency of urine, which may indicate superinfection or toxicity

       5) Maintain adequate fluid intake (2–3 liters/day)

> **_Practice to Pass_**
>
> The client states, "I don't know why the doctor wants me to have the vancomycin every 6 hours now instead of every 8 hours as I had been getting it. It seems as though I am so tied down." How do you respond?

4. Telithromycin

    a. Actions and uses

        1) Sole drug in a class of antibiotics called *ketolides*; blocks protein synthesis of bacteria, similar to macrolides

        2) Approved for use in acute bacterial exacerbation of chronic bronchitis and community-acquired pneumonia from *Streptococcus pneumoniae*

    b. Administration considerations: only available in oral tablets

    c. Contraindications

        1) May cause hepatotoxicity; use cautiously in those with impaired liver function

        2) Contraindicated in myasthenia gravis

        3) May cause prolonged QT intervals; avoid use in clients with a history of *torsade de pointes*

    d. Significant drug interactions

        1) Avoid concurrent administration with simvastatin, lovastatin, atorvastatin; may cause increased drug levels of "statins"

        2) Administration with Class IA or III antiarrhythmics may lead to life-threatening dysrhythmias

        3) Increases peak levels of digoxin by 73%

        4) Potential for numerous other drug interactions

    e. Significant food interactions: more than 0.9 liters (1 qt) per day of grapefruit juice may increase drug levels and side effects

    f. Significant laboratory studies: elevated liver enzymes, BUN, creatinine, potassium

    g. Side effects

        1) Diarrhea, nausea and vomiting, headache, dizziness, loose stools, dysgeusia

        2) May cause blurred or double vision and difficulty focusing, which may necessitate discontinuation of drug

    h. Adverse reactions/toxicity: increased risk for ventricular dysrhythmias in clients with history of prolonged QT interval

    i. Client-centered nursing care: see Box 11-1 again; assess liver and renal function prior to administration

    j. Client education (see Box 11-2 again)

        1) Stop taking drug and notify provider if dizziness or fainting occurs

        2) Report signs of jaundice, unexplained fatigue, loss of appetite, nausea, dark urine, or clay-colored stools

        3) If visual changes occur, avoid quick changes in viewing between close and distant objects

5. Linezolid

    a. Actions and uses: inhibits bacterial protein synthesis; the first antibacterial drug in a class known as oxazolidinones; treats infections associated with vancomycin-resistant *Enterococcus faecium* or VRE, pneumonias, infections of skin and skin structures

    b. Administration considerations: has excellent oral absorption

    c. Contraindications: hypersensitivity to linezolid; concurrent use with monoamine oxidase inhibitors (MAOIs)

    d. Significant drug interactions

        1) May increase effect of vasopressor drugs, such as dopamine

        2) May lead to serotonin syndrome when given with other serotonergic drugs, such as selective serotonin reuptake inhibitors (SSRIs) and MAOIs

    e. Significant food interactions: tyramine-containing foods, such as soy sauce, aged cheeses, wines, smoked foods, and fish, can raise blood pressure

    f. Significant laboratory studies: monitor electrolytes, liver and renal function tests, WBC with differential, and CBC

    g. Side effects: headache, nausea and vomiting, diarrhea

    h. Adverse reactions/toxicity

        1) Serotonin syndrome may occur if given with serotonin reuptake inhibitors, tricyclic antidepressants, serotonin 5ht1-receptor agonists, meperidine, or buspirone

        2) Myelosuppression, including anemia, leukopenia, pancytopenia, and thrombocytopenia (long-term use)

    i. Client-centered nursing care (see Box 11-1 again)

        1) Monitor client for signs of low platelets, such as easy bruising, prolonged bleeding

        2) Monitor for signs of pseudomembranous colitis

    j. Client education (see Box 11-2 again)

        1) Report diarrhea, easy bruising, or bleeding to prescriber

        2) Avoid foods and beverages high in tyramine, such as aged, fermented, pickled, or smoked foods

        3) Avoid use of OTC cold remedies or decongestants containing pseudoephedrine

6. Daptomycin

    a. Actions and uses

        1) Drug in a class known as *cyclic lipopeptides*

        2) Binds to gram-positive cells in a calcium-dependent process, which causes rapid depolarization of cell membrane potential, leading to inhibition of protein, DNA, and RNA synthesis

        3) Used for complicated skin and soft tissue infections caused by gram-positive bacteria, including MRSA and VRE; bloodstream infection with *Staphyloccocus aureus*

    b. Administration considerations

        1) Only available IV

        2) Safe use in infants and children less than 18 years is not known

        3) Use cautiously in presence of renal or hepatic impairment, peripheral neuropathy, history of rhabdomyolysis

    c. Contraindications: pseudomembranous colitis, myopathy, allergy to daptomycin

    d. Significant drug interactions: potential increased risk for myopathy if given with HMG-COa reductase inhibitors ("statins")

    e. Significant food interactions: none identified

    f. Significant laboratory studies

        1) Liver and renal function tests

        2) PT/INR during first few days of therapy if client taking warfarin

        3) Weekly creatine phosphokinase (CPK) levels

        4) Daily blood glucose in clients with diabetes mellitus

        5) Serum electrolytes if signs of hypokalemia or hypomagnesemia appear

    g. Side effects

        1) Hypotension and hypertension

        2) Headache, dizziness, rash, GI discomfort

        3) Dyspnea

        4) Thrombocytopenia, anemia, fever

    h. Adverse reactions/toxicity: elevated liver enzymes, renal failure, fungal infection

    i. Client-centered nursing care (see Box 11-1 again)

        1) Monitor LFTs and for signs of impaired liver function such as anorexia, abdominal pain, dark urine

          2) Withhold drug if signs of myopathy appear (muscle pain or weakness) or CPK is elevated greater than 1,000 units

          3) Monitor serum electrolytes; monitor blood glucose in clients with diabetes mellitus

  j. Client education: see Box 11-2 again; report muscle pain, weakness, unusual tiredness; numbness or tingling; difficulty breathing or shortness of breath; severe diarrhea or vomiting; skin rash or itching

7. Metronidazole

  a. Action and use

          1) The protype antiprotozoal medication for amebiasis, giardiasis (off label), and trichomoniasis

          2) Has both antiprotozoal and anti-infective properties against anaerobioc bacteria

          3) Frequently used to treat pseudomembranous colitis, Crohn disease, and colitis (off-label)

          4) In combination with bismuth and tetracycline, it is FDA-approved to treat *Helicobacter pylori* infection

          5) Used to treat intra-abdominal and gynecologic infections caused by anaerobes *Eubacterium spp.*, *Bacteroides spp.*, and *Clostridium spp.*

          6) Topical drug form is used to treat rosacea

          7) Binds to DNA and RNA of intracellular proteins, causing cell death

  b. Administration considerations

          1) Available in PO, IV, topical skin and vaginal creams

          2) In 2011, Pregnancy Risk Category was changed from a C to a D for high dose (400–800 mg daily); long-term administration during first trimester may be associated with birth defects

  c. Contraindications: allergy to metronidazole; blood dyscrasias (may cause bone marrow depression)

  d. Significant drug interactions

          1) May cause disulfiram-like reaction if taken with alcohol

          2) May increase toxicity of lithium, benzodiazepines, cyclosporine, calcium channel blockers, warfarin, and antidepressants

          3) Phenytoin and phenobarbital may reduce effects of metronidazole

  e. Significant food interactions: none reported

  f. Significant laboratory studies: monitor liver function in clients with alcoholism or hepatic impairment

  g. Side effects

          1) Dizziness, headache, nasal congestion

          2) GI discomfort, anorexia, nausea and vomiting, diarrhea

          3) Reversible neutropenia, thrombocytopenia

          4) Dry mouth, unpleasant metallic taste

  h. Adverse reactions/toxicity

          1) Bone suppression may occur

          2) Dosage adjustment needed if client on warfarin or has hepatic impairment

  i. Client-centered nursing care (see Box 11-1 again)

          1) Discontinue therapy if client develops seizures or peripheral neuropathy

          2) Monitor total and differential WBC counts before, during, and after therapy

          3) Monitor for lithium toxicity if client is taking lithium

  j. Client education (see also Box 11-2)

          1) Instruct client to avoid alcohol consumption 24 hours before beginning therapy and for 36 hours after cessation of therapy

          2) Avoid use of OTC products containing alcohol, such as cold and cough remedies

3) Refrain from sexual intercourse during therapy when treatment is for trichomoniasis; sexual partner should also be treated

4) Report symptoms of candidiasis, including vaginitis, milky vaginal discharge, proctitis, furry tongue, glossitis, or stomatitis

5) Do not breastfeed without permission of healthcare provider

II. ANTIMYCOBACTERIALS

A. Antituberculins

1. Action and use

  a. Inhibit cell wall synthesis or mycocolic acid coat of bacteria (INH); protein synthesis, DNA or RNA synthesis (rifampin and rifapentine), or cell wall division (ethionamide)

  b. Effects limited primarily to *Mycobacterium tuberculosis* and then certain other mycobacterium strains; for prophylaxis or treatment of pulmonary tuberculosis (TB) or extrapulmonary TB

  c. Often used in combination with other antituberculin agents

  d. Used to prevent or delay onset of *Mycobacterium avium* bacteremia in clients with advanced AIDS, in combination with other antituberculins

  e. Rifampin also eradicates meningococci from nasopharynx of asymptomatic *Neisseria meningitides* carriers when there is increased risk for infection outbreaks among a community, and is used prophylactically with exposure to *Haemophilus influenzae* Type B (hib) infection

  f. Antituberculins are used in combination to treat leprosy

  g. Used in combination to treat mycobacterial infections including TB

  1) Effective treatment requires compliance and therapy over months to years

  2) Common antituberculin medications (Table 11-11)

2. Administration considerations

  a. Effectiveness depends on correct drug, correct combination therapy, adequate dosing, adequate duration of therapy, and compliance

  b. Empiric treatment is initiated with isoniazid, rifampin, pyrazinamide, and ethambutol or streptomycin

  c. TB medications are classified as first- or second-line drugs (see Table 11-11); multicombination drug therapy decreases risk or rate of developing resistance to any single drug

  d. Give isoniazid 1 hour before meals on empty stomach

3. Contraindications

  a. Hypersensitivity to drug

  b. Variable by specified drug: caution in pregnancy unless risk is significant

  c. Caution in renal or liver dysfunction, history of seizures, ethanol abuse, or CNS dysfunction

  d. Caution in older clients, children, diabetics, those with gout or blood dyscrasias, and optic neuritis or defects

4. Significant drug interactions

  a. Increased effect of antituberculin drug with antigout drugs such as probenecid and sulfinpyrazone, glucocorticosteroids such as methylprednisolone and prednisolone, nonsteroidal anti-inflammatory drugs (NSAIDs), aminoglycosides, and testosterone agents

  b. Decreased effect of antituberculin drug with quinidine, metoprolol, propranolol, oral anticoagulants, oral contraceptives, phenytoin, methadone, verapamil, cyclosporine, and ketoconazole

Table 11-11   **Antituberculin Drugs**

Generic Name	Route
First-Line Drugs	
Isoniazid	PO
Ethambutol	PO
Pyrazinamide	PO
Rifampin	PO, IV
Rifapentine	PO
Rifabutin	PO
Rifater: combination of pyrazinamide, isoniazid, rifampin	PO
Second-Line Drugs	
Amikacin (also an aminoglycoside)	IV/IM
Aminosalicylic acid	PO
Bedaquiline	PO
Capreomycin	IM
Ciprofloxacin or ofloxacin (fluoroquinolones)	PO/IV; IV
Cycloserine	PO
Ethionamide	PO
Kanamycin (also an aminoglycoside)	IM
Streptomycin (also an aminoglycoside)	IM

    c. Increased toxicity
        1) Salicylates, other antitubercular agents, nephrotoxic and hepatotoxic drugs, alcohol
        2) Increased neurotoxicity: cycloserine, isoniazid, ethionamide, and phenytoin
    d. Hyperkalemia with potassium-sparing diuretics and angiotensin-converting enzyme (ACE) inhibitors
    e. Crystalluria with ascorbic acid (vitamin C)
    f. Decreased efficacy of oral contraceptives
  5. Significant food interactions: decreased rate or extent of absorption of isoniazid when taken with food (take 1 hour before meals)
  6. Significant laboratory studies

    a. Monitor for hepatic dysfunction with ALT, AST, alkaline phosphatase, bilirubin
    b. Purified protein derivative (PPD) tuberculin skin test to check for positive reaction indicating prior exposure to *M. tuberculosis* and T-lymphocyte production; cellular response to tubercle bacillus occurs 3–10 weeks after infection and does not diagnose active infection; chest x-rays and sputum tests for tubercle bacillus are done to clarify actual status

    c. Chest x-ray if PPD positive
    d. Sputum smear culture to confirm diagnosis if chest x-ray positive
  7. Side effects
    a. Fairly well tolerated
    b. Nausea and vomiting, anorexia, constipation, diarrhea, dyspepsia
    c. Headache, dizziness, malaise, fever, chills, arthralgia, flulike symptoms, weakness

      d. Skin rash, dry skin, peripheral paresis, photophobia, photosensitivity, vision changes

      e. Dysrhythmias

      f. Urinary retention (in males)

      g. Change in color to orange-red of excretions or secretions as urine, tears, feces, perspiration (with rifampin and rifabutin)

      h. Electrolyte imbalances

      i. Metallic taste with ethionamide

      j. Disulfiram-like effect with alcohol ingestion

    8. Adverse effects/toxicity

      a. Nephrotoxicity, hepatotoxicity, or ototoxicity (tinnitus, hearing loss)

      b. Hematologic disorders: agranulocytosis, thrombocytopenia, eosinophilia, anemia

      c. Seizure, depression, confusion, ataxia, paresis, paresthesias, drowsiness

    9. Client-centered nursing care (see Box 11-1 again)

      a. Assess for shortness of breath, numbness, tingling, or hallucinations

      b. Assess for pregnancy; instruct female clients of ineffectiveness of oral contraceptives

      c. Coadminister pyridoxine (vitamin B_6) and/or cyanocobalamin (vitamin B_{12}) to prevent seizures and to correct metabolic acidosis

      d. Encourage food high in B-complex vitamins (especially pyridoxine), such as meat (chicken, beef, and pork), liver, soybeans, baked potato with skin, raw avocado

      e. Evaluate client compliance; ensure full course of therapy is completed to lessen risk of reinfection or development of drug resistance; directly observed therapy (DOT) may be required for some clients

      f. Encourage sufficient hydration and good nutrition with high-quality protein

    10. Client education

      a. See Box 11-2 for universal teaching points for anti-infectives

      b. Take isoniazid 1 hour before meals

      c. Report adverse reactions, especially signs of hepatic, renal, or ototoxicity; teach signs and symptoms of neurotoxicity and importance of increased intake of foods rich in vitamin B_6

      d. Rifampin: may discolor urine, tears, saliva, and stain contact lenses and undergarments

      e. Keep follow-up appointments with healthcare provider and for tests

      f. Use infection control measures to protect self and others

      g. Avoid alcohol because of increased risk for hepatitis or disulfiram-like effect; if taking isoniazid, avoid foods high in tyramine

      h. Use alternative contraception during therapy and for at least 1 month after therapy is discontinued if using oral contraceptives

      i. For dry skin, use emollients or oils

      j. Explain pharmacotherapy noncompliance is most common cause of treatment failure; explain need to treat close contacts prophylactically due to infectiousness of tuberculosis

  B. Leprostatics

    1. Action and use

      a. Treat leprosy and *Pneumocystis jiroveci* pneumonia, an AIDS-related opportunistic infection

      b. Dapsone is bacteriostatic against *Mycobacterium leprae, Pneumocystis jiroveci, Plasmodium, Mycobacterium tuberculosis*

Table 11-12	Leprostatics
Generic Name	**Route**
Dapsone	PO
Clofazimine	PO
Thalidomide	PO
Rifampin	PO

  c. Clofazimine is bactericidal against *Mycobacterium leprae* and *Mycobacterium avium*
  d. Rifampin, clofazimine, and dapsone are used in combination to prevent development of resistant strains
2. Common leprostatic medications (Table 11-12)
3. Administration considerations: give clofazimine with food
4. Contraindications
  a. Hypersensitivity to dapsone and possible sulfonamides
  b. Use cautiously in clients with hepatic disease or glucose-6-phosphate dehydrogenase (G6PD) deficiency (an inherited hemolytic anemia associated with stress or certain drug interactions)
  c. Not established for safe use in pregnant and lactating clients
5. Significant drug interactions: trimethoprim, a urinary tract anti-infective, and pyrimethamine, an anti-infective and antimalarial, increase levels and risk for adverse effects
6. Significant food interactions: none reported
7. Significant laboratory studies: monitor CBC for hemoglobin decline and reticulocyte count increase
8. Side effects
  a. Skin pigmentation changes, as pink to brownish-black color; may resolve in weeks to months
  b. Dry skin
  c. Nausea and vomiting, diarrhea, abdominal pain
  d. Headache, insomnia, malaise, paresthesias, nervousness, tinnitus, vertigo, vision changes, neuritis
9. Adverse effects/toxicity
  a. Agranulocytosis, hepatotoxicity, phototoxicity
  b. Dose-related hemolysis (increased in G6PD deficiency)
  c. Methemoglobinemia may occur resulting in rhinitis, fatigue, difficulty breathing, cyanosis
  d. Male infertility with dapsone
10. Client-centered nursing care (see Box 11-1 again)
  a. Ensure pregnancy test is negative
  b. Monitor laboratory tests for hemoglobin and reticulocyte count
  c. Assess concurrent medication regimen to avoid or minimize drug–drug interactions, such as with rifampin and trimethoprim
11. Client education
  a. See Box 11-2 for universal teaching points for anti-infectives
  b. Take clofazimine with meals; skin discoloration may be pink to brownish-black; resolves months to years after drug is discontinued
  c. Keep follow-up appointments with healthcare provider and for tests
  d. Ensure infection control measures are used
  e. Encourage adequate hydration and good nutrition with complete or complementary proteins for tissue healing

III. ANTIVIRALS

A. **Medications to treat herpesvirus and cytomegalovirus**

   1. Action and use

      a. Virustatic; prevents viral replication by inhibiting DNA replication; virus must be in living cell to survive and replicate

      b. Drug has little effect on host cells; effective only during acute phase of infection, not during latent phase

      c. Used to treat broad spectrum of diseases including cold sores, viral encephalitis, shingles, and genital infection

      d. Viruses include **herpes simplex** virus-1 (HSV-1) in oral herpes or herpes labialis, herpes simplex virus-2 (HSV-2) in genital herpes, **herpes zoster** in shingles, **herpes varicella** zoster virus (VZV) in chickenpox, **cytomegalovirus** (CMV), and some Epstein-Barr viruses

   2. Common antiviral medications and uses (Table 11-13)

   3. Administration considerations

      a. Hydrate client to decrease risk or extent of nephrotoxicity

      b. Administer as soon as possible to improve effectiveness

      c. Wear gloves for topical application to limit exposure to drug or lesions

      d. Preferred central venous access when given IV

      e. Foscarnet: precipitates with many drugs when given IV; use with D_5W or NaCl solutions

   4. Contraindications

      a. Hypersensitivity to drug

      b. Use caution in clients with preexisting hepatic or renal dysfunction, concurrent use of nephrotoxic drugs, and during pregnancy or lactation

Table 11-13 Antivirals: Medications to Treat Herpesvirus and Cytomegalovirus (CMV)

Generic Name	Route	Uses
Acyclovir	PO, IV, topical	Herpes zoster, varicella zoster, CMV (most strains resistant), varicella pneumonia, herpes simplex infection, disseminated primary eczema herpeticum
Cidofovir	IV	Cytomegalovirus retinitis clients with HIV who have failed on ganciclovir or foscarnet
Docosanol	Topical	Herpes simplex cold sores and fever blisters
Famciclovir	PO	Acute herpes zoster, recurrent orolabial or genital herpes simplex infections
Foscarnet	IV	CMV retinitis in clients with HIV; monocutaneous acyclovir-resistant herpes simplex virus infections; varicella zoster
Ganciclovir	PO, IV, ophthalmic gel, ocular implant	CMV retinitis, prevention of CMV disease in transplant recipients or immunocompromised clients, acute herpetic keratitis
Penciclovir	Topical	Herpes labialis (cold sores) on lips and face
Trifluridine	Ophthalmic	Herpes simplex 1 and 2; primary keratoconjunctivitis; recurrent epithelial keratitis
Valacyclovir	PO	Herpes zoster, recurrent genital herpes, cold sores, varicella
Valganciclovir	PO	CMV retinitis, prevention of CMV disease in immunocompromised clients
Vidarabine	Ophthalmic, IV	Acute keratoconjunctivitis and recurrent epithelial keratitis from herpesvirus

5. Significant drug interactions
   a. Increased drowsiness with zidovudine
   b. Nephrotoxic drugs potentiate renal effects
   c. Probenecid can prolong effects of antiviral agent
6. Significant food interactions: none reported
7. Significant laboratory studies
   a. CBC including WBC with differential, T-cell count, and platelet count
   b. Tests of liver function (ALT, AST, alkaline phosphatase, and bilirubin) and renal function (serum creatinine, BUN, creatinine clearance)
8. Side effects
   a. Anemia, headache, mood changes, depression, seizures
   b. Nausea and vomiting, diarrhea
   c. Local irritation including phlebitis at IV site; inflammation with topical application
   d. Neutropenia; often dose-dependent because of bone marrow suppression
   e. Fever, hypocalcemia, hypomagnesemia, hypokalemia, metabolic acidosis, dysrhythmias
   f. Increased risk for CNS disturbances and fluid overload in clients with impaired hepatic or renal function
   g. Ocular hypotony
9. Adverse effects/toxicity
   a. Additive neutropenia with zidovudine
   b. Infertility in males and females: ganciclovir
   c. Nephrotoxicity or hepatotoxicity, pancreatitis
   d. Thrombocytopenic purpura
10. Client-centered nursing care (see Box 11-1 again)
   a. Use protective gloves to administer topical antivirals
   b. Hydrate to decrease risk of nephrotoxicity (e.g., 2,000–3,000 mL/fluids per day if not contraindicated by other conditions)
   c. Offer small, frequent high-protein meals, and monitor nutritional status, especially if GI side effects occur
   d. Assess for neutropenic infection if immunosuppressed
   e. Monitor I&O and renal and hepatic function as noted in previous section
   f. Collaborate with prescriber if dosage needs adjustment for hepatic or renal dysfunction
   g. Evaluate CBC with differential, CD4 count, platelet count to monitor bone marrow activity and for effectiveness of drug therapy
   h. Preexisting CNS disturbances may be exacerbated; assess orientation and reflexes; implement safety measures to protect against injury if CNS disturbances exist
   i. Assess skin and lesions regularly; monitor for relief of pain and infection and of pain
   j. Monitor platelets and evidence of petechiae or increased risk of bleeding
   k. Monitor nutritional status, especially if GI side effects occur; ensure adequate protein intake
11. Client education
   a. See Box 11-2 for universal client teaching points
   b. Self-administration techniques if indicated; wear gloves for topical applications
   c. Clinical manifestations to report: severe side effects; evidence of increased bleeding, edema, fatigue; severe rash, especially if accompanied by blisters, fever, and other indications of infection to avert serious complications
   d. Avoid sexual intercourse if genital herpes being treated

e. Avoid touching lesions (by self and others) to avoid spreading infection to new sites

f. Avoid hazardous tasks and driving if drowsiness, dizziness, seizure activity occurs

g. Follow-up labs and appointments with healthcare provider are important

h. It is important to drink 2,000–3,000 mL/day and eat a nutritious, high-protein diet

i. Female clients should have annual Papanicolaou smear since there is increased risk of cervical cancer with genital herpes infection

j. Antiviral agents do not cure herpes and CMV infections

k. Notify healthcare provider if lesions recur or do not heal

B. **Medications for HIV and AIDS**

1. Antiretroviral protease inhibitors (PIs)

a. Action and use

1) Most potent of antiviral agents; inhibit cell protein synthesis that interferes with viral replication; block protease activity in HIV, thus preventing final maturation of virions

2) Not curative but slows progression of disease and prolongs life

3) Used prophylactically because viral replication peaks before clinical manifestations emerge and antiviral efficacy is then more limited; virus relies on using resources within live host cell and there is increased risk for toxicity to host cell

4) Used in AIDS, AIDS-related complex (ARC), and possibly hepatitis B and C to decrease viral load and opportunistic infections

5) Used in combination with other antiretroviral drug classes to decrease viral load, increase CD4 counts, and decrease incidence or rate of development of drug resistance

6) Rapidly absorbed from GI tract

b. Common protease inhibitor medications (Box 11-3)

c. Administration considerations

1) Saquinavir: take with high-fat meals or within 2 hours of full meal

2) Ritonavir: unpalatable; take with chocolate milk, nutritional supplement, or food

3) Indinavir requires an acidic gastric environment for absorption; take 1 hour before or 2 hours after a light, low-fat snack; drink greater than 1.5 liters of fluid daily

d. Contraindications: hypersensitivity; not recommended for children or pregnant or lactating women

e. Significant drug interactions

1) To decrease risk of resistance, drug may be combined with reverse transcriptase agents

2) Rifampin and rifabutin lower blood levels of protease inhibitors; mycobacterium prophylaxis may be changed to clarithromycin

3) All PIs inhibit P450 and can cause other drugs to accumulate to dangerous levels; drugs that inhibit P450 can slow metabolism of PIs, thereby increasing their levels; drugs that induce P450 can accelerate metabolism of PIs and reduce their levels

4) Always use a drug interaction checker to verify safety before administering protease inhibitors with other drugs

Box 11-3	Amprenavir	Lopinavir/ritonavir
Oral Antiretroviral Drugs for HIV and AIDS: Protease Inhibitors	Atazanivir	Nelfinavir
	Darunavir	Ritonavir
	Fosamprenavir	Saquinavir
	Indinavir	Tipranavir

      f. Significant food interactions (see section on administration considerations)

      g. Significant laboratory studies

        1) Aminotransferase and triglyceride levels may be elevated with ritonavir

        2) ALT, AST, alkaline phosphatase, bilirubin

        3) CBC; CD4 cell count; viral load measurement

        4) Creatinine, BUN, creatinine clearance

      h. Side effects

        1) Common to all PIs: fat redistribution, hyperlipidemia, hyperglycemia, possible increased risk of bleeding in clients with hemophilia, bone loss, elevation of serum transaminase

        2) Headache, fatigue, nausea and vomiting, diarrhea, abdominal discomfort, anemia, taste perversion, asthenia, circumoral paresthesia with ritonavir

        3) Reversible hyperbilirubinemia and nephrolithiasis with indinavir: greater than 1.5 liters fluid daily are needed to prevent nephrolithiasis

      i. Adverse effects/toxicity: hepatotoxicity; reduce dose in liver dysfunction

      j. Client-centered nursing care (see Box 11-1 again)

        1) Monitor for hepatotoxicity: increased liver function tests, nausea and vomiting, jaundice, upper right abdominal quadrant enlargement and tenderness

        2) Monitor for nephrotoxicity: creatinine, BUN, creatinine clearance, urinalysis; keep accurate I&O

        3) Monitor CBC for blood dyscrasias such as neutropenia, thrombocytopenia, or anemia and for improvement as evidenced by increased T-cell count

        4) If neutropenic, employ neutropenic precautions as appropriate; observe for occult signs of infection (e.g., low back, flank, or suprapubic pain, normal temperature or low-grade fever related to UTI)

        5) See specific administration guidelines for PIs; taking with food may increase or decrease bioavailability; ritonavir oral solution diluted to mask taste but food does not affect absorption; indinavir requires at least 1,500 mL/day of fluids to prevent nephrolithiasis

      k. Client education

        1) See Box 11-2 for universal teaching points for anti-infectives

        2) Ensure fluid intake of at least 1,500 mL/day

        3) Follow drug specific guidelines regarding taking with or without food

        4) Eat small, frequent meals with complete or complementary proteins

        5) Keep appointments for follow-up examinations and laboratory testing

        6) Use neutropenic precautions as indicated by provider

   2. Reverse transcriptase inhibitors

      a. Action and use

        1) Block viral reverse transcriptase; stop replication and growth

        2) Used for all symptomatic, HIV clients with a CD4 count less than $500/mm^3$ and some with higher counts

        3) Penetrate blood–brain barrier

        4) Possible prophylaxis for known occupational HIV exposure

        5) Effectiveness diminishes over time

        6) AZT is used to prevent maternal transmission of HIV

        7) A major advantage of non-nucleoside reverse transcriptase inhibitors is that they do not adversely affect development of blood cells

        8) Significant cross-resistance between nucleoside reverse transcriptase inhibitors (NRTIs); no cross-resistance between nucleoside and nonnucleoside reverse transcriptase inhibitors (NNRTIs)

        9) Used in combination because resistant strains rapidly evolve if used as single-agent therapy

    b. Common oral antiretroviral reverse transcriptase inhibitors for HIV and AIDS (Box 11-4); note that zidovudine ia also available for IV use

    c. Administration considerations

        1) Crush or chew buffered tablets that are chewable because drug has acid lability

        2) May administer at bedtime for better tolerance of CNS adverse effects

    d. Contraindications

        1) Concurrent use of drugs that cause peripheral neuropathy, such as choramphenicol, vinca alkaloids (vincristine, vinblastine, etoposide, cisplatin), dapsone, hydralazine, isoniazid, metronidazole, nitrofurantoin, phenytoin, and ribavirin

        2) Avoid or use with caution drugs that can increase toxicity, such as probenecid, acetaminophen, lorazepam, indomethacin, and cimetidine

        3) If neurotoxic signs occur, discontinue drug until signs are resolved

    e. Significant drug interactions

        1) Many drug class interactions; see individual product literature; drugs that are myelosuppressive, nephrotoxic, or directly toxic to circulating blood cells increase risk of hematologic toxicity

        2) Antivirals will decrease effect of oral contraceptives

        3) Tenofovir can increase serum level of didanosine

        4) May be given with other drugs to enhance antiviral effect: acyclovir, interferon, didanosine, granulocyte colony-stimulating factor (GCSF) such as epoetin alfa

    f. Significant food interactions: decreased absorption of didanosine when taken with food; most other NRTIs can be taken without regard to meals but NNRTIs vary; check drug-specific literature

    g. Significant laboratory studies

        1) Amylase, cholesterol, liver function tests (ALT, AST, alkaline phosphatase, bilirubin)

        2) CBC (including WBC with differential), platelet count, CD4 cell count, and viral load measurement

        3) Electrolytes

        4) Serum creatinine, BUN, creatinine clearance

    h. Side effects

        1) Neurologic side effects of insomnia, confusion, peripheral neuropathies, and seizures

        2) Diarrhea, nausea and vomiting, headache, and fatigue are common during first few weeks of therapy with NRTIs; rash is common with NNRTIs and, though rare, can progress to Stevens–Johnson syndrome

        3) Hypermagnesemia

        4) Discolored fingernails, rash

Box 11-4 **Oral Antiretroviral Drugs for HIV and AIDS: Reverse Transcriptase Inhibitors**	*Nucleoside and Nucleotide Reverse Transcriptase Inhibitors*	*Nonnucleoside Reverse Transcriptase Inhibitors*
	Abacavir	Delavirdine
	Didanosine	Efavirenz
	Emtricitabine	Etravirine
	Lamivudine	Nevirapine
	Stavudine	Rilpivirine
	Tenofovir	
	Zidovudine	

         5) Myalgias, numbness and tingling of extremities, altered taste sensations, dizziness, anxiety, tremors

         6) Cough

   i. Adverse effects/toxicity

         1) Pancreatitis

         2) Lactic acidosis and hepatic steatosis are potential risks with all NRTIs; risk is higher with use of combination NRTIs during pregnancy

         3) Anemia, leukopenia, thrombocytopenia with nucleosides

         4) Nevirapine: severe hepatotoxicity and dermatologic effects such as Stevens–Johnson syndrome

   j. Client-centered nursing care (see Box 11-1 again)

         1) Assess baseline and periodic renal and liver function tests

         2) Ensure client takes complete course and all drugs included in regimen to improve effectiveness and retard risk for resistant strains emerging

         3) Administer around the clock as needed to maintain therapeutic levels

         4) Stop administration if severe rash or other hypersensitivity reaction occurs

         5) Assess client for complications of HIV infection (e.g., opportunistic infections, cancer, neurologic disease)

         6) Monitor level of consciousness (LOC), strength, appropriateness of activity, short-term memory, ability to follow complex commands, reasoning and calculation abilities, and peripheral sensation

         7) Assess for compromised respiratory or cardiovascular status

         8) Provide safety measures to protect from injury if CNS adverse effects occur

         9) Assess nutritional intake and tolerance, I&O, daily weight

        10) Monitor skin and mucous membranes frequently

        11) Monitor for alleviation of clinical manifestations of AIDS or ARC and for increase in CD4 count and decrease in viral load

   k. Client education

         1) See Box 11-2 for universal teaching points for anti-infectives

         2) Caution about risks of dizziness or altered mentation; do not drive or perform hazardous tasks

         3) Avoid crowds and persons with infections

         4) Practice good personal hygiene and employ safe-sex practices

         5) Hair loss possible with zidovudine

         6) Drug does not cure but helps manage infection; reduces viral load, decreases risk for complications, and extends survival

         7) Explain use of combination of drugs that work by different mechanisms; improves client's survival by reducing viral resistance to drug therapy

3. Entry inhibitors (see Table 11-14)

   a. Two drugs are currently available in this relatively new class and work in different ways

   b. Enfurvitide binds to viral envelope and blocks fusion of virus to bilipid layer of CD4 cell membrane; administered subcutaneously twice daily; indicated in clients resistant to other antiretroviral classes; injection site reactions may include erythema, severe pain, pruritis, cysts, abscesses, and cellulitis; other common side effects are nausea, diarrhea and fatigue; clients should be monitored for pneumonia secondary to increased risk of lung infections

   c. Maraviroc is a *chemokine coreceptor 5 antagonist* (CCR5 antagonist), which reversibly binds to chemokine coreceptor on CD4 cells; is used in combination with other antiretroviral drugs; it may cause hepatotoxicity and caution should be used in clients with preexisting cardiac disease due to risk for cardiac ischemia

Practice to Pass

The client with HIV states, "I quit taking the acyclovir. I don't have any symptoms. I don't want to take it now and risk becoming resistant to it when I may really need it." How do you respond?

Table 11-14 **Other Antiretroviral Medications**

Classification	Generic Name	Route
Entry inhibitors	Enfuvirtide	Subcut
	Maraviroc	PO
Integrase inhibitors	Dolutegravir	PO
	Elvitegravir	PO
	Raltegravir	PO

or infarction; other side effects include upper respiratory tract infection, cough, dizziness, fever, and rash

4. Integrase inhibitors (see Table 11-14 again)
   a. Also among newest drug classes for treatment of HIV infection
   b. Inhibit activity of integrase enzyme, needed by HIV to insert viral DNA into human chromosome
   c. Current drugs in this category are dolutegravir, elvitegravir, and ralategravir; may be used in combination therapy with other antiretrovirals
   d. Most common side effects are nausea, diarrhea, fatigue, insomnia, and headache; myopathy and rhabdomyolysis have also been reported
5. Chronic hepatitis pharmacotherapy
   a. Treatment of chronic hepatitis B may include use of interferon alfa or PEG interferon (see Immune chapter) and antivirals lamivudine, adefovir, tenofovir, and entecavir
   b. Treatment of chronic hepatitis C includes use of interferon and ribavirin, as well as HCV protease inhibitors boceprevir and telaprivir; triple therapy with three agents has significantly higher efficacy levels; most common adverse effects are fatigue, nausea and vomiting, altered taste, chills, insomnia, anemia, and neutropenia; boceprevir and telaprevir have many drug interactions

C. **Medications for influenza and respiratory viruses**
   1. Action and use
      a. Virustatic
      b. Most viral replication occurs before clinical evidence appears; bacterial replication occurs as clinical manifestations of infection emerge; antibacterial agents are more effective against bacterial infections than antiviral agents are against viral infections, since drug therapy relies on viral replication for effectiveness
      c. Ribavirin
         1) Aerosolized administration for respiratory syncytial virus (RSV) or severe infections of respiratory tract secondary to RSV
         2) May decrease length of infection
         3) Efficacy demonstrated in influenza A and B and in hepatitis A
      d. Amantadine and rimantadine
         1) Used prophylactically for influenza A; increased efficacy if initiated at time of exposure or at least within 48 hours
         2) Adjunctive therapy for temporary immunization of influenza A
         3) May limit severity of clinical manifestations of influenza and/or decrease length or duration
   2. Common influenza and respiratory viral medications (Table 11-15)
      a. Amantadine: prophylactically and therapeutically used for respiratory viral infections such as influenza; also used to treat Parkinson disease; recommendations for use of amantadine change yearly based on type of influenza that is prevalent;

Table 11-15 Medications for Influenza and Respiratory Viruses

Generic Name	Route	Uses
Amantadine	PO	Respiratory viral infections Decrease Parkinson-related symptoms No longer recommended for influenza as most strains are resistant
Oseltamivir	PO	Prevention and treatment of uncomplicated influenza
Palivizumab	IM	Monoclonal antibody for preventing respiratory syncytial virus in premature infants and young children with chronic lung disease
Peramivir	IV	Treatment of influenza
Ribavirin	PO, inhalation	Chronic hepatitis C in clients who relapse after interferon alpha therapy; treatment of influenza A and B, severe respiratory syncytial virus pneumonia, and herpes virus infections
Vaccinations		Discussed in Chapter 10 (Immune System Medications)
Zanamivir	Inhalation	Treatment of uncomplicated influenza

refer to Centers for Disease Control and Prevention website for most current information
  - **b.** Ribavirin: treat influenza A, RSV, and herpes infections
  - **c.** Rimantadine: used prophylactically against influenza A
  - **d.** Oseltamivir and zanamivir used to prevent and treat influenza; dosing must begin within 2 days after symptom onset
3. Administration considerations
  - **a.** Initiate drug therapy as soon as possible to enhance effectiveness and to deter complications of infection
  - **b.** Administer before flu season for prophylactic purpose as indicated, but do not use as substitute for influenza vaccination
  - **c.** If given within 48 hours of onset of symptoms, the neuraminidase inhibitors, oseltamivir, and zanamivir will shorten the normal 7-day duration of symptoms
4. Contraindications
  - **a.** Known hypersensitivity
  - **b.** Ribavirin contraindicated in pregnancy (teratogenic); use cautiously in lactating clients and children
  - **c.** Caution in clients with renal or liver dysfunction
  - **d.** Caution in clients with psychotic disorders or seizures
5. Significant drug interactions
  - **a.** Stop neuraminidase inhibitors (oseltamivir and zanamivir) 2 days before giving a live, attenuated influenza vaccine and do not resume until after 2 weeks
  - **b.** Ribavirin with digoxin increases risk for digitalis toxicity
6. Significant food interactions: none reported
7. Significant laboratory studies
  - **a.** CBC with WBC differential
  - **b.** Possible C&S of pharynx or of sputum
  - **c.** Liver and renal function studies
8. Side effects
  - **a.** Nausea and vomiting most common with influenza treatment agents; give with food to reduce nausea
  - **b.** Inhaled drugs may cause cough or throat irritation
9. Adverse effects/toxicity: rare reactions include severe hypersensitivity reactions and neuropsychiatric effects

10. Client-centered nursing care (see Box 11-1 again)
    a. Assess for preexisting hepatic and renal dysfunction
    b. Assess baseline neurologic status (e.g., orientation, affect, coordination, reflexes)
    c. Maintain hydration with 2,000–3,000 mL fluids/day if not contraindicated by other conditions
    d. Initiate drug therapy as soon as possible after exposure
    e. Ensure complete course of therapy taken to enhance drug effectiveness
    f. Monitor for adverse effects; monitor for respiratory deterioration in infants; assess for adventitious breath sounds in all clients
    g. Provide safety precautions if CNS adverse effects develop

11. Client education
    a. See Box 11-2 for universal teaching points for anti-infectives
    b. Initiate therapy as soon as possible when prescribed
    c. Report increased respiratory distress or severe adverse effects to healthcare provider
    d. If drowsiness, dizziness, light-headedness, confusion, ataxia, or blurred vision occurs, do not drive or perform hazardous tasks
    e. If improvement is not noted within 2–3 days, notify healthcare provider
    f. Drink at least six to eight glasses of fluids a day
    g. Keep appointments with healthcare provider and for tests
    h. Obtain influenza A vaccine before flu season begins

D. **Locally active antiviral agents**
    1. Action and use: not absorbed systemically; interfere with viral replication and metabolic processes
    2. Common locally active antiviral medications (Table 11-16)
    3. Administration considerations
        a. Wash hands well before applying medication
        b. Wear gloves and may use cotton-tip applicator to apply to skin lesions, being cautious not to contaminate drug or other sites on skin
        c. Stop drug if severe local adverse effect or open lesions develop
    4. Contraindications: caution if known hypersensitivity, pregnancy, lactation; fomivirsen should not be used if treated with cidofovir in last 2–4 weeks
    5. Significant drug interactions: do not apply other topical agents to same lesions
    6. Significant food interactions: none reported
    7. Significant laboratory studies: none reported
    8. Side effects
        a. Local burning, stinging, discomfort may occur at time of application but usually resolve without intervention
        b. Temporary visual impairment possible with ophthalmic application

Practice to Pass

The client taking amantadine reports symptoms of xerostomia. What is this complaint? What intervention or teaching would you provide?

Table 11-16 Locally Active Antiviral Agents

Generic Name	Route	Uses
Docosanol	Topical	Herpes simplex cold sores and fever blisters
Fomivirsen	Injected into affected eye	CMV retinitis
Ganciclovir	Implanted into eye	CMV retinitis
Idoxuridine	Topical	Herpes simplex keratitis
Imiquimod	Topical	Genital and perianal warts
Penciclovir	Topical	Herpes labialis
Trifluridine	Ophthalmic	Herpes simplex of eye
Vidarabine	Ophthalmic	Herpes simplex of eye that does not respond to idoxuridine

9. Adverse effects/toxicity: skin eruptions; hypersensitivity
10. Client-centered nursing care (see Box 11-1 again)
    a. See previous administration considerations
    b. Assess site prior to administration to evaluate effectiveness of previous dose(s)
    c. Monitor for therapeutic response and adverse effects and for client comfort, safety, and compliance
11. Client education
    a. See Box 11-2 for universal teaching points for anti-infectives
    b. Use proper administration technique
    c. Does not cure but alleviates pain and discomfort and prevents extended damage to uninvolved tissue
    d. Report severe local discomfort or reaction to healthcare provider

IV. ANTIFUNGALS

A. Antifungals for systemic mycoses
   1. Action and use
      a. Systemic mycoces are those affecting internal organs, typically lungs, brain, and digestive organs; less common but sometimes fatal to immunosuppressed clients; drug-resistant forms becoming more common
      b. Fungistatic or fungicidal depending on therapeutic serum levels and sensitivity to fungi
   2. Common systemic antifungal medications (Table 11-17)
   3. Administration considerations
      a. Administer carefully as prescribed, especially IV dosages
      b. Combination of antifungal agents may deter or retard drug resistance; several months of therapy may be required for a complete cure
      c. Amphotericin B
         1) May premedicate with an antipyretic such as acetaminophen, an antihistamine such as diphenhydramine, an antiemetic, and meperidine to reduce severity of

Table 11-17	Systemic Antifungal Medications	
Generic Name	**Route**
Classification Polyene Antifungals	
Amphotericin B preparations	IV
Classification Azoles	
Fluconazole	PO, IV
Itraconazole	PO, IV
Ketoconazole	PO, topical
Voriconazole	PO, IV
Posaconazole	PO, IV
Classification Echinocandins or Beta-Glucan Synthesis Inhibitors	
Anidulafungin	IV
Caspofungin acetate	IV
Micafungin	IV
Classification Pyrimidine Analog	
Flucytosine	PO

fever or chills response; heparin or hydrocortisone added to IV solutions may reduce risk for thrombophlebitis at IV site

> 2) Give with heparin or hydrocortisone and over 4–6 hours to avert clinical manifestations of hypersensitivity or drug toxicity

> 3) Hydrate with IV fluids usually 2 hours before and 2 hours after drug administration to decrease risk for nephrotoxicity

> 4) To test for hypersensitivity prior to administration, deliver 1 mg/20 mL D_5W IV over 10–30 minutes; if hypersensitivity response occurs, a lipid preparation such as amphotericin B liposomal complex may minimize severe fever, shaking, and chills; premedicate as discussed earlier

> 5) Mix in D_5W only; precipitates form in any solution containing sodium chloride

> 6) Amphotericin B liposomal complex: shake gently to distribute drug particles; use 5-micrometer filter needle to inject agent into container of D_5W and thoroughly disperse drug throughout solution; redisperse drug in solution every 2 hours if infusion time extends beyond 2 hours; no in-line filter used

4. Contraindications
    a. Hypersensitivity
    b. If IV test dose of amphotericin B elicits hypersensitivity response, lipid preparations (more expensive) may be given to avoid severe response of fever, shaking, chills
    c. Avoid histamine$_2$ (H$_2$)antagonists unless scheduled so not to interfere with absorption of antifungals
    d. Use caution with IV administration of miconazole because of risk of cardiotoxicity
    e. Use caution in pregnant and lactating clients
    f. Use caution with amphotericin B agents in renal impairment and/or severe bone marrow depression

5. Significant drug interactions
    a. Increased risk for bleeding with concurrent administration of anticoagulants or corticosteroids
    b. Increased risk for nephrotoxicity if given concurrently with other nephrotoxic drugs
    c. Antidiabetic agents given concurrently with miconazole, fluconazole, and itraconazole may exaggerate hypoglycemia effect
    d. Ketoconazole and itraconazole depend on acid environment; give antifungal agent 1 hour before or 2 hours after administration of antacid
    e. Ketoconazole and fluconazole prolong effect of cyclosporine
    f. Ketoconazole: rifampin decreases effect of antifungal
    g. Fluconazole: increases phenytoin level and decreases serum levels of fluconazole with administration of rifampin; interacts with benzodiazepines, anticoagulants, and oral contraceptives; should use aspirin instead of acetaminophen for pain relief
    h. Amphotericin B: synergistic effect with tetracyclines, rifampin, or 5-flucytosine; do not administer with any other nephrotoxic drugs or with conticosteroids, digoxin, or thiazide diuretics

6. Significant food interactions
    a. Itraconazole: take with food to enhance absorption
    b. Ketoconazole: take with food to decrease nausea and vomiting

7. Significant laboratory studies
    a. Baseline and periodic liver and renal function studies
    b. PT and INR if taking oral anticoagulants
    c. Electrolytes, especially potassium, magnesium, and sodium
    d. Monitor metabolic acidosis development during amphotericin B therapy
    e. Monitor CBC with hemoglobin and hematocrit, RBC indices, and platelet count

8. Side effects
   a. Thrombophlebitis with administration through peripheral vein
   b. Fever, chills, shaking, headache
   c. Anorexia, nausea and vomiting during or after administration, heartburn, diarrhea, flatulence, diminished taste acuity or unpleasant taste in mouth
   d. Myalgia, arthralgia, weakness, hypotension
   e. Insomnia, vertigo, confusion, photosensitivity
   f. Rash, pruritus, dry skin, urticaria
   g. Hypokalemia, hypomagnesemia, especially with concurrent use of glucocorticosteroids or diuretics
   h. Furry tongue with griseofulvin
   i. Ketoconazole: sexual impotency, hair loss, and gynecomastia
9. Adverse reactions/toxicity (newer azole drugs are much safer)
   a. Bone marrow depression resulting in neutropenia, thrombocytopenia, anemia
   b. Ototoxicity and nephrotoxicity with amphotericin B preparations
   c. Superinfections
   d. Drug toxicity or hypersensitivity: fever, chills, shaking, piloerection, headache, anorexia, nausea and vomiting
   e. Stevens–Johnson syndrome
   f. Renal dysfunction with amphotericin B may result in severe hypokalemia
   g. Cardiovascular collapse with too-rapid infusion
   h. Hepatic necrosis: rare
10. Client-centered nursing care (see Box 11-1 again)
   a. Assess concurrent medications to avoid drug interactions; check for incompatibility of solutions as there are many
   b. Assess for pregnancy, lactation, liver or renal dysfunction; monitor liver and renal laboratory studies throughout therapy
   c. Monitor serum levels of antifungal agents
   d. Monitor WBC for improvement and for early detection of developing neutropenia, thrombocytopenia, anemia
   e. Give potassium supplements if hypokalemia occurs
   f. Amphotericin B (IV)
      1) Use in-line filter with pores greater than 1 micron
      2) Premedicate with acetaminophen, diphenhydramine, an antiemetic, corticosteroids, and opioid analgesics as indicated
      3) Assess vital signs and for adverse reactions every 15 minutes twice, then every 30 minutes for 4 hours with initial administration and thereafter as indicated; administer IV over 2–6 hours
      4) Hydrate with 2,000–3,000 mL/day unless contraindicated by other conditions; keep accurate I&O
      5) Protect drug solution from light with foil covering
      6) Closely monitor for hypokalemia and hypomagnesemia and impaired renal function
11. Client education
   a. See Box 11-2 for universal teaching points for anti-infectives
   b. Amphotericin B may be given over weeks or months
   c. Explain administration procedure
   d. Report adverse effects such as burning at IV site, increased bleeding or bruising, or evidence of superinfection
   e. Febrile reaction may decrease over time
   f. Maintain fluid intake of 2,000–3,000 mL/day if not contraindicated by other conditions

Practice to Pass

The client with AIDS is to be given a first dose of amphotericin B intravenously after a central line is inserted. The client states, "I'm scared to get this stuff. The doctor told me all the bad things that can happen." How would you respond?

    g. Eat frequent, small meals with high-quality protein

    h. Take oral agents with food to minimize GI distress

B. Antifungals for superficial mycoses

  1. Action and use

    a. Local infections of skin and mucous membranes of oropharnyx, vagina, or intestines caused by *Candida* species; infections of **tinea** pedis (athlete's foot), tinea cruris (in scrotal, crural, anal, and genital areas, called "jock itch"), tinea corporis (skin), tinea unguium or onychomycosis (nail fungus), tinea manus, tinea versicolor (infection of skin with yellow- or beige-colored brawny patches)

    b. Use vaginal tablets up to 6 weeks prior to delivery to prevent newborn thrush

  2. Common antifungal medications for superficial mycoses (Box 11-5); most are topical; some are available as lozenges, shampoo, or vaginal suppository or cream; see individual product literature

  3. Administration considerations

    a. Oral tablets or lozenges or troches are not to be chewed or swallowed whole; swallow saliva as lozenge or troche dissolves slowly over 5–30 minutes; avoid food or drink during and for 30 minutes after dose

    b. For oral infections in client with dentures, remove dentures at bedtime; with oral suspension, remove dentures before each rinse or before each oral lozenge or troche

    c. For application to skin: wear latex gloves, cleanse area with tepid water (soap if prescribed), dry thoroughly (without application of heat), and apply to infected area sparingly; do not cover with an occlusive dressing or tight clothing; wash hands well after removing gloves

    d. For treatment of tinea pedis (athlete's foot), apply antifungal powder such as nystatin to inside of shoes and stockings

    e. For vulvovaginal use: insert one applicator full or one vaginal tablet into vagina at bedtime as instructed; continue therapy during menstruation

    f. Avoid contact of antifungal with eyes; with certain agents, avoid contact with mucous membranes

    g. Do not apply occlusive dressing unless prescribed; client to avoid restrictive clothing in areas of infection

    h. Store creams, vaginal application, and topical preparation at room temperature; if specified for vaginal tablets and troches, refrigerate but do not freeze

  4. Contraindications: hypersensitivity (skin blistering, burning)

  5. Significant drug interactions: do not apply other preparations on same surface area

  6. Significant food interactions: none reported

Box 11-5	*Azole Type*	*Others*
Antifungal Medications for Superficial Mycoses	Butaconazole	Butenafine
	Clotrimazole	Ciclopirox
	Econazole	Griseofulvin
	Ketoconazole	Naftifine
	Miconazole	Nystatin
	Oxiconazole	Terbinafine
	Sertaconazole	Tolnaftate
	Sulconazole	Undecylenic acid
	Terconazole	

7. Significant laboratory studies: liver enzymes in hepatic impairment
8. Side effects
    a. Topical: stinging, burning, erythema, edema, dry skin, vesication, pruritus, urticaria, desquamation, skin fissures
    b. Vaginal: slight burning, lower abdominal discomfort, bloating, erythema, itching, vaginal soreness during intercourse
    c. Oral troches or swish and swallow: nausea and vomiting
9. Adverse effects/toxicity: possible hepatotoxicity in client with liver impairment
10. Client-centered nursing care (see Box 11-1 again)
    a. Observe for clinical evidence of liver dysfunction, such as upper right quadrant tenderness, abdominal discomfort or bloating, lethargy, mentation changes, icterus, enlarged liver, elevated liver enzymes (ALT, AST, alkaline phosphatase, bilirubin)
    b. Stop application if severe burning or exacerbation of lesions occur and collaborate with prescriber
11. Client education
    a. See Box 11-2 for universal teaching points for anti-infectives
    b. Explain how to apply or instill dose
    c. Observe for resolution of signs or symptoms within first week of therapy; some infections require 2–4 weeks of treatment; notify prescriber if condition worsens or no improvement is noted in 1–2 weeks
    d. Store in tightly covered container at room temperature; if vaginal tablet or suppository, store as recommended, usually in refrigerator or above 15°C (59°F); avoid freezing or excess heat of all products
    e. If taken vaginally, refrain from sexual intercourse or have partner wear condom to avoid burning or irritation of penis or urethra
    f. Wash clothing and linens in contact with infectious sites with soap and water after each treatment; ointments may be removed from fabric with commercial cleaning products
    g. If severe burning, stinging, or eruptions occur, discontinue use and notify prescriber
    h. Avoid or eliminate alcohol while on antifungals to avoid hepatic complications
    i. Dissolve oral antifungal lozenges (troches) in mouth or rinse with liquids after meals and at bedtime; if dentures are worn, remove them before using drug and leave out overnight; swish liquid drug around mouth and hold in mouth at least 2 minutes before expectorating; do not swallow unless instructed to do so by provider and do not rinse mouth afterward

V. ANTIPROTOZOALS

A. Antimalarials (schizonticides)

1. Action and use
    a. Therapeutic use to treat acute episodes or prophylaxis to prevent malarial infection and/or relapse
    b. Chloroquine treatment for **giardiasis** (a protozoan intestinal infection) and amebiasis outside GI tract, as well as rheumatoid arthritis and discoid lupus erythematosus
    c. Primaquine and pyrimethamine: treat toxoplasmosis and used with other medications against malaria infection
2. Common antiprotozoal medications (Table 11-18)
3. Administration considerations
    a. Separate drug from antacid administration by 4 hours (before or after)
    b. Take quinine sulfate with food to decrease gastric distress and mask bitter taste; do not crush capsule

Table 11-18		Antiprotozoal Medications
Generic Name	**Route**	**Uses**
Chloroquine	PO	*Plasmodium* malaria; extraintestinal amebiasis
Atovaquone/proguanil	PO	*Plasmodium* malaria
Hydroxychloroquine sulfate	PO	*Plasmodium* malaria
Mefloquine	PO	*Plasmodium* malaria
Primaquine (generic)	PO	Toxoplasmosis; prevent relapses of *Plasmodium* malaria in combination with other agents to suppress transmission
Pyrimethamine	PO	Toxoplasmosis; prevent relapses of *Plasmodium* malaria in combination with other agents to suppress transmission
Pyrimethamine and sulfadoxine	PO	Toxoplasmosis
Quinine	PO	Chloroquine-resistant *Plasmodium* infections
Tinidazole	PO	Amebiasis, giardiasis, trichomonas infection

    c. Primaquine: take dose with food to minimize GI distress

    d. Chloroquine, hydroxychloroquine, and pyrimethamine: take with food to minimize gastric distress

    e. For prophylaxis, take as prescribed, such as same day every week when entering high-risk area and for 10 weeks after departing

    f. Mefloquine: take with at least 8 ounces of water; separate by at least 8 hours from dose of quinine or quinidine, an antidysrhythmic

  4. Contraindications

    a. Quinine sulfate: tinnitus, optic neuritis, myasthenia gravis, G6PD deficiency, pregnancy; use caution with dysrhythmias and cardiac disorders

    b. Pyrimethamine: caution with antiseizure agents

    c. Mefloquine: hypersensitivity; with calcium channel blockers; in dysrhythmias, psychotic or seizure disorders; in pregnancy and in infants

    d. Chloroquine: renal disease; caution in hepatic dysfunction, alcohol abuse, eczema, G6PD deficiency, blood dyscrasias, GI and neurologic disorders, psoriasis, porphyria (may precipitate attacks) or children

    e. Primaquine: administer cautiously to clients of Eastern Mediterranean or African origins (pharmacogenetics) and clients with preexisting hematologic conditions

  5. Significant drug interactions

    a. Quinine sulfate: may increase digoxin levels; increased vagolytic effects with anticholinergics; decreased effectiveness if concurrent use of rifampin, antiseizure agents, or barbiturates; increased risk for toxicity with systemic and oral antacids; increased anticoagulant effects with oral anticoagulants; decreased mefloquine levels; increased risk for seizures from possible lowered levels of valproic acid

    b. Disulfiram-like effects with alcohol and some antimalarials

    c. Pyrimethamine: decreased effectiveness against **toxoplasmosis** (protozoan systemic infection transmitted by contact with oocysts in feces of domesticated animals) with concurrent use of folic acid or para-aminobenzoic acid (PABA)

    d. Chloroquine: interacts with cimetidine, digoxin, penicillamine, and rabies vaccine; has decreased absorption if taken with kaolin or magnesium-containing antacids

    e. Mefloquine: beta blockers, calcium blockers, and digoxin can prolong cardiac conduction

    f. Decreased absorption with antacids or laxatives containing aluminum or magnesium

    g. May interfere with rabies vaccine

6. Significant food interactions: none reported

7. Significant laboratory studies

    a. ALT, AST, alkaline phosphatase, bilirubin

    b. CBC with differential, reticulocyte count, red blood cell indices, hemoglobin, hematocrit, platelet count

    c. Evaluate electrolytes affected by GI side effects

    d. Prior to therapy, test for G6PD deficiency in African Americans and clients of Mediterranean descent

8. Side effects

    a. Dizziness, vertigo, headache, visual impairment, angina

    b. Nausea and vomiting, diarrhea, gastric distress, abdominal cramps

    c. Confusion, apprehension, insomnia, nightmares, syncope, delirium

    d. Cutaneous flushing, pruritus, rash, paresthesia, dyspnea, weight loss, fatigue

    e. Pyrimethamine: symptoms of folic acid deficiency (at high dose), ulcerative stomatitis, atrophic glossitis, pharyngitis, and diarrhea

    f. Chloroquine and hydroxychloroquine sulfate: alopecia, bleaching of scalp or hair (including eyebrows and body hair) and freckles; bluish-black hue of skin or mucous membranes, rash, pruritis; photophobia

9. Adverse effects/toxicity

    a. Tinnitus, hearing loss

    b. Cardiotoxicity in clients with atrial fibrillation

    c. Leukopenia, thrombocytopenia, agranulocytosis, hypoprothrombinemia, hemolytic anemia

    d. Hypotension, tachypnea, tachycardia, hypothermia

    e. Seizures, coma, cardiovascular collapse, blackwater fever (extensive intravascular hemolysis with renal failure), death

    f. Visual halos, blurring, inability to focus

10. Client-centered nursing care (see Box 11-1 again)

    a. Assess hepatic and cardiac function at intervals

    b. Assess for electrolyte disturbances, blood disorders as anemia, thrombocytopenia

    c. If taking antiepileptics, monitor drug levels of these agents

    d. Ensure regular ophthalmic exams, electrocardiograms, and lab tests as prescribed

    e. Assess for muscle weakness, CNS side effects, and depressed deep tendon reflexes periodically

11. Client education

    a. See Box 11-2 for universal teaching points for anti-infectives

    b. If weekly, take on same day every week

    c. Do not drive or perform hazardous tasks if drowsiness, dizziness, vertigo, or visual disturbances occur

    d. Report fever, sore throat, myalgias, visual disturbances, anxiety, mental changes, hallucinations

    e. Chloroquine: sunglasses may decrease risk of photophobia or ocular changes; urine may become rusty yellow or brown; do not take OTC antacids or laxatives containing magnesium

B. Other antiprotozoals
  1. Action and use
      a. Amebic dysentery, hepatic amebiasis, or abscess
      b. Some are bactericidal as well as amebicidal, especially in GI tract
      c. Destroy intestinal bacteria that forms nitrogen to decrease ammonia in hepatic disease and coma
      d. Pentamidine isoethionate: treat ***Pneumocystis jiroveci pneumonia***, an opportunistic infection in client with AIDS
      e. Kills insects and parasites and their ova as in head lice, body lice, and scabies
  2. Common medications: metronidazole, paromomycin, pentamidine isoethionate, lindane, atovaquone
  3. Administration considerations
      a. Pentamidine isoethionate: decreased doses in renal dysfunction
      b. Rotate IM injection sites
      c. Administer atovaquone with high-fat meal greater than 23 grams to increase absorption
  4. Contraindications
      a. Caution in pregnancy and lactation
      b. Hypersensitivity to drug or to iodine, iodoquinol, or primaquin
  5. Significant drug interactions: none reported
  6. Significant food interactions: none reported
  7. Significant laboratory studies
      a. Electrolytes including potassium, magnesium, and calcium if GI problems
      b. CBC with WBC and differential: check for infection and blood disorders such as leukopenia, anemia, neutropenia, thrombocytopenia if indicated
      c. Blood glucose for hypoglycemia if pancreatitis develops
  8. Side effects
      a. Hypotension, tachycardia, precordial stiffness, dizziness, headache, syncope
      b. Flushing, pruritis, dyspnea
      c. Abdominal cramps, diarrhea, nausea and vomiting, epigastric distress, unpleasant taste
      d. Myalgia, tremors, restlessness
  9. Adverse effects/toxicity
      a. Nephrotoxicity: mild and reversible
      b. Leukopenia, neutropenia, anemia, thrombocytopenia
      c. Dysrhythmias
      d. Hypoglycemia related to pancreatitis
      e. Large doses can cause abscess, cellulitis, or lesion in muscle in GI tract, heart, liver, and kidneys
      f. Pain at injection site
      g. Lindane topical shampoo can cause CNS problems such as seizures or eczematous eruptions
  10. Client-centered nursing care (see Box 11-1 again)
      a. Assess skin for scabies, tracking, lesions, nits
      b. For scabies: warm (not hot) shower and apply topical lindane, then rinse off after 24 hours
      c. For lice: massage lindane into head or area infected; leave on for 5 minutes and shampoo out; do not get agent into eyes or on face; do not repeat treatment in less than 1 week

      11. Client education

        a. See Box 11-2 for universal teaching points for anti-infectives

        b. Report side or adverse effects to healthcare provider

        c. Wash clothes and linens after treatment and use hot setting on dryer to prevent reinfection; place nonwashable items in sealed airtight plastic bags for 2 weeks

        d. Know clinical manifestations of infections to recognize and report

VI. ANTIHELMINTHICS

A. Action and use

    1. Effective against *Ascaris lumbricoides* (intestinal roundworm infestation)**,** *Enterobius vermicularis* (pinworm), *Ancytostoma duodenale* (hookworm)**,** *Necator americanus* (hookworm), and *Trichostrongylus* (intestinal worm infestation)

    2. Most antihelminthics work by inhibiting glucose transport and uncoupling metabolism in parasite's mitochondria

B. Common oral antihelminthic medications (Box 11-6)

C. Administration considerations

    1. Mebendazole: may be chewed, swallowed whole, crushed, mixed with food

    2. Pyrantel: may take with food

    3. Thiabendazole: take after meals

D. Contraindications

    1. Known hypersensitivity

    2. Piperazine citrate: in renal or hepatic impairment, seizure disorders

    3. Mebendazole: use cautiously in inflammatory bowel disease; contraindicated with liver disease or during pregnancy

    4. Use cautiously with other anthelmintics in clients with hepatic or renal dysfunction

    5. Safety not established in pregnancy and lactation

E. Significant drug interactions

    1. Piperazine citrate: may decrease pyrantel pamoate levels

    2. Phenothiazines: may increase extrapyramidal effects or risk for seizures

    3. Carbamazepine and phenytoin can increase metabolism of mebendazole, therefore decreasing blood levels

F. Significant food interactions: high-fat foods may increase absorption of mebendazole

G. Significant laboratory studies

    1. Liver and renal function studies

    2. Stool for ova and parasites (O & P) for accurate diagnosis of **helminths** (disease-producing parasites)

Box 11-6 **Antihelminthics for Worm Infestations**	Albendazole Ivermectin Mebendazole Praziquantel Pyrantel Thiabendazole

H. Side effects
1. Nausea and vomiting, diarrhea, abdominal cramps, anorexia
2. Rash, urticaria, erythema multiforme, photosensitivity, purpura, lacrimation, rhinorrhea
3. Dizziness, drowsiness, vision changes
4. Fever, productive cough, anemia
5. Thiabendazole: urinary odor

I. Adverse effects/toxicity
1. Low toxicity; adverse effects usually with large doses
2. Neurotoxicity: headache, vertigo, ataxia, tremors, jerking movements, muscle weakness, paresthesia, depressed reflexes, mental changes, abnormal ECG, seizures
3. Dose-related neutropenia; reversed with discontinuation of drug

J. Client-centered nursing care (see Box 11-1 again)
1. Assess laboratory findings for hepatic, renal, or blood disorders and to verify diagnosis
2. Collect stool specimen for O & P for baseline and follow-up to verify eradication of infectious agents

K. Client education
1. See Box 11-2 for universal teaching points for anti-infectives
2. Recognize and report evidence of effectiveness as well as adverse effects that may require discontinuation of drug
3. Agents may be taken with or after food to minimize gastric disturbances
4. Store drug at room temperature protected from light and heat
5. Do not repeat drug therapy for continued infection until 1 week after initial treatment
6. Practice personal hygiene to prevent transmission
7. Urine odor may occur with thiabendazole
8. Mebendazole may be chewed, swallowed whole, crushed, or mixed with food
9. Do not drive or operate machinery after dose of praziquantel

Case Study

A 25-year-old married female client has tested positive for group A Streptococcus of the oropharyngeal area. The sensitivity report is not yet available. Amoxicillin PO is to be initiated as empiric drug therapy.

1. What baseline assessment, including laboratory findings, is indicated prior to administering the first dose of amoxicillin?
2. How should you evaluate drug effectiveness?
3. If the client developed diarrhea, how would you differentiate the diarrhea from pseudomembranous colitis? What interventions would you implement to manage the diarrhea? For what fluid and electrolyte imbalance would you monitor?
4. Why is it important to ensure completion of the antibiotic therapy? What two infectious sequela may occur with inadequate therapy against group A streptococcus?
5. What client education would be appropriate?

For suggested responses, see pages 542–543.

POSTTEST

1 While teaching the client about newly prescribed oral metronidazole, what information would be most important for the nurse to include?

1. Avoid intake of alcoholic beverages.
2. Headache may accompany drug ingestion.
3. Drug may cause constipation.
4. Drug may cause vaginal dryness.

2 Which statement by an immunocompromised client to the nurse best indicates that the client understands self-application of the topical drug acyclovir?

1. "I need to wash my hands for at least 10 seconds before and after applying the drug."
2. "I need to apply several thin layers of the medication on the lesions."
3. "I need to avoid touching the lesions and opening the container with the same finger cot."
4. "I should not allow anyone else to use this drug."

3 A nurse is assigned to a client who has received amphotericin B 0.3 mg/kg/day IV for 5 days. The nurse should place priority on reviewing the client's record for which data?

1. Alanine aminotransferase (ALT) and aspartate aminotransferase (AST) levels
2. Sodium level and serum protein
3. Blood urea nitrogen (BUN) and creatinine
4. Number and consistency of stools in the past 24 hours

4 A client is receiving combination drug therapy of isoniazid, rifampin, and pyrazinamide for treatment of tuberculosis. What information should the nurse include in client education? Select all that apply.

1. Treatment will take 2 weeks.
2. Finish taking all doses of isoniazid before starting ethambutol.
3. Eliminate alcohol intake during drug therapy.
4. Aluminum-containing antacids decrease the absorption of isoniazid.
5. Vitamin B_6 may help prevent side effects such as seizures and metabolic acidosis.

5 The nurse is teaching a group of clients who are infected with HIV about the various available drug treatments. Which point of information would be important for the nurse to explain during the discussion using appropriate terminology?

1. Entry inhibitors enhance release of reverse transcriptase.
2. Protease inhibitors are the most potent anti-HIV drugs.
3. Nonnucleoside reverse transcriptase inhibitors (NNRTIs) prevent replication of HIV.
4. Nucleoside transcriptase inhibitors (NRTIs) suppress production of reverse transcriptase.

6 The nurse should include which information when instructing a client who has been started on mebendazole for the treatment of pinworms?

1. Do not chew or crush the tablets.
2. Take the medication with fatty food.
3. Use sunscreen when going outdoors.
4. The drug may cause constipation.

7 A client is scheduled to receive fidaxomicin. What information should the nurse include in client teaching? Select all that apply.

1. Because the drug is not absorbed, it is effective against *Clostridium difficile*.
2. This is one of the medications used for combination therapy of tuberculosis.
3. This medication is not effective for treatment of systemic infections.
4. Do not stop taking until the full course of treatment is completed.
5. Do not take if allergic to erythromycin.

8 When hanging an intravenous dose of vancomycin, the nurse administers the drug over 90 minutes to prevent which speed-related adverse drug effect?

1. Hypertension
2. Projectile vomiting
3. Flushing of face, neck, and chest
4. Pseudomembranous colitis

9 After liquid tetracycline is prescribed for a 2-year-old child, the nurse provides which most important instruction to the licensed practical or vocational nurse (LPN/LVN) who is administering the medication?

1. "Have the client drink the dose through a straw."
2. "Withhold the dose until I telephone the prescriber."
3. "Monitor the client for diarrhea."
4. "Administer with 6–8 ounces of milk."

10 A client has been prescribed to take both a tetracycline and a sulfonamide drug. When providing client teaching, what priority information should the nurse give the client related to adverse drug effects?

1. "Avoid exposure to upper respiratory infections."
2. "Use protective measures when exposed to the sun."
3. "Report problems with constipation to your provider."
4. "Change position slowly to avoid orthostatic hypotension."

➤ *See pages 386–387 for Answers and Rationales.*

ANSWERS & RATIONALES

Pretest

1 **Answers: 1, 3, 4, 5 Rationale:** Isoniazid can be hepatotoxic and aspartate aminotransferase (AST) levels reflect liver inflammation or damage. The client should be monitored for elevated levels. Antacids interfere with absorption of isoniazid when taken within 1–2 hours of the isoniazid, so the nurse should ensure that ingestion of the antacid dose is separated from the isoniazid dose by 2 hours. Vitamin B_6 should be administered with isoniazid therapy to reduce the incidence of peripheral neuritis. Thrombocytopenia is an adverse effect of isoniazid, which can lead to the potential for bleeding and excessive bruising. Isoniazid can cause hypocalcemia, not hypercalcemia. **Cognitive Level:** Applying **Client Need:** Pharmacological and Parenteral Therapies **Integrated Process:** Nursing Process: Assessment **Content Area:** Pharmacology **Strategy:** Correlate

major drug side effects with the client's signs and symptoms and also consider drug interactions (antacids and vitamin B_6). **References:** Wilson, B. A., Shannon, M. T., & Shields, K. M. (2017). *Pearson nurse's drug guide 2017.* New York, NY: Pearson, pp. 856–858; Adams, M. P., & Urban, C. (2015). *Pharmacology: Connections to nursing practice* (3rd ed.). New York, NY: Pearson, pp. 558, 563.

2 **Answers: 4, 2, 5, 1, 3 Rationale:** The client is manifesting indications of an infiltrated IV line. The nurse should first stop the infusion. After stopping the infusion, the nurse should remove the peripheral catheter. After discontinuing the catheter, the nurse should apply a sterile dressing. Once the line is removed and the site is dressed, the nurse should elevate extremity. The last step is to apply a warm compress to help reabsorb IV fluid that has infiltrated into the tissue. **Cognitive Level:** Applying **Client Need:** Pharmacological and Parenteral

Therapies **Integrated Process:** Nursing Process: Implementation **Content Area:** Pharmacology **Strategy:** Note the question is asking for the correct sequence of actions. Visualize the procedure to aid in answering correctly. **References:** Ignatavicius, D. D., & Workman, M. L. (2016). *Medical-surgical nursing: Patient-centered collaborative care* (8th ed.). Philadelphia, PA: Elsevier, p. 207; Berman, A., Snyder, S., & Frandsen, G. (2016). *Kozier & Erb's fundamentals of nursing: Concepts, process, and practice* (10th ed.). New York, NY: Pearson, p. 1355.

3 **Answer: 2 Rationale:** A common side effect of oseltamivir is diarrhea; others include nausea and vomiting and dizziness. Stevens–Johnson syndrome is a rare side effect of peramivir. Urinary frequency is not associated with oseltamivir. Nephrotoxicity is not associated with oseltamivir, although it is an adverse effect of aminoglycoside antiobiotics. **Cognitive Level:** Applying **Client Need:** Pharmacological and Parenteral Therapies **Integrated Process:** Nursing Process: Assessment **Content Area:** Pharmacology **Strategy:** Specific knowledge of drug side effects is needed to answer the question. Consider that GI symptoms are common side effects of many medications. **Reference:** Adams, M. P., Holland, N., & Urban, C. (2017). *Pharmacology for nurses: A pathophysiologic approach* (5th ed.). New York, NY: Pearson, p. 604.

4 **Answer: 4 Rationale:** Acyclovir can be nephrotoxic and so it is important to ensure high fluid intake to keep the client well hydrated and perfuse the kidneys. Acyclovir is not hepatotoxic. It would not be necessary to avoid sexual intercourse while taking this medication. Acyclovir drug may cause headaches and nausea and vomiting, but not insomnia. **Cognitive Level:** Applying **Client Need:** Pharmacological and Parenteral Therapies **Integrated Process:** Nursing Process: Implementation **Content Area:** Pharmacology **Strategy:** To answer this question correctly, it is necessary to know specific information about this drug. Determine nursing interventions according to knowledge of drug characteristics. **Reference:** Wilson, B. A., Shannon, M. T., & Shields, K. M. (2017). *Pearson nurse's drug guide 2017.* New York, NY: Pearson, pp. 21–24.

5 **Answer: 1 Rationale:** A full course of antibiotic therapy must be taken in order to decrease the risk of resistance to the antibiotic or recurrence of the infection. Missed doses should be taken as soon as they are remembered and the dose should not be doubled. Antibiotic doses are to be taken at regular intervals spaced throughout the 24 hours, without interrupting sleep when possible, to maintain effective therapeutic blood level of the antibiotic. Chewable tablets must be crushed or chewed or the drug may not absorb adequately. Attempting to swallow chewable tablets could also put the client at risk for airway obstruction. **Cognitive Level:** Analyzing **Client Need:** Pharmacological

and Parenteral Therapies **Integrated Process:** Nursing Process: Evaluation **Content Area:** Pharmacology **Strategy:** The core issue of the question is knowledge that antibiotic therapy needs to be taken for the full course of therapy to effectively eradicate infection and prevent development of drug resistance. Apply knowledge of client compliance issues and potential outcomes. **Reference:** Adams, M. P., & Urban, C. (2015). *Pharmacology: Connections to nursing practice* (3rd ed.). New York, NY: Pearson, pp. 559–561.

6 **Answers: 1, 4 Rationale:** The client is at risk for developing metabolic acidosis because of increased loss of bowel contents that consist primarily of alkaline fluids. Excessive watery stools or stools that contain blood may indicate pseudomembranous colitis, caused by the toxins released by *C. difficile.* A stool specimen should be collected as a priority measure. If the cause of the diarrhea is *C. difficile,* the toxin needs to be eliminated. Antiperistaltic agents or antidiarrheal agents can promote retention of toxins and should not be given. Some fruit juices could further exacerbate diarrhea and would not be encouraged. **Cognitive Level:** Applying **Client Need:** Pharmacological and Parenteral Therapies **Integrated Process:** Nursing Process: Implementation **Content Area:** Pharmacology **Strategy:** Correlate the most life-threatening side effects exhibited by GI alterations with the specific drug and the specific microorganism. This will allow you to systematically select the options that should be anticipated by the nurse. **Reference:** Adams, M. P., & Urban, C. (2015). *Pharmacology: Connections to nursing practice* (3rd ed.). New York, NY: Pearson, pp. 541, 696–697.

7 **Answers: 2, 5 Rationale:** Aminoglycosides, such as tobramycin, can cause ototoxicity and nephrotoxicity. The nurse should review the client's creatinine level to detect onset of nephrotoxicity. The nurse should assess for ringing in the ears as an indicator of ototoxicity. Hand strength is a routine neurologic assessment that is not required during aminoglycoside therapy. ALT levels are an indicator of liver function. Amylase levels are an indicator of pancreatic function. **Cognitive Level:** Applying **Client Need:** Pharmacological and Parenteral Therapies **Integrated Process:** Nursing Process: Evaluation **Content Area:** Pharmacology **Strategy:** Recall that aminoglycosides tend to cause ototoxicity and nephrotoxicity. Evaluate each option in relation to these toxicities to select the correct options. **Reference:** Adams, M. P., Holland, N., & Urban, C. (2017). *Pharmacology for nurses: A pathophysiologic approach* (5th ed.). New York, NY: Pearson, pp. 548–550.

8 **Answers: 3, 5 Rationale:** The tablets should not be crushed because it can alter drug release for absorption. Erythromycin can cause severe diarrhea with life-threatening pseudomembranous colitis, so the provider should be notified if this occurs. Erythromycin should be taken with a full glass of water for best absorption. Fruit juices and some carbonated beverages can interfere with complete absorption and so should be avoided. Abdominal fullness is a vague symptom that is not expected during therapy with erythromycin; abdominal pain would be more common. Hearing loss (from ototoxicity) does not occur with erythromycin therapy, because it is a macrolide antibiotic, not an aminoglycoside. **Cognitive Level:** Applying **Client Need:** Pharmacological and Parenteral Therapies **Integrated Process:** Nursing Process: Evaluation **Content Area:** Pharmacology **Strategy:** Recall the toxicities and drug interactions that could occur with erythromycin to choose the correct options. **Reference:** Adams, M. P., Holland, N., & Urban, C. (2017). *Pharmacology for nurses: A pathophysiologic approach* (5th ed.). New York, NY: Pearson, pp. 547–548.

9 **Answer: 4 Rationale:** There is a small chance that the client may have a cross-allergenicity with penicillin, and it is worth discussing with the prescriber, who may choose a drug from another category. The BUN is within normal limits. It is expected that granulocytosis (such as elevated neutrophils) would occur in response to a bacterial infection. It is common practice to collect the specimen for culture and sensitivity (C&S), then begin therapy with a broad-spectrum antibiotic, which can be changed if the C&S reveals that a different drug would be more appropriate. **Cognitive Level:** Analyzing **Client Need:** Pharmacological and Parenteral Therapies **Integrated Process:** Nursing Process: Planning **Content Area:** Pharmacology **Strategy:** Identify common, life-threatening side effects of antibiotics, such as hypersensitivity. Next, associate this risk with the appropriate nursing action. **Reference:** Adams, M. P., Holland, N., & Urban, C. (2017). *Pharmacology for nurses: A pathophysiologic approach* (5th ed.). New York, NY: Pearson, pp. 544–546.

10 **Answer: 1 Rationale:** Gram stain testing is a method of classifying bacteria. Bacteria with a thick cell wall retain a purple color after staining and are called gram-positive bacteria. Bacteria with thinner cell walls lose the violet stain and are called gram-negative bacteria. Some antibiotics are only effective for gram-positive or gram-negative bacteria, so this is necessary information. Gram stain has no use in determining drug therapy for acute viral infection, parasitic infection, or fungal infection. **Cognitive Level:** Analyzing **Client Need:** Pharmacological and Parenteral Therapies **Integrated Process:** Nursing Process: Planning **Content Area:** Pharmacology **Strategy:** Use knowledge of assessing types of microorganisms. The words *gram stain* constitute a critical phrase. **Reference:** Adams, M. P., Holland, N., & Urban, C. (2017). *Pharmacology for nurses: A pathophysiologic approach* (5th ed.). New York, NY: Pearson, p. 536.

Posttest

1 **Answer: 1 Rationale:** Ingesting alcoholic beverages with metronidazole can result in a *disulfiram reaction*, including exaggerated sympathomimetic signs/symptoms. Headache, constipation, and vaginal dryness may occur and can be easily managed, but are not as significant as tachycardia and flushing. **Cognitive Level:** Analyzing **Client Need:** Pharmacological and Parenteral Therapies **Integrated Process:** Teaching and Learning **Content Area:** Pharmacology **Strategy:** Note the critical words *most important* in the question. Evaluate each option and select the one that will likely have the greatest negative effect on the client. **Reference:** Adams, M. P., Holland, N., & Urban, C. (2017). *Pharmacology for nurses: A pathophysiologic approach* (5th ed.). New York, NY: Pearson, p. 580.

2 **Answer: 3 Rationale:** A different gloved finger or a different finger cot should be used to apply acyclovir to each lesion not only to prevent spread on client's own body, but also to prevent spread of the virus. Hand hygiene is a standard precaution associated with infection control for all clients. One thin layer of medication is sufficient. Not sharing medication with others is a universal principle associated with drug therapy. **Cognitive Level:** Applying **Client Need:** Pharmacological and Parenteral Therapies **Integrated Process:** Nursing Process: Evaluation **Content Area:** Pharmacology **Strategy:** Correlate the characteristics of the target microorganism with the client's needs. **Reference:** Wilson, B. A., Shannon, M. T., & Shields, K. M. (2017). *Pearson nurse's drug guide 2017.* New York, NY: Pearson, pp. 21–24.

3 **Answer: 3 Rationale:** Since this drug can be nephrotoxic, it would be most important to check BUN and creatinine as indicators of renal function. Alanine aminotransferase (ALT) and aspartate aminotransferase (AST) reflect liver function and damage and would be assessed prior to beginning drug therapy as a general routine measure. Serum sodium levels could indirectly reflect renal function, but are not as important as checking direct indicators of kidney function. Monitoring serum protein is not necessary. Diarrhea can be a side effect but the priority assessment is the client's renal function. **Cognitive Level:** Applying **Client Need:** Pharmacological and Parenteral Therapies **Integrated Process:** Nursing Process: Assessment **Content Area:** Pharmacology **Strategy:** Associate the drug with nephrotoxicity. From this point, determine which option *best* reflects kidney function. **Reference:** Adams, M. P., Holland, N., & Urban, C. (2017). *Pharmacology for nurses: A pathophysiologic approach* (5th ed.). New York, NY: Pearson, p. 570.

4 **Answers: 3, 4, 5 Rationale:** Drug therapy for tuberculosis lasts 6–24 months. The medications are taken concurrently, not one after another. Alcohol intake can cause hepatotoxicity when ingested in combination with these drugs. Aluminum-containing antacids decrease the absorption of isoniazid. Vitamin B_6 is used to prevent seizures and to prevent or correct metabolic acidosis. The dose may be repeated several times. **Cognitive Level:** Analyzing **Client Need:** Pharmacological and Parenteral Therapies **Integrated Process:** Nursing Process: Diagnosis **Content Area:** Pharmacology **Strategy:** Note first that tuberculosis requires prolonged treatment and that combination therapy means at the same time. Apply knowledge of the administration guidelines for the specific drugs. **Reference:** Adams, M. P., Holland, N., & Urban, C. (2017). *Pharmacology for nurses: A pathophysiologic approach* (5th ed.). New York, NY: Pearson, p. 558.

5 **Answer: 4 Rationale:** NRTIs suppress production of reverse transcriptase, which prevents conversion of viral RNA to DNA similar to human DNA. Entry inhibitors work by blocking attachment of the HIV virus to the host cell. Protease inhibitors block protease (which is needed for cell replication) and are used in conjunction with other drugs to reduce the viral load in HIV. NNRTI drugs work by reducing the synthesis of reverse transcriptor A. **Cognitive Level:** Applying **Client Need:** Pharmacological and Parenteral Therapies **Integrated Process:** Teaching and Learning **Content Area:** Pharmacology **Strategy:** Compare and contrast the major elements existing among the drug categories. Associate the conclusions with the disease process. **Reference:** Burchum, J. (2016). *Lehne's pharmacology for nursing care* (9th ed.). St. Louis, MO: Elsevier, p. 1128.

6 **Answer: 2 Rationale:** Taking mebendazole with fatty food will help to improve absorption. The tablets may be chewed for maximum effectiveness, swallowed whole, crushed, or mixed with food. Mebendazole does not cause photosensitivity so sunscreen is not necessary because of this drug. It may cause abdominal cramping and diarrhea, but not constipation. **Cognitive Level:** Applying **Client Need:** Pharmacological and Parenteral Therapies **Integrated Process:** Teaching and Learning **Content Area:** Pharmacology **Strategy:** Recall that mebendazole is an antihelminthic and recall specific information about this medication. **Reference:** Adams, M. P., Holland, N., & Urban, C. (2017). *Pharmacology for nurses: A pathophysiologic approach* (5th ed.). New York, NY: Pearson, p. 582.

7 **Answers: 1, 3, 4, 5 Rationale:** Fidaxomicin is a macrolide antibiotic that does not absorb and therefore is effective against *Clostridium difficile* or pseudomembranous colitis. It is not used for tuberculosis. It is not effective for treatment of systemic infections. As with other antibiotics, the client should not stop taking until the full course of treatment is completed. Because it is a macrolide antibiotic, it should not be taken if the client is allergic to erythromycin, another macrolide antibiotic. **Cognitive Level:** Applying **Client Need:** Pharmacological and Parenteral Therapies **Integrated Process:** Nursing Process: Implementation **Content Area:** Pharmacology **Strategy:** First recognize the drug classification. The wording of the question indicates that more than one answer is correct, so evaluate each one as a true-false statement. **Reference:** Wilson, B. A., Shannon, M. T., & Shields, K. M. (2017). *Pearson nurse's drug guide 2017.* New York, NY: Pearson, pp. 673–674.

8 **Answer: 3 Rationale:** Flushing of the face, neck, and chest, which is known as "red man syndrome" or "red neck syndrome," is associated with too-rapid administration of vancomycin. Hypotension, not hypertension, is associated with vancomycin administration. Vancomycin may cause nausea, but not projectile vomiting. Vancomycin is often used to treat *Clostridium difficile*, associated with pseudomembranous colitis. This complication is not associated with speed of the transfusion. **Cognitive Level:** Applying **Client Need:** Pharmacological and Parenteral Therapies **Integrated Process:** Nursing Process: Assessment **Content Area:** Pharmacology **Strategy:** Recall that "red neck syndrome" or "red man syndrome" occurs with rapid infusion and use this to choose from the available options. **Reference:** Adams, M. P., Holland, N., & Urban, C. (2017). *Pharmacology for nurses: A pathophysiologic approach* (5th ed.). New York, NY: Pearson, p. 556.

9 **Answer: 2 Rationale:** Tetracycline is contraindicated in children less than 8 years of age because it causes permanent tooth discoloration. The prescription should be questioned by the nurse. Drinking through a straw is necessary when administering liquid iron preparations, but not tetracycline. Tooth discoloration is caused by systemic absorption, not direct contact. The drug may cause diarrhea, but this is not the most important consideration. Milk and other dairy products will decrease the absorption of tetracycline. **Cognitive Level:** Applying **Client Need:** Pharmacological and Parenteral Therapies **Integrated Process:** Nursing Process: Planning **Content Area:** Pharmacology **Strategy:** Associate this drug with staining of teeth in children less than 8 years old and use this information to eliminate the incorrect options. **Reference:** Wilson, B. A., Shannon, M. T., & Shields, K. M. (2017). *Pearson nurse's drug guide 2017.* New York, NY: Pearson, pp. 536–537.

10 **Answer: 2 Rationale:** Photosensitivity is a side effect of both classes of antibiotics. The client should avoid sun exposure and tanning beds. These drugs would not increase the client's risk for upper respiratory infections. Orthostatic hypotension and constipation are not side effects of either drug. **Cognitive Level:** Applying **Client Need:** Pharmacological and Parenteral Therapies **Integrated Process:** Teaching and Learning **Content Area:** Pharmacology **Strategy:** Look for the option that illustrates teaching associated with an adverse drug effect that occurs with both drugs. In this case, the correct option relates to photosensitivity. **Reference:** Wilson, B. A., Shannon, M. T., & Shields, K. M. (2017). *Pearson nurse's drug guide 2017.* New York, NY: Pearson, pp. 556–558, 1481–1484.

References

Adams, M. P., Holland, N., & Urban, C. (2017). *Pharmacology for nurses: A pathophysiologic approach* (5th ed.). New York, NY: Pearson.

Adams, M. P., & Urban, C. (2015). *Pharmacology: Connections to nursing practice* (3rd ed.). New York, NY: Pearson.

Berman, A., Snyder, S., & Frandsen, G. (2016). *Kozier & Erb's fundamentals of nursing: Concepts, process, and practice* (10th ed.). New York, NY: Pearson.

Burchum, J. & Rosenthal, L. (2016). *Lehne's pharmacology for nursing care* (9th ed.). St. Louis, MO: Elsevier.

Drug Facts & Comparisons (Updated monthly). St. Louis, MO: A. Wolters Kluwer.

Holland, L., Adams, M., & Brice, J. (2018). *Core concepts in pharmacology* (5th ed.). New York, NY: Pearson.

Ignatavicius, D. D., & Workman, M. L. (2016). *Medical-surgical nursing: Patient-centered collaborative care* (8th ed.). Philadelphia, PA: Elsevier.

Kee, J. L. (2017). *Pearson handbook of laboratory and diagnostic tests with nursing implications* (8th ed.). New York, NY: Pearson.

LeMone, P., Burke, K., Bauldoff, G., & Gubrud, P. (2015). *Medical surgical nursing: Clinical reasoning in patient care* (6th ed.). New York, NY: Pearson.

Wilson, B. A., Shannon, M. T., & Shields, K. M. (2017). *Pearson nurse's drug guide 2017.* New York, NY: Pearson.

Antineoplastic Medications

12

Chapter Outline

Alkylating Agents
Antimetabolites
Antitumor Antibiotics
Plant-Based Antineoplastic
   Agents

Hormones and Hormone
   Modulators
Other Antineoplastics
Safe Handling of
   Chemotherapeutic Agents

Nursing Management of
   Treatment Side Effects

Objectives

➤ Describe the general goals of antineoplastic therapy.
➤ Describe the common side effects of antineoplastic medications.
➤ Identify primary toxic effects associated with antineoplastic therapy.
➤ Identify nursing interventions for the client with depressed white blood cell production, bleeding tendencies, or stomatitis.
➤ List the significant client education points related to antineoplastic medications.

NCLEX-RN® Test Prep

Access the NEW Web-based app that provides students with additional practice questions in preparation for the NCLEX experience.

Review at a Glance

acral erythema red palms
alopecia partial or complete hair loss
anticipatory nausea conditioned response resulting from repeated association of chemotherapy-induced nausea and vomiting and a stimulus from the environment
cell-cycle nonspecific chemotherapy agent that exhibits its cytotoxic effect regardless of the stage of cell division

cell-cycle specific chemotherapy agent that exhibits its cytotoxic effect at a certain stage of cell division
chemotherapy-induced nausea and vomiting (CINV) severe nausea associated with the use of highly emetogenic chemotherapy agents
hemorrhagic cystitis chemical irritation of bladder that causes bleeding and hematuria
irritant a chemotherapy agent that causes redness and irritation of

skin upon extravasation, but without sloughing
nadir lowest point to which blood counts will drop after chemotherapy administration
myelosuppression decrease in blood counts usually related to chemotherapy
vesicant medication that causes severe skin and tissue necrosis if it extravasates from the vein

1 A client with cancer is receiving vincristine. The nurse should assess for which finding as an early indicator of neurotoxicity from vincristine?

1. Confusion
2. Short-term memory loss
3. Depression of the Achilles reflex
4. Decreased hand-grasp strength

2 The nurse should focus on which set of nursing interventions that are most likely to prevent cardiotoxicity in a client receiving doxorubicin?

1. Exercise and smoking cessation
2. Smoking cessation and oxygen (O_2) administration
3. Exercise and administration of dexrazoxane
4. O_2 administration and a low-fat diet

3 A client is experiencing manifestations of pulmonary toxicity related to chemotherapy. To maximize the client's respiratory potential, the nurse should teach the client to take which actions? Select all that apply.

1. Elevate head of the bed.
2. Exhale through pursed lips.
3. Perform shallow, slow breathing during activity.
4. Exhale using accessory muscles.
5. Plan rest and exercise periods.

4 The nurse should include management of pulmonary toxicity in the plan of care for clients receiving which antineoplastic agent?

1. 5-fluorouracil
2. Bleomycin
3. Etoposide
4. Paclitaxel

5 A nurse is caring for a client receiving chemotherapy. The nurse explains that taking measures to reduce mucositis should have which effect for the client?

1. Increased comfort
2. Decreased risk of infection
3. Maintenance of self-image
4. Reduced risk of cancer recurrence

6 Several clients have received chemotherapy in an outpatient clinic. Which client should the nurse expect to have increased episodes of nausea and vomiting?

1. Mother of two who experienced severe morning sickness during both of her pregnancies
2. Navy pilot who experienced motion sickness as a child
3. 38-year-old male who has alcoholism
4. Young woman with no significant history of emesis

7 The nurse should plan to include which nursing intervention in the care of a client experiencing neutropenia?

1. Insert an indwelling urinary catheter to maintain accurate intake and output.
2. Leave all wounds open to the air for better healing.
3. Encourage regular oral care and perianal care after each stool.
4. Flush all lumens of the long-term intravenous catheter with heparinized saline every 8 hours.

8 A client with cancer has breakdown of oral mucous membranes because of side effects of fluorouracil, an antimetabolite. The nurse should plan to implement which optimal nursing intervention?

1. Schedule oral hygiene every 2 hours during the day with warm saline rinses.
2. Rinse mouth every 2 hours during the day and every 4 hours at night with a baking soda and peroxide rinse.
3. Schedule oral care every 2 to 4 hours with a soft-bristle toothbrush and fluorinated toothpaste, followed by a dilute baking soda rinse.
4. Continue oral hygiene twice daily with baking soda and rinse with commercial mouthwash.

9 A client receiving vincristine is at risk for developing constipation. In order to reduce this risk, the nurse should help the client to make which lifestyle changes? Select all that apply.

1. Increase physical activity.
2. Add fiber to the diet.
3. Use laxative of choice.
4. Increase fluid intake.
5. Ingest antiflatulent of choice.

10 The nurse should share with a client who has cancer which important advantage of combination chemotherapy over single-drug regimens?

1. Reduce potential for nausea and vomiting.
2. Reduce potential for tumor resistance.
3. Spare normal cells from severe toxicity.
4. Decrease likelihood of drug-induced gonadal sterility.

➤ *See pages 418–420 for Answers and Rationales.*

I. ALKYLATING AGENTS

A. Action and use

1. Interfere with DNA replication through cross-linking of DNA strands, DNA strand breaking, and abnormal base pairing proteins
2. Most agents are **cell-cycle nonspecific**, which means that they exhibit a cytotoxic effect in multiple phases of cell cycle; most effective in the G_0 phase

3. Major toxicities occur in hematopoietic, gastrointestinal (GI), and reproductive systems
4. There are three major types of alkylating agents:
   a. Nitrogen mustards: commonly cyclophosphamide, ifosfamide
   b. Platinum compounds: commonly cisplatin, carboplatin
   c. Nitrosoureas: commonly carmustine, streptozocin

B. Common alkylating medications: see Table 12-1

C. Administration considerations

1. Nitrogen mustards
   a. Hydrate with oral or intravenous (IV) fluids before administering dose

   b. Administer by mouth on an empty stomach; if nausea and vomiting are severe it may be taken with food; antiemetic agent should be given before the drug is administered
   c. Administer intravenous piggyback (IVPB) dose over 60–90 minutes
2. Mechlorethamine
   a. Potent **vesicant** (causes severe skin and tissue necrosis if medication extravasates from vein)
   b. Should be administered through side-arm portal of a freely running intravenous to avoid extravasation

Table 12-1 Common Alkylating Agents	
Generic Name	**Route**
Nitrogen Mustards	
Bendamustine	IV
Chlorambucil	PO
Cyclophosphamide	PO, IV
Estramustine	PO
Ifosfamide	IV
Mechlorethamine	IV, IT, T
Melphalan	PO, IV
Nitrosoureas	
Carmustine	IV
Lomustine	PO
Streptozocin	IV
Platinum Compounds	
Carboplatin	IV
Cisplatin	IV
Oxaliplatin	IV
Miscellaneous Alkylating Agents	
Busulfan	PO, IV
Dacarbazine	IV
Procarbazine	PO
Temozolomide	PO, IV
Thiotepa	PO, IC

    c. If drug should extravasate, subcutaneous and intradermal injection with isotonic sodium thiosulfate and application of ice compresses may reduce local irritation

    d. Short **nadir** period (6–8 days), which is the lowest point to which blood counts will drop after chemotherapy administration

    e. Wear surgical gloves during preparation and avoid inhalation of powder and vapors

3. Platinum compounds

    a. General information

        1) Plan to administer a parenteral antiemetic agent before therapy is instituted and give it on a scheduled basis throughout day and night as long as necessary

        2) Needles or intravenous sets containing aluminum should not be used

    b. Cisplatin

        1) Does not cause significant myelosuppression, unlike other alkylating agents

        2) Provide hydration with 1–2 liters of intravenous fluid before and after administration

        3) Obtain baseline electrocardiogram (ECG) and cardiac monitoring during therapy

  c. Carboplatin
   1) First-line palliative treatment of advanced ovarian cancer; less toxic than cisplatin
   2) Do not repeat dosage until neutrophil count is at least 2,000/mm^3
   3) Monitor closely for anaphylaxis during first 15 minutes of infusion
  d. Nitrosourea: carmustine
   1) One of the few drugs that can penetrate blood–brain barrier; used for brain tumors
   2) Administer over 1–2 hours by slow intravenous infusion with constant monitoring if given peripherally
   3) Vesicant: if possible, avoid starting intravenous in dorsum of hand, wrist, or antecubital veins, since extravasation may cause damage to underlying tissues

D. Contraindications
1. Nitrogen mustards
  a. Cyclophosphamide
   1) Use with extreme caution in men and women of childbearing years because of effects on reproductive system
   2) Serious infections including chickenpox and herpes zoster
   3) Immunosuppression
   4) Pregnancy and nursing mothers
  b. Ifosfamide
   1) Severe bone marrow suppression or known hypersensitivity to ifosfamide
   2) Cautious use in clients with impaired renal function, prior radiation therapy, or prior cytotoxic agents
   3) Cautious use in pregnancy (Category D) and nursing mothers
  c. Mechlorethamine
   1) **Myelosuppression**: a decrease in blood counts usually related to chemotherapy
   2) Infectious granuloma
   3) Known infectious diseases, including herpes zoster
   4) Pregnancy (Category D) and lactation
2. Platinum compounds
  a. General
   1) History of sensitivity to platinum-containing compounds
   2) Cautious use in pregnancy (Category D) and with other nephrotoxic drugs
   3) Impaired renal function and/or hearing
  b. Cisplatin: history of gout and urate renal stones
  c. Carboplatin: severe bone marrow depression (thrombocytopenia, leukopenia, and neutropenia)
3. Nitrosourea: carmustine
  a. History of pulmonary function impairment
  b. Decreased platelets, leukocytes, or erythrocytes
  c. Safe use during pregnancy (Category D) not established

E. Significant drug interactions
1. Nitrogen mustards
  a. Cyclophosphamide
   1) Multiple interactions, including a decreased serum level of digoxin if used concurrently
   2) Doxorubicin: may increase cardiotoxicity

    b. Ifosfamide

        1) Barbiturates, phenytoin, and chloral hydrate may increase hepatic conversion of ifosfamide to active metabolite

        2) Corticosteroids may inhibit conversion to active metabolite

  2. Mechlorethamine: may reduce effectiveness of antigout agents by raising serum uric acid levels

  3. Platinum compounds

    a. General

        1) Nephrotoxic drugs such as aminoglycosides, amphotericin-B, and vancomycin increase risk of nephrotoxicity

        2) Aminoglycosides and furosemide increase risk of ototoxicity

        3) Incompatible with 5% dextrose solutions, sodium bicarbonate, and metoclopramide

    b. Carboplatin may decrease phenytoin levels

  4. Carmustine: cimetidine may potentiate neutropenia and thrombocytopenia

F. Significant food interactions

  1. Are primarily for the miscellaneous alkylating agent procarbazine

  2. Avoid foods high in tyramine (e.g., avocado, beer, wine, salami, cheese, brewer's yeast, chicken livers, and bananas) while taking procarbazine, since it may lead to hypertension and possible intracranial hemorrhage

  3. A disulfiram-like reaction can occur if client consumes alcohol and procarbazine

G. Significant assessment parameters

  1. Nitrogen mustards

    a. Cyclophosphamide

        1) Determine total differential leukocyte count, platelet count, and hematocrit initially and at least every 2 weeks thereafter

        2) Obtain baseline and periodic determinations of liver and kidney function in addition to serum electrolytes

        3) Microscopic urine examinations are recommended after large doses

    b. Ifosfamide

        1) Monitor complete blood count (CBC) with differential before each dose; hold dose if WBC is below $2,000/\text{mm}^3$ or platelet count is below $50,000/\text{mm}^3$

        2) Monitor urine before and during each dose for microscopic hematuria

        3) Hydrate with at least 3,000 mL of fluid daily to reduce risk of **hemorrhagic cystitis** (excessive bleeding from bladder due to chemical irritation)

  2. Platinum compounds

    a. Cisplatin

        1) Pretreatment ECG is indicated because of possible myocarditis or focal irritation

        2) Monitor urine output (UO) and specific gravity for 4 consecutive hours before therapy and for 24 hours after; report UO less than 100 mL/hr or a specific gravity of greater than 1.030; a UO of less than 75 mL/hr requires medical intervention

        3) Audiometric testing should be performed before initial dose

        4) Anaphylactic reactions may occur within minutes of drug administration

        5) Assess BUN, serum uric acid, serum creatinine, and urinary creatinine clearance before initiating therapy and every subsequent course

        6) Nephrotoxicity usually occurs within 2 weeks after drug administration and becomes more severe and prolonged with repeated courses

        7) Suspect ototoxicity if client manifests tinnitus or difficulty hearing in the high-frequency range

        8) Assess blood pressure (BP), mental status, pupils, and optic fundi every hour during therapy since hydration increases risk of elevated intracranial pressure

        9) Monitor and report abnormal bowel patterns since constipation may be an early sign of neurotoxicity

    b. Carboplatin

        1) Frequently monitor peripheral blood counts; nadir usually occurs at day 21

        2) Periodically monitor kidney function and creatinine clearance, although it has less renal toxicity than cisplatin

        3) Monitor for peripheral neuropathy, ototoxicity, and visual disturbances, although they occur less frequently than with cisplatin

        4) Monitor clients on diuretic therapy closely since carboplatin may also decrease serum sodium, potassium, calcium, and magnesium levels

3. Nitrosourea: carmustine

    a. Persistent nausea and vomiting may occur 2 hours after drug administration and persist up to 6 hours; prior administration of an antiemetic will help

    b. Monitor blood counts prior to beginning drug therapy and weekly for at least 6 weeks after last dose

    c. Assess results of pulmonary function studies prior to therapy and periodically thereafter

    d. Report symptoms of lung toxicity, such as cough, dyspnea, and fever

    e. Be alert to hepatic and renal insufficiency

H. Side effects/toxicity

1. Nitrogen mustards

    a. Cyclophosphamide

        1) Cardiotoxicity, acute cardiomegaly with high dose; prior radiation therapy and prior anthracycline therapy increases risk

        2) Hemorrhagic cystitis (occasionally chronic and severe)

        3) Metallic taste on administration

        4) Acute myelosuppression

        5) Acral erythema (palmar redness) and sloughing of skin on palms of hands and feet

        6) Decreased sperm production, which may be permanent

        7) Nausea and vomiting

    b. Ifosfamide

        1) Hemorrhagic cystitis, occasionally chronic and severe; mesna is a chemoprotectant used with ifosfamide to minimize bladder damage

        2) Neutropenia and thrombocytopenia

        3) Nausea and vomiting

        4) Hepatic dysfunction and renal toxicity

        5) Somnolence, confusion, and hallucinations

2. Platinum compounds

    a. General

        1) Renal and hepatic toxicity

        2) Peripheral neuropathy; neurotoxicity

        3) Auditory toxicity: 8th cranial nerve damage

        4) Myelosuppression with pronounced thrombocytopenia

        5) Intense nausea and vomiting

3. Nitrosourea: carmustine

    a. Severe nausea and vomiting

    b. Ocular infarctions, retinal hemorrhage, suffusion of conjunctiva

    c. Delayed myelosuppression

    d. Pulmonary infiltration or fibrosis

Practice to Pass

List three measures to assist in the prevention of renal toxicity secondary to cisplatin administration.

I. Client and family education

1. Nitrogen mustards
   a. Cyclophosphamide
      1) Because of the drug's mutagenic potential, teach client to use adequate contraception during and for at least 4 months after termination of drug therapy
      2) Instruct client to void frequently and maintain hydration with oral fluids to at least 3,000 mL/24 hours for 4–5 days before and after therapy
   b. Ifosfamide
      1) Instruct client to void frequently and to maintain hydration
      2) Advise client that susceptibility to infection will increase
      3) Teach client to report any unusual bleeding or bruising
2. Platinum compounds
   a. Cisplatin
      1) Continue maintenance of adequate hydration with oral fluids to at least 3,000 mL/24 hr; report reduced UO, anorexia, nausea and vomiting uncontrolled by antiemetics, fluid retention, and weight gain
      2) Keep vestibular stimulation to a minimum to avoid dizziness or falling
      3) Tingling, numbness, tremors of extremities, loss of position sense and taste, and constipation are early warning signs of neurotoxicity
   b. Carboplatin
      1) Give special attention to strategies to prevent nausea
      2) Explain risk for infection and for hemorrhagic complications related to bone marrow suppression
   c. Instruct client to report paresthesias, visual disturbances, or symptoms of ototoxicity (hearing loss/tinnitus)
3. Nitrosoureas
   a. Myelosuppression is severe and may be cumulative; teach neutropenic precautions and symptoms of sepsis
   b. Teach signs and symptoms of hypoglycemia when administering streptozocin
   c. Teach signs and symptoms of pulmonary toxicity when administering carmustine
   d. Stress need for central venous catheter (CVC) to prevent vascular damage, provide access for laboratory studies (blood draws), and promote ease of providing high-volume IV fluids with antineoplastic drugs

II. ANTIMETABOLITES

A. Action and use
   1. Inhibit protein synthesis, substitute erroneous metabolites or structural analogues during DNA synthesis, and inhibit DNA synthesis
   2. Cancer cells require nutrients to grow; use of antimetabolites disrupt these pathways causing cell death or slowed growth
   3. Most agents are **cell-cycle specific**; that is, they exhibit a cytotoxic affect during a specific phase of the cell cycle, such as the S phase
   4. Used to treat leukemia, solid tumors, and lymphoma
   5. Most toxicity occurs in hematopoietic and GI systems; bone marrow toxicity is the primary adverse effect of drugs in this class
B. **Common antimetabolite medications:** see Table 12-2
C. Administration considerations
   1. Fluorouracil (5FU): usually for palliative treatment for inoperable neoplasms
   2. Cytarabine: blocks DNA synthesis, treating acute myelocytic leukemia
   3. Methotrexate
      a. A powerful immunosuppressant
      b. Avoid skin exposure and inhalation of drug during preparation

Table 12-2 **Common Antimetabolites**

Generic Name	Route
Folic Acid Analogs	
Methotrexate	IV, PO
Pemetrexed	IV
Pralatrexate	IV
Purine Analogs	
Cladribine	IV
Clofarabine	IV
Fludarabine	IV
Mercaptopurine	PO
Nelarabine	IV
Pentostatin	IV
Thioguanine	PO
Pyrimidine Analogs	
Capecitabine	PO
Cytarabine	IV, IT, SQ
Floxuridine (FUDR)	Intra-arterial
Fluorouracil	IV
Gemcitabine	IV

    c. Pregnancy Risk Category X

    d. Treatment of overdose: Leucovorin, which is a reduced form of folic acid

D. Contraindications

    1. Myelosuppression

    2. Pregnancy (Category D) and nursing women

    3. Concurrent administration of hepatotoxic drugs and hematopoietic depressants

    4. Cautious use in clients with hepatic, renal, or immune system impairment

E. Significant drug interactions

    1. Fluorouracil (5FU): cimetidine increases pharmacological effects; thiazide diuretics increase risk of myelosuppression; leucovorin increases cytotoxicity

    2. Cytarabine: decreases bioavailability of digoxin

    3. Methotrexate

      a. Protein-bound drugs (i.e., aspirin, phenytoin, and tetracycline) increase toxicity

      b. Nonsteroidal inflammatory drugs (NSAIDs) increase and prolong methotrexate levels

    4. Mercaptopurine

      a. Allopurinol increases 6-mercaptopurine levels

      b. Warfarin affects prothrombin time (PT) levels

      c. Nondepolarizing muscle relaxants: decreased neuromuscular blockade

    5. Fludarabine: fatal pulmonary toxicity can occur if administered concurrently with pentostatin

    6. Capecitabine: increased risk of excessive bleeding with anticoagulants; increased capecitabine levels and toxicity when combined with leucovorin

F. Significant food interactions: none known

Practice to Pass

What measures should the nurse take to prevent or decrease the severity of stomatitis secondary to the administration of fluorouracil?

    G. Significant assessment parameters
1. Assess baseline CBC, WBC differential, and platelet count prior to administration
2. Notify healthcare provider if WBC is less than 3,500/mm^3 or platelet count less than 100,000/mm^3
3. Assess for signs and symptoms of infection or bleeding

    H. Side effects/toxicity
1. General toxicities for this drug group
   a. Myelosuppression
   b. Nausea and vomiting
   c. Mucosal inflammation: stomatitis
   d. Photosensitivity with or without hyperpigmentation
   e. Diarrhea (most commonly associated with antimetabolites)
2. Fluorouracil: specific side effects/toxicity
   a. Cardiotoxicity mimicking an acute myocardial infarction (MI), angina, cardiogenic shock
   b. Photosensitivity and hyperpigmentation
   c. Cerebellar toxicity
3. Methotrexate: specific side effects/toxicity
   a. Fatal bone marrow toxicity at high doses
   b. Low platelet counts can cause hemorrhage and bruising
   c. Use caution with OTC vitamins due to possibility of folic acid, which decreases response to methotrexate
4. Cytarabine: specific side effects/toxicity
   a. Maculopapular rash, with or without fever
   b. Cytarabine syndrome (rash with or without fever, myalgia, bone pain, malaise)
   c. Chemical conjunctivitis
   d. Acute neurotoxicity: cerebellar toxicity; clients over age 50 are at highest risk
   e. Hepatotoxicity
   f. Acral erythema

    I. Client and family education
1. Self-care measures are important to avoid infection and bleeding
   a. Avoid large crowds
   b. Avoid proximity to people with infections
   c. Avoid over-the-counter (OTC) aspirin-containing medications
   d. Report elevated temperature, fatigue, and other symptoms of infection
2. Perform an oral assessment, maintain scheduled mouth care, and report development of stomatitis to prescriber
3. Maintain a low-residue diet after discharge and report excessive diarrhea (more than three loose stools in 24 hours) to prescriber
4. Darkening of veins, mucous membranes, and fingernails may occur
5. Follow photosensitivity precautions year-round
   a. Use sunscreen with a sun protection factor (SPF) of at least 15
   b. Avoid sun exposure between 10:00 A.M. and 2:00 P.M.
   c. Wear long sleeves and a large-brimmed hat

III. ANTITUMOR ANTIBIOTICS

    A. Action and use
1. Interfere with nucleic acid synthesis and function, inhibit ribonucleic acid (RNA) synthesis, and inhibit DNA synthesis
2. Most agents are cell-cycle nonspecific and treat only a few specific types of cancer
3. Major toxicities occur in hematopoietic, GI, reproductive, and cardiac systems (cumulative doses)

4. Similar in action to alkylating agents, and side effects are also similar
5. All antitumor antibiotics are administered intravenously or directly into a body cavity
B. Common antitumor antibiotic medications: see Table 12-3
C. Administration considerations
1. Most antitumor antibiotics are severe vesicants except for bleomycin (see signs and symptoms of extravasation in Table 12-4 and antidotes for vesicant drugs in Table 12-5)
2. General principles of safe administration
 a. Administer slowly by intravenous push (IVP) via side-arm portal of a freely flowing intravenous line
 b. Maintain clear view of injection site during administration
 c. Intravenous catheter should have an excellent blood return, be recently placed, and not more than 48 hours old before administering vesicant therapy

Table 12-3 Antitumor Antibiotics

Generic Name	Route
Bleomycin	IV
Dactinomycin	IV
Daunorubicin	IV
Doxorubicin	IV
Epirubicin	IV
Idarubicin	IV
Mitomycin	IV
Mitoxantrone	IV
Valrubicin	IC

Table 12-4 Signs and Symptoms of Extravasation

Assessment Parameter	Immediate Manifestations	Delayed Manifestations	Irritation of Vein	Flare Reaction
Pain	Severe pain or burning that lasts minutes to hours and eventually subsides; usually occurs while drug is being given around needle site	Up to 48 hours	Aching and tightness along vein	No pain
Redness	Blotchy redness around needle site; not always present at time of extravasation	Later occurrence	Full length of vein may be reddened or darkened	Immediate blotches or streaks along vein, which usually subside within 30 minutes with or without treatment
Ulceration	Develops insidiously; usually occurs 48–96 hours later	Later occurrence	Not usually	Not usually
Swelling	Severe swelling; usually occurs immediately	Up to 48 hours	Not likely	Wheals may appear along vein line
Blood return	Inability to obtain a blood return	Good blood return during drug administration	Usually	Usually
Other	Change in quality of infusion	Local tingling and sensory deficits	NA	Urticaria

Table 12-5	Antidotes for Vesicant Therapy
Chemotherapeutic Drug	**Antidote**
Nitrogen mustard, cisplatin	Thiosulfate
Dactinomycin	Apply ice and elevate, heat may enhance tissue damage
Doxorubicin	Cold pack with circulating ice water first 24–48 hours
Vinblastine, vincristine, vinorelbine	Hyaluronidase; apply warm pack for first 24–48 hours
Paclitaxel	Hyaluronidase; apply ice for first 24 hours

   d. If possible, avoid use of antecubital veins, wrist or dorsum of hand, where extravasation could damage underlying tendons and nerves
   e. Avoid venous access in an extremity with compromised venous or lymphatic drainage
3. Doxorubicin: extravasation, which can cause severe tissue damage and pain, should be treated with ice packs to the infiltrated area
4. Valrubicin
   a. Used to treat bladder cancer by instilling directly into the bladder
   b. Use aseptic technique to insert urinary catheter to maintain bladder drainage; use gravity to instill valrubicin slowly over several minutes intravesically
   c. Provide increased fluid intake (at least 2L daily) to prevent urate calculi formation
D. Contraindications
   1. General
   a. Myelosuppression increasing the risk of bleeding and coagulation disorders
   b. Use cautiously in clients with compromised hepatic, renal, or pulmonary function or previous cytotoxic drug or radiation therapy
   c. Extreme caution with pregnant or lactating women and women of childbearing age
   d. Hypersensitivity reactions
   2. Valrubicin: perforated bladder and urinary tract infection
E. Significant drug interactions
   1. Serum digoxin levels and phenytoin levels decreased with concurrent use
   2. Multiple incompatibilities, including other chemotherapeutic agents, antibiotics, and other commonly prescribed medications
F. Significant food interactions: none known
G. Significant assessment parameters
   1. General
   a. Assess hepatic, renal, hematopoietic, and cardiac function prior to administration and at regular intervals thereafter and report early signs of dysfunction
   b. Begin a flowchart to establish baseline data, including temperature, pulse, respiration, blood pressure, body weight, laboratory values, intake and output (I&O) ratio and pattern, and cardiac ejection fraction
   c. Closely assess for symptoms of extravasation frequently during administration
   2. Doxorubicin
   a. Give prompt attention to reports of stinging or burning sensation at injection site
   b. Stomatitis is greatest at 2 weeks following therapy; begins with a burning sensation
   c. Nadir usually occurs 10–14 days after administration
   d. Radiation recall, erythema that develops in previously irradiated field, is common
   3. Valrubicin
   a. Assess I&O, reporting urine output less than 30 mL/hour
   b. Monitor temperature because fever could indicate beginning of infection

    4. Bleomycin

       a. Inject a test dose of 2 units or less deeply into muscle to assess anaphylactic response before intravenous administration

       b. Assess vital signs; a febrile reaction is relatively common

       c. Bone marrow toxicity is rare with bleomycin

       d. Pulmonary toxicity occurs in about 10% of clients, most usually in clients over age 70 and when cumulative dose reaches 400 units (also called "Bleo lung")

       e. Radiation recall is common

H. Side effects/toxicity

    1. General

       a. Bone marrow suppression (neutropenia, anemia, thrombocytopenia)

       b. Severe gastrointestinal issues, including severe nausea and vomiting, mucositis, stomatitis, and diarrhea

       c. Cardiotoxicity and pulmonary toxicity

          1) Cardiotoxicity leading to degenerative cardiomyopathy occurs over time

          2) Prior radiation therapy to chest wall may predispose client to enhanced cardiotoxicity

       d. Vesicant: flare reaction is common and may be difficult to distinguish from an extravasation

    2. Bleomycin

       a. Pulmonary toxicity that is dose and age related

       b. Anaphylactic reaction may occur

       c. Mild febrile reaction commonly occurs

       d. Diffuse **alopecia**, skin hyperpigmentation, vesiculation, acne, thickening of skin and nail beds

I. Client and family education

    1. General

       a. Alopecia, which may also involve eyelashes, eyebrows, beard and mustache, and pubic and axillary hair; regrowth of hair usually begins 2–3 months after completion of administration

       b. Report signs and symptoms of infection (e.g., fever and upper respiratory symptoms) and decreased platelet count (e.g., hemorrhage or bleeding)

       c. Use caution with over-the-counter medications including herbal extracts

    2. Bleomycin: notify for changes in breathing, including shortness of breath

    3. Valrubicin: report bladder irritation and passage of red-colored urine; increase fluid intake for 48 hours after administration

IV. PLANT-BASED ANTINEOPLASTIC AGENTS

A. Action and use

    1. Plant-based drugs that arrest or inhibit mitosis

    2. Most agents are cell-cycle specific, M phase

    3. Major toxicities occur in hematopoietic, integumentary, neurologic, and reproductive systems; hypersensitivity reactions may also occur

    4. Bone marrow suppression is the major dose-limiting factor

B. Common plant-based antineoplastic medications: see Table 12-6

C. Administration considerations

    1. Etoposide

       a. Inhibits an enzyme that helps repair DNA damage, thus damaging the tumor's DNA

       b. Administer by slow IV piggyback to avoid hypotension and bronchospasm

---

Practice to Pass

Before administration of a vesicant, list at least three steps the nurse should complete.

Table 12-6	Plant-Based Antineoplastic Agents
Generic Name	**Route**
Vinca Alkaloids	
Vinblastine	IV
Vincristine	IV
Vinorelbine	IV
Taxanes	
Cabazitaxel	IV
Docetaxel	IV
Paclitaxel	IV
Topoisomerase Inhibitors	
Etoposide	IV
Irinotecan	IV
Teniposide	IV
Topotecan	IV
Miscellaneous	
Eribulin	IV

2. Paclitaxel
   a. Generally used for metastatic ovarian and breast cancer
   b. Do not use equipment or devices containing polyvinyl chloride (PVC)
   c. Administer via nitroglycerin tubing with an in-line filter of 0.22 micron or less
   d. Tissue necrosis occurs with extravasation
   e. Requires strict premedication (preferably with dexamethasone, diphenhydramine, and either cimetidine or ranitidine) per protocol order set before administration to prevent anaphylaxis
3. Vincristine
   a. Major advantage: causes minimal immunosuppression
   b. Commonly used for pediatric leukemias, lymphomas, and other solid tumors
   c. Vesicant
      1) Administer into side arm portal of a freely flowing IV
      2) Hyaluronidase is the antidote should extravasation occur; also apply moderate heat to disperse drug and minimize sloughing
D. **Contraindications**
   1. General
      a. Prior allergic reaction to any drugs in this class
      b. Pregnancy: Risk Category D–X
      c. Use cautiously in clients with hepatic, cardiac, or renal impairment
      d. Severe bone marrow depression including baseline neutropenia of less than 1,500 cells/mm^3
   2. Vincristine
      a. Obstructive jaundice
      b. Demyelinating neurologic diseases, preexisting neuromuscular disease
E. **Significant drug interactions**
   1. Etoposide
      a. Anticoagulants, antiplatelet agents, NSAIDs, and aspirin increase risk of bleeding
      b. Do not administer live vaccines

2. Paclitaxel
   a. Increased myelosuppression when administered with cisplatin
   b. Avoid using PVC bags and infusion sets due to leaching of DEPH (plasticizer)
3. Docetaxel: possible interaction with cyclosporine, erythromycin, ketoconazole, terfenadine, or troleandomycin
4. Vincristine: bronchospasm may occur in clients previously treated with mitomycin; hepatic metabolism of vincristine may be decreased when given with asparaginase (doses must be separated by 12–24 hours)

F. **Significant food interactions:** none known

G. **Significant assessment parameters**
   1. General
      a. Assess intravenous site before and after infusion; extravasation can cause thrombophlebitis and necrosis
      b. Assess frequently for symptoms of anaphylaxis
      c. Assess CBC, WBC and differential, and hepatic and renal function before administration and periodically during treatment
   2. Etoposide: monitor VS during and after infusion; if hypotension occurs, stop infusion
   3. Paclitaxel
      a. Monitor for sensitivity reaction during first and second administration of drug; development of angioedema and generalized urticaria requires immediate discontinuation
      b. Monitor VS frequently; bradycardia occurs in 12% of clients who receive the drug
      c. Assess for peripheral neuropathy
   4. Vincristine
      a. Assess for leukopenia, which occurs in a significant number of clients
      b. Perform frequent neurologic checks
         1) Symptoms of toxicity include numbness and tingling in limbs, loss of reflexes
         2) Assess hand grasps and deep tendon reflexes; depression of Achilles reflex is the earliest sign of neuropathy

H. **Side effects/toxicity**
   1. General
      a. Severe myelosuppression, including leukopenia, thrombocytopenia, neutropenia
      b. Severe mucositis and alopecia
   2. Etoposide
      a. Acral erythema and sloughing of skin on palms and soles
      b. Fever and chills during infusion
   3. Paclitaxel
      a. Transient bradycardia
      b. Peripheral neuropathy
      c. Neutropenia, thrombocytopenia
      d. Hypersensitivity reaction including hypotension, bronchospasm, urticaria, and angioedema
   4. Vincristine
      a. Neurotoxicity; loss of sensation on soles of feet and fingertips
      b. Severe constipation and paralytic ileus

I. **Client and family education**
   1. General
      a. Inspect mouth daily for ulcerations and bleeding and avoid obvious **irritants**
      b. Avoid use of products containing aspirin or ibuprofen, razors, or commercial mouthwash to decrease risk of bleeding

Practice to Pass

Constipation is a concern when administering vinca or plant alkaloid medications. What can the nurse do to prevent this treatment side effect?

    c. Use nonhormonal contraceptive measures during therapy and more than 4 months after

    d. Inform of high probability of developing alopecia, which is reversible when therapy is completed

2. Etoposide: make position changes slowly, particularly if client is rising from a recumbent position

3. Paclitaxel

    a. Report dyspnea, chest pain, palpitations, or angioedema

    b. Be aware of and report signs of peripheral neuropathy

4. Vincristine

    a. Maintain a prophylactic regimen against constipation and paralytic ileus

    b. Report a change in bowel habits

    c. Report depression, double vision, paresthesias, pain, and motor problems

V. HORMONES AND HORMONE MODULATORS

A. Action and use

1. Corticosteroids: lyse lymphoid malignancies and have an indirect effect on malignant cells

2. Estrogens: suppress testosterone production in males and alter response of breast cancers to prolactin

3. Progestins: promote palliation and tumor cell regression; exact mechanism of action is unknown

4. Antiestrogens: compete with estrogens for binding with estrogen receptor sites on malignant cells

5. Androgens: hormone therapy that has palliative use in metastatic/advanced carcinoma of breast; used if surgery and irradiation deemed inappropriate; otherwise, tamoxifen is drug of choice for this purpose

6. Androgen antagonists: inhibit binding of androgens at androgen receptor sites in target tissues; indicated for use in metastatic/advanced prostate cancer

B. Common hormones and hormone modulator medications: see Table 12-7

C. Administration considerations

1. Corticosteroids

    a. Oral forms should be administered with meals and may be crushed

    b. IV form should be given slowly by IV piggyback to prevent vaginal and anal burning

2. Estrogens

    a. Give orally immediately after solid food

    b. An exception is estramustine, which is a combination estrogen and nitrogen mustard compound; must be taken with water an hour before meals, and requires that no dairy products or other calcium-containing products be used concurrently

3. Progestins: give orally without regard to meals

4. Estrogen antagonists: give orally; dosage may be decreased if side effects are severe

5. Androgens and anti-androgens: give orally

D. Contraindications

1. Corticosteroids

    a. Systemic infections

    b. Ulcerative colitis, diverticulitis, active or latent peptic ulcer disease

    c. Safe use in pregnancy (Category C) and nursing mothers has not been established

Table 12-7	Hormones and Hormone Modulators		
Generic Name		**Route**	**Uses**
Corticosteroids			
Prednisone		PO	Inflammatory, allergic, and debilitating conditions related to
Dexamethasone		PO, IV	autoimmune disorders, asthma, allergic reactions, and malignancies
Hydrocortisone		PO	
Methylprednisolone		IV	
Estrogens			
Diethylstilbestrol (DES)		PO	Hormone replacement therapy, oral contraceptive, atrophic vaginitis,
Ethinyl estradiol		PO	female hypogonadism, primary ovarian failure, palliation of prostatic and mammary cancers
Antiestrogens			
Tamoxifen Toremifene Anastrozole		PO	Treatment of breast cancer in postmenopausal women, women
Exemestane		PO	without ovarian function, and treatment of prostatic cancer
Fulvestrant		PO	
Letrozole		IM	
Raloxifene			
Progestins			
Medroxyprogesterone acetate		PO, IM	Contraceptive, treatment of amenorrhea, palliative cancer therapy, fertility
Megestrol acetate		PO	Appetite stimulant for anorexia
Anti-androgens (Androgen Receptor Blockers)			
Bicalutamide		PO	Advanced and metastatic prostate cancer, breast cancer,
Flutamide		PO	management of endometriosis
Nilutamide		PO	
Androgens			
Testosterone (generic)		PO	Breast cancer in pre- and postmenopausal women
Fluoxymesterone (generic)		PO	

2. Estrogens
   a. Known or suspected pregnancy
   b. Estrogen-dependent neoplasms
   c. History of thromboembolic disorders
3. Progestins
   a. Severe dysrhythmias possible if client also takes a calcium-channel blocker
   b. Psychiatric depression
   c. Pregnancy (Category C); cautious use in lactation
4. Antiestrogens: first trimester of pregnancy (Category C)

E. **Significant drug interactions**
   1. Corticosteroids
      a. Phenytoin and rifampin increase steroid metabolism
      b. Increased doses may be required when given with amphotericin-B
      c. Diuretics increase potassium loss
      d. May inhibit antibody response to vaccines and toxoids
   2. Estrogens: phenytoin and rifampin decrease estrogen effect by increasing its metabolism

    3. Progestins

        a. Can prolong cardiac conduction in clients taking beta blockers, calcium channel blockers, and possibly digoxin

        b. Quinine may decrease plasma levels

        c. Chloroquine may increase risk of seizures

    4. Antiestrogens: may enhance hypoprothrombinemic effect of warfarin

F. Significant food interactions: none known

G. Significant assessment parameters

    1. Corticosteroids

        a. Establish baseline and continuing data on blood pressure, I&O, weight, and sleep patterns

        b. Measure 2-hour postprandial blood glucose, serum potassium, and serum calcium prior to therapy and at regular intervals thereafter

        c. Watch for changes in mood, emotional stability, and sleep patterns

    2. Estrogens

        a. Spotting or breakthrough bleeding may occur

        b. Severe hypercalcemia may occur

    3. Progestin

        a. Assess weight periodically

        b. Assess for allergic reactions, rash, urticaria, anaphylaxis, and tachypnea

    4. Antiestrogens: assess CBC, including platelet count, periodically

    5. Androgens: monitor serum calcium levels; hypercalcemia can result, requiring temporary termination of drug therapy and administration of large volumes of intravenous fluid

    6. Anti-androgens: monitor liver function studies periodically to detect rare complication of hepatitis

H. Side effects/toxicity

    1. Corticosteroids

        a. Euphoria, headache, insomnia, psychosis

        b. Edema

        c. Muscle weakness, delayed wound healing, osteoporosis, spontaneous fractures

        d. Hyperglycemia

    2. Estrogens

        a. Thromboembolic disorders

        b. Nausea

    3. Progestins

        a. Vaginal bleeding and breast tenderness

        b. Abdominal pain and nausea and vomiting

        c. Increased appetite and weight gain

    4. Antiestrogens

        a. Thrombosis

        b. About 25% of clients experience nausea and vomiting

        c. Hot flashes, weight gain, changes in menstrual cycle, leaking from breasts

    5. Androgens

        a. Virilization, including clitoral enlargement, increases in facial and body hair, deepened voice, increased libido, and male-pattern baldness

        b. Hypercalcemia

    6. Anti-androgens

        a. Gynecomastia

        b. GI disturbances (nausea and vomiting, constipation, and diarrhea)

        c. Hepatitis

I. Client and family teaching: for all drug groups, teach clients about adverse effects and when to report them

VI. OTHER ANTINEOPLASTICS

A. Action and use

1. Asparaginase depletes extracellular supply of asparagine, an amino acid essential to DNA synthesis
2. Hydroxyurea blocks incorporation of thymidine into DNA and may damage already formed DNA molecules

B. Common medications: asparaginase (also referred to as L-asparaginase) and hydroxyurea

C. Administration considerations

1. Asparaginase
   a. Administer intradermal (ID) skin test before initial dose because of the potential for anaphylaxis; a negative skin test does not preclude the possibility of an allergic reaction
   b. Fiber-like particles may develop in vial after reconstitution; use a 5-micron filter to remove particles (will not affect potency); do not use cloudy solutions
2. Hydroxyurea: capsule may be opened and mixed with water if client has difficulty swallowing

D. Contraindications

1. Asparaginase
   a. History of or existing pancreatitis
   b. Safe use during pregnancy (Category C) and nursing mothers is not established
2. Hydroxyurea: pregnancy (Category D)

E. Significant drug interactions

1. Asparaginase
   a. Causes decreased hypoglycemic effects of sulfonylureas and insulin
   b. Antitumor effect is blocked if administered concurrently with vincristine or methotrexate
2. Hydroxyurea: none established

F. Significant food interactions: none known

G. Significant assessment parameters

1. Asparaginase
   a. Prepare for anaphylaxis and have personnel, emergency medications, oxygen, and airway equipment readily available
   b. During administration, monitor vital signs and be alert for hypersensitivity or anaphylactic reaction, which usually occurs 30–60 minutes after medication administration
   c. Assess laboratory values prior to treatment and routinely thereafter, including CBC, amylase, serum calcium, coagulation factors, hepatic and renal function studies, and ammonia and uric acid levels
2. Hydroxyurea
   a. Determine status of kidney, liver, and bone marrow function before and periodically during therapy
   b. Monitor I&O and increase fluid intake, especially in clients with high-serum uric acid levels

H. Side effects/toxicity

1. Asparaginase
   a. Severe anaphylaxis is possible; crash cart should be readily available
   b. Severe nausea and vomiting
   c. Potential for bleeding because of reduced clotting factors, decreased circulating platelets, and decreased fibrinogen levels
2. Hydroxyurea
   a. Bone marrow suppression
   b. Stomatitis

        c. Maculopapular rash

        d. Hyperuricemia

VII. SAFE HANDLING OF CHEMOTHERAPEUTIC AGENTS

A. Drug preparation and administration

1. All individuals preparing and administering cytotoxic drugs should be specially trained in safety procedures for handling of chemotherapeutic drugs and comply with agency standards, which in turn comply with government and professional practice standards
2. Chemotherapy doses are generally individualized according to body weight (kg) or body surface area (m^2)
3. Most chemotherapy protocol order sets consist of short, intermittent, high-dose courses of drugs (often in combination) to maximize cancer cell kill while allowing normal cells time to heal and recover
4. Chemotherapy drugs should be prepared for use in an air-vented space, such as a clean-air workstation or biohazard cabinet; access to this area should be limited
5. Wear a disposable, leak-proof gown, surgical latex gloves, a mask, and eye protection when preparing chemotherapeutic agents
6. Do not prepare or administer intravenous chemotherapy if pregnant because of possible risk to fetus; almost all chemotherapeutic agents are Pregnancy Risk Category D or X

B. Safe handling of antineoplastic agents and spill management

1. Use leak-proof, puncture-resistant containers to dispose of antineoplastic drugs and associated vials, needles, syringes, tubing, and other equipment; use double-bagging technique and identify container with a "biohazard" label
2. Do not separate needle from syringe or break needles to avoid leaking medication from them
3. If drug accidentally touches a nurse or client, wash area well with soap and water; immediately remove any contaminated clothing; copiously flush eyes if involved while keeping eyelids open
4. Double-glove to clean a drug spill, washing hands before and after
5. For powdered medications, wear a mask and eye protection as well
6. Place spilled substance in a plastic bag; wipe remaining area with a damp cloth and place it in same bag; place this bag into another plastic bag (double-bag) and label it as biohazardous
7. All materials used for drug preparation and administration must be disposed of by incineration

C. Disposal of client's body fluids

1. Handle all body substances cautiously, such as blood, urine, vomitus, stool, and others; carefully follow standard precautions and other procedures as designated by agency policy
2. Wear gloves when in contact with all body substances; carefully dispose of them in toilet; clean containers carefully and thoroughly

VIII. NURSING MANAGEMENT OF TREATMENT SIDE EFFECTS

A. Myelosuppression

1. Neutropenia
      a. Assessment
         1) Neutropenia is defined as an absolute neutrophil count of 1,500/mm^3 or less
         2) Nadir (lowest point in WBC count reached after chemotherapy) most commonly occurs 7–14 days following chemotherapy administration

       3) Fever of more than 38°C (100.4°F) is the most reliable and often only sign of infection in clients with neutropenia

   b. Management

       1) Avoid exposure to these substances:

         a) Fresh fruits, vegetables, flowers, and live plants

         b) People recently vaccinated with live organisms or viruses

         c) Pet excreta including fish tanks and aquariums

       2) Instruct clients to avoid contact with people who have a contagious illness

       3) Teach people who come in contact with client to wash hands prior to touching client

       4) Encourage client to practice good personal hygiene

       5) Prevent trauma to skin and mucous membranes

       6) Culture urine, peripheral blood, all lumens of CVCs, and suspected sources of infection; obtain chest x-ray (CXR); administer antibiotics as prescribed for empiric therapy

       7) Institute neutropenic precautions for hospitalized clients whose absolute neutrophil count drops as described above using previously described measures

       8) Administer filgrastim, a granulocyte colony-stimulating factor (G-CSF) that increases production of neutrophils, either intravenously or subcutaneously as prescribed; client may report bone pain 1–3 days before blood count increases; may be controlled with nonopioid analgesics

   c. Client and family education

       1) Report temperature greater than 38°C (100.4°F), shaking chills, dysuria, dyspnea, sputum production, or pain

       2) Reinforce need for meticulous hygiene

       3) Teach self-administration of G-CSF for neutropenia or granulocyte/macrophage colony-stimulating factor (GM-CSF) for treatment of blood-forming organ cancers as prescribed

  2. Thrombocytopenia

   a. Bone marrow suppression decreases platelet production

   b. Circulating platelets are diminished gradually because platelet lifespan is only 10 days

   c. Chemotherapy drugs accelerate platelet destruction

   d. Assessment

       1) Platelet count below 50,000/mm^3; risk significantly increases when platelet count falls below 20,000/mm^3

       2) Petechiae, bruising, and hemorrhage

       3) Neurologic changes that may indicate intracranial bleeding

       4) Hypotension and tachycardia

   e. Management

       1) Institute bleeding precautions

       2) Decrease activity to prevent falls and maintain a safe environment

       3) Discourage heavy lifting and Valsalva maneuver, which may increase risk of intracranial bleeding

       4) Encourage client to eat a high-fiber diet and drink adequate liquids

       5) Daily care

         a) Avoid use of straight-edge razors; use an electric razor instead

         b) Avoid using nail clippers; use a nail file instead

         c) Avoid using vaginal douches, rectal suppositories, or enemas

         d) Use water-soluble lubricant for sexual intercourse

         e) Avoid intercourse when platelet count is below 50,000/mm^3

Practice to Pass

What measures should the nurse teach the client to decrease the potential for infection after chemotherapy administration?

    f) Instruct menstruating women to monitor pad count and amount of saturation; tampon use should be avoided

    g) Encourage client to blow nose gently

    h) Instruct client to avoid dental floss and oral irrigation and to use a soft-bristle toothbrush or sponge-tipped applicator for mouth care

    i) Avoid administration of aspirin or aspirin-containing products as well as NSAIDs

    j) Apply pressure for 5–10 minutes following venipuncture, bone marrow biopsy, or other invasive procedures; platelet transfusion prior to procedure may be indicated

  f. Client and family education

    1) Notify MD of symptoms of bleeding

    2) Test urine and stool for occult blood

    3) Teach other safety recommendations for daily management

B. Nausea and vomiting

  1. Anticipatory nausea: a conditioned response resulting from repeated association of **chemotherapy-induced nausea and vomiting (CINV)** and stimulus from environment

  2. Acute nausea: occurs 0–24 hours after chemotherapy administration

  3. Delayed nausea: persistent vomiting lasting 1–4 days after chemotherapy administration

  4. Assessment parameters

    a. Women have a higher incidence than men

    b. Younger clients experience more nausea than their older counterparts

    c. A history of motion sickness can predispose some to experience chemotherapy-induced nausea

    d. Dehydration may accelerate nausea and vomiting

  5. Administer antiemetics to cover the emetogenic period (see Table 12-8); these may include (but are not limited to) ondansetron and metoclopramide, a prokinetic GI stimulant

  6. Provide additional antiemetics to manage breakthrough nausea

  7. Dexamethasone may be most effective agent in preventing anticipatory nausea and vomiting

  8. Client and family education

    a. Eat frequent, small meals and avoid fatty, sweet, salty, or spicy foods

    b. Notify healthcare professional if vomiting persists more than 24 hours and client is unable to take oral hydration

    c. Maintain antiemetic schedule for 48–72 hours to avoid delayed nausea

C. Diarrhea

  1. Chemotherapy affects rapidly dividing cells of villi and microvilli in gastrointestinal mucosa

  2. Combination chemotherapy and radiation therapy to pelvis can lead to additional cellular destruction

  3. Monitor number of stools, amount, and consistency

  4. Replace fluid and electrolytes, including potassium

  5. Administer antidiarrheal medication to reduce peristalsis and frequency and volume of stools

  6. Client and family education

    a. Consume low-residue, high-protein, high-calorie diet to promote bowel rest

    b. Eliminate irritating foods, such as alcohol, coffee, cold liquids, popcorn, and raw fruits and vegetables

    c. Drink six to eight glasses of water per 24-hour period

Table 12-8	Emetogenic Potential, Onset, and Duration of Selected Chemotherapeutic Agents		
Incidence	**Agent**	**Onset**	**Duration**
Very high	Cisplatin	1–6	24–72+
	Dacarbazine	1–3	1–12
	Mechlorethamine	0.5–2	8–24
	Melphalan	3–6	6–12
	Dactinomycin	1–2	4–20
High	Carmustine	2–4	4–24
	Cyclophosphamide	4–12	12–24
	Procarbazine	24–27	Variable
	Etoposide	4–6	24+
	Methotrexate	1–12	24–72
Moderate	Doxorubicin	4–6	6+
	Mitoxantrone	4–6	6+
	Fluorouracil	3–6	24+
	Mitomycin	1–4	48–72
	Carboplatin	4–6	12–24
	Ifosfamide	3–6	24–72
	Cytarabine	6–12	3–12
Low	Bleomycin	3–6	–
	Daunorubicin	1–2	–
	6-Mercaptopurine	4–8	–
	Methotrexate	4–12	–
	Vinblastine	4–8	–
	Lomustine	2–6	2–24
Very low	Vincristine	4–8	–
	Paclitaxel	4–8	–

    d. Implement a liquid diet if diarrhea is severe

    e. Avoid milk products and chocolate

    f. Decrease activity when diarrhea is severe to provide rest and decrease peristalsis

    g. Clean rectal area with mild soap after each bowel movement and apply moisture barrier

    h. Take warm sitz baths

D. Stomatitis

    1. Epithelial cells of oral mucosa are destroyed, causing an inflammatory response and wearing-away of oral mucosa

    2. Initial presentation: burning sensation with no physical changes in oral mucosa, sensitivity to heat and cold, and sensitivity to salty and spicy foods

    3. Promote a well-balanced intake, including a protein intake of greater than 1 gram/kg of body weight

    4. Promote consistent, thorough oral hygiene after each meal and at hour of sleep

    5. Administer antifungal or antiviral medication for prophylaxis as directed

    6. Client and family education

        a. Instruct in consistent oral hygiene

        b. Avoid using lemon/glycerin swabs, hydrogen peroxide, and products containing alcohol, which promote dryness and irritation

E. Constipation

    1. Neurotoxic effects of chemotherapy can decrease peristalsis or cause paralytic ileus

    2. Assess patterns of elimination including amount and frequency

    3. Assess usual fiber and fluid intake

    4. Determine laxative and cathartic use, including frequency and amounts taken

    5. Initiate a bowel maintenance program for clients receiving neurotoxic chemotherapeutic agents or those at high risk for constipation

    6. Recognize complications associated with constipation, such as fecal impaction

    7. Client and family education

        a. Drink warm liquids to stimulate bowel movement

        b. Increase fiber intake to increase peristalsis and stool bulk

        c. Drink at least eight glasses of water per day

        d. Exercise regularly

        e. Develop a regular bowel program, avoiding use of laxatives if possible

F. Alopecia

    1. Cells responsible for hair growth have a high mitotic rate and are affected to some degree by most chemotherapeutic agents

    2. Hair loss begins approximately 2 weeks after drug administration and will continue until 3–5 months after last chemotherapy treatment is completed

    3. Devices to decrease circulation to scalp are contraindicated since they can also promote micrometastasis

    4. Provide emotional support to client who is experiencing body image change

    5. Client and family education

        a. Rationale and expected time frame of hair loss and regrowth

        b. Provide gentle hair care, avoiding permanent waves, coloring, peroxide, electric rollers, and curling irons until regrowth has been reestablished long enough for two haircuts

        c. Hair prosthesis (wig)

        d. Emotional support strategies to cope with changing body image

G. Cardiotoxicity

    1. May occur within 24 hours to up to 4–5 weeks after drug administration; self-limiting; warrants immediate drug discontinuation

    2. Higher doses over a shorter period of time increase its incidence

    3. Baseline ejection fraction should be assessed before administration of cardiotoxic agents

    4. Characteristics of cardiotoxicity are outlined in Table 12-9

    5. Maintain ongoing documentation of client's cumulative dose

    6. Cardioprotective iron chelating agents (e.g., dexrazoxane) may be administered to prevent cardiotoxicity in clients that have received three-fourths of their lifetime dosage

    7. Client and family education

        a. Cardiotoxicity is an expected side effect of some chemotherapy medications

        b. It is important to recognize signs of congestive heart failure and report them to healthcare provider as directed

        c. Chronic cardiotoxicity is dose-related and possibly irreversible

H. Pulmonary toxicity

    1. Lung tissue is sensitive to toxic effects of chemotherapy, causing direct damage to alveoli and capillary endothelium

    2. Dyspnea is the cardinal symptom

    3. Deteriorating creatinine clearance (renal dysfunction) is an important predictor for pulmonary pneumonitis

    4. High oxygen concentrations can enhance pulmonary toxicity of bleomycin

    5. Risk of pulmonary toxicity increases significantly after age 70

    6. Monitor pulmonary function studies as indicated

    7. Client education

        a. Provide education regarding symptoms associated with pulmonary toxicity (e.g., dyspnea, chest pain, shallow breathing, chest wall discomfort)

Table 12-9	Cardiotoxicity	
Drug	**Characteristics**	**Comments**
DNA Intercalators		
Doxorubicin Daunorubicin Dactinomycin Mitoxantrone	EKG changes, nonspecific ST-T wave changes; premature ventricular and atrial contractions; low-voltage QRS changes	Chronic effects seen with cumulative dosages greater than recommended
High-Dose Therapy		
Cylcophosphamide	Diminished QRS complexes on EKG, cardiomegaly, pulmonary congestion	May result in acute lethal pericarditis, hemorrhagic myocardial necrosis
Fluorouracil	Angina, palpitations, sweating, and syncope	May treat prophylactically or therapeutically with long-acting nitrates or calcium channel blockers
Taxanes		
Paclitaxel	Asymptomatic bradycardia, hypotension, asymptomatic ventricular tachycardia, and atypical chest pain	A baseline EKG, client history, and cardiac assessment should be performed before treatment; routine cardiac monitoring not warranted

   b. Teach pursed-lipped breathing and use a small fan to decrease symptoms of dyspnea
   c. Encourage use of opioid analgesia as prescribed to decrease fear of air hunger
   d. Review safety issues related to oxygen administration
   e. Explore with client and significant other their wishes for intubation and resuscitation; breastfeeding should be discontinued
I. Hemorrhagic cystitis
   1. Bladder mucosal irritation and inflammation results from contact with acrolein, the metabolic by-product of cyclophosphamide and ifosfamide
   2. Prior radiation therapy to pelvis or bladder increases risk
   3. Presents with dysuria, frequency, burning upon urination, and hematuria
   4. A chemo-protectant agent (mesna) may be given to bind to acrolein in bladder, inactivating it and allowing excretion from bladder
   5. Client education
   a. Instruct that hemorrhagic cystitis is a possible side effect of cyclophosphamide and ifosfamide therapy
   b. Report signs and symptoms of hemorrhagic cystitis
   c. Void every 4–6 hours and take medication early in the day
   d. Drink a minimum of six to eight glasses of fluid daily
J. Hepatotoxicity
   1. Caused by direct toxic effect on liver when drugs are metabolized; see Table 12-10 for incidence
   2. Prior liver infection, tumor involvement in liver, advanced age, total bilirubin greater than 2 mg/100 dL, or cirrhosis increase incidence
   3. Clinical manifestations include jaundice, ascites, fatigue, anorexia, nausea, hyperpigmentation, upper-right quadrant pain, hepatomegaly, and changes in urine and stool
   4. Avoid hepatotoxic drugs if liver function tests are abnormal
   5. Client and family education
   a. Client should avoid alcohol-containing beverages
   b. Hepatotoxicity is a possible side effect of some chemotherapeutic medications
   c. Be aware of and report signs and symptoms of liver failure

Table 12-10	Hepatotoxicity	
Classification	**Incidence**	**Comments**
Alkylating Agents		
Nitrogen Mustards		
Cyclophosphamide	Rare	Exception is greater than 3 grams used in bone marrow transplant (BMT)
Nitrosoureas		
Carmustine (BCNU) Lomustine Streptozocin	26% at low doses 26% 15–67%	Usually not clinically significant; however, may be associated with veno-occlusive disease when used in BMT
Antimetabolites		
Methotrexate	24% with oral administration	Cumulative dose is important; seen only when cumulative dosages exceed 2 mg/kg/day
Fluorouracil Cytarabine	Rare Unknown	
Antitumor Antibiotics		
Doxorubicin	Rare	May be lower than other anthracyclines
Mitoxantrone	Rare	
Bleomycin	Rare	
Plicamycin	16%	
Plant-Based Agents		
Vincristine Etoposide Paclitaxil	Rare Rare 7–22%	Rarely seen with standard dosages, higher dosages can cause irreversible liver enzyme changes
Miscellaneous		
Asparaginase	42–67%	Increases with higher doses

K. Nephrotoxicity

1. Caused by direct damage to glomerulus, renal blood vessels, different parts of nephron, and/or precipitation of metabolites in acid environment of urine; leads to obstructive nephropathy
2. Advancing age, preexisting renal disease, poor nutritional status, and administration of other nephrotoxic agents predispose client to nephrotoxicity
3. Manifested by increasing serum creatinine, declining creatinine clearance, hypomagnesemia, proteinuria, and hematuria
4. Continuation of nephrotoxic agents should be reviewed if blood urea nitrogen (BUN) is greater than 22 mg/dL and/or creatinine is >2 mg/dL
5. Institute hydration of 3,000 mL/day to prevent or minimize renal damage
6. Induce diuresis with mannitol or furosemide when administering cisplatin
7. Administer allopurinol to decrease uric acid production from high tumor-cell kill (e.g., leukemia, lymphoma, small-cell lung cancer)
8. Maintain alkalinization of urine with sodium bicarbonate to a pH level greater than 8 to prevent renal damage when giving high-dose methotrexate
9. Avoid administration of aspirin and NSAIDs
10. Client and family education
    a. Instruct that nephrotoxicity is a possible side effect of selected chemotherapeutic agents

      b. Reinforce importance of compliance with measures to prevent nephrotoxicity
        1) Accurately obtain 12- or 24-hour urine for creatinine clearance
        2) Increase fluid intake
        3) Comply with instructions to alkalinize urine, complete leucovorin rescue, and/or allopurinol therapy

L. Neurotoxicity
  1. Caused by direct toxicity on nervous system, metabolic encephalopathy, or intracranial hemorrhage related to chemotherapy-induced coagulopathy
  2. Risk factors
    a. Administration of agents that cross blood–brain barrier
    b. Specified chemotherapeutic agents, especially cumulative doses of vinca alkaloids
    c. Concurrent radiation therapy to brain
    d. Incidence increases with age
    e. Impaired renal function
  3. Use assessment guidelines to determine fine motor losses, numbness, tingling, gait disturbance, constipation, and change in mentation, which are early warning signs
  4. Use measures outlined in Table 12-11 for collaborative management of neurotoxicity
  5. Client and family education
    a. Neurotoxicity is a possible side effect of some chemotherapy agents
    b. Be aware of early warning signs of neurotoxicity and importance of notifying provider if they occur

M. Sexual and reproductive dysfunction
  1. Infertility occurs in men primarily through depletion of germinal epithelium that lines seminiferous tubules
  2. Women experience reproductive dysfunction primarily as a result of hormonal alterations or direct effects that cause ovarian fibrosis and follicular destruction

Table 12-11 Neurotoxicity

Area Affected	Chemotherapy Agent	Assessment	Collaborative Management
Cerebrum	Asparaginase Cisplatin Carboplatin Ifosfamide	Assess for confusion, memory loss, and level of consciousness	1. Use positive support and encouragement 2. Maintain a consistent schedule
Sensory	Cisplatin Carboplatin Cytarabine Etoposide Paclitaxil Vincristine	Assess for decreased deep tendon reflexes, numbness, decreased sensation, jaw pain, paresthesia of hands or feet	1. Avoid extreme temperatures 2. Use assistive devices as required 3. Use opioids, antidepressants, and antiepileptics for neuropathic pain
Autonomic	Vincristine	Assess for abdominal pain, constipation, ileus, bladder atony	1. Recommend a high-fiber diet 2. Increase fluid intake 3. Administer stool softeners and laxatives as required 4. Initiate a bowel management program 30 minutes after meals 5. Monitor for bladder infection with urinary retention
Auditory	Cisplatin Prednisone	Assess for tinnitus, hearing loss	1. Report auditory changes 2. Reduce or discontinue chemotherapy

3. Chemotherapy compromises fertility by exerting cytotoxic effects on gametogenesis; degree is related to therapeutic agent and duration of treatment
4. Approximately 40–100% of clients experience some sexual dysfunction following treatment; it is frequently underreported because it is often not assessed by health-care personnel
5. Males should be encouraged to bank sperm before starting treatment
6. Although expensive (and not always successful), females should be informed of opportunities to bank oocytes or cryopreserve embryos
7. Water-based lubricants or estrogen supplements may help to decrease vaginal dryness
8. Client education and counseling
   a. Provide an unbiased, sexually neutral environment that promotes open discussion
   b. Identify whether sexual issues pose a problem for client and/or partner
   c. Explain implications of treatments on sexuality
   d. Provide information related to contraception
   e. Discourage pregnancy during treatment
   f. Advise client of possible long-term side effects on reproductive function
   g. Encourage communication between client and significant other

Case Study

A 64-year-old male client is admitted for his first dose of chemotherapy. His wife died 6 months ago of a massive heart attack. He has two daughters who live out of state; one is a lawyer, while the other is a pediatrician. The client is the chief executive officer (CEO) of his own electronics business, is self-insured, and has no oncology supplement.

Chemotherapy orders include:
- Cyclophosphamide 800 mg intravenous piggyback
- Methotrexate 160 mg intravenous piggyback
- Adriamycin 40 mg in 1,000 mL normal saline IV infusion over 24 hours times two doses
- Leucovorin 75 mg intravenous piggyback q6 hours times four doses; begin Leucovorin 24 hours after methotrexate
- 5-FU 80 mg intravenous piggyback after second dose of leucovorin

Other medication orders include:
- Ondansetron 35 mg intravenous piggyback prior to starting chemotherapy and prior to the second liter of Adriamycin
- Ondansetron 15 mg intravenous piggyback 4 and 8 hours after each 35 mg loading dose

For suggested responses, see pages 534–535.

- Diphenhydramine 12.5 mg, metoclopramide 5 mg, and dexamethasone 2 mg intravenous piggyback q6 hours around the clock

Diagnostic studies include MUGA scan, ultrasound of the liver, CBC, and chemistry profile.

1. What are the most important priority nursing concerns, and what is your rationale for prioritizing them the way you did?
2. What important diagnostic and assessment values need to be obtained before initiating the chemotherapy?
3. Outline a pretreatment teaching plan for this client.
4. What orders need further clarification with the healthcare provider?
5. How will you prepare the client for discharge from the hospital?

POSTTEST

1 A client is receiving chemotherapy with carmustine, a nitrosourea, as treatment for cancer. The intravenous line infiltrates and extravasation occurs. The nurse should perform the following interventions in which order?

1. Discontinue carmustine infusion.
2. Consult plastic surgeon.
3. Treat site with local injections of sodium carbonate and normal saline.
4. Choose new site for continuation of administration.

2 The nurse makes it a priority to assess for hematuria and dysuria when a client is receiving which cancer chemotherapy agent?

1. Cyclophosphamide
2. Methotrexate
3. Streptozocin
4. Cisplatin

3 Prior to administering 5-fluorouracil, the nurse teaches the client that which unique long-term disabling side effect may persist after administration ends?

1. Myelosuppression
2. Cerebellar syndrome
3. Nausea and vomiting
4. Alopecia

4 Prior to initiating chemotherapy, the nurse teaches clients the most common side effects associated with chemotherapy. In which order should the side effects be addressed?

1. Cardiotoxicity
2. Neurotoxicity
3. Myelosuppression
4. Hepatotoxicity

5 When preparing a client who has cancer and the client's family for the initiation of chemotherapy, in which order would the nurse complete the following interventions?

1. Clarify information and dispel misconceptions.
2. Obtain informed consent.
3. Evaluate client for chemotherapy-induced anemia and neutropenia.
4. Choose an appropriate venous access.
5. Demonstrate safe gloving, gowning, and administration of prescribed chemotherapy.

6 A client receiving chemotherapy who overheard the healthcare team use the term *cell-cycle specific* in reference to drug therapy asks for an explanation of the term. Which response is best?

1. "It is medical jargon that is not related to your care."
2. "Chemotherapy drugs are lethal to certain types of cells."
3. "These drugs are aimed at cells that are growing."
4. "This means the drugs work best after the cells have been through several cycles."

7 Several weeks after a healthcare provider changed the type of chemotherapy from an antimetabolite to an alkylating agent, the client is very anxious because of worsened fatigue, nausea and vomiting, and symptoms of peripheral neuropathy. What is the best response by the nurse to the client's concern?

1. "The new drug does not differentiate between normal and abnormal cells as well as the first drug."
2. "You are experiencing the side effects of both drugs."
3. "The lesion may not have responded to the first drug."
4. "I will obtain medication to relieve the signs and symptoms."

8 The nurse is providing care for several clients receiving chemotherapy. Which client is most likely to experience cardiotoxicity?

1. Female client receiving vincristine
2. Older adult receiving doxorubicin
3. A reproductive-age male receiving mechlorethamine
4. Native American receiving cisplatin

9 A client receiving chemotherapy has a serum neutrophil level of less than 2,300/mm^3. The nurse should expect to complete which collaborative and nursing interventions? Select all that apply.

1. Administer filgrastim 5 mg/kg/day intravenously.
2. Prepare client for administration of whole-blood transfusion.
3. Administer epoetin alfa 500 units/kg three times weekly subcutaneously.
4. Educate regarding proper hand hygiene techniques and food preparation.
5. Teach client to limit exposure to groups of people and those with any illness.

10 A client wants the dosage of chemotherapy doubled to ensure maximum impact on a large inoperable lesion. Which is the most appropriate response by the nurse?

1. "I'll check with the healthcare provider."
2. "I don't know if this is realistic based on your history of previous treatments."
3. "The prescriber will gradually increase the dose as the lesion shrinks."
4. "The dosage is predetermined by the effect of the drug on the body."

➤ *See pages 420–421 for Answers and Rationales.*

ANSWERS & RATIONALES

Pretest

1 Answer: 3 Rationale: The most profound adverse effects of plant (vinca) alkaloids such as vincristine lie in the peripheral nervous system. A decreased Achilles reflex is the earliest sign of neuropathy. There is no evidence of a significant change in level of consciousness or memory. Foot and hand drop (which would interfere with motor ability), along with paresthesia, occur later than impairment of the Achilles tendon. **Cognitive Level:** Analyzing **Client Need:** Pharmacological and Parenteral Therapies **Integrated Process:** Nursing Process: Assessment **Content Area:** Pharmacology **Strategy:** The core issue of the question is the ability to recognize an adverse effect of the plant alkaloids. Take time to review this information if this question was difficult. **Reference:** Adams, M. P., Holland, N., & Urban, C. (2017). *Pharmacology for nurses: A pathophysiologic approach* (5th ed.). New York, NY: Pearson, p. 626.

2 Answer: 3 Rationale: The combination of exercise and dexrazoxane are the best interventions. Since the outcome of the toxicity results in decreased strength of the cardiac muscle, exercise is the best intervention because it strengthens cardiac muscle. Dexrazoxane protects the cardiac muscle against the toxic effects of doxorubicin.

It interferes with iron-mediated free radicals thought to cause cardiomyopathy. Exercise and cessation of smoking would contribute to general health maintenance but would not protect the heart from cardiotoxicity. Smoking cessation and O_2 administration would be appropriate if the client developed congestive heart failure. A low-fat diet has no known contributory effects. **Cognitive Level:** Applying **Client Need:** Pharmacological and Parenteral Therapies **Integrated Process:** Nursing Process: Implementation **Content Area:** Pharmacology **Strategy:** A critical word in the question is *prevention*. Identify the category of dexrazoxane as a cytoprotective agent and associate it with outcomes of the drug. **Reference:** Wilson, B. A., Shannon, M. T., & Shields, K. M. (2017). *Pearson nurse's drug guide 2017.* New York, NY: Pearson Education, pp. 533–536.

3 Answer: 1, 2, 5 Rationale: Elevating the head of the bed will decrease the work of breathing. Pursed-lip breathing is the best respiratory technique because it creates a back pressure that keeps the airways open longer, resulting in prolonged exhalation. This also facilitates removal of secretions from the bronchial tree. To manage normal life activities, the client needs to plan exercise and rest periods. Shallow, slow breathing would not maximize the client's pulmonary potential. Clients with hypoxia are likely to use accessory muscles in an attempt to "get more air in," rather than to exhale. The method is tiring and should not be taught; it is not as efficient as pursed-lip breathing. **Cognitive Level:** Analyzing **Client Need:** Pharmacological and Parenteral Therapies **Integrated Process:** Teaching and Learning **Content Area:** Pharmacology **Strategy:** Select the options most likely to promote perfusion and cellular ventilation as well as maximize utilization of available oxygen. **Reference:** LeMone, P. T., Burke, K. M., Bauldoff, G., & Gubrud, P. (2015). *Medical surgical nursing: Clinical reasoning in patient care* (6th ed.). New York, NY: Pearson, pp. 1034–1143.

4 **Answer: 2** **Rationale:** Pulmonary toxicity is a known adverse effect of bleomycin. Primary side effects of 5-fluorouracil are GI (nausea and vomiting) and immune (leucopenia). Primary side effects of etoposide are myelosuppression, anaphylaxis, and bronchospasms. Primary side effects of paclitaxel are neutropenia, thrombocytopenia, and peripheral neuropathy. **Cognitive Level:** Analyzing **Client Need:** Pharmacological and Parenteral Therapies **Integrated Process:** Nursing Process: Assessment **Content Area:** Pharmacology **Strategy:** It is helpful to think of "blue for bleomycin" to recall that it has significant respiratory adverse effects. **Reference:** Wilson, B. A., Shannon, M. T., & Shields, K. M. (2017). *Pearson nurse's drug guide 2017.* New York, NY: Pearson, pp. 193–195.

5 **Answer: 2** **Rationale:** Clients receiving chemotherapy have reduced immunity and are at greater risk for opportunistic infections. Intact skin and mucous membranes are the body's first defense against infection. The nurse should also work to prevent any alteration that could result in significant discomfort or change in body image, but they do not override the risk of an infection. Occurrence of mucositis has no relationship to cancer recurrence. **Cognitive Level:** Applying **Client Need:** Pharmacological and Parenteral Therapies **Integrated Process:** Nursing Process: Diagnosis **Content Area:** Pharmacology **Strategy:** Select the option that places the client at greatest risk. **Reference:** LeMone, P. T., Burke, K. M., Bauldoff, G., & Gubrud, P. (2015). *Medical surgical nursing: Clinical reasoning in patient care* (6th ed.). New York, NY: Pearson, p. 613.

6 **Answer: 1** **Rationale:** Being female as well as having a positive history of non-disease-oriented nausea indicates the mother of two is more likely to experience chemotherapy-induced nausea and vomiting (CINV). Because the pilot presents with only one of the predisposing factors (childhood motion sickness), this client is at risk to a lesser degree than a client with non-disease-oriented nausea. Since alcoholism predisposes to dehydration, the 38-year-old client presents with one predisposing factor. The female client without a history of non-disease-producing nausea is less likely to experience chemotherapy-induced nausea than a client with a history of morning sickness. **Cognitive Level:** Analyzing **Client Need:** Pharmacological and Parenteral Therapies **Integrated**

Process: Nursing Process: Diagnosis **Content Area:** Pharmacology **Strategy:** Apply knowledge of characteristics of nausea experiences to clients receiving chemotherapy. **Reference:** Adams, M. P., Holland, N., & Urban, C. (2017). *Pharmacology for nurses: A pathophysiologic approach* (5th ed.). New York, NY: Pearson, p. 178.

7 **Answer: 3** **Rationale:** Any activity that increases the potential for infection should be avoided. Since most clients become septic from organisms on their skin and in their environment, meticulous hygiene is the best way to prevent infection. An indwelling catheter is a source of infection and should only be used if the client is immobile and has a high risk for skin breakdown. Dressings should cover all open wounds to prevent contamination. Long-term catheters should be flushed after use or every 8 hours to prevent clotting; however, this will not decrease the client's risk for infection. **Cognitive Level:** Applying **Client Need:** Pharmacological and Parenteral Therapies **Integrated Process:** Nursing Process: Planning **Content Area:** Pharmacology **Strategy:** Associate the function of neutrophils (fighting infection) with the nursing care activity that also best fights infection. **Reference:** LeMone, P. T., Burke, K. M., Bauldoff, G., & Gubrud, P. (2015). *Medical surgical nursing: Clinical reasoning in patient care* (6th ed.). New York, NY: Pearson, p. 1049.

8 **Answer: 3** **Rationale:** Once stomatitis develops, meticulous oral hygiene must continue with a soft-bristle toothbrush and fluoride-containing toothpaste and rinsing with a dilute baking soda solution. The nurse should provide cleansing along with rinsing during the night as well as during the day. Dilute hydrogen peroxide mouthwashes are not recommended since they can dry the mouth and inhibit granulation tissue formation. Commercial mouthwashes are never recommended since they usually contain alcohol, which is drying and can burn. **Cognitive Level:** Applying **Client Need:** Pharmacological and Parenteral Therapies **Integrated Process:** Nursing Process: Planning **Content Area:** Pharmacology **Strategy:** Evaluate each of the options in terms of how well they provide cleansing to reduce the bacteria count in the mouth, and by the gentleness of the products used to reduce the risk of further tissue breakdown. **Reference:** Adams, M. P., Holland, N., & Urban, C. (2017). *Pharmacology for nurses: A pathophysiologic approach* (5th ed.). New York, NY: Pearson, p. 616.

9 **Answer: 1, 2, 4** **Rationale:** Increasing fiber in the diet increases bulk and gastric motility, thereby decreasing constipation. Increasing activity alone is likely to prevent constipation. Increased fluid intake could help reduce the occurrence by increasing the intestinal volume, which increases peristalsis. The use of stool softeners should be encouraged, but laxative usage should be kept to a minimum to prevent becoming laxative dependent. Clients receiving chemotherapy are at risk for nutritional imbalance and should avoid ingesting anything that would increase loss of nutrients. The purpose of an antiflatulent is to reduce bloating, but this will not prevent constipation, although it would be helpful for clients following a meal high in gas-producing foods. **Cognitive Level:** Applying **Client Need:** Pharmacological and Parenteral Therapies **Integrated Process:** Nursing Process: Implementation **Content Area:** Pharmacology **Strategy:** Associate requirements for normal intestinal functioning with the threat of constipation. **Reference:** Wilson, B. A., Shannon, M. T., & Shields, K. M. (2017). *Pearson nurse's drug guide 2017.* New York, NY: Pearson Education, pp. 1647–1649.

10 **Answer: 2** **Rationale:** Single-category chemotherapy leads to major tumor drug resistance. Most malignant tumors are comprised of cells at various stages of development. Because combination chemotherapy can attack cells at various stages of development, it has proven to be more successful in reducing tumor size and tumor resistance. Combined therapy can compound the nausea and vomiting response. The primary goal is to reduce tumor size and treat any parallel side effects. Depending on the drugs, the effect on normal cells can be greater, but this is less relevant than tumor reduction. If drugs have an affinity for gonadal tissue, this will not be reduced by combination chemotherapy. **Cognitive Level:** Applying **Client Need:** Pharmacological and Parenteral Therapies **Integrated Process:** Nursing Process: Diagnosis **Content Area:** Pharmacology **Strategy:** Correlate the nature of cancerous growths with the nature and purpose of chemotherapy. **Reference:** Adams, M. P., Holland, N., & Urban, C. (2017). *Pharmacology for nurses: A pathophysiologic approach* (5th ed.). New York, NY: Pearson, p. 617.

Posttest

1 **Answer: 1, 3, 4, 2** **Rationale:** Discontinuation of medication is the first priority in order to minimize the damage caused to the tissue. Vesicant therapy will cause tissue irritation with eventual sloughing without the appropriate antidote, which should be utilized immediately after discontinuing the infusion. Protocols should be in place to administer the antidote promptly to neutralize the vesicant and minimize tissue trauma. The priority is not choosing a new site for administration, but preventing tissue damage. However, the infusion should be completed at another intravenous site once the site is cared for. The site should be observed for 3–4 weeks, but a plastic surgeon need only be consulted if tissue damage actually occurs. **Cognitive Level:** Applying **Client Need:** Pharmacological and Parenteral Therapies **Integrated Process:** Nursing Process: Implementation **Content Area:** Adult Health **Strategy:** Recall that cancer chemotherapeutic drugs are more likely to be vesicants because of the nature in which they work. When an IV line infiltrates, consider this risk the priority and order the options that minimize local tissue damage. **Reference:** Adams, M. P., Holland, N., & Urban, C. (2017). *Pharmacology for nurses: A pathophysiologic approach* (5th ed.). New York, NY: Pearson, p. 435.

2 **Answer: 1** **Rationale:** Cystitis can occur in the urinary bladder after administration of cyclophosphamide or ifosfamide. This could lead to hematuria and dysuria. Damage to the renal tubules is more likely to occur after the administration of methotrexate, streptozocin, and cisplatin, and signs would then reflect renal impairment rather than bladder symptoms. **Cognitive Level:** Analyzing **Client Need:** Pharmacological and Parenteral Therapies **Integrated Process:** Nursing Process: Assessment **Content Area:** Pharmacology **Strategy:** The core issue of the question is being able to identify which drug is most likely to cause damage to the urinary bladder. Associate the *cy* in the beginning of the word *cystitis* and the name *cyclophosphamide* as a strategy to remember the adverse effects of this drug. **Reference:** Wilson, B. A., Shannon, M. T., & Shields, K. M. (2017). *Pearson nurse's drug guide 2017.* New York, NY: Pearson, pp. 402–404.

3 **Answer: 2** **Rationale:** Cerebellar syndrome characterized by headache, disorientation, and nystagmus may persist after administration ceases. Myelosuppression is *not* unique to 5-fluorouracil. Nausea and vomiting are common to most antineoplastic drugs and generally cease after administration ends. Alopecia is not unique to this drug and will resolve after treatment is completed. **Cognitive Level:** Applying **Client Need:** Pharmacological and Parenteral Therapies **Integrated Process:** Teaching and Learning **Content Area:** Pharmacology **Strategy:** Specific drug knowledge is needed to answer this question. Focus on the critical word *unique* in the question and select the most unusual adverse effect from those listed. **Reference:** Wilson, B. A., Shannon, M. T., & Shields, K. M. (2017). *Pearson nurse's drug guide 2017.* New York, NY: Pearson Education, pp. 689–692.

4 **Answer: 1, 4, 3, 2** **Rationale:** Cardiotoxicity is ranked first because this impaired the most relevant life-sustaining body function. Hepatotoxicity is ranked second because of the risk of bleeding and possible hemorrhage; also, the liver performs many life-sustaining activities. Myelosuppression ranks third because infection and generalized bleeding are important after heart function and the risk of hemorrhage are addressed. Neurotoxicity is not as common as myelosuppression and this toxic effect is not as life-threatening, making it fourth in priority. **Cognitive Level:** Analyzing **Client Need:** Pharmacological and Parenteral Therapies **Integrated Process:** Nursing Process: Planning **Content Area:** Pharmacology **Strategy:** Select the most significant side effect that could occurs with antineoplastic agents (remember there is only one heart). Then rank the adverse effects according to the immediacy and magnitude of the effect(s) on the client. **Reference:** Adams, M. P., Holland, N., & Urban, C. (2017). *Pharmacology for nurses: A pathophysiologic approach* (5th ed.). New York, NY: Pearson, pp. 619–626.

5 **Answer: 1, 2, 4, 5, 3** **Rationale:** Since fear and anxiety are commonly associated with management of a cancer diagnosis, clarifying information and dispelling the myths that surround cancer and cancer treatment should be the initial step in client and family education. Informed consent helps the client anticipate the outcomes of the chemotherapy; the form must be completed after initial education is performed. An IV access site is chosen third to be ready for drug infusion. Safe gowning and gloving are nursing procedures that should be performed with administration of the chemotherapy to prevent injury to both the client and nurse. Bone marrow suppression, as evidenced by decreased platelet, WBC, and RBC counts, should be evaluated last at the nadir postchemotherapy, which occurs at different times depending on the chemotherapeutic agent administered. **Cognitive Level:** Analyzing **Client Need:** Safety and Infection Control **Integrated Process:** Nursing Process: Implementation **Content Area:** Adult Health **Strategy:** Visualize the sequence of events in order to administer chemotherapy safely. **Reference:** LeMone, P. T., Burke, K. M., Bauldoff, G., & Gubrud, P. (2015). *Medical surgical nursing: Clinical reasoning in patient care* (6th ed.). New York, NY: Pearson, pp. 333–370.

6 **Answer: 3 Rationale:** Drugs that are cell-cycle specific act preferentially on cells that are proliferating (growing). Cells that are rapidly growing tend to be more sensitive to these drugs. The statement about medical jargon that is not related to care violates a standard of practice that requires the nurse to provide clients with a reasonable response to their questions. The term addresses the phase of cell development rather than specific type. Cells move through one cycle rather than several. **Cognitive Level:** Applying **Client Need:** Pharmacological and Parenteral Therapies **Integrated Process:** Teaching and Learning **Content Area:** Pharmacology **Strategy:** Select the option that best describes the term *cell-cycle specific* as it relates to chemotherapy. **Reference:** Adams, M. P., Holland, N., & Urban, C. (2017). *Pharmacology for nurses: A pathophysiologic approach* (5th ed.). New York, NY: Pearson, pp. 612–632.

7 **Answer: 1 Rationale:** Because non-cell-cycle-specific drugs do not differentiate between normal and abnormal cells as well as cell-cycle-specific drugs, they tend to be more toxic. The side effects mentioned often cease after administration of the drugs end. There is no evidence that worsening of the signs and symptoms is related to the response of the lesion. This may unnecessarily increase the anxiety level. Because of the high level of anxiety, the nurse should help the client understand the reason for the change in the intensity of the signs and symptoms. **Cognitive Level:** Applying **Client Need:** Pharmacological and Parenteral Therapies **Integrated Process:** Communication and Documentation **Content Area:** Pharmacology **Strategy:** Compare and contrast the significant differences between the two drug groups. **Reference:** Adams, M. P., Holland, N., & Urban, C. (2017).

Pharmacology for nurses: A pathophysiologic approach (5th ed.). New York, NY: Pearson, pp. 615–635.

8 **Answer: 2 Rationale:** Doxorubicin has a dose-limiting cardiotoxic effect that is more pronounced in older adult and pediatric clients. The major side effect of vincristine is peripheral neuropathy. There is no evidence that the side effect is gender related. The major side effects of nitrogen mustard are severe nausea and vomiting and thrombocytopenia. There are no known gender-related side effects. The major side effects of cisplatin are severe nausea and vomiting and nephrotoxicity. There are no known culture-related side effects. **Cognitive Level:** Analyzing **Client Need:** Pharmacological and Parenteral Therapies **Integrated Process:** Nursing Process: Assessment **Content Area:** Pharmacology **Strategy:** Correlate client demographics, the antineoplastic category, and cardiotoxicity. **Reference:** Wilson, B. A., Shannon, M. T., & Shields, K. M. (2017). *Pearson nurse's drug guide 2017.* New York, NY: Pearson Education, pp. 355–357, 533–536, 966–968, 1647–1649.

9 **Answer: 1, 4, 5 Rationale:** Filgrastim is a hematopoietic growth factor that increases the production of neutrophils. A client with a decreased neutrophil count does need to be educated about proper infection control practices. Also, exposure should be limited, since exposure to even a mild illness may cause sepsis and death in a client with decreased neutrophils. Whole-blood transfusion contains RBCs and is not indicated at this time. Epogen is a hematopoietic growth factor that stimulates the production of RBCs and is not indicated based on the information given. **Cognitive Level:** Analyzing **Client Need:** Pharmacological and Parenteral Therapies **Integrated Process:** Nursing Process: Implementation **Content Area:** Adult Health **Strategy:** Correlate the drug with the remedy most likely to reverse or reduce the problem. **Reference:** Wilson, B. A., Shannon, M. T., & Shields, K. M. (2017). *Pearson nurse's drug guide 2017.* New York, NY: Pearson Education, pp. 589, 674–676.

10 **Answer: 4 Rationale:** Although a client's physical well-being and response to previous treatments are important to know, toxicities of the drug commonly determine the maximum amount of the drug that can be administered safely. The number of cancer cells in the body has little to do with the dose limitations of the medications. Checking with the healthcare provider will not resolve the problem. The primary health history feature most likely to determine dosage is influenced more by organs involved in metabolism and elimination. Because chemotherapy is systemic and can have a whole-body effect, size of the lesion will not determine the maximum dosage. **Cognitive Level:** Applying **Client Need:** Pharmacological and Parenteral Therapies **Integrated Process:** Communication and Documentation **Content Area:** Pharmacology **Strategy:** Apply knowledge of the criteria used to determine chemotherapy dosages. **Reference:** Adams, M. P., Holland, N., & Urban, C. (2017). *Pharmacology for nurses: A pathophysiologic approach* (5th ed.). New York, NY: Pearson, p. 617.

ANSWERS & RATIONALES

References

Adams, M. P., Holland, N., & Urban, C. (2017). *Pharmacology for nurses: A patho-physiologic approach* (5th ed.). New York, NY: Pearson.

Adams, M. P., & Urban, C. (2016). *Pharmacology: Connections to nursing practice* (3rd ed.). New York, NY: Pearson.

Burchum, J., & Rosenthal, L. (2016). *Lehne's pharmacology for nursing care* (9th ed.). St. Louis, MO: Elsevier.

Drug Facts & Comparisons (2017; updated monthly). St. Louis, MO: Wolters Kluwer.

Karch, A. M. (2016). *Focus on nursing pharmacology* (7th ed.). Philadelphia, PA: Lippincott Williams & Wilkins.

Kee, J. L. (2017). *Pearson's handbook of laboratory and diagnostic tests* (8th ed.). New York, NY: Pearson.

LeMone, P. T., Burke, K. M., Bauldoff, G., & Gubrud, P. (2015). *Medical surgical nursing: Clinical reasoning in patient care* (6th ed.). New York, NY: Pearson.

Lewis, S., Dirksen, S., Heitkemper, M., & Bucher, L. (2017). *Medical-surgical nursing: Assessment and management of clinical problems* (10th ed.). St. Louis, MO: Elsevier.

Lilley, L. L., Rainforth Collins, S., & Snyder, K. M. (2017). *Pharmacology and the nursing process* (8th ed.). St. Louis, MO: Mosby.

Vallerand, A. H., Sanoski, C. A., & Deglin, J. H. (2017). *Davis's drug guide for nurses* (8th ed.). Philadelphia, PA: F.A. Davis.

Wilson, B. A., Shannon, M. T., & Shields, K. M. (2017). *Pearson nurse's drug guide 2017.* New York, NY: Pearson.

Endocrine System Medications

13

Chapter Outline

Medications Affecting the
   Pituitary Gland
Medications Affecting the
   Adrenal Glands

Medications Affecting the
   Thyroid Gland
Medications Affecting the
   Parathyroid Glands

Medications Used to Treat
   Diabetes Mellitus

Objectives

➤ Describe the general goals of therapy when administering
   endocrine system medications.
➤ Describe the action, use, and nursing considerations related to the
   administration of medications used to treat diabetes insipidus.
➤ Identify the nursing considerations related to the administration of
   thyroid replacement medications.
➤ Identify the medications used to treat hyperthyroidism.
➤ List the client teaching points related to the administration of
   calcium and vitamin D supplements.
➤ Identify the characteristics of various types of insulin.
➤ Outline the side effects and complications associated with the use
   of glucocorticoids.
➤ Identify the nursing considerations related to the administration
   of insulin.
➤ Describe the significant client teaching points related to the
   administration of medications used to treat diabetes mellitus.
➤ List the significant client education points related to various
   endocrine system medications.

NCLEX-RN® Test Prep

Access the NEW Web-based app
that provides students with additional
practice questions in preparation
for the NCLEX experience.

Review at a Glance

Addison disease life-threatening
disease caused by partial or complete
failure of adrenocortical function
adrenal crisis an acute, life-threatening
state of profound adrenocortical insufficiency requiring immediate therapy
adrenal insufficiency a condition
in which adrenal glands are unable to
produce adequate amounts of adrenocortical hormones
catecholamine any one of a group of
sympathomimetic compounds composed
of a catechol molecule and the aliphatic

portion of an amine; some are produced
naturally by body and function as key
neurologic chemicals
cushingoid state having the habitus
and facies characteristic of Cushing
disease, including fat deposits on upper
back and face, ruddy complexion, striae
on trunk, thin legs, and excess facial hair
glucocorticoid an adrenocortical
steroid hormone that increases glyco-
genesis, exerts an anti-inflammatory
effect, and influences many body
functions

glycosylated hemoglobin concentration representative of average
blood glucose level over previous several
weeks
Graves' disease a disorder characterized by pronounced hyperthyroidism
usually associated with an enlarged
thyroid gland and exophthalmos; also
called *thyrotoxicosis*
hypercalciuria presence of
abnormally large amounts of calcium in
urine resulting from conditions characterized by augmented bone resorption

PRETEST

hyperglycemia a greater than normal amount of glucose in blood most frequently associated with diabetes mellitus, postadministration of glucocorticoids, and with excessive infusion of glucose-containing intravenous solutions

hyperthyroidism a condition characterized by hyperactivity of thyroid gland, which is usually enlarged, secreting higher than normal amounts of thyroid hormones, and metabolic processes of body are accelerated

hypoglycemia a less than normal amount of glucose in blood, usually caused by administration of too much insulin, excessive secretion of insulin by islet cells of the pancreas, or dietary deficiency

hypoparathyroidism a condition of insufficient secretion of parathyroid glands caused by primary parathyroid dysfunction or by elevated serum calcium level

hypothyroidism a condition characterized by decreased activity of thyroid gland caused by atrophy of thyroid gland, surgical removal of all or part of thyroid gland, excess dosage of antithyroid medication, decreased effect of thyroid-releasing hormone secreted by hypothalamus, or decreased secretion of thyroid-stimulating hormone by pituitary gland

lipodystrophy any abnormality in metabolism or deposition of fats

mineralocorticoid a steroid hormone that acts on kidney to promote retention of sodium and water and excretion of potassium and hydrogen

myxedema most severe form of hypothyroidism characterized by swelling of hands, face, feet, and periorbital tissues and may lead to coma and death

osteomalacia an abnormal condition of lamellar bone, characterized by a loss of calcification of matrix resulting in softening of bone; accompanied by weakness, fracture, pain, anorexia, and weight loss

osteoporosis a disorder characterized by abnormal reduction in bone density most frequently seen in postmenopausal women, sedentary or immobilized clientss, and those receiving long-term corticosteroid therapy

Paget disease a common nonmetabolic disease of bone of unknown cause, usually affecting middle-aged people and older adults, characterized by excessive bone destruction and unorganized bone repair

PRETEST

1 Parents are concerned that their 5-year-old son is not growing fast enough and ask the nurse if he should be receiving growth hormone (GH). Which response by the nurse would be most appropriate?

1. "Growth hormone will only affect your child's short bones."
2. "Can your son swallow pills easily?"
3. "Scientific evidence is required before growth hormone can be administered to children."
4. "How tall do you think your son should be?"

2 After ingesting high dosages of glucocorticoids for several weeks, the client asks the nurse about stopping drug therapy. Which statement would be the nurse's best response?

1. "Even at high doses, adverse reactions are unlikely if the medication is abruptly withdrawn."
2. "It is dangerous for steroids to be withdrawn suddenly."
3. "You may experience severe psychological symptoms when the medication is withdrawn."
4. "Tapering of the medication requires daily bloodwork to measure serum chemistries."

3 A nurse is providing client education regarding prescribed intranasal desmopressin (DDAVP). What items of information should the nurse include during the teaching session? Select all that apply.

1. Shake the drug rigorously prior to use.
2. Keep a record of each night's sleep and record incidents of bed-wetting.
3. Angle the tip of the nasal spray low into the cavity when administering this drug.
4. Report a rapid weight gain to the prescriber immediately.
5. Report drowsiness to the prescriber.

4 A client is taking a high dose of fludrocortisone to treat Addison disease. The nurse should provide which instruction to the client?

1. Keep a log of weekly early-morning weights.
2. Report weight loss greater than 2.3 kg (5 lb) per week.
3. There will be reduced ability to resist infection.
4. It is important to measure postural blood pressures.

- -

5 The nurse is reviewing a client's medication record and notes that levothyroxine is prescribed. The nurse considers that the client may have which condition? Select all that apply.

1. Cretinism
2. Thyroid cancer
3. Myxedema coma
4. Adrenal insufficiency
5. Type 2 diabetes mellitus

- -

6 Liotrix is prescribed for a client with hypothyroidism. The nurse should include which important statement as part of client teaching prior to discharge?

1. "Measure the body temperature every morning."
2. "Report chest pain or palpitations to your healthcare provider immediately."
3. "You may experience sleepiness while taking this drug."
4. "You may experience nervousness while taking this drug."

- -

7 After taking propylthiouracil for 6 weeks, a client with Graves disease reports a sore throat and fever. What should the outpatient clinic nurse do next as a priority?

1. Ask client about exposure to the common cold.
2. Measure client's body temperature and ask about history of fever over last few weeks.
3. Review laboratory report for client's white blood cell (WBC) count with differential.
4. Ask about current mental stressors that could be weakening the immune system.

- -

8 Several weeks ago calcitonin was prescribed for a client with Paget disease. To determine therapeutic effectiveness, the nurse should review which follow-up testing results for this client?

1. Decreased alkaline phosphatase levels
2. Increased serum calcium levels
3. Bone x-rays for return of bones to normal
4. Magnetic resonance imaging (MRI) results of skull deformities

- -

9 When making a home visit to a male client who has been receiving insulin for 2 weeks, the nurse should include which statements in follow-up client teaching? Select all that apply.

1. "A family member also needs to learn how to administer insulin injections."
2. "Visual changes can occur over time if blood glucose is not sufficiently controlled with insulin."
3. "You may experience impotence as an effect of the disease process."
4. "Loss of sight and toe or leg amputation are common in clients with diabetes who take insulin."
5. "A high glucose level is not always an indication for an increase in insulin dosage."

- -

10 The nurse is evaluating a client's knowledge of the treatment of an insulin reaction. The nurse would place highest priority on determining that the client understands which point?

1. Symptoms indicating the need to notify the healthcare provider
2. When to schedule fasting (serum) blood glucose level
3. When to ingest orange juice and crackers with peanut butter
4. Importance of maintaining sufficient oral fluid intake

➤ *See pages 449–451 for Answers and Rationales.*

I. MEDICATIONS AFFECTING THE PITUITARY GLAND

A. Growth hormone (GH) or GH suppressants

1. Action and use of GH
   a. Stimulates growth and metabolism of all body cells
   b. Action: determines adult physical size by regulating growth of organs and tissues, specifically length of long bones
   c. Use: approved only for use in children to treat GH deficiency or inadequate GH secretion related to documented lack of GH
2. Action and use of GH suppressants: reduce GH levels; bromocriptine may manage amenorrhea associated with prolactinemia, symptoms of Parkinson disease, or acromegaly
3. Common growth hormone medications: see Table 13-1
4. Administration considerations
   a. Only given parenterally (IM or subcut); oral route is inactivated by digestive enzymes
   b. Packaged in powder form and is reconstituted for administration with 1–5 mL of approved diluent; mixture must be clear and not cloudy or contain any undissolved particles; label date of reconstitution and discard refrigerated drug according to manufacturer's directions
   c. Rotate IM sites and use appropriate needle length to inject into muscle layer
5. Contraindications
   a. To stimulate growth in children who are short unrelated to GH deficiency; during or after closure of epiphyseal plates in long bones; or with secondary intracranial tumors
   b. Use cautiously if there is diabetes or family history of same, hypothyroidism, or concurrent or previous use of thyroid hormones in males before puberty
   c. Known sensitivity to benzyl alcohol (a preservative in bacteriostatic water that may also be harmful to newborns); preferred diluent is sterile water, especially for newborns
6. Significant drug interactions
   a. Adrenocorticotropic hormone (ACTH) or corticosteroids may slow the action of growth hormone
   b. Octreotide acetate may decrease cyclosporine levels
   c. Thyroid hormone, anabolic steroids, androgens, or estrogens may hasten closure of epiphyseal plates of long bones

Table 13-1   Drugs that Influence Growth Hormone

Generic Name	Route	Uses
Growth Hormone Suppressants		
Bromocriptine	PO	Suppresses growth hormone levels in acromegaly
Octreotide	subcut, IM, IV	Suppresses intestinal peptide hormones, insulin, glucagons, and growth hormone; promotes fluid and electrolyte reabsorption
Lanreotide	subcut	Suppresses GH level in clients with acromegaly who have not responded to radiation therapy or are unable to tolerate surgery
Pegvisomant	subcut	GH receptor antagonist
Growth Hormone		
Mecasermin	subcut	Recombinant DNA insulin-like growth factor (IGF) with same actions as GH; used for growth failure in children only (before bone epiphyses close)
Somatropin	IM, subcut	Used as replacement therapy

7. Significant food interactions: none
8. Significant laboratory studies
   a. Plasma GH levels to confirm deficiency (less than 5–7 ng/mL)
   b. Regular measurement of thyroid levels to detect undiagnosed hypothyroidism
   c. Blood or urine glucose levels to detect glucose intolerance in diabetic clients or those with significant family history of diabetes
9. Side effects
   a. Metabolic: glucose intolerance, ACTH deficiency, or hypothyroidism
   b. Renal: **hypercalciuria** (excess calcium excretion in urine) during first 2–3 months of treatment; risk of renal calculi (signs include flank pain, colic, GI upset, urinary frequency, chills, fever, and hematuria)
   c. Other: recurrent intracranial tumor growth or presence of GH antibodies
10. Adverse effects/toxicity
   a. Local allergic reaction: pain and edema at injection site
   b. Systemic allergic reaction: peripheral edema, headache, myalgia, and weakness
   c. Excess dosage: diabetes mellitus, atherosclerosis, enlarged organs, hypertension, and features related to acromegaly
11. Nursing considerations
   a. Make sure growth rate has been documented for at least 6–12 months prior to initiating treatment
   b. Assess client for any adverse effects or toxicities related to drug administration
   c. Make sure annual bone age assessments are performed, especially for clients undergoing thyroid, androgen, or estrogen replacement therapy
12. Client education
   a. Advise parents or caregivers to have regular bone age assessments done at specific times
   b. Tell parents or caregivers that a 7.6- to 12.7-cm (3–5-in.) growth rate is expected during first year and less in second year, with normal growth rate in subsequent years; subcutaneous fat is diminished during treatment, but will return later
   c. Teach parents or caregivers how to accurately measure and document monthly height and weight and to report any less-than-expected growth to prescriber
   d. Teach parents or caregivers signs and symptoms of slipped femoral epiphysis (hip or knee pain and limp) and to notify prescriber of same
   e. Advise parents or caregivers that treatment is discontinued when adequate adult height reached, when epiphyseal plates are fused, or when client fails to respond to growth hormone
   f. Instruct client and caregivers how to administer subcut or IM injections

B. **Antidiuretic hormone (ADH)**
   1. Action and use
      a. Action: promotes reabsorption of water in renal tubules; vasopressor effect due to constriction of smooth muscle; increases aggregation of platelets
      b. Use: a posterior pituitary hormone for replacement therapy for clients with diabetes insipidus; for use in hemophilia A, von Willebrand disease Type 1; nocturnal enuresis
   2. Common medications for diabetes insipidus: see Table 13-2
   3. Administration considerations
      a. Give intranasally, intravenously (IV), subcutaneously (subcut), intramuscularly (IM), or intra-arterially according to prescription and preparation
      b. Infusion pump is needed for intravenous or intra-arterial routes

Table 13-2	Drugs to Treat Diabetes Insipidus (DI)	
Generic Name	**Route**	**Uses**
Desmopressin	Intranasal, IV, subcut, PO	Used as replacement therapy in DI; relieve polyuria and polydipsia associated with trauma or pituitary surgery
Vasopressin	IM, IV, subcut, intra-arterial	Used as replacement therapy in DI or dispel gas in abdominal x-ray

4. Contraindications: clients with coronary artery or vascular disease; blood pressure (BP) elevation is caused by vasoconstriction

5. Significant drug interactions
  a. Demeclocycline and lithium carbonate may inhibit action and promote continuation of diuresis
  b. Carbamazepine, chlorpropamide, and clofibrate may also extend action of antidiuretics
  c. Epinephrine, heparin, and phenytoin may decrease ADH effects of vasopressin
  d. Guanethidine and neostigmine increase vasopressor actions

6. Significant food interactions: none known

7. Significant laboratory studies
  a. Serum osmolality and plasma osmolality with diabetes insipidus
  b. Factor VIII coagulation level for hemostasis

8. Side effects
  a. CNS: drowsiness, headache, lethargy
  b. EENT: nasal congestion and irritation; rhinitis
  c. GI: abdominal cramps, nausea, and heartburn
  d. GU: pain in vulva
  e. CV: elevated BP

9. Adverse effects/toxicity
  a. IV route may cause anaphylaxis
  b. Overdose may produce symptoms of water intoxication

10. Nursing considerations
  a. Check client's alertness to rule out water intoxication disorientation, lethargy, and behavioral changes
  b. Initial dose is given in evening and amount is increased until uninterrupted sleep is noted
  c. Check vital signs (BP and pulse) before giving by IV and subcut routes
  d. Measure daily I&O to monitor water retention and sodium depletion; assess edema in extremities
  e. Weigh daily to monitor water retention
  f. For nasal spray, make sure nasal mucosa is intact by inspecting nares prior to dose; use alternate nares for alternate doses
  g. IV dose may be given undiluted over 1 minute
  h. Store nasal spray at room temperature; all other solutions need refrigeration

Practice to Pass

A female client who is taking antidiuretic hormone (ADH) intranasally calls to tell you that she has a cold and flulike symptoms. What will you advise her to do?

11. Client education
  a. Proper technique for nasal instillation (tube inserted into nostril to instill)
  b. Avoid over-the-counter (OTC) meds containing epinephrine that can decrease drug's action
  c. Avoid alcohol use when taking drug
  d. Wear medic alert identification
  e. Do not double-dose if dose missed; may take skipped dose up to 1 hour before next dose
  f. Report any nasal congestion or upper respiratory tract infection

II. MEDICATIONS AFFECTING THE ADRENAL GLANDS

A. Mineralocorticoids

1. Action and use

    a. A **mineralocorticoid** is a steroid hormone that acts on kidneys to retain sodium and water and release potassium

    b. Synthesis is regulated by renin-angiotensin system

    c. Hormone therapy is required to replace missing mineralocorticoid, which is deficient when there is adrenal gland failure or hypofunction

2. Common medications for adrenal replacement (mineralocorticoids): see Table 13-3; fludrocortisone acetate is drug of choice for mineralocorticoid activity; note that not all corticosteroids have strong mineralocorticoid action; others may be cortisone and hydrocortisone

3. Administration considerations: fludrocortisone is given orally from 0.1 mg 3 times/week to 0.2 mg/day

4. Contraindications: hypersensitivity to glucocorticoids; idiopathic thrombocytopenic purpura (ITP); acute glomerulonephritis; viral or bacterial skin infections or infections not being treated with antibiotics; amebiasis; Cushing syndrome; vaccinations and immunologic procedures, osteoporosis

5. Drug interactions

    a. Hypokalemic effect may potentiate action of other drugs

    b. Hypernatremia may result if given with high-sodium drugs

Table 13-3	Corticosteroid Drugs	
Generic Names	**Route**	**Uses**
Betamethasone	PO	Has little or no mineralocorticoid action; used for hypercalcemia associated with cancer, reduction of inflammatory and immune responses from a variety of causes, prevention of respiratory distress syndrome in premature neonates
Cortisone	PO	Has both glucocorticoid and mineralocorticoid properties; used for replacement therapy in adrenal cortical insufficiency, and to reduce inflammatory and immune responses from a variety of causes, hypercalcemia related to cancer
Dexamethasone	PO, IV	Has strong glucocorticoid action but little mineralocorticoid action; used to suppress inflammation in a variety of disorders
Fludrocortisone	PO	Strong mineralocorticoid action; used for replacement therapy in primary and secondary adrenocortical insufficiency, treatment of salt-losing adrenogenital syndrome, management of orthostatic hypotension
Hydrocortisone	PO	Has both glucocorticoid and mineralocorticoid properties; used for replacement therapy in adrenal cortical insufficiency, to reduce inflammatory and immune responses from a variety of causes
Methylprednisolone	PO; IV, IM	Has little mineralocorticoid activity; in addition to adrenal replacement therapy, used to treat a variety of non-endocrine conditions requiring suppression of inflammatory and immune system responses
Prednisolone	PO, IM, IV	Has little mineralocorticoid activity; in addition to adrenal replacement therapy, used to treat a variety of non-endocrine conditions requiring suppression of inflammatory and immune system responses
Prednisone	PO	Has little mineralocorticoid activity; in addition to adrenal replacement therapy, used to treat a variety of non-endocrine conditions requiring suppression of inflammatory and immune system responses
Triamcinolone	PO, topical, inhalation	Has little mineralocorticoid activity; used most often for asthma and other non-endocrine conditions requiring suppression of inflammatory and immune system responses

        c. Higher dosage may be needed if given with drugs, such as rifampin and phenytoin, affecting hepatic metabolic enzymes

        d. Decreased steroid blood levels with phenytoin, phenobarbital, and rifampin

  6. Food interactions: high-sodium foods

  7. Significant laboratory studies: monitor serum electrolyte levels

  8. Side effects: sodium and fluid retention, nausea, acne, and impaired wound healing

  9. Adverse effects/toxicity

        a. Adverse reactions occur rarely, but use cautiously in clients with heart disease, congestive heart failure (CHF), or hypertension

        b. Thromboembolism

        c. Aggravation or masking of infection

        d. Anaphylactoid reactions are rare but may occur in clients hypersensitive to glucocorticoids

  10. Nursing considerations

        a. Is used with glucocorticoids for replacement therapy

        b. Monitor serum electrolyte levels

        c. Monitor weight and I&O and report weight gain of 2.3 kg (5 lb)/week

        d. Monitor and record BP daily and more frequently during periods of dosage adjustment

        e. Check for signs of overdosage related to hypercorticism (psychosis, excess weight gain, edema, CHF, increased appetite, severe insomnia, and elevated BP)

        f. Give daily doses before 9:00 A.M. to mimic peak corticosteroid blood levels

        g. Check for signs of underdosage: weight loss, poor appetite, nausea and vomiting, diarrhea, muscular weakness, increased fatigue, and low BP

  11. Client education

        a. Report signs of low potassium associated with high sodium (muscle weakness, paresthesias, circumoral numbness, fatigue, anorexia, nausea, depression, delirium, diminished reflexes, polyuria, irregular heart rate, CHF, ileus)

        b. Utilize range-of-motion exercises to decrease musculoskeletal effects

        c. Eat foods high in potassium

        d. Salt intake regulates drug's effect, so report signs of edema

        e. Weigh self daily and report consistent weight gain

        f. Report any infections, trauma, or unexpected stress

        g. Wear or carry medical alert identification including drug use and MD's name

        h. Call prescriber to increase dosage if client is under stress

B. Glucocorticoids

  1. Action and use

        a. A **glucocorticoid** is a steroid hormone that affects carbohydrate, protein, and fat metabolism and has anti-inflammatory and immunosuppressive activity; its synthesis is regulated by pituitary gland via negative feedback loop; may regulate metabolism of skeletal and connective tissues

        b. Used in acute **adrenal insufficiency** (inability of adrenal glands to produce sufficient adrenocortical hormones) caused by trauma or thrombosis; chronic primary adrenal insufficiency (also known as **Addison disease**); and secondary adrenal insufficiency (diseased or destroyed adenohypophysis with inadequate production of ACTH)

        c. Used in allergic conditions (asthma, angioedema, transfusion reactions, and serum sickness)

        d. Used in dermatologic conditions, such as dermatitis and pemphigus

        e. Used in inflammatory GI disorders, such as Crohn disease and ulcerative colitis

        f. Used in hematologic disorders, such as autoimmune hemolytic anemia and thrombocytopenia

Practice to Pass

A client taking mineralocorticoid therapy tells you that she has gained 2.5 kg (5½ lb) in the last 2 days. What action will you take?

   g. Used in joint inflammation, bursitis

   h. Used with antineoplastic agents in leukemias and lymphomas

   i. Used in ophthalmic diseases, such as allergic conjunctivitis, chorioretinitis, iritis, iridocyclitis, and keratitis

   j. Used in rheumatic disease (acute inflammatory states of arthritis and systemic lupus erythematosus)

2. Common medications for adrenal replacement (glucocorticoids): see Table 13-3 again

3. Administration considerations

   a. Routes of administration for systemic use to treat inflammatory conditions include IV, IM, and PO

   b. Routes of administration for nonsystemic use include inhalation, nasal, ophthalmic, otic, and topical

4. Contraindications: systemic fungal infections and known hypersensitivity

5. Significant drug interactions

   a. Antibiotics, cyclosporine, estrogen, and ketoconazole slow metabolism or clearance of glucocorticoids

   b. Aminoglutethimide, carbamazepine, cholestyramine, phenobarbital, phenytoin, and rifampin increase metabolism

   c. Anti-anxiety agents, antipsychotics, anticholinesterases, anticoagulants, antihypertensives, hypoglycemics, vaccines, pancuronium, salicylates, and sympathomimetics also affect metabolism or clearance

6. Significant food interactions: none identified

7. Significant laboratory studies

   a. CBC and differential, serum electrolytes, and blood glucose

   b. With long-term therapy monitor hypothalamic–pituitary–adrenal axis to check adrenal function

8. Side effects: few if high doses given for only a few days

9. Adverse effects/toxicity

   a. Higher doses and prolonged therapy may alter metabolism of tissues and organs leading to muscle wasting and increased fat deposits in face and central portion of body; emotional lability or changes in behavior and personality may also occur

   b. Prolonged therapy may cause growth suppression in children and osteoporosis in adults; impaired glucose tolerance and diabetes mellitus may also result

   c. Prolonged therapy can suppress the hypothalamic–pituitary–adrenal axis; **adrenal crisis** (an acute, life-threatening state of profound adrenocortical insufficiency) may result if drug is withdrawn abruptly, so always taper doses

   d. Toxicity may include anaphylactoid reactions, hypertriglyceridemia, peptic ulcers, acute pancreatitis, aseptic necrosis of bone, cataracts, glaucoma, hypertension, and opportunistic infections

10. Nursing considerations

   a. Check vital signs including BP, lung sounds, weight (including history of gain or loss), nausea and vomiting, and signs of dependent edema

   b. Conduct mental status exam and assess for signs of depression, withdrawal, insomnia, and anorexia

   c. Check skin for striae, thinning, bruising, change in color, change in hair growth, and acne

   d. In children on prolonged therapy, monitor height and growth pattern

   e. Advise regular ophthalmic examinations with long-term therapy

   f. Check stool for occult blood periodically

   g. With prolonged therapy, move and reposition immobilized clients carefully and limit use of adhesive tape on skin because skin may become fragile and damaged more easily

11. Client education
   a. Benefits and possible side effects with long-term use; report any new side effects
   b. Take oral doses with meals and avoid use of alcohol
   c. If prescribed every other day, take any missed dose as soon as remembered if on same day; if remembered the next day, then take dose and readjust schedule to be every other day; do not double up missed doses
   d. Implement weight reduction diet, limit sodium intake, and increase potassium intake if excessive weight gain occurs
   e. For clients with diabetes mellitus, carefully monitor blood glucose levels for elevation
   f. Report any blood in stool or black, tarry stools, mood changes or insomnia, vision changes or headache, weight gain of more than 5 pounds per week, irregular menses or pregnancy, irregular heart rate, excessive fatigue, severe abdominal pain, serious injury, or infection
   g. Avoid strenuous activities if skin is fragile and bruises easily
   h. With long-term therapy, take prescribed doses every day and do not discontinue medication without notifying prescriber; do not increase or decrease dose on own; tapering of dose is necessary
   i. Avoid immunizations during therapy and for 3 months after; avoid contact with anyone with measles or chickenpox or anyone receiving oral polio vaccine
   j. Avoid skin testing during therapy
   k. Wear specific medical alert identification during therapy
   l. With long-term therapy, report any fever, cough, sore throat, malaise, and unhealed injuries; avoid contact with anyone who has an active infection
   m. Review drug and teach specific administration and that client should not share drug with others

C. **Adrenocorticotropic hormone (ACTH)**
   1. Action and use
      a. Directly stimulates adrenal cortex to synthesize adrenal steroids
      b. Used to diagnose adrenal disorders such as Addison disease and secondary adrenal insufficiency caused by pituitary dysfunction
      c. Used in treatment of adrenocorticoid-responsive diseases, such as MS
      d. Limited use in treatment of adrenal insufficiency
   2. Common drugs for diagnosing adrenal gland disorders: see Table 13-4
   3. Administration considerations
      a. Agents may be given IV, IM, subcut, or PO
      b. Administer drug according to manufacturer's instructions
      c. Incompatible if mixed with aminophylline or sodium bicarbonate
   4. Contraindications
      a. Ocular herpes simplex; recent surgery
      b. Disorders such as CHF, scleroderma, osteoporosis, systemic fungoid infections, hypertension
      c. Sensitivity to porcine proteins
      d. Conditions related to adrenocortical insufficiency or hyperfunction
   5. Significant drug interactions: aspirin, nonsteroidal anti-inflammatory drugs (NSAIDs), barbiturates, phenytoin, rifampin, estrogens, amphotericin B, and diuretics
   6. Significant food interactions: none
   7. Significant laboratory studies: baseline electrolyte levels and baseline plasma cortisol level
   8. Side effects: nausea and vomiting, dizziness, drowsiness, or light-headedness

Practice to Pass

A client taking glucocorticoid therapy asks the nurse about wearing some sort of medic alert identification. How should the nurse respond?

Table 13-4	Drugs Used in Diagnosing Adrenal Gland Disorders	
Generic Name	**Route**	**Uses**
Corticotropin	IV, subcut	Evaluates adrenal function, nonsuppurative thyroiditis, hypercalcemia related to cancer, MS, trichinosis, tuberculosis meningitis, leukemia, lymphoma, infantile spasms, or rheumatic, collagen, or allergic reaction
Cosyntropin	IV, IM, subcut	Assists in diagnosing adrenocortical insufficiency, bronchial asthma, bronchospasm, allergic rhinitis, allergic disorders of the eye, mastocytosis (orphan drug use), prevention of GI and systemic food allergies
Metyrapone	PO	Evaluates hypothalamic and pituitary function; blocks cortisol synthesis in adrenals (may cause acute adrenal insufficiency)

9. Adverse effects/toxicity
   a. Hypersensitivity including urticaria, pruritus, dizziness, vomiting, and anaphylactic shock
   b. Cataracts or glaucoma; peptic ulcer with perforation; hirsutism and amenorrhea
   c. Sodium and water retention, potassium and calcium loss, and hyperglycemia
   d. Acne, impaired wound healing, fragile skin, petechiae, ecchymosis
   e. **Osteoporosis** (abnormal loss of bone density), decreased muscle mass, **cushingoid state** (having the appearance and facies characteristic of Cushing disease), activation of latent tuberculosis or diabetes mellitus, vertebral compression fractures

10. Nursing considerations
    a. Individualized dosage and gradual dosage changes should be made only after apparent full effect from drug is seen
    b. Shake liquid drug well before injecting into deep gluteal muscle; after administration observe closely for 15 minutes for any hypersensitivity reactions; prolonged treatment may increase risk of hypersensitivity reactions
    c. Monitor vital signs and BP and assess for dizziness, fever, flushing, rash, and urticaria
    d. Monitor plasma or urinary cortisol levels and serum electrolytes
    e. Be aware that agents may suppress signs and symptoms of chronic disease; new infections may appear during treatment
    f. At high dosage levels, drug must be gradually tapered
    g. Carefully monitor growth and development in children
    h. Clients with diabetes mellitus may require increased doses of oral antidiabetic agents or insulin during corticosteroid therapy

11. Client education
    a. Do not discontinue drug before notifying prescriber
    b. Low-salt or potassium-rich diet if prescribed
    c. Take oral doses with food, milk, or meals
    d. If dizziness, drowsiness, or light-headedness occurs, avoid driving or operating hazardous equipment
    e. Avoid exposure to communicable diseases or people with infections

III. MEDICATIONS AFFECTING THE THYROID GLAND

A. Thyroid hormones
1. Action and use
   a. As replacement hormone therapy for **hypothyroidism** (decreased activity of thyroid gland with a variety of specific causes); have same action as thyroid hormones produced in body to increase metabolic rate

b. Used to diagnose and treat thyroid deficiency and **myxedema** (most severe form of hypothyroidism characterized by swelling of face, feet, and periorbital tissues; may lead to coma and death) and to control goiter or thyroid carcinoma

2. Common drugs for thyroid disorders: see Table 13-5
3. Administration considerations
   a. May be given IV, IM, subcut, or PO
   b. Administer drug according to manufacturer's instructions
4. Contraindications
   a. Thyrotoxicosis, acute MI and cardiovascular disease, morphologic hypogonadism, nephrosis, and uncorrected hypoadrenalism
   b. Cautious use with angina pectoris; hypertension; older adults with cardiac disease; renal insufficiency; pregnancy; concurrent use of **catecholamines** (drugs that mimic effects of sympathetic nervous system); diabetes mellitus; **hyperthyroidism** (hyperactivity of thyroid gland), and malabsorption states
5. Significant drug interactions: thyroid hormones given with oral anticoagulants, insulin and sulfonylureas, epinephrine, and cholestyramine
6. Significant food interactions: soybean flour, walnuts, and dietary fiber may bind and decrease absorption of levothyroxine
7. Significant laboratory studies: serum T_4, free thyroxine, T_3 uptake, serum T_3, serum thyroid-stimulating hormone (TSH), protirelin test, thyroid uptake of radioiodine, TSH test, and thyroid suppression test
8. Side effects: weight loss, vomiting, and tachycardia
9. Adverse effects/toxicity
   a. Angina pectoris, coronary occlusion, or stroke in elderly or predisposed clients
   b. Relative adrenal insufficiency in clients with inadequate pituitary function related to secondary hypothyroidism and secondary adrenal insufficiency; adrenal crisis
   c. Overdosage causing signs of hyperthyroidism related to thyroid storm with shock and coma; thyrotoxicosis with CHF, angina, cardiac dysrhythmias, and shock
   d. Reactions to thioamides include fever, itching, and skin rash; blood dyscrasias and peripheral neuropathy; pain and swelling of joints or lupus-like syndrome; dizziness; or alterations in taste
   e. Overdosage of thioamides causes hypothyroidism
10. Nursing considerations
   a. Assess vital signs, BP, weight and history of weight change, normal diet, energy level, mood, subjective feeling, and response to temperature
   b. In children, check height
   c. Monitor thyroid function test results and blood glucose levels

Practice to Pass

A client taking thyroid hormone is also receiving sodium warfarin. What laboratory test should the nurse monitor?

Table 13-5	Drugs to Diagnose or Treat Hypothyroidism	
Generic Name	**Route**	**Uses**
Levothyroxine	PO, IV	Chemically pure form of T_4 and preferred therapy for hypothyroidism; given IV for myxedema coma
Liothyronine	PO, IV	Chemically pure form of T_3; for adult hypothyroidism; not used for cretinism since T_3 does not cross blood–brain barrier as well as T_4 does
Liotrix	PO	Chemically pure T_4 and T_3 in 4:1 ratio; used for hypothyroidism
Thyrotropin	IM, subcut	Natural TSH extracted from animals; used diagnostically to differentiate primary hypothyroidism from secondary hypothyroidism

      d. TSH may be frequently checked, high TSH indicates hormone replacement level is low; low TSH may indicate hormone replacement is too high

      e. Start older adults on lower doses of thyroid hormones and increase dose by small increments; assess for symptoms of stress that could lead to angina or stroke

  11. Client education

      a. How to monitor pulse, weight, and height

      b. Adhere to hormone replacement dosage schedule and intervals; realize that therapy is life-long; do not change brand of thyroid medication without discussing with prescriber because of differences in bioavailability

      c. Immediately report any chest pain or other signs of aggravated cardiovascular disease

      d. With juvenile hypothyroidism therapy, dramatic weight loss and catch-up growth may occur

      e. Do not discontinue drug and do carry medical alert identification

      f. Explain side effects and related treatment if changes in insulin or anticoagulants are needed

B. Antithyroid medications

  1. Action and use: treatment of hyperthyroidism and **Graves' disease** (pronounced hyperthyroidism often associated with enlarged thyroid gland and exophthalmos; also called *thyrotoxicosis*)

  2. Common medications for hyperthyroidism and Graves' disease: see Table 13-6

  3. Administration considerations: given orally according to manufacturer's instructions

  4. Contraindications

      a. Previous allergic or other severe reactions to thioamides

      b. Impaired hepatic function may require reduced doses

  5. Significant drug interactions

      a. Thioamides given with any iodine preparations including amiodarone, iodine solution, potassium iodide, and some contrast imaging dyes or radioactive iodine uptake

      b. Coumarin and other anticoagulants; digitalis

  6. Significant food interactions: none noted

  7. Significant laboratory studies: serum T_4, serum T_3, free T_4, free T_3, T_3, resin uptake, serum thyroid uptake of radioiodine, and thyroid suppression test; TSH diagnoses primary versus secondary hypothyroidism

  8. Side effects: fever, itching, and skin rash

Table 13-6   Drugs Used to Treat Hyperthyroidism and Graves Disease

Generic Name	Route	Notes
Thioamides		
Methimazole	PO	Inhibits thyroid hormone synthesis but not release
Propylthiouracil	PO	Inhibits thyroid hormone synthesis but not release; in peripheral tissues inhibits conversion of T_4 to T_3
Iodine		
Potassium Iodide and Iodine	PO	Has direct action on thyroid and used for short-term inhibition of thyroid hormone synthesis
Radioactive iodide (I-131)	PO	Radionuclide concentrated in thyroid; releases radiation and destroys tissue
Beta-Adrenergic Blockers		
Propranolol	PO	Does not lower T_4 and T_3 release from thyroid; treats symptoms of rapid pulse and increased BP related to hyperthyroidism

9. Adverse effects/toxicity
   a. Blood dyscrasias and peripheral neuropathy
   b. Pain and swelling of joints or lupus-like syndrome
   c. Dizziness and alteration in taste
   d. Overdosage results in hypothyroidism
   e. Rare instances of agranulocytosis
10. Nursing considerations
    a. Assess for tingling of fingers and toes
    b. Monitor weight and check for hair loss and skin changes
    c. Check CBC, differential count, and thyroid and liver function tests

    d. Dilute oral iodine solutions well in milk, juice, or other beverage
    e. Assess for metallic taste in mouth, sneezing, edematous thyroid, vomiting, and bloody diarrhea
11. Client education
    a. Explain need to wear medical alert identification tag or bracelet
    b. Explain goals and side effects of medications (side effects may not appear for days or weeks after treatment begun)

    c. Advise to report any fever, chills, sore throat, and unusual bleeding or bruising
    d. Instruct to take med at same time of day and with meals or snack; space additional daily doses throughout the day

IV. MEDICATIONS AFFECTING THE PARATHYROID GLANDS

A. Medications to treat hypocalcemia

1. Action and use
   a. Consist of calcium supplements
   b. Replaces calcium to supply body's metabolic needs

   c. Helps prevent calcium loss from bones and maintain bone strength
   d. Used to treat mild hypocalcemia and supplementation of dietary calcium
   e. Has additional use as an antacid
2. Common medications for calcium deficiency: see Table 13-7
3. Administration considerations
   a. Oral route
   b. Dosage differs among different oral calcium salts
   c. Must be taken with large glass of water with or after meals
   d. When used as antacid, should be taken 1 hour after meals and at bedtime
4. Contraindications: hypercalcemia, renal calculi, and hypophosphatemia
5. Significant drug interactions
   a. Glucocorticoids reduce calcium absorption
   b. Absorption of tetracyclines and quinolones is reduced if given with calcium

Table 13-7	Drugs Used to Treat Mild Calcium Deficiency	
Generic Name	**Route**	**Calcium Content**
Calcium acetate	PO	25%
Calcium carbonate	PO	40%
Calcium citrate	PO	21%
Calcium glubionate	PO	6.6%
Calcium phosphate tribasic	PO	39%

c. Thiazide diuretics decrease renal excretion of calcium

d. May enhance inotropic and toxic effects of digoxin

6. Significant food interactions: spinach, Swiss chard, beets, and bran and whole-grain cereals can reduce calcium absorption

7. Significant laboratory studies: serum calcium level

8. Side effects: constipation and flatulence

9. Adverse effects/toxicity

a. Hypercalcemia may occur if frequent or high doses

b. May also occur in clients being treated with calcium as part of renal dysfunction therapy

10. Nursing considerations

a. Take 1–1½ hours after meals

b. Space additional daily doses throughout day

c. Note number and consistency of stools; if constipation a problem, then a laxative or stool softener may be prescribed

d. With prolonged therapy, monitor weekly serum and urine calcium levels

e. Observe for signs of hypercalcemia if receiving frequent or high doses

f. Monitor for acid rebound if used as an antacid on repeated basis for more than 1–2 weeks

11. Client education

a. Signs of hypercalcemia; report any nausea and vomiting, constipation, frequent urination, lethargy, or depression

b. Do not take with cereals or other foods high in oxalates that form insoluble, nonabsorbable compounds with calcium

c. Potential dangers of repeated use as an antacid for more than 2 weeks

B. Vitamin D

1. Action and use

a. Vitamin D is needed for proper absorption of calcium; a fat-soluble vitamin that can accumulate in body

b. Used to help treat hypocalcemia or vitamin D deficiency

c. Used to treat rickets, **osteomalacia** (abnormal loss of calcification of matrix in lamellar bone, leading to bone softening and fracture) and **hypoparathyroidism** (insufficient secretion of parathyroid glands caused by primary parathyroid dysfunction or elevated serum calcium level)

2. Common medications for vitamin D deficiency: see Table 13-8

3. Administration considerations

a. Given orally (all) or IV (calcitriol)

b. Adequate calcium is needed for optimal response to treatment

4. Contraindications: clients with hypercalcemia or vitamin D toxicity and malabsorption syndrome

5. Significant drug interactions

a. Antacids or other preparations containing magnesium may cause high serum magnesium levels

b. Digitalis glycosides

Practice to Pass

A client taking long-term calcium supplements also takes digoxin. What type of drug interaction should the client be prepared to monitor for?

Table 13-8	**Drugs Used to Treat Vitamin D Deficiency**	
Generic Name	**Route**	**Uses**
Calcitriol	PO, IV	Hypoparathyroidism or chronic renal failure
Doxercalciferol	PO	Hypoparathyroidism or chronic renal failure
Ergocalciferol	PO	Hypoparathyroidism and to treat and prevent vitamin D deficiency

6. Significant food interactions: none noted
7. Significant laboratory studies
   a. Serum calcium and phosphorus levels
   b. BUN, serum creatinine levels, serum alkaline phosphatase
   c. Urinary calcium and urinalysis
8. Side effects: hypercalcemia related to overdosage; signs include ataxia, fatigue, irritability, seizures, somnolence, tinnitus, hypertension, GI tract distress or constipation, and hypotonia in infants
9. Adverse effects/toxicity
   a. Vitamin D hypercalcemia may lead to dysrhythmias in clients taking digoxin
   b. Hypervitaminosis D caused by large therapeutic doses may lead to hypercalcemia, hypercalciuria, bone decalcification, and calcium deposits in soft tissues
10. Nursing considerations
    a. Assess for any CNS problems
    b. Monitor BP, pulse, and I&O
    c. Monitor BUN, serum creatinine levels, serum calcium and phosphorus levels, serum alkaline phosphatase, and urinalysis
    d. If vitamin D toxicity occurs, make sure client stops drug immediately, forces fluid, and eats a low-calcium diet
11. Client education
    a. Make sure oral dose is swallowed intact without crushing or chewing tablet
    b. Do not increase or decrease dosage before notifying prescriber
    c. Check with prescriber before taking any OTC meds containing calcium, phosphorus, or vitamin D and any excessive amounts of any substances containing vitamin D
    d. Do not drive or use heavy equipment if client develops fatigue, somnolence, vertigo, or weakness
    e. Avoid magnesium-containing antacids

C. **Medications to treat hypercalcemia**
1. Action and use
   a. Promote urinary excretion of calcium
   b. Decrease mobilization of calcium from bone
   c. Decrease intestinal absorption of calcium
   d. Form complexes with free calcium in blood
   e. Achieve rapid lowering of blood calcium levels
   f. Used in emergency treatment of hypercalcemia, and to control hypercalcemia resulting from malignancies of the bone
2. Common medications for hypercalcemia: see Table 13-9
3. Administration considerations
   a. May be given subcut, IM, IV, or PO
   b. Give IM doses at bedtime to minimize effects of flushing following injection
   c. In emergency situations, dilute IV dose before administration to prevent extravasation; infuse over prescribed period of time
4. Contraindications: known hypersensitivity or with impaired renal function
5. Significant drug interactions
   a. Antacids, mineral supplements, calcium salts, and vitamin D
   b. Decreased effects of digoxin when serum calcium is reduced
   c. Nephrotoxic medications
6. Significant food interactions: calcium-rich dairy products
7. Significant laboratory studies
   a. CBC with differential count
   b. Serum electrolytes, alkaline phosphatase, and creatinine

Table 13-9		Drugs Used to Treat Hypercalcemia
Generic Name	**Route**	**Uses**
Edetate disodium	IV	Strong chelating agent; used on short-term basis to remove excess calcium
Gallium nitrate	IV	Used for hypercalcemia caused by cancer
Pamidronate	IV	Acts directly on bone by slowing bone reabsorption and lowering release of calcium; also used for Paget disease

Practice to Pass

A client with osteoporosis is reporting severe bone pain. What assessment criteria should the nurse employ?

      c. Liver function tests
      d. Urinalysis
8. Side effects
      a. Nausea and vomiting, diarrhea, and dyspepsia with oral route
      b. Facial flushing and occasional inflammatory reaction at injection site
      c. Transient influenza-like symptoms with IV route
      d. Nasal dryness and irritation with intranasal spray
9. Adverse effects/toxicity
      a. Allergic reactions with calcitonin salmon
      b. IV administration may cause venous irritation, thrombophlebitis, and nephrotoxicity
      c. Varying effects of hypocalcemia
      d. Toxicity with higher doses causes more severe GI distress, such as esophagitis, severe nephrotoxicity, and severe hypocalcemia
10. Nursing considerations
      a. Assess for hypercalcemia and hypocalcemia
      b. Monitor weight and I&O if vomiting and diarrhea occur
      c. Monitor serum electrolytes, serum alkaline phosphatase, serum creatinine, BUN, and liver function tests
      d. Monitor vital signs and assess for dysrhythmias with IV infusion
      e. Provide emotional support as needed
11. Client education
      a. How to self-administer subcut injection (use return demonstration)
      b. Do not discontinue therapy without notifying prescriber
      c. Taking doses in evening may lessen flushing
      d. Take oral doses on empty stomach
      e. Wear medical alert identification if on long-term therapy
      f. Reduced-calcium and reduced–vitamin D diet (e.g., decrease in dairy products)
      g. Drink sufficient fluids (at least six to eight glasses of water per day and possibly more if not contraindicated by other health problems)
   D. Medications to treat osteoporosis and Paget disease
      1. Action and use
         a. Reduce calcium release from bone
         b. Slow bone resorption and remodeling
         c. Prevent high-serum calcium concentrations
         d. Used long-term for **Paget disease** (a nonmetabolic disease of bone) and postmenopausal osteoporosis (abnormal loss of bone density)
         e. Also used to treat heterotropic ossification after spinal cord injury and hip replacement
      2. Common medications for bone disorders: see Table 13-10
      3. Administration considerations
         a. Given subcut, IM, PO, IV, and intranasal
         b. Nasal spray is given once daily in alternate nostrils

Table 13-10	Drugs Used to Treat Osteoporosis and Other Bone Disorders

Generic Name	Route
Bisphosphonates	
Alendronate	PO
Etidronate	PO
Ibandronate	PO, IV
Pamidronate	IV
Risedronate	PO
Tiludronate	PO
Zolendronate	IV
Miscellaneous Agents	
Bazedoxifene with conjugated estrogens	PO
Calcitonin salmon	IM, subcut
Cinacalcet	PO
Raloxifene	PO
Teriparatide	Subcut

4. Contraindications: do not give to clients with known hypersensitivity to salmon calcitonin or fish products, esophageal disorders, or during lactation; use cautiously with renal insufficiency, osteoporosis, and pernicious anemia

5. Significant drug interactions: antacids, mineral supplements, calcium salts, and vitamin D

6. Significant food interactions: calcium-rich dairy products

7. Significant laboratory studies
   a. Serum electrolytes, serum alkaline phosphatase, calcium and phosphorus and 24-hour urinary hydroxyproline prior to therapy, during first 3 months and then every 3–6 months
   b. Baseline values of bone mineral density (BMD) in hip, vertebrae, and forearm

8. Side effects
   a. Nausea and vomiting, diarrhea, and dyspepsia with oral route
   b. Facial flushing and occasional inflammatory reaction at injection site
   c. Transient influenza-like symptoms with IV route
   d. Muscle spasms, leukopenia with chills, fever, or sore throat
   e. Nasal dryness and irritation with intranasal spray

9. Adverse effects/toxicity
   a. Allergic reactions with calcitonin salmon
   b. IV administration may cause venous irritation, thrombophlebitis, and nephrotoxicity
   c. Varying effects of hypocalcemia
   d. Toxicity with higher doses causes more severe hypocalcemia, GI distress such as severe esophagitis with ulceration, and severe nephrotoxicity

10. Nursing considerations
   a. Assess for hypercalcemia and hypocalcemia
   b. Monitor weight and I&O if vomiting and diarrhea occur
   c. Monitor serum electrolytes, serum alkaline phosphatase, calcium and phosphorus, and 24-hour urinary hydroxyproline
   d. Monitor BMD values; in some clients therapy may be discontinued when symptoms are relieved

        e. Monitor bone pain in clients with Paget disease

        f. Ensure parenteral calcium is available to treat hypocalcemic tetany if it occurs

11. Client education

        a. How to self-administer subcutaneous injection (obtain return demonstration) and rotate sites

        b. Do not discontinue therapy without notifying prescriber

        c. Taking doses in evening may lessen flushing

        d. Take PO doses on empty stomach and remain upright for 30 minutes after taking

        e. Recognize signs of esophagitis and discontinue drug and notify prescriber if difficulty swallowing or worsening heartburn occur

        f. Wear medic alert identification if on long-term therapy

        g. How to follow low-calcium and low–vitamin D diet

        h. Sufficient fluid intake is important

        i. How to activate and administer metered-dose pump for nasal spray use

V. MEDICATIONS USED TO TREAT DIABETES MELLITUS

A. Insulin

1. Action and use

        a. Restores ability of cells to use glucose as an energy source

        b. Corrects **hyperglycemia** (higher than normal amount of glucose circulating in blood)

        c. Corrects many associated metabolic derangements

        d. Used to treat both type 1 and type 2 diabetes mellitus and diabetic ketoacidosis

        e. Also lowers plasma potassium levels and used as emergency treatment of hyperkalemia

2. Types of insulin: see Table 13-11

3. Administration considerations

        a. Given only by injection; inactivated by digestive system enzymes if given orally

        b. May be given subcut, IM, or IV; only *regular insulin* may be given IV

        c. Injection sites include upper arms, thighs, abdomen, and scapular area of back (scapular area rarely used because inaccessible, but may be used if dose is not self-administered)

        d. One general location is used at one time to maintain consistent absorption rates, although sites within each general location are used only once each month; American Diabetes Association (ADA) currently recommends rotating on abdominal sites

        e. Only mix insulins that are compatible with one another and use according to manufacturer's guidelines

        f. Store unopened vials in refrigerator; opened vials can remain at room temperature for up to 1 month; label vial with date and time opened and/or due to expire according to agency policy

        g. Alternate methods of delivery include jet injectors, pen injectors, portable insulin pumps, implantable pumps, and insulin by inhalation; an intranasal form is undergoing study

        h. Dosage must be monitored and linked with insulin needs

        i. A variety of insulin administration schedules, including multiple dosing schedules, are available to maintain euglycemia

4. Contraindications: previous allergic response to local or systemic use of drug

5. Significant drug interactions

        a. Hypoglycemic agents that lower blood glucose levels, such as sulfonylureas; acute use of alcohol; and beta-adrenergic blocking agents

Practice to Pass

A male client newly diagnosed with type 1 diabetes mellitus is going camping for 6 weeks and asks the nurse how he can store his insulin. What advice should the nurse give?

Table 13-11	Types of Insulin Preparations	
Insulin Type	**Action**	**Notes**
Lispro	**Onset:** 5–15 min **Peak:** 0.5–1 hr **Duration:** 3–4 hr	Rapid-acting
Aspart	**Onset:** 10–20 min **Peak:** 1–3 hr **Duration:** 3–5 hr	Rapid-acting
Glulisine	**Onset:** 15–30 min **Peak:** 1 hr **Duration:** 3–4 hr	Rapid-acting
Regular	**Onset:** 0.5–1 hr **Peak:** 2–4 hr **Duration:** 5–7 hr	Short-acting
Isophane (NPH)	**Onset:** 1–2 hr **Peak:** 4–12 hr **Duration:** 18–24 hr	Intermediate-acting
Insulin detemir	**Onset:** gradual over 24 hr **Peak:** none **Duration:** 24 hr	Long-acting
Insulin glargine	**Onset:** gradual over 24 hr **Peak:** none **Duration:** 24 hr	Long-acting
NPH/Regular Mixture (70–30%)	**Onset:** 0.5–1 hr **Peak:** 5–10 hr **Duration:** 6–8 hr	Combination isophane insulin suspension and regular insulin

    b. Hyperglycemic agents that increase blood glucose levels, such as thiazide diuretic agents, glucocorticoids, and sympathomimetics

    c. Beta-adrenergic blocking agents that delay response of insulin-related hypoglycemia and mask signs of sympathetic nervous system stimulation (tachycardia and palpitations)

6. Significant food interactions: moderate to high alcohol consumption without food enhances hypoglycemic action

7. Significant laboratory studies: random blood glucose (BG), fasting BG, glucose tolerance test, **glycosylated hemoglobin** A1c (a blood test representative of the average BG level over the past 2–3 months), urinary glucose and ketones, and serum electrolytes

8. Side effects

    a. Hypoglycemic reactions when blood glucose levels drop below 50 mg/dL

    b. Signs of hypoglycemic reaction include anxiety, confusion, nervousness, hunger, diaphoresis, and cool, clammy skin

9. Adverse effects/toxicity

    a. Somogyi phenomenon: a rapid decrease in blood glucose level at night

    b. Coma related to inadequate dosage caused by uncontrolled diabetic derangements with high blood glucose levels and ketoacidosis

    c. Hyperosmolar coma (nonketotic hyperglycemia)

    d. Coma related to insulin overdosage caused by inadequate food intake, excessive exercise, or excessive insulin administration; may be life-threatening if prolonged

10. Complications
    a. Presence of insulin antibodies that can lead to insulin resistance
    b. **Lipodystrophy** (abnormal deposition of subcutaneous fat at injection sites)
    c. Local allergic reaction related to a contaminant in the insulin preparation
    d. Systemic allergic reaction related to insulin itself and not to any contaminant
11. Nursing considerations
    a. Assess vital signs, weight, condition of skin and nails, serum and urine glucose levels, and glycosylated hemoglobin (and electrolyte and arterial blood gas levels) when appropriate
    b. Assess for long-term complications related to acceleration of atherosclerosis (hypertension, heart disease, stroke); retinopathy leading to possible blindness, nephropathy leading to possible renal failure; neuropathy leading to lower-limb ulcerations and amputation, impotence, and gastroparesis
    c. Consult with prescriber regarding insulin management when there is insufficient food intake or when client is NPO for surgery
    d. Adhere to agency policy regarding insulin administration
12. Client education
    a. Individualized teaching plan regarding insulin management
    b. All aspects of insulin administration including syringe use, mixing of insulins, stability of mixture, injection technique and sites
    c. Do not switch type or source of insulin or brand of syringe and avoid taking any new drug before notifying prescriber
    d. Signs and symptoms of hyperglycemia and hypoglycemia (client and family)
    e. How to test blood glucose levels
    f. Dietary restrictions and weight control; refer to dietitian for individualized instruction and meal planning
    g. Regular exercise helps achieve euglycemia
    h. Foot care and related aspects of personal hygiene
    i. Sick-day management of diabetes and insulin administration (continue to eat and take liquids as able, check blood glucose, maintain insulin schedule, and call prescriber if blood glucose is >250 mg/dL)
    j. Obtain and wear a medic alert tag or bracelet
    k. Avoid smoking or drinking alcoholic beverages
    l. Female clients should consult with healthcare provider before conceiving
    m. Refer to local home care agency and to ADA for additional follow-up and access to community-based resources

B. **Oral antidiabetic (hypoglycemic) agents—sulfonylureas**
    1. Action and use
        a. Stimulate release of insulin from pancreatic islets and increase sensitivity of insulin receptors on cells
        b. Used as an adjunct to nondrug therapy to reduce BG levels in type 2 diabetes mellitus
    2. Common oral antidiabetic medications (sulfonylureas: see Table 13-12; note tolbutamide has shortest duration of action and is quickly converted to inactive metabolites
    3. Administration considerations
        a. Dose is given orally one to three times a day
        b. Different agents possess different durations of action
        c. May be used alone or in combination with insulin
    4. Contraindications
        a. During pregnancy related to teratogenicity in animals
        b. In women who are nursing or lactating
        c. In clients with allergy to sulfa or urea

Practice to Pass

A client with type 2 diabetes mellitus has been sick at home for several days with a fever and flulike symptoms. What instructions should the nurse give to the client regarding sick-day diabetes management?

Table 13-12	Oral Antidiabetics/Hypoglycemics (Sulfonylureas)
Generic Name	**Duration of Action**
First-Generation	
Tolbutamide	6–12 hours
Tolazamide	12–24 hours
Chlorpropamide	24–72 hours
Second-Generation	
Glipizide Standard	12–24 hours
Glipizide Sustained release	24 hours
Glyburide	12–24 hours
Glyburide Micronized	24 hours
Glimepiride	24 hours

5. Significant drug interactions
   a. Nonsteroidal anti-inflammatory drugs (NSAIDs), sulfonamide antibiotics, acute use of ethanol, salicylates, phenothiazines, thiazides, ranitidine, and cimetidine
   b. Beta-adrenergic blocking agents can suppress insulin release and delay response to hypoglycemia
6. Significant food interactions: none noted
7. Significant laboratory studies
   a. CBC with differential, platelet count
   b. Liver function tests
   c. Blood glucose
8. Side effects: GI distress and neurologic symptoms such as dizziness, drowsiness, or headache
9. Adverse effects/toxicity
   a. Alcohol may cause a disulfiram-like reaction causing flushing, palpitations, and nausea
   b. Allergy related to skin reaction
   c. Hypoglycemia related to drug overdosage, drug interactions, altered drug metabolism, or inadequate food intake
   d. Hypoglycemic reactions are most likely to occur in presence of renal or hepatic dysfunction
10. Nursing considerations
    a. Assess vital signs, weight, condition of skin and nails, serum and urine glucose levels, glycosylated hemoglobin, and electrolyte and arterial blood gas levels when appropriate
    b. Assess for long-term complications of diabetes as noted in previous section regarding nursing considerations with insulin
    c. Consult with prescriber regarding management when client has insufficient food intake or is NPO for surgery
    d. Discuss psychosocial factors and lifestyle as they relate to adherence with therapy
11. Client education
    a. Individualized teaching plan based on client's previous knowledge, educational level, motivation to learn, and cultural considerations
    b. All aspects of drug therapy; take with food if GI upset occurs
    c. Take medication even if not feeling well

d. Take dose with first daily meal and take any missed dose as soon as remembered unless time for next dose; do not double-dose

e. Signs and symptoms of hypoglycemia (client and family) and notify prescriber if they occur

f. How to test blood glucose levels

g. Dietary restrictions and weight control; refer to dietitian (very helpful for developing effective meal and weight management plans)

h. Regular aerobic exercise in amount suited to client's health and abilities will help control BG levels

i. Foot care and related aspects of personal hygiene

j. Sick-day management of diabetes and prn insulin administration

k. Obtain and wear medic alert tag or bracelet

l. Avoid smoking or drinking alcoholic beverages

m. Female clients should consult with prescriber before conceiving and discontinue drug during pregnancy and lactation

n. Refer to local home care agency and to ADA for additional follow-up and access to community-based resources

C. Oral antidiabetics (hypoglycemic) agents—nonsulfonylureas

1. Action and use

   a. Alpha-glucosidase inhibitors block an intestinal enzyme that breaks down carbohydrates into more simple sugars; this action delays absorption of dietary carbohydrates and reduces blood glucose

   b. Biguanide (metformin) lowers blood glucose by decreasing production of glucose by liver

   c. Incretin mimetics (GLP-1 agonists) target a glucagonlike peptide to stimulate insulin release and inhibit glucagon release

   d. Incretin enhancers (DPP-4 inhibitors) prevent breakdown of natural incretins, leading to rising insulin levels and a greater antidiabetic response

   e. Meglitinides stimulate release of insulin from pancreas

   f. Sodium-glucose co-transporter (SGLT) inhibitors block enzyme SGLT2 in kidney tubule, leading to more glucose excretion in urine

   g. Thiazolidinediones (also called "glitazones") decrease insulin resistance and inhibit hepatic production of glucose, leading to reduced blood glucose levels

2. Common oral antidiabetic medications (nonsulfonylureas): Table 13-13

3. Administration considerations

   a. Orally one to three times a day depending on drug

   b. Metformin is used alone or in combination with a sulfonylurea

   c. Alpha-glucose inhibitors are used alone or in combination with insulin or a sulfonylurea

4. Contraindications: renal insufficiency and kidney disease

5. Significant drug interactions: vary depending on drug; see individual drug product insert

6. Significant food interactions: alcohol may increase risk of hypoglycemia or lactic acidosis

7. Significant laboratory studies

   a. CBC with differential, platelet count

   b. Liver function tests

   c. Blood glucose

8. Side effects

   a. Alpha-glucosidase inhibitors cause flatulence, cramps, abdominal distention, borborygmus ("stomach growling"), and diarrhea; also may decrease absorption of iron, leading to anemia

Table 13-13	Oral Antidiabetic Agents (Nonsulfonylureas)
Classification	**Generic Names**
Alpha-glucosidase inhibitors	Acarbose, miglitol
Biguanide	Metformin (immediate and extended release)
Incretin mimetics (GLP-1 agonists)	Albiglutide, exenatide, dulaglutide, liraglutide
Incretin inhibitors (DPP-4 inhibitors)	Alogliptin, linagliptin, saxagliptin, sitagliptin
Meglitinides	Nateglinide, repaglinide
Sodium-glucose co-transporter (SGLT) inhibitors	Canaglifozin, dapaglifozin, empaglifozin
Thiazolidinedione	Pioglitazone, rosiglitazone

    b. Biguanide (metformin) may cause decreased appetite, nausea, and diarrhea that usually subside over time; also, increased absorption of vitamin B_{12} and folic acid may occur

    c. Incretin mimetics may cause nausea, diarrhea, headaches, and dizziness in response to falling insulin levels

    d. Thiazolidinediones may lead to anemia and edema

  9. Adverse effects/toxicity

    a. Biguanide (metformin) with hypoglycemia and lactic acidosis result in a mortality rate of 50%

    b. Alpha-glucosidase inhibitors may lead to hypoglycemia if given with insulin or a sulfonylurea

    c. Thiazolidinediones (rosiglitazone) may cause CHF or angioedema

  10. Nursing considerations

    a. Assess vital signs, weight, condition of skin and nails, serum and urine glucose levels, glycosylated hemoglobin, and electrolyte and arterial blood gas levels when appropriate

    b. Assess renal function and evidence of renal insufficiency

    c. Assess for early signs of lactic acidosis (metformin)

    d. Assess for long-term complications of diabetes mellitus

    e. Consult with prescriber regarding management when client has insufficient food intake or is NPO for surgery

  11. Client education

    a. All aspects of diabetic management as outlined in previous client education section for sulfonylureas

    b. Early signs of hypoglycemia and lactic acidosis (hyperventilation, myalgia, malaise, unusual somnolence) and notify prescriber immediately if occur

D. Glucose-elevating medications—glucagon

  1. Action and use

    a. Promotes breakdown of glycogen, reduces glycogen synthesis, and stimulates synthesis of glucose

    b. Emergency treatment of severe **hypoglycemia** (lower than normal circulating glucose level) in unconscious clients or those unable to swallow and in clients receiving insulin shock therapy

  2. Common medication: glucagon

  3. Administration considerations

    a. Reconstitute according to manufacturer's directions

    b. Given subcut, IM, or direct IVP; flush IV line with 5% dextrose instead of NaCl solution

    c. Incompatible in syringe with any other medication

Practice to Pass

A client who has been experiencing frequent hypoglycemic (insulin) reactions at home calls and says that he cannot afford to buy any more blood glucose testing equipment. What should the nurse do?

4. Contraindications
   a. Hypersensitivity to glucagon or protein compounds
   b. Cautious use in insulinoma and pheochromocytoma
 ! 5. Significant drug interactions: incompatible with sodium chloride solutions or additives
6. Significant food interactions: none noted
7. Significant laboratory studies: blood glucose levels
8. Side effects: nausea and vomiting
9. Adverse effects/toxicity: hypersensitivity reactions, hyperglycemia and hypokalemia
10. Nursing considerations
    a. Client usually responds or awakens within 5 to 20 minutes after administration
 ! b. Give 50% glucose IV if no response to glucagon
    c. After client awakens and is able to swallow, give oral carbohydrate
    d. After recovery assess for persistent headache, nausea, and weakness
11. Client education
    a. How to test blood glucose levels
 ! b. Teach responsible family member how to administer subcut or IM if client unable to swallow oral glucose source during hypoglycemic reaction
    c. Notify prescriber immediately after reaction to determine cause

Case Study

A 20-year-old female is newly diagnosed with type 1 diabetes mellitus (DM). She is hospitalized to manage her presenting symptoms, establish a schedule for insulin therapy, and learn initial information on diabetic self-management. She has been prescribed a 2,000-calorie diabetic diet with three meals and two snacks. She is physically active and takes dance classes twice weekly.

1. What should you teach this client about the onset and pathophysiology of type 1 DM?

2. How should you explain the clinical manifestations of DM?

3. What should you teach the client about hyperglycemia and hypoglycemia and the treatment for each condition?

4. What should you teach the client about managing insulin therapy to prevent hyperglycemia and hypoglycemia?

5. What teaching should you provide about the interrelationships among diet, exercise, and insulin therapy in maintaining normal blood glucose levels?

For suggested responses, see pages 543–544.

POSTTEST

1 Before a child begins drug therapy with growth hormone, the nurse should stress which teaching point with the parents?

1. "Your child's expected growth rate is 7.6 to 12.7 cm (3–5 in.) during the first year of treatment."
2. "You need to measure your child's height and weight daily."
3. "Growth hormone therapy, once started, must be taken until the child reaches the age of 21."
4. "The amount of subcutaneous fat your child has will increase during the treatment period."

2 When the nurse teaches a client about insulin administration, what information about the client alerts the nurse that special instruction is needed?

1. Client closely restricts foods high in carbohydrates.
2. Client wants spouse to learn to administer insulin.
3. Client performs 30 minutes of aerobic exercise every other day.
4. Client takes nap each day in the afternoon.

3 A client recently diagnosed with type 2 diabetes mellitus is beginning drug therapy with tolbutamide. The nurse should conduct a drug history with special emphasis on which drugs? Select all that apply.

1. Ginseng, which increases hypoglycemic effects
2. Alcoholic beverages, which cause a disulfiram-like reaction
3. Thiazide diuretics, which increase risk for aplastic anemia
4. Beta blockers, which mask signs and symptoms of hypoglycemic reaction
5. Garlic, which increases risk of bleeding

4 A female client with a tumor on the posterior pituitary gland is taking cabergoline 0.25 mg by mouth twice weekly. The nurse should monitor for which of the following therapeutic outcomes?

1. Normal serum calcium levels
2. Reduced number of hot flashes per day
3. Lowering of blood pressure
4. Relief from inappropriate lactation

5 A client who has received metyrapone experiences an adrenal crisis. The nurse considers that which condition most likely predisposed the client to this occurrence?

1. Hyperaldosteronism
2. Adrenal insufficiency
3. Pheochromocytoma
4. Type 1 diabetes mellitus

6 A client with adrenal insufficiency is prescribed to take hydrocortisone three times daily on a long-term basis. What should the nurse include in client teaching? Select all that apply.

1. "Immediately stop taking this medication if weight gain or diarrhea occurs."
2. "Alcohol and caffeine should be avoided while taking this medication."
3. "You will likely notice an improvement in your daily blood glucose levels and hemoglobin A1C levels."
4. "Report symptoms of persistent heartburn or indigestion."
5. "Report any wound that will not heal or is healing very slowly."

7 A client who recently started taking desmopressin reports onset of a headache, lethargy, and drowsiness. The nurse should make which assessment of the client next?

1. History of recent streptococcal infection
2. Whether client also takes carbamazepine
3. If client has developed hypertension
4. Signs and symptoms of dehydration

8 Before surgery, propranolol is prescribed for a client with hyperthyroidism. The nurse should assess for which set of intended outcomes?

1. Change in heart rate, reduced anxiety, reduced sweating
2. Regrowth of scalp hair, increased tolerance of extreme temperature changes
3. Weight gain, improved respiratory status
4. Decreased insomnia, decreased restlessness

9 A client taking digoxin is scheduled to receive an injection of intravenous calcium. The nurse should prepare to intervene if which sign(s) of drug interaction occur(s)?

1. Hypertension and tingling around the mouth
2. Sustained, significant bradycardia
3. Nausea and vomiting and diarrhea
4. Sloughing of tissue at the injection site

. . . .

10 Because a client with hypocalcemia needs to increase the level of calcium absorption, which activity should the nurse perform as part of the therapeutic plan of care?

1. Administer magnesium sulfate PO.
2. Encourage increase in exercise.
3. Administer verapamil 80 mg PO q8h.
4. Administer ergocalciferol (vitamin D).

➤ *See pages 449–452 for Answers and Rationales.*

ANSWERS & RATIONALES

Pretest

1 **Answer: 3 Rationale:** Growth hormone (GH) is only approved for use in children to treat a documented lack of growth hormone. It is available as a parenteral medication only, to be given IM or subcutaneously. Only long bones are affected. The nurse should answer the parent's question before exploring other areas. **Cognitive Level:** Analyzing **Client Need:** Pharmacological and Parenteral Therapies **Integrated Process:** Communication and Documentation **Content Area:** Pharmacology **Strategy:** Recall first the guidelines for prescribing growth hormone. Then compare this information to the statement in each option and use the process of elimination to make a selection. **Reference:** Wilson, B. A., Shannon, M.T., & Shields, K. M. (2017). *Pearson nurse's drug guide 2017.* New York, NY: Pearson, pp. 1424–1426.

2 **Answer: 2 Rationale:** Abrupt cessation of long-term steroid therapy can cause acute adrenal insufficiency, which could lead to death. Signs and symptoms include nausea and vomiting, lethargy, confusion, and coma. Because long-term glucocorticoid therapy results in shrinkage of the adrenal gland, it cannot produce an adequate level of the hormone. Abrupt withdrawal can cause problems. Central nervous system symptoms such as confusion and psychosis are adverse effects of steroids such as prednisone. Gradual reduction of dosages decreases the severity of the withdrawal signs and symptoms without bloodwork. **Cognitive Level:** Applying **Client Need:** Pharmacological and Parenteral Therapies **Integrated Process:** Communication and Documentation **Content Area:** Pharmacology **Strategy:** Determine the time frame associated with safe withdrawal of corticosteroids. Then select the option that best matches this information. **Reference:** Wilson, B. A., Shannon, M. T., & Shields, K. M. (2017). *Pearson nurse's drug guide 2017.* New York, NY: Pearson, p. 1281.

3 **Answer: 2, 4, 5 Rationale:** A record of nocturnal enuresis should be maintained and discussed with the prescriber. Rapid increases in weight, heart rate, blood pressure, and shortness of breath should be reported to the prescriber because they may indicate water retention. Drowsiness, lethargy, or confusion may be signs of water intoxication and should be reported to the prescriber. The drug should not be shaken, as this may lead to drug breakdown. Desmopressin (DDAVP) nasal spray should be administered high up into the nasal cavity and not down the throat. **Cognitive Level:** Applying **Client Need:** Pharmacological and Parenteral Therapies **Integrated Process:** Nursing Process: Implementation **Content Area:** Pharmacology **Strategy:** Specific drug information is needed to answer the question. Consider all aspects of drug administration and note the wording of the question indicates that more than one option will be correct. **Reference:** Adams, M. P., & Koch, R. W. (2010). *Pharmacology: Connections to nursing practice.* Upper Saddle River, NJ: Pearson, p. 1115.

4 **Answer: 1 Rationale:** High doses of fludrocortisone may result in excess retention of sodium and water, resulting in excessive weight gain. Because outcomes include sodium and fluid retention, the client is more likely to gain weight than lose it. A reduced ability to resist infection is associated with Cushing disease rather than Addison disease. Because of the risk of excess fluid retention, the client is not likely to experience hypovolemia. **Cognitive Level:** Applying **Client Need:** Pharmacological and Parenteral Therapies **Integrated Process:** Nursing Process: Planning **Content Area:** Pharmacology **Strategy:** Recall first that the drug is a mineralocorticoid. Therefore, the drug's action will involve sodium retention. Next recall that sodium retention leads to water retention and associate this with the need to measure weight as an indicator of fluid volume status. **Reference:** Wilson, B. A., Shannon, M. T., & Shields, K. M. (2017). *Pearson* *nurse's drug guide 2017*. New York, NY: Pearson, pp. 659–661.

5 **Answer: 1, 2, 3 Rationale:** Levothyroxine is indicated for use in clients with cretinism, congenital hypothyroidism, and for some types of thyroid cancer that contribute to hypothyroidism. Myxedema coma occurs in clients who have very low thyroid hormone levels. The use of levothyroxine and other forms of thyroid hormone replacement would be indicated. Glucocorticoid and mineralocorticoid replacement is expected for adrenal insufficiency. Oral and injectable hypoglycemic agents are used to treat type 2 diabetes mellitus. **Cognitive Level:** Analyzing **Client Need:** Pharmacological and Parenteral Therapies **Integrated Process:** Nursing Process: Planning **Content Area:** Pharmacology **Strategy:** Consider options that have some relationship to the thyroid gland to make your selections. Note the wording of the question indicates that more than one option is correct. **Reference:** Adams, M. P., & Urban, C. (2015). *Pharmacology: Connections to nursing practice* (3rd ed.). New York, NY: Pearson, p. 1152.

6 **Answer: 2 Rationale:** Symptoms of adverse effects of liotrix include tachycardia and angina. Without treatment, these symptoms can result in cardiac damage. Assessing the heart rate is the most important assessment. Toxicity can result in slight hyperthermia, but this will have minimal impact on the client's health. Thus, temperature does not have to be monitored. Sleepiness is a sign or symptom of the disease, which should decrease or resolve once drug therapy is started. Nervousness is a side effect of this drug, but this is less threatening than cardiac alterations. **Cognitive Level:** Applying **Client Need:** Pharmacological and Parenteral Therapies **Integrated Process:** Communication and Documentation **Content Area:** Pharmacology **Strategy:** Select the option that could place the client at risk the most rapidly and the most significantly. Oxygenation and circulation should be considered first when the items ask for priority-setting. As a separate strategy to eliminate sleepiness being a side effect, differentiate the disease profile from the characteristics of the drug. **Reference:** Wilson, B. A., Shannon, M. T., & Shields, K. M. (2017). *Pearson nurse's drug guide 2017*. New York, NY: Pearson, pp. 908–909.

7 **Answer: 3 Rationale:** Agranulocytosis is the most serious toxic effect of this drug, and it can predispose the client to a variety of infections. Attempts to determine the risk for infection are important, but are not as important as reviewing the white blood cell count as an indicator of current ability to fight infection. Although stress can predispose the client to infection, the immediate concern is the client's actual condition and ability to combat infection, as evidenced by the WBC count. **Cognitive Level:** Applying **Client Need:** Pharmacological and Parenteral Therapies **Integrated Process:** Nursing Process: Implementation **Content Area:** Pharmacology **Strategy:** To answer the question correctly, it is necessary to be aware of the risk for agranulocytosis with this drug. From there, associate the drug side effects with the option that directly assesses this parameter. **Reference:** Wilson, B. A., Shannon, M. T., & Shields, K. M. (2017). *Pearson nurse's drug guide 2017*. New York, NY: Pearson, pp. 1312–1314.

8 **Answer: 1 Rationale:** Paget disease is characterized by overactive osteoblasts (cells that break down the bone), which stimulates an increase in alkaline phosphatase levels. Calcitonin decreases the cell turnover. This is evident in the reduced alkaline phosphate level. Calcitonin would decrease the calcium level rather than increase it. Bone deformity is permanent, not temporary, so bones will not return to normal. Skull deformities are common with Paget but are unrelated to therapeutic effectiveness. **Cognitive Level:** Applying **Client Need:** Pharmacological and Parenteral Therapies **Integrated Process:** Nursing Process: Implementation **Content Area:** Pharmacology **Strategy:** The critical words in the question are *therapeutic effectiveness*. This tells you that the correct option is one that illustrates the expected effect of the drug. Use this knowledge and the process of elimination to make a selection. **Reference:** Wilson, B. A., Shannon, M. T., & Shields, K. M. (2017). *Pearson nurse's drug guide 2017*. New York, NY: Pearson, pp. 217–219.

9 **Answer: 2, 3, 5 Rationale:** Visual changes can occur because of diabetic retinopathy, particularly in clients whose blood glucose is not well controlled. Changes in penile vasculature may cause impotence prior to diagnosis of diabetes mellitus; initial insulin therapy may increase this problem. Some clients experience a rebound hyperglycemia (Somogyi effect). It is helpful for a family member to be able to inject insulin, but the initial focus should be on teaching the client. With control of serum glucose levels, complications such as vision loss and loss of limbs due to accelerated atherosclerosis can be prevented or delayed. **Cognitive Level:** Applying **Client Need:** Pharmacological and Parenteral Therapies **Integrated Process:** Teaching and Learning **Content Area:** Pharmacology **Strategy:** The wording of the question indicates that the correct responses are true statements. Read each statement and determine whether it is a true or false statement and use the process of elimination to make your selections, using knowledge of the disease process of diabetes mellitus and information about insulin and its effects on the body. **Reference:** Wilson, B. A., Shannon, M. T., & Shields, K. M. (2017). *Pearson nurse's drug guide 2017*. New York, NY: Pearson, pp. 802–813.

10 **Answer: 3 Rationale:** The priority learning need in treatment of an insulin reaction is that the client understands to take some form of oral glucose, such as orange juice or crackers with peanut butter. The protein prevents a rebound hypoglycemia. This is the most appropriate action because it fixes the problem within a reasonable time frame. The problem can be remedied most of the time without notifying the prescriber, so this is a lesser priority. Scheduling serum glucose levels would be routine and not in relation to an insulin reaction; instead, the client would monitor finger-stick glucose at home. Ingesting fluid would not contribute to the recovery from drug-induced hypoglycemia. **Cognitive Level:** Analyzing **Client Need:** Pharmacological and Parenteral Therapies **Integrated Process:** Teaching and Learning **Content Area:** Pharmacology **Strategy:** Recall that an insulin reaction is a critical event and the priority action needs to focus on reversing the low blood glucose. With this in mind, easily eliminate each of the incorrect options. **Reference:** LeMone, P., & Burke, K. M., Bauldoff, G., & Gubrud, P. (2015). *Medical-surgical nursing: Clinical reasoning in patient care.* (6th ed.). New York, NY: Pearson, pp. 1232–1238.

Posttest

1 **Answer: 1 Rationale:** The expected growth rate with growth hormone therapy is 3–5 inches in the first year. Height and weight is measured monthly. Growth hormone is discontinued when optimum adult height is attained, fusion of epiphyseal plates has occurred, or when there is no response to growth hormone. Growth hormone is related to growth of long bones, not fat deposition. **Cognitive Level:** Analyzing **Client Need:** Pharmacological and Parenteral Therapies **Integrated Process:** Teaching and Learning **Content Area:** Pharmacology **Strategy:** Correlate the action of the drug with the expected outcome. Parents may expect a more rapid rate of growth than is typical. Eliminate two options because of the words *daily* and *must*, respectively. Use knowledge of growth hormone to make the final selection. **Reference:** Adams, M. P., & Urban, C. (2015). *Pharmacology: Connections to nursing practice* (3rd ed.). Upper Saddle River, NJ: Pearson, pp. 1106–1112.

2 **Answer: 1 Rationale:** Insulin contributes to the metabolism of fats, proteins, and carbohydrates. The client should ingest a balanced diet, not just restrict carbohydrates. It is appropriate for the spouse to learn to administer the insulin if the client becomes unable to. Regular exercise can increase peripheral use of glucose. Napping in the afternoon would have no significant impact on insulin administration. **Cognitive Level:** Applying **Client Need:** Pharmacological and Parenteral Therapies **Integrated Process:** Nursing Process: Assessment **Content Area:** Pharmacology **Strategy:** Select the option most closely associated with the function of insulin. **Reference:** LeMone, P., & Burke, K. M., Bauldoff, G., & Gubrud, P. (2015). *Medical-surgical nursing: Clinical reasoning in patient care.* (6th ed.). New York, NY: Pearson, p. 536.

3 **Answer: 1, 2, 4 Rationale:** Ginseng lowers glucose levels. Tolbutamide interacting with alcohol can lead to a *disulfiram-like* reaction, causing complaints of headache and flushing of the skin. This is an important teaching point for the client who has a history of alcoholism, even if currently not drinking. Beta blockers reduce the sympathomimetic response to hypoglycemic

reactions. Hence, signs and symptoms of hypoglycemia are less likely to occur. Aplastic anemia is a side effect of tolbutamide, not thiazide diuretics. Garlic does not interact with tolbutamide to increase the risk of bleeding. **Cognitive Level:** Analyzing **Client Need:** Pharmacological and Parenteral Therapies **Integrated Process:** Teaching and Learning **Content Area:** Pharmacology **Strategy:** Presume the major focus will be on increasing the risk of hypoglycemia as well as the disulfiram-like (Antabuse) reaction. **Reference:** Wilson, B. A., Shannon, M. T., & Shields, K. M. (2017). *Pearson nurse's drug guide 2017.* New York, NY: Pearson, p. 1528.

4 **Answer: 4 Rationale:** The primary purpose of the cabergoline is to reduce or eliminate lactation related to hyperprolactinemia. The drug has no effect on calcium levels. Hot flashes are a side effect of the drug. Hypotension is a common side effect. **Cognitive Level:** Analyzing **Client Need:** Pharmacological and Parenteral Therapies **Integrated Process:** Nursing Process: Evaluation **Content Area:** Pharmacology **Strategy:** Specific knowledge of this medication is needed to answer the question. Align the drug's action with the client's health needs and the disease process. **Reference:** Wilson, B. A., Shannon, M. T., & Shields, K. M. (2017). *Pearson nurse's drug guide 2017.* New York, NY: Pearson, p. 217.

5 **Answer: 2 Rationale:** In the presence of adrenal insufficiency, metyrapone may cause an adrenal crisis by reducing the synthesis of cortisol. The drug is utilized for diagnosis of Cushing disease. Aldosterone is a mineralocorticoid, while metyrapone influences glucocorticoids. Pheochromocytoma is related to excessive secretion of catecholamines and would not cause an adrenal crisis, which is related to decreased glucocorticoid level. Diabetes is more likely to develop with high levels of glucocorticoids. **Cognitive Level:** Applying **Client Need:** Pharmacological and Parenteral Therapies **Integrated Process:** Nursing Process: Diagnosis **Content Area:** Pharmacology **Strategy:** First recall that an adrenal crisis results from insufficient amounts of hormones produced by the adrenal cortex. With this in mind, look for the option that identifies hypofunction of the adrenal gland. Alternatively, determine the relationship between adrenal function and the function of the drug. **Reference:** Adams, M. P., & Urban, C. (2015). *Pharmacology: Connections to nursing practice* (3rd ed.). Upper Saddle River, NJ: Pearson, p. 1171.

6 **Answer: 2, 4, 5 Rationale:** Alcohol and caffeine should be avoided during long-term hydrocortisone therapy because they contribute to the development of peptic ulcer disease. Heartburn or indigestion should be reported; they are adverse effects of this medication and may signal peptic ulcer disease. Corticosteroids inhibit the inflammatory and immune response. A slow-healing wound should be reported to the healthcare provider. Replacement steroids should not be abruptly discontinued. If needed, the client should be tapered off the medication to avoid withdrawal symptoms and/or adrenal insufficiency. Replacement corticosteroids may contribute to secondary diabetes. It is unlikely that an improvement of blood glucose or hemoglobin A1C will occur. **Cognitive Level:** Applying **Client Need:** Pharmacological and Parenteral Therapies **Integrated Process:** Teaching and Learning **Content Area:** Pharmacology **Strategy:** The wording of the question indicates that more than one option is correct. Choose the options that contain true statements based on the wording of the question. **Reference:** Adams, M. P., & Urban, C. (2015). *Pharmacology: Connections to nursing practice* (3rd ed.). Upper Saddle River, NJ: Pearson, p. 1168.

7 **Answer: 2 Rationale:** Desmopressin is a drug used to treat diabetes insipidus. The manifestations listed are all signs of water intoxication, which could occur as an excessive effect of the medication. Carbamazepine prolongs the effect of desmopressin and could lead to water retention. The drug has no known effects on the immune system. Hypertension may develop with overhydration, but the headache is related more to the swelling of the brain cells. The client's symptoms are not related to dehydration. **Cognitive Level:** Applying **Client Need:** Pharmacological and Parenteral Therapies **Integrated Process:** Nursing Process: Assessment **Content Area:** Pharmacology **Strategy:** Associate the drug with antidiuretic hormone and note that the symptoms are related to fluid overload. Use the process of elimination to choose the option that seems most likely to pose a risk of fluid retention. **Reference:** Wilson, B. A., Shannon, M. T., & Shields, K. M. (2017). *Pearson nurse's drug guide 2017*. New York, NY: Pearson, p. 439.

8 **Answer: 1 Rationale:** The excessive levels of thyroxine in hyperthyroidism lead to symptoms such as tachycardia, anxiety, and diaphoresis. Propranolol is a beta-adrenergic blocker and is used to treat sympathetic nervous system responses. Although the disease affects the volume of hair and heat tolerance, propranolol has no direct effect on heat tolerance or scalp hair. Because of the excessive thyroxine secretion, the metabolic process is increased, which results in dyspnea without exertion. The purpose of the propranolol is to reduce the cardiovascular signs and symptoms, not respiratory symptoms. Because propranolol reduces tachycardia and palpitations, the insomnia and restlessness may decrease,

but this is not the primary purpose for the administration of the drug. **Cognitive Level:** Applying **Client Need:** Pharmacological and Parenteral Therapies **Integrated Process:** Nursing Process: Evaluation **Content Area:** Pharmacology **Strategy:** The critical words in the question are *intended outcomes*. Associate the signs and symptoms of the disease profile along with the actions of propranolol and use the process of elimination to make a selection. **Reference:** Wilson, B. A., Shannon, M. T., & Shields, K. M. (2017). *Pearson nurse's drug guide 2017*. New York, NY: Pearson, pp. 1302–1306.

9 **Answer: 2 Rationale:** Because calcium influences cardiac contractility and neural transmission, it can potentiate the actions of digoxin. The nurse should monitor for severe bradycardia. Hypotension is more likely to occur than hypertension, and tingling around the mouth is more indicative of hypocalcemia. Nausea and vomiting are side effects associated with digoxin, but not diarrhea. Neither is related to a drug interaction between calcium and digoxin. Sloughing of tissue at the site is associated with injection of calcium, but this is not a drug interaction. **Cognitive Level:** Applying **Client Need:** Pharmacological and Parenteral Therapies **Integrated Process:** Nursing Process: Planning **Content Area:** Pharmacology **Strategy:** Correlate the potential combined effect of both drugs on the heart. Eliminate two options first because they are least related to the heart, and then eliminate a third option because it contains a symptom of hypocalcemia. **Reference:** Wilson, B. A., Shannon, M. T., & Shields, K. M. (2017). *Pearson nurse's drug guide 2017*. New York, NY: Pearson, pp. 471–475.

10 **Answer: 4 Rationale:** Ergocalciferol (vitamin D) regulates calcium and phosphorus metabolism and increases blood levels of both elements. Magnesium may reduce calcium absorption. Exercise contributes to bone maintenance. Calcium may reduce the effects of verapamil. Absorption of calcium is not affected. **Cognitive Level:** Applying **Client Need:** Pharmacological and Parenteral Therapies **Integrated Process:** Nursing Process: Implementation **Content Area:** Pharmacology **Strategy:** Determine the relationship between the elements most likely to enhance absorption of calcium. **Reference:** Wilson, B. A., Shannon, M. T., & Shields, K. M. (2017). *Pearson nurse's drug guide 2017*. New York, NY: Pearson, pp. 219–220.

References

Adams, M., Holland, L., & Urban, C. (2017). *Pharmacology for nurses: A pathophysiologic approach* (5th ed.). New York, NY: Pearson.

Adams, M. P., & Urban, C. (2015). *Pharmacology: Connections to nursing practice* (3rd ed.). Upper Saddle River, NJ: Pearson.

Burchum, J. & Rosenthal, L. (2016). *Lehne's Pharmacology for Nursing Care*. (9th ed.). St. Louis, MO: Elsevier.

Drug Facts & Comparisons (updated monthly). St. Louis, MO: Wolters Kluwer.

Karch, A. M. (2016). *Focus on nursing pharmacology* (7th ed.). Philadelphia, PA: Lippincott Williams & Wilkins.

Kee, J. L. (2017). *Handbook of laboratory and diagnostic tests with nursing implications*. (8th ed.). New York, NY: Pearson.

LeMone, P. T., Burke, K. M., Bauldoff, G., & Gubrud, P. (2015). *Medical-surgical nursing: Clinical reasoning in patient care*. (6th ed.). New York, NY: Pearson.

Reproductive System Medications

14

Chapter Outline

Estrogens
Progestins
Androgens
Anabolic Steroids

Medications for Erectile
    Dysfunction
Contraceptives
Fertility Medications

Medications for Labor and
    Delivery
Emergency Contraceptives

Objectives

➤ Describe general goals of therapy when administering medications associated with the reproductive system.

➤ Identify side effects and adverse effects of estrogens, progestins, and androgens.

➤ Describe client-centered nursing care related to medications used to treat erectile dysfunction.

➤ Describe effects of oxytocin on the uterus.

➤ Identify indications, contraindications, side effects, and adverse reactions of ergonovine and methylergonovine.

➤ Identify action and use for ritodrine.

➤ Identify indications, contraindications, side effects, and adverse reactions of magnesium sulfate.

➤ Describe specific client-centered nursing care when administering magnesium sulfate.

➤ List significant client education points related to reproductive system medications.

NCLEX-RN® Test Prep

Access the NEW Web-based app that provides students with additional practice questions in preparation for the NCLEX experience.

Review at a Glance

anabolic steroid an androgen with anabolic properties, rarely prescribed but often abused by athletes to increase muscle mass

androgen a medication that induces or increases male hormone-like effects

cryptorchidism a congenital condition characterized by failure of testis to descend into the scrotum

hypogonadism underdevelopment of gonads

priapism painful penile erection that does not spontaneously subside

PRETEST

1 The healthcare provider at an outpatient clinic is considering prescribing sildenafil for a 61-year-old client. The nurse would make it a priority to discuss which item in the client's health history with the prescriber?

1. Coronary artery disease (CAD) with nitroglycerin use
2. Renal impairment with elevated creatinine level
3. Blurred vision of unknown etiology
4. Gout managed with allopurinol

2 A pregnant client is being prepared for labor induction with oxytocin. The nurse concludes that the client has adequate understanding when the client verbalizes the medication will have which action? Select all that apply.

1. Cause an increase in blood pressure to provide adequate oxygen for the baby
2. Cause the uterus to contract harder and more often
3. Start contractions that will be almost continuous until the baby is born
4. Be given through the intravenous line (IV) in small continuous amounts that can be adjusted as needed
5. Cause the client to be in real labor

3 The client with preterm labor is receiving magnesium sulfate (generic) intravenously. To detect an early side effect, the nurse should perform which assessments?

1. Check deep tendon reflexes.
2. Auscultate lung sounds every 15 minutes.
3. Ask the client to report sudden flank pain.
4. Percuss the suprapubic area every hour.

4 To better help a client understand the action of clomiphene, the nurse should include which information in the teaching plan for a female client who will begin taking the drug?

1. Teach normal process of conception.
2. Explain uterine involution process.
3. Teach the client to keep a record of daily temperatures.
4. Explain function of female hormones.

5 The client taking an estrogen–progestin combination oral contraceptive calls the clinic reporting that she has forgotten her pills for the last 2 days. What medication directions should the nurse provide?

1. "Take two pills today and two pills tomorrow, then one pill daily for the rest of the pill pack."
2. "Take two pills today and then one each day until the pill pack is finished."
3. "Notify your healthcare provider of the missed dosage."
4. "Stop taking the pills and have your partner use condoms until the next menses, then restart a new pill pack."

6 The perinatal nurse is assigned to several clients. The nurse anticipates that which client is most likely to be a candidate for drug therapy with terbutaline?

1. Client at 27 weeks' gestation who has regular uterine contractions
2. Client at 41 weeks' gestation with irregular uterine contractions
3. Client with postpartum hemorrhage following delivery
4. Client at 38 weeks' gestation with hypertension and seizures

7 Because a hypertensive client is experiencing postpartum hemorrhage, the nurse anticipates that the healthcare provider will most likely prescribe which drug to treat the hemorrhage?

1. Ergonovine
2. Methylergonovine
3. Oxytocin
4. Carboprost tromethamine

8 The nurse is reviewing the health history of a client who is to begin therapy with a combined oral contraceptive drug. Which findings in the client's history should the nurse address with the client? Select all that apply.

1. Use of St. John's wort for depression
2. Smoking cessation over 10 years ago
3. Frequent migraine headaches
4. Follows a vegan diet
5. Cholecystectomy 3 months ago

9 After testosterone cypionate is prescribed for a 16-year-old male client diagnosed with hypogonadism, the client asks, "Why do I need these hormones, anyway?" The nurse should provide which description of the relationship between hypogonadism and this drug?

1. "Testosterone is necessary to prevent your muscles from atrophying."
2. "This medication is a form of testosterone. Your doctor can best explain it to you."
3. "Testosterone prevents your body from becoming feminine-looking."
4. "This medication will increase your testosterone to a normal level."

10 The nurse determines a client with endometriosis understands the purpose of the newly prescribed danazol when the client makes which statement?

1. "It suppresses pituitary output of the follicle-stimulating hormone (FSH)."
2. "I'll need to take this medication for the rest of my life."
3. "I have to administer injections weekly."
4. "This medication will relieve hot flashes."

➤ *See pages 476–478 for Answers and Rationales.*

I. ESTROGENS

A. Action and use
1. Hormone replacement therapy (HRT) after spontaneous or surgically induced menopause
2. Relieves symptoms of menopause such as hot flashes, night sweats, sleep disturbances, and vaginal dryness; protects against coronary heart disease and osteoporosis
3. Used to treat female **hypogonadism**, a condition characterized by underdevelopment of the gonads
4. Adjunctive therapy for osteoporosis (oral or transdermal forms only)
5. Used in men to decrease the progression of prostate carcinoma

B. Common estrogen medications: see Table 14-1

C. Administration considerations
1. Report symptoms of menopause to provider for dosage adjustment
2. Dose should be given with food to reduce nausea
3. Intravenous (IV) estrogen is given slowly by direct IV injection at a rate of 5 mg/min
4. Rapid IV injection may cause skin flushing
5. Estradiol transdermal should be applied to clean, dry area on the trunk of the body (including buttocks and abdomen)
6. Replace patch according to schedule
7. Cream form of the medication should be applied deeply into vagina, to assist in retention
8. Intravaginal ring should be placed near cervix and checked for placement periodically

D. Contraindications
1. Current undiagnosed vaginal bleeding
2. History of breast cancer

Table 14-1 Common Estrogens

Generic Name	Route	Uses	Adverse Effects
Estradiol	PO, IM, transdermal patch, intravaginal	Vasomotor symptoms, hypoestrogenism from hypogonadism, castration, primary ovarian failure, atrophic vaginitis, kraurosis vulvae, palliative therapy for advanced inoperable breast or prostate cancer, osteoporosis prevention	Thromboembolism, increased risk of breast or endometrial cancer, hepatic adenoma, breast changes, gynecomastia, abnormal Pap smear, increased appetite, weight gain, jaundice, gallbladder disease, nausea and vomiting, diarrhea, bloating, cervical erosion, altered cervical secretions, uterine fibromas, breakthrough bleeding, testicular atrophy, impotence, hypercalcemia, urticaria, melasma (dark skin discoloration), hair loss, dermatitis
Conjugated estrogens, synthetic	PO	Hormonal imbalance with bleeding, vaginal atrophy, castration, primary ovarian failure, palliative therapy for inoperable prostate cancer, palliative therapy for breast cancer, osteoporosis prevention	Breast tenderness, bloating, fluid retention, edema, abdominal cramps, increased risk of endometrial cancer in postmenopausal women, symptoms of liver problems, vision changes, severe or persistent dizziness or headache, nausea and vomiting, severe stomach pain, pulmonary embolism, myocardial infarction, thromboembolism
Estropipate	PO, intravaginal	Vulvar and vaginal atrophy, ovarian failure, castration, hypogonadism, osteoporosis prevention	Depression, seizures, headache, dizziness, pulmonary embolism, myocardial infarction, thromboembolism, cerebrovascular accident, edema, nausea and vomiting, abdominal cramps, bleeding, endometrial cancer, breast cancer, erythema multiforme, breast engorgement, porphyria, breast enlargement, hirsutism
Esterified estrogens	PO	Inoperable prostate cancer, metastatic breast cancer, hypogonadism, castration, ovarian failure, vasomotor menopausal symptoms, atrophic vaginitis, urethritis, osteoporosis prevention	Headache, dizziness, seizure, depression, edema, thromboembolism, hypertension, thrombophlebitis, pulmonary embolism, stroke, breast and endometrial cancer, amenorrhea, abnormal menstrual flow, hirsutism, hepatic adenoma, gallbladder disease, gynecomastia, weight changes, breast changes, breakthrough bleeding, pancreatitis, myopia, astigmatism, testicular atrophy, uterine fibromas

3. Cautious use in smokers
4. Cautious use in women with history of deep vein thrombosis (DVT) or thrombophlebitis
5. Use cautiously with severe renal or hepatic disease

E. **Significant drug interactions**
1. May create need to increase doses of warfarin, oral hypoglycemic agents, or insulin
2. Increased risk of hepatotoxicity when estrogens are taken with drugs that are hepatotoxic
3. May increase risk of toxicity with cyclosporine
4. Barbiturates, St. John's wort, and rifampin may decrease effectiveness of estrogens
5. Increased effects possible with ginseng
6. Red clover and black cohosh may interfere with estrogen therapy (have weak estrogenic effects)

F. **Significant food interactions:** none reported

G. Significant laboratory studies

1. May increase levels of high-density lipoproteins (HDL), phospholipids, and triglycerides in blood
2. May decrease low-density lipoprotein (LDL) and total cholesterol levels
3. May increase bone density

H. Side effects

1. Increased skin pigmentation when exposed to sunlight; chloasma
2. Weight gain and fluid retention
3. Nausea (oral forms)
4. Change in libido and increased breast tenderness
5. Headaches, moodiness, and hypertension
6. Amenorrhea, breakthrough bleeding

I. Adverse effects/toxicity

1. May increase risk of breast cancer
2. Endometrial cancer risk increases if uterus is intact and there is no concurrent progestin use

J. Client-centered nursing care

1. Assess blood pressure (BP) prior to and periodically during use
2. Monthly breast self-exams and annual mammograms as recommended
3. In clients with breast cancer and bone metastasis, severe hypercalcemia (greater than 15 mg/dL) may be caused by estradiol therapy
4. Nausea frequently occurs in the morning, but disappears after 1–2 weeks of treatment; administer dose with meals or at bedtime to decrease nausea
5. Monitor for thromboembolic events
6. Monitor blood glucose in clients with diabetes mellitus

K. Client education

1. Correct dosage and route of administration, including how often to change transdermal patches
2. Take medication with food if nausea occurs, usually at beginning of therapy
3. Cigarette smoking increases risk of thrombus formation
4. Report signs of fluid retention (edema, weight gain)
5. When taken cyclically, vaginal bleeding will likely occur during the week each month when the estrogen is withheld
6. Remain lying down for 30 minutes after administration of vaginal creams
7. Place cream deep into vagina, avoid douching, and wash applicator with warm, soapy water after use
8. Use panty liners or mini-pads, but avoid use of tampons with vaginal creams
9. Instruct client to report calf pain on dorsiflexion of the foot, possibly caused by formation of clots in the vein; also assess for limited leg movement
10. Caution client that risk of blood clot formation is high with use of morning-after pill; teach signs of thrombophlebitis such as tenderness, swelling, redness in extremity, and pain; assess for sudden severe chest pain that could indicate pulmonary embolism
11. Instruct client to take medications exactly as prescribed
12. Encourage smoking cessation (smoking increases risk of cardiovascular events)

II. PROGESTINS

A. Action and use

1. Cause the endometrium to change from proliferative to secretory in the latter half of the menstrual cycle in preparation for implantation of an embryo
2. Decrease midcycle bleeding in peri- and postmenopausal women or in women with dysfunctional uterine bleeding

Practice to Pass

The client has been started on estradiol and asks how to use this medication. How do you respond?

Table 14-2	Common Progestins		
Generic Name	**Route**	**Therapeutic Indications**	**Adverse Effects**
Medroxyprogesterone	PO, IM, subcut	Abnormal uterine bleeding caused by hormonal imbalance, endometrial or renal cancer, contraception, paraphilia	Dizziness, migraine headache, depression, nervousness, pulmonary embolism, jaundice, tremors, gallbladder disease, thrombophlebitis, hypertension, edema, breakthrough bleeding, intolerance to contact lenses, hyperglycemia, weight gain, rash, pain, decreased libido, breast tenderness, breast enlargement, hypersensitivity reaction, uterine fibromas, nausea and vomiting
Norethindrone acetate	PO	Amenorrhea, abnormal uterine bleeding, endometriosis, pregnancy prevention	Headache, changes in vaginal bleeding, depression, edema, jaundice, melasma
Megestrol acetate	PO	Breast, renal cell, and endometrial cancer, severe weight loss, anorexia, and cachexia in clients with HIV/AIDS and cancer	Vaginal bleeding, breast tenderness, headache, increased appetite, weight gain, abdominal pain, nausea and vomiting
Progesterone	IM	Primary and secondary amenorrhea, functional uterine bleeding, contraception, premenstrual syndrome, prevention of premature labor	Loss of vision, migraine headaches, depression, dizziness, insomnia, rash, acne pruritis, breakthrough bleeding, amenorrhea, cervical erosion, thromboembolism, thrombotic disease, decreased glucose tolerance, hepatic adenoma, edema, breast enlargement or tenderness, increase in sodium and chloride excretion, photosensitivity, jaundice, bradycardia, somnolence, syncope, spontaneous abortion, pelvic infection

   3. Used to treat postmenopausal syndrome
   4. Used to treat amenorrhea, breast cancer, and renal cancer
   B. Common progestin medications: see Table 14-2; **common estrogen-progestin medications:** see Table 14-3
   C. Administration considerations
   1. Must be discontinued immediately if pregnancy is suspected
   2. Intramuscular (IM) injection should be given deeply; injection site may be irritated
   3. Oral capsules contain peanut oil; they should not be given to clients with allergy to peanuts

Table 14-3	Common Estrogen-Progestin Hormone Replacement Medications		
Generic Name	**Route**	**Therapeutic Indications**	**Adverse Effects**
Conjugated estrogens with medroxyprogesterone	PO	Relief of menopausal symptoms, osteoporosis prevention	Breakthrough bleeding, breast tenderness, weight gain, hypertension, nausea and vomiting, dysmenorrhea, vaginal candidiasis, thromboembolic disease
Ethinyl estradiol and norethindrone acetate	PO or transdermal patch		
Estradiol with norgestimate	PO		

    D. **Contraindications**
        1. Pregnancy
        2. Cautious use with current or past history of depression
    E. **Significant drug interactions:** decreased effectiveness when taken concomitantly with antiepileptic medications; decreased medroxyprogesterone levels with aminoglutethimide, barbiturates, primidone, rifampin, rifabutin, and topiramate
    F. **Significant food interactions:** increased caffeine levels if caffeine is ingested; use with St. John's wort may cause bleeding between menses and reduced efficacy
    G. **Significant laboratory studies**
        1. Increased LDL
        2. Decreased HDL
        3. Abnormal liver function tests
        4. May affect coagulation, thyroid, and endocrine function
    H. **Side effects**
        1. Depression
        2. Male-pattern baldness
        3. Increased or decreased libido
        4. Insomnia and somnolence
        5. Fluid retention, edema, weight gain
        6. Nausea and vomiting
        7. Amenorrhea, changes in menstrual flow
    I. **Adverse effects/toxicity**
        1. Change in menstrual flow, amenorrhea, and breast changes
        2. Edema
        3. Cholestatic jaundice
    J. **Client-centered nursing care**
        1. Prior to administration in clients with current or history of depression, make certain a plan is in place to deal with worsening or recurrent depressive symptoms
        2. A thorough physical examination should be done with special attention to pelvic organs, breasts, and hepatic function
        3. A Pap test should be done prior to initiation of therapy and every 6 to 12 months while client is taking the medication
        4. Monitor vital signs, including blood pressure (BP)
        5. Monitor intake and output (I&O)
    K. **Client education**
        1. How to use medication and the timing of use
        2. Possible side effects and symptoms to report, such as sudden severe headache, vomiting, dizziness, fainting, pain in calves, acute chest pain, and dyspnea
        3. Postmenopausal women might resume cyclical vaginal bleeding
        4. Perform routine breast self-examinations
        5. Monitor blood pressure and I&O
        6. Avoid exposure to ultraviolet (UV) light
        7. Diabetic clients should monitor glucose levels closely
        8. Client should take medication with food if gastrointestinal upset occurs
        9. Smoking increases risk of cerebrovascular and cardiovascular adverse effects

III. ANDROGENS

    A. **Action and use**
        1. **Androgens** are steroids that stimulate the action of endogenous hormones
        2. Used primarily to treat male androgen (testosterone) deficiency in men with delayed puberty, hypogonadism, oligospermia, **cryptorchidism** (a congenital condition characterized by failure of the testis to descend into the scrotum), or orchiectomy

Practice to Pass

A 16-year-old male client with hypogonadism is starting testosterone enanthate therapy. You are developing a plan of care for this client. What information should be included in the plan regarding the effects of this medication?

3. Used for hormone replacement therapy in women who experience decreased energy and libido
4. Used to suppress tumor growth in androgen-sensitive breast cancer
5. Danazol is used to treat endometriosis and fibrocystic breast disease in women

B. **Common androgen medications:** see Table 14-4
C. **Administration considerations**
   1. Medically indicated androgen use will often result in virilization and side effects must be monitored closely
   2. Buccal tablets should not be chewed or swallowed
   3. Transdermal testosterone should be applied to scrotal skin; dry-shave the area
   4. Transdermal testosterone patch should be applied to nonscrotal skin; apply to clean, dry area of back, abdomen, upper arms, or thighs
   5. Use very cautiously in children because of the bone maturation effects
   6. Can reduce blood glucose levels, thus reducing insulin requirements in the diabetic client
   7. Intramuscular preparations may crystallize at low temperatures; therefore the vial may need warming and gentle agitation to redissolve crystals

D. **Contraindications**
   1. Pregnancy and lactation
   2. Heart failure (HF), renal and liver failure
   3. Enlarged prostate

E. **Significant drug interactions**
   1. Increased action of warfarin can cause bleeding
   2. Increased action of oral hypoglycemic agents, insulin, and glucocorticoids
   3. Additive hepatotoxicity (toxic to liver) when administered with other hepatotoxic medications
   4. Increase the effect of imipramine (increased paranoid symptoms)

Practice to Pass

A client has admitted to using illegally obtained anabolic steroids IM with his athletic teammates for the past 2 years. How would you explain to the client the laboratory studies that the healthcare provider will likely order, and why they are needed?

Table 14-4 **Common Androgens**

Generic Name	Route	Uses	Adverse Effects
Danazol	PO	Endometriosis, fibrocystic breast disease, hereditary angioedema, precocious puberty, gynecomastia, hemolytic anemia, thrombocytopenia	Pseudotumor cerebri, hirsutism, dizziness, headache, sleep disorder, menstrual disturbances, hepatic damage (rare), thrombophlebitis, thromboembolism, fluid retention, weight gain, hypoestrogenic effects
Fluoxymesterone	PO	Hypogonadism, inoperable breast cancer in women	Aggressiveness, hirsutism, insomnia, irritability
Methyltestosterone	PO, buccal	Primary hypogonadism, testicular failure, delayed puberty	
Testosterone	Gel, transdermal, buccal, pellets	Hypogonadism, hypogonadotropic hypogonadism, delayed puberty, inoperable breast cancer, metastatic mammary cancer	Dizziness, sleep disorders, fatigue, headache, rash, dermatitis, acne, hirsutism, deepening of voice, weight gain, clitoral hypertrophy, testicular atrophy, nausea, hepatocellular carcinoma, fluid retention, polycythemia, leucopenia, hypercalcemia, chills, premature closure of epiphyses
Testosterone cypionate	IM, subcut implant, transdermal		
Testosterone enanthate	IM, subcut implant, transdermal patch		

   F. **Significant food interactions:** none reported
   G. **Significant laboratory studies**
      1. Complete blood count (CBC): hemoglobin (Hgb) and hematocrit (Hct) will increase in women
      2. Decrease in HDL and increase in LDL levels
   H. **Side effects**
      1. In both genders are dose-related, including lowered voice, edema, acne, change in libido, increased facial hair growth, and increase in aggressive tendencies
      2. In male: gynecomastia, oligospermia, impotence, decreased ejaculatory volume, and urinary urgency
      3. In female: menstrual irregularities, enlarged clitoris, breast size decrease, male-pattern baldness, deepening of voice, and increase in oiliness of skin
   I. **Adverse effects/toxicity**
      1. Androgens will increase male sex characteristics in prepubertal boys; x-ray examination of the epiphyseal growth plate must be done every 6 months in pre-pubescent boys
      2. **Priapism** (painful penile erection) may also occur
      3. Polycythemia may develop
   J. **Client-centered nursing care**
      1. Assess client for edema, weight gain, and any changes in skin
      2. Assess lung and heart sounds
      3. Assess client for signs of liver dysfunction
      4. Evaluate client for signs of depression
      5. Assess client for the presence of secondary sexual characteristics
   K. **Client education**
      1. Apply transdermal patches to shaved skin
      2. Monitor weight twice weekly and report increase
      3. Notify prescriber if fluid retention develops
      4. Be aware of signs of virilization as side effects
      5. Women who are sexually active should use a nonhormonal (barrier) contraceptive while on therapy
      6. Take medication with meals or a snack

IV. ANABOLIC STEROIDS

   A. **Action and use:** developed to replace androgens
   B. **Common anabolic steroid medications:** see Table 14-5
   C. **Administration considerations**
      1. **Anabolic steroids** are androgens with anabolic properties and are rarely prescribed but are commonly abused by athletes in an attempt to enhance performance
      2. Medically indicated androgen use will often result in virilization, and side effects must be monitored
      3. High doses of androgen are occasionally used to treat breast cancer
   D. **Contraindications**
      1. During pregnancy and lactation
      2. Contraindicated with HF, renal and liver failure, and enlarged prostate
   E. **Significant drug interactions**
      1. Increased action of warfarin, oral hypoglycemic agents, insulin, and glucocorticoids
      2. Additive hepatotoxicity when administered with other hepatotoxic medications
   F. **Significant food interactions:** none reported

Table 14-5		Common Anabolic Steroids	
Generic Name	**Route**	**Uses**	**Adverse Effects**
Oxandrolone	PO	Adjuvant therapy to enhance weight gain in debilitated clients, offset protein catabolism when administering corticosteroids, short stature associated with Turner syndrome	Insomnia, confusion, phallic enlargement, hirsutism, inhibition of testicular function, clitoral enlargement, epididymitis, liver failure, intra-abdominal hemorrhage, increased blood lipid levels, sodium and water retention, acne, premature closure of epiphyses, abdominal fullness, loss of appetite, burning of tongue, increased risk of benign prostatic hyperplasia (BPH)
Oxymetholone	PO	Anemia related to deficiency in red blood cell production, acquired or congenital aplastic anemia, myelofibrosis and hypoplastic anemia due to myelotoxic drugs	Swelling, rapid weight gain, priapism, problems with urination, nausea and vomiting, stomach pain, anorexia or loss of appetite, jaundice

G. Significant laboratory studies
1. May cause increase in serum aspartate aminotransferase (AST)
2. May increase bilirubin level
3. May suppress clotting factors II, V, VII, and X
4. Hgb and Hct will increase in female
5. HDL cholesterol level will decrease and LDL cholesterol level will increase

H. Side effects
1. In both genders: lowered voice, edema, acne, change in libido, increased facial hair growth, and increase in aggressive tendencies
2. In male: gynecomastia, oligospermia, impotence, and decreased ejaculatory volume
3. In female: menstrual irregularities, enlarged clitoris, decreased breast size, male-pattern baldness; voice changes and hair growth patterns are not reversible after discontinuation of use

I. Adverse effects/toxicity
1. Hepatotoxicity, especially when used with other hepatotoxic effects
2. Abusers of anabolic steroids often share needles, increasing the incidence of hepatitis B and C and human immunodeficiency virus (HIV) transmission

J. Client-centered nursing care
1. Assess client athletes from junior high through adulthood (especially football players, bodybuilders, weightlifters, sprinters, and endurance sport participants) for anabolic steroid abuse
2. Assess client for edema, weight gain, and skin changes
3. Assess lung and heart sounds
4. Assess clients for signs of liver dysfunction
5. Evaluate clients for signs of depression
6. Assess client for the presence of secondary sexual characteristics

K. Client education
1. Risks of using anabolic steroids if obtained and used illegally
2. Risks of sharing needles if illegal use
3. Risks of contamination when using non-U.S.–manufactured or veterinary quality substances
4. Notify healthcare provider if using these medications
5. Anabolic steroids raise cholesterol level and lower male sperm counts
6. Females may experience menstrual irregularities

V. MEDICATIONS FOR ERECTILE DYSFUNCTION

A. Actions and use

1. Enhance normal erectile response to sexual stimuli through inhibition of phosphodiesterase type 5 (PDE5)
2. Increase corpus cavernosus arterial inflow and decrease venous outflow, resulting in erection
3. Used for erectile dysfunction

B. Common erectile dysfunction medications: see Table 14-6

C. Administration considerations

1. Sildenafil should not be used more than once per day
2. Alprostadil should not be used more than once per 24 hours and no more than three times per week
3. Alprostadil: reconstitute using 1 mL of diluent of bacteriostatic or sterile water
4. Alprostadil should not be used more than twice in 24 hours

D. Contraindications

1. Clients with cardiovascular diseases, myocardial infarction (MI), cerebrovascular accident (CVA), or dysrhythmias within 6 months
2. Heart failure (HF) and unstable angina (UA)
3. Use of nitroglycerin or other nitrates
4. Hypertension (BP greater than 170/110) or hypotension (BP less than 90/50)

E. Significant drug interactions

1. Life-threatening hypotension can occur with concurrent use of nitroglycerin or nitroprusside
2. Increased adverse effects with antidepressants
3. Alprostadil increases risk of bleeding if used concurrently with warfarin
4. Do not take alpha blockers within 4 hours of anti-impotency medications
5. Erythromycin, itraconazole, and ketoconazole will increase vardenafil levels
6. Nitrates enhance hypotensive effects and should not be used concurrently
7. Levodopa and papaverine may interfere with levodopa in clients with Parkinson disease

F. Significant food interactions: grapefruit juice may increase levels but delay absorption, high-fat meals reduce peak drug levels, hawthorne (herb) increases vasodilator effects

G. Significant laboratory studies: none reported

H. Side effects

1. Ecchymosis and painless fibrotic nodules in the corpus cavernosus may occur with injections

Practice to Pass

The client has *!* been experiencing erectile dysfunction. He asks if sildenafil is the only medication that can be used to treat his condition. How should you answer?

Table 14-6	Common Medications for Erectile Dysfunction	
Generic Name	**Route**	**Adverse Effects**
Sildenafil citrate	PO	Sudden cardiac arrest, ventricular dysrhythmias, hemorrhagic stroke, transient ischemic attack, flushing, hypotension, temporary vision loss, ocular redness, increased intraocular pressure (IOP), retinal bleeding, diarrhea, dyspepsia, respiratory infection, flulike syndrome
Tadalafil	PO	Headache, flushing, nasal congestion, dyspepsia, back pain, limb pain, myalgia
Vardenafil hydrochloride	PO	Headache, dizziness, flushing, rhinitis, sinusitis, dyspepsia, nausea, back pain, flulike symptoms
Alprostadil	IV, transurethral pellets	Cardiac arrest, seizures, penile pain, rash, fibrosis, erection, priapism, apnea, respiratory distress

2. With transurethral administration: a dull penile pain, prolonged erection (4–6 hours)
3. Sildenafil: headache, blurred vision, flushing, dyspepsia, and nasal congestion

I. Adverse effects/toxicity

1. Priapism may occur and must be treated as a medical emergency
2. Upper respiratory infection and urinary tract infection (UTI)
3. Urethral bleeding
4. Increased motor activity

J. Client-centered nursing care

1. Obtain a thorough medical history of clients experiencing erectile dysfunction, especially history of cardiovascular disease
2. Obtain accurate history of onset of the problem to assess for possible psychological cause since not all cases of sexual dysfunction are truly erectile dysfunction
3. Sildenafil is the most prescribed medication in the United States and has been presented as a panacea for all sexual problems in the population
4. Sildenafil is usually taken 1 hour prior to sexual activity

K. Client education

1. How to inject papaverine into corpus cavernosum using a ⅜-inch 27- or 28-gauge needle 1-mL syringe
2. Instruct client to insert transurethral pellets with a plastic introducer about 1½ inches into the urethra
3. Maximum use of the medication in a 24-hour time block and in each week
4. Take sildenafil 1 hour prior to sexual activity
5. Report chest pain or palpitations immediately if taking sildenafil
6. Eating a high-fat meal before taking sildenafil may delay onset of drug action

7. Do not take these medications with other drugs containing nitrates
8. Eliminate grapefruit from diet because of interaction with medications for erectile dysfunction

VI. CONTRACEPTIVES

A. Action and use

1. Decrease incidence of ovulation to prevent conception
2. Thin endometrial lining of uterus, reducing incidence of implantation if fertilization takes place
3. Decrease fallopian tube ciliary peristalsis, which decreases likelihood of an ovum meeting a sperm
4. Thicken cervical mucus, preventing sperm from penetrating into uterine cavity
5. Used as a means of birth control
6. NuvaRing is the only vaginal contraceptive containing estrogen and progesterone; it is a 5-cm diameter ring inserted for 3 weeks, followed by a ring-free week allowing for withdrawal bleeding
7. Two intrauterine devices (IUDs) are available
   a. Nonhormonal T-shaped IUD (ParaGard) creates an ionic charge in uterus, making it deadly to sperm; it can be left in place up to 10 years
   b. Hormonal levonorgestrel-releasing system IUD (Mirena, Liletta, Skyla, Kyleena) thickens cervical mucus, making it impenetrable to sperm; depending on brand, can be left in place for 3–6 years

B. Common contraceptive medications: see Table 14-7

C. Administration considerations

1. If an adolescent has not yet attained maximum growth, estrogen may cause epiphyseal plates to close
2. Estrogen may decrease milk supply

Type	Estrogen	Progestin	Brand Name
Combination orals	Ethinyl estradiol, mestranol	Norethindrone, ethynodiol acetate, levonorgestrel, desogestrel, norgestrel, norgestimate	Triphasil, Tri-Cyclen, Tri-Norinyl, Desogen, Demulen, Ovrette, Mircette, LoEstrin, Ovcon, Nordette, Lybrel, Seasonale, Nordette, Yasmin, Yaz
Progestin-only orals	N/A	Norethindrone	Micronor, Nor-QD
Combination injectable	Estradiol cypionate	Medroxyprogesterone acetate	Lunelle
Progestin-only injectable	N/A	Medroxyprogesterone acetate	Depo-Provera
Spermicidal agents: creams, foams, jellies, sponge, and suppositories	N/A	Non-oxynol-9	Today sponge
Levonorgestrel-releasing IUD	N/A	N/A	Mirena, Liletta, Skyla, Kyleena
Nonhormonal IUD	N/A	N/A	ParaGard

Table 14-7   Common Contraceptives

3. Smokers older than 35 years of age are recommended to either quit smoking or use another method of birth control due to increased risk of DVT
4. Dosing schedule is usually based on a 28-day menstrual cycle
5. Infertility and amenorrhea may persist as long as 18 months after repeated injections of progestin-only injectables
6. Progestin-only injectables such as medroxyprogesterone acetate have black box warnings that users may lose significant bone mineral density, which may be greater with increasing duration of use
7. Spermicides are available in creams, foams, jellies, suppositories, and sponges; Nonoxynol-9 has a 1-hour duration of action; reapply if coitus extends beyond this time; the sponge releases the drug slowly and provides up to 24 hours of protection

D. **Contraindications**
1. Estrogen-containing and progestin-only methods are contraindicated in females with a history of cerebral vascular accident (CVA), DVT, and known or suspected breast, ovarian, or endometrial cancer
2. Postpartum women should avoid use of combined hormonal contraceptives during the first 21 days after delivery due to a high risk for venous thromboembolism (VTE); women with a risk for VTE should wait until more than 42 days postpartum

E. **Significant drug interactions**
1. Progestin efficacy decreases in presence of antiepileptic medications
2. Most antibiotics such as ampicillin, isoniazid, nitrofurantoin, rifampin, penicillin V, sulfonamides, and tetracyclines will decrease effectiveness of contraceptives
3. Increased effects of benzodiazepines, beta blockers, caffeine, corticosteroids, and theophylline occur

F. **Significant food interactions:** none reported

G. **Significant laboratory studies**
1. Progestin other than desogestrel increases total cholesterol and LDL
2. Desogestrel decreases total cholesterol and increases HDL
3. Thyroid-stimulating hormone (TSH) will become slightly elevated while on combination oral contraceptive therapy (OCT)

H. Side effects

1. Estrogen-containing methods: cyclical weight gain, increased skin pigmentation, breast enlargement and tenderness, and irritability
2. Progestin-containing methods: decreased libido, depression, acne, and male-pattern baldness
3. The symptoms of possible complications of combination OCT form the acronym ACHES: **A**bdominal pain (liver tumor formation), **C**hest pain, **H**eadache, **E**ye problems (embolus), and **S**evere leg pain (thrombophlebitis)
4. Loss of bone mineral density with progestin-only injectables such as medroxyprogesterone acetate
5. Vaginal dryness, vaginitis, and toxic shock syndrome with contraceptive sponge

I. Adverse effects/toxicity

1. Spotting, change in menstrual flow, amenorrhea
2. Nausea and vomiting, abdominal cramps, bloating
3. Headaches, depression, edema

J. Client-centered nursing care

1. No single hormonal contraceptive method works best for all females
2. Finding the right combination and dosage of hormones may occur by trial-and-error
3. Encourage smokers to quit because of increased risk of DVT, especially after age 35
4. Monitor for signs and symptoms of thrombophlebitis (calf pain, possible redness and warmth, and possible edema in affected leg)
5. Administer intramuscular progestin-only injectables deep into a large muscle

K. Client education

1. Take oral contraceptive exactly as directed
2. Methods of using different oral contraceptives
   a. Combination orals: take one pill daily at same time each day; the last 5–7 days of the pills are inert; withdrawal bleeding may occur during last 5–7 days
   b. Progestin-only orals: take one pill each day at exactly the same time; each pill is a medicated pill; there is no week off hormones; bleeding will be irregular or may not occur
   c. Medroxyprogesterone acetate: bleeding will be irregular until second or third dose is given; after third dose, most females develop amenorrhea
3. Do not miss doses
4. Follow schedule below for missed dose
   a. If one dose is missed, take two tablets the next day
   b. If two doses are missed, take two tablets as soon as remembered with the next pill or take two tablets daily for the next 2 days; use a backup method such as condom for the rest of the pill pack
   c. If three doses are missed, begin a new compact of tablets starting on day one of the cycle after the last pill was taken; use a backup contraceptive method
5. Report prolonged vaginal bleeding or amenorrhea
6. Wait at least three months before becoming pregnant after stopping oral contraceptives
7. Conduct breast self-examination monthly
8. Instruct clients taking medroxyprogesterone injections to increase intake of calcium-containing foods
9. Spermicides have low levels of effectiveness when used alone; use with barrier method such as condom or diaphragm
10. When using a contraceptive sponge, moisten with water to activate spermicide; insert high into vagina to cover cervix; leave in place for 6 hours after intercourse; may provide protection for up to 24 hours, but remove by 30 hours after insertion to avoid toxic shock syndrome

Practice to Pass

The client is considering beginning combination oral contraceptive pills. What questions do you need to ask as part of her medical history?

VII. FERTILITY MEDICATIONS

A. Action and use

1. Used when an infertility workup determines that the cause of an inability to conceive after 12 months of unprotected intercourse is due to lack of ovulation
2. Will stimulate ovulation or follicular maturation

B. Common female infertility medications: see Table 14-8

C. Administration considerations

1. Ovulation induction agents are expensive and can cost over $1,000 per cycle
2. Multifetal pregnancy will occur in 12–20% of cases, mostly twins
3. Clients should start with smaller doses, and then increasing dosages will be used if the cycle does not achieve ovulation

D. Contraindications

1. Inability to keep track of the dosing schedule
2. Lack of access to emergency medical care
3. Primary ovarian failure
4. Hepatic dysfunction

E. Significant drug interactions

1. Butyrophenones, phenothiazines, and methyldopa may increase prolactin levels, which may interfere with fertility

F. Significant food interactions: none reported

G. Significant laboratory studies: none reported

H. Side effects

1. Ovarian hyperstimulation syndrome is more common in female with polycystic ovaries
2. Nausea and vomiting, constipation, bloating, abdominal pain
3. Transient blurring, diplopia, photophobia
4. Vasomotor flushes, breast discomfort
5. Headache, fatigue, dizziness, vertigo

Table 14-8	Common Medications for Female Infertility
Generic Name	**Route**
Bromocriptine	PO
Clomiphene	PO
Danazol	PO
FSH- and LH-Enhancing Drugs	
Chorionic gonadotropin HCG	IM
Follitropin alfa, follitropin beta	Subcut
Menotropins	Subcut
Urofollitropin	Subcut
GnRH Antagonists	
Cetrorelix acetate	Subcut
Ganirelix (generic)	Subcut
GnRH Analogs/Agonists	
Goserelin	Subcut implant (endometriosis and advanced carcinoma)
Leuprolide	Subcut infertility; IM endometriosis
Nafarelin	Intranasal

      6. Tachycardia, phlebitis

      7. Blurred vision, diplopia, photophobia

  I. Adverse effects/toxicity

      1. Ovarian enlargement resulting in lower abdominal or pelvic pressure or pain

      2. Tenderness or infection of injection site

      3. Heavy menses, exacerbation of endometriosis

      4. Mental depression

      5. Insomnia

  J. Client-centered nursing care

      1. Make certain that the client understands the potential for multifetal pregnancy

      2. Full diagnostic measures are important if abnormal bleeding occurs

      3. Client should have an ophthalmic examination at regular intervals if clomiphene is prescribed more than 1 year

      4. Client with pelvic pain should be assessed carefully

  K. Client education

      1. Techniques for medication administration

      2. Take medication at same time every day

      3. Be aware of side effects and the importance of reporting them

      4. If there is a response, ovulation usually occurs 4–10 days after last day of treatment

      5. The incidence of multiple births is increased as high as six times normal

      6. Be aware of treatment regimen including probable office visits for ultrasound examination of the ovaries

      7. Client should have intercourse at least every other day beginning on the fifth day after the last dose of clomiphene, or the day prior to chorionic gonadotropin administration and 3 days following

      8. If a medication dose is missed:

         a. Take medication as soon as possible

         b. If not remembered until time for next dose, double the dose, then resume regular dosing schedule

         c. If more than one dose is missed, notify the prescriber

VIII. MEDICATIONS FOR LABOR AND DELIVERY

  A. Oxytocics

      1. Action and use

         a. Initiate or improve uterine contraction at term

         b. Facilitate involution in treatment or prevention of postpartum hemorrhage

         c. Used to stimulate letdown reflex in nursing mothers and relieve pain from breast engorgement

      2. Common oxytocic medications: see Table 14-9

      3. Administration considerations

         a. Only oxytocin is Food and Drug Administration (FDA) approved for use during labor

         b. Methylergonovine is used only for postpartum control of excessive bleeding and hemorrhage

         c. Oxytocin should never be administered by more than one route at a time

         d. Diluted IV oxytocin solution should be administered continuously

         e. Oxytocin IV preparation: for inducing labor, 10 units (1 mL) of oxytocin in 1 liter of D_5W or normal saline (NS) to give 10 milliunits/mL; for postpartum bleeding, 10–40 units in 1 liter of D_5W or NS provides 10–40 milliunits/mL

         f. Nurse should have a clear understanding of when medication is to be administered in relation to delivery

Table 14-9	Common Oxytocic Medications			
Generic Name	**Route**	**Therapeutic Indications**		**Adverse Effects**
Oxytocin	IV	Induce or stimulate labor, reduce postpartum bleeding, incomplete abortion, oxytocin challenge test to assess fetal distress in high-risk pregnancy		Subarachnoid bleed, seizures, coma, water intoxication, hypertension, arrhythmias, tetanic uterine contractions, abruption placentae, impaired uterine blood flow, increased uterine motility, anaphylaxis, anoxia, asphyxia, bradycardia
Methylergonovine	IM, IV, PO	Management of delivery of the placenta, postpartum atony and hemorrhage, uterine stimulation in the second stage of labor		Dizziness, headache, tinnitus, diaphoresis, transient hypertension, palpitations, chest pain, dyspnea, nausea and vomiting

4. Contraindications
    a. Methylergonovine is contraindicated with hypertension and should be avoided, if possible, in clients planning to breastfeed, as they inhibit lactation
    b. Contraindicated in unfavorable fetal position or presentations that are undeliverable
    c. Fetal distress in which delivery is not imminent
    d. Prematurity, placenta previa
    e. Previous surgery of uterus or cervix including cesarean section
5. Significant drug interactions: oxytocin and vasoconstrictors may cause severe hypertension
6. Significant herbal/food interactions: ephedra use with oxytocin may cause hypertension
7. Significant laboratory studies: oxytocin intrapartum increases unconjugated fetal bilirubin
8. Side effects
    a. Methylergonovine: significant increase in systolic and diastolic BP, chest pain
    b. In fetus: bradycardia or other dysrhythmias, hypoxia, intracranial hemorrhage, trauma from too-rapid propulsion through pelvis
    c. In mother: nausea and vomiting, postpartum hemorrhage, pelvic hematoma
    d. All oxytocics will cause uterine cramping when administered postpartum
9. Adverse effects/toxicity
    a. Uterine tetany leading to fetal demise
    b. Uterine rupture has been documented with overdose
    c. Newborns exposed to oxytocin *in utero* have higher incidence of hyperbilirubinemia
10. Client-centered nursing care
    a. Antepartum and intrapartum: monitor uterine contraction pattern, fetal heart rate (FHR), and blood pressure
    b. Postpartum: monitor lochia and blood pressure
    c. Massage injection site after deep injection of oxytocin into deltoid muscle to assist quick absorption
    d. Obtain baseline tracing of uterine contraction and fetal heart rate prior to medication
    e. Increase IV dosage of oxytocin only after assessing contraction, fetal heart rate, maternal blood pressure and heart rate
    f. Do not increase rate of oxytocin once the desired contraction pattern is achieved (contraction frequency of 2–3 minutes lasting 60 seconds)

          g. Oxytocin should be discontinued if contraction frequency is less than 2 minutes or duration is more than 90 seconds

          h. Breastfeeding should be delayed by at least 24 hours after oxytocin is discontinued

          i. Oxytocin has antidiuretic action; monitor client for water intoxication

    11. Client education

          a. Indication for administration

          b. Route of administration and possible side effects

          c. Report sudden headache

B. Ergot alkaloids

    1. Action and use

          a. Used to control postpartum hemorrhage

          b. Cause clonic contractions

    2. Common medication: ergonovine, 0.2 mg IV over 60 seconds only in emergency, more commonly given by IM route

    3. Administration considerations: causes rebound uterine relaxation

    4. Contraindications

          a. Contraindicated in hypersensitivity to ergot medication

          b. Cautious use with hypertension, unstable angina, recent myocardial infarction

    5. Significant drug interactions: none reported

    6. Significant food interactions: none reported

    7. Significant laboratory studies: none reported

    8. Side effects

          a. Significant increase in systolic and diastolic BP

          b. Uterine cramping

          c. Decreased milk production

    9. Adverse effects/toxicity

          a. Hypertension

          b. Ergotism or overdose: nausea and vomiting, weakness, muscle pain, insensitivity to cold, paresthesia of extremities

    10. Client-centered nursing care: closely monitor lochia and blood pressure after administration

    11. Client education

          a. Indication for administration

          b. Route of administration and possible side effects, such as cramping

          c. Report increased blood loss, increased temperature, or foul-smelling lochia

          d. Perform pad count to monitor bleeding

          e. Do not smoke because of increased/additive vasoconstriction with ergonovine use

C. Prostaglandins

    1. Action and use

          a. To terminate pregnancy from 12th week through second trimester

          b. Dinoprostone has FDA approval only for cervical ripening prior to labor induction

          c. Carboprost tromethamine has FDA approval only for control of postpartum bleeding

    2. Common prostaglandin medications: see Table 14-10

    3. Administration considerations

          a. Client should remain in supine position for 10 minutes after administration of dinoprostone

          b. Before dinoprostone, client should receive antiemetic and antidiarrheal medications

    4. Contraindications

          a. Use with caution in hypertension and with history of asthma

          b. Use of dinoprostone during labor has been documented to cause uterine rupture and fetal demise

Table 14-10	Common Prostaglandins Used During Pregnancy		
Generic Name	**Route**	**Therapeutic Indications**	**Adverse Effects**
Carboprost tromethamine	IM	Pregnancy termination 13–20 weeks, evacuation of uterus for missed abortion or fetal death during second trimester, postpartum hemorrhage	Flushing, hypotension, nausea, cough, dyspnea, perforated uterus, vaginal and uterine pain, endometriosis, incomplete abortion
Dinoprostone (prostaglandin E2 or PGE2)	Vaginal suppository, gel, or insert	Termination of pregnancy, cervical ripening	Headache, dizziness, syncope, hypotension, nausea and vomiting, diarrhea, perforated uterus, uterine rupture, uterine and vaginal pain, coughing, dyspnea, endometriosis, incomplete abortion
Misoprostol	PO	Prevention of nonsteroidal anti-inflammatory induced gastric ulcers, abortifacient	Nausea, diarrhea, abdominal pain, flatulence, dyspepsia, miscarriage, cramping, spotting, dysmenorrhea, hypermenorrhea, headache

  c. Acute pelvic inflammatory disease
  d. History of pelvic surgery
 5. Significant drug interactions: none reported
 6. Significant food interactions: none reported
 7. Significant laboratory studies: none reported
 8. Side effects
  a. Diarrhea, nausea and vomiting, possible increase in BP
  b. Uterine cramping
  c. Tension headache
  d. Flushing, cardiac dysrhythmias
 9. Adverse effects/toxicity
  a. Hypertension
  b. Uterine tetany may develop with prelabor or intrapartum administration
  c. Uterine rupture
 10. Client-centered nursing care
  a. Prenatal: follow manufacturer's instructions for placement of medication; client must remain recumbent for up to 20–30 minutes after administration and have fetal monitoring during this time
  b. Postpartum: monitor lochia and BP; be prepared for client to develop diarrhea
  c. Ensure adequate hydration when administering dinoprostone
  d. When administering carboprost, arrange pretreatment for nausea and vomiting prior to drug administration
 11. Client education
  a. Prenatal: report long or continuous contractions, as uterine tetany may develop; count fetal movement as an indicator of fetal well-being; monitor uterine tone and client temperature
  b. Postpartum: route of administration and possible side effects
D. Uterine relaxants
 1. Action and use
  a. Inhibit contractions and therefore arrest labor for at least 48 hours so that corticosteroids (betamethasone) can be given to facilitate fetal lung maturity
  b. Used for cessation of contractions to allow intrauterine fetal resuscitation when uterine hyperstimulation is present
  c. Used to delay delivery in preterm labor

2. Common uterine relaxant medications: see Table 14-11
3. Administration considerations
   a. Medication is started at lowest possible dose and increased as indicated until contractions cease
   b. Be certain about recommended dose
   c. If gastrointestinal symptoms occur, advise client to take the medications with food
   d. Dilute IV terbutaline by adding each 5 mg to 1,000 mL D_5W or NS to yield a concentration of 5 mcg/mL
   e. Infuse the medication via microdrip and infusion pump
4. Contraindications
   a. Known fetal anomaly incompatible with life
   b. Beta-adrenergics contraindicated in presence of pulmonary edema
   c. Cautious use if cervix is dilated greater than 5 cm or if gestational age is less than 20 or greater than 36 weeks
   d. Severe hypertension and coronary artery disease (CAD)
5. Significant drug interaction
   a. Increased incidence of pulmonary edema when used concurrently with corticosteroids (betamethasone) for fetal lung maturity acceleration
   b. Additive cardiovascular effects when given with sympathomimetic drugs
   c. Antagonistic effects when given with beta blockers
6. Significant food interactions: caffeine will increase side effects of beta-adrenergics
7. Significant laboratory studies: beta-adrenergics will cause hyperglycemia, worse with concomitant corticosteroid use
8. Side effects
   a. Beta-adrenergics: maternal and fetal tachycardia, palpitations, tremors, jitteriness, anxiety, hypertension
   b. May cause or exacerbate constipation
   c. Nausea and vomiting, anorexia
   d. Hyperglycemia, hypokalemia
9. Adverse effects/toxicity
   a. Beta-adrenergics: pulmonary edema
   b. Nifedipine and indomethacin can cause oligohydramnios
   c. Indomethacin can cause premature closure of the ductus arteriosus leading to fetal death
10. Client-centered nursing care
    a. Beta-adrenergics: if client continues on to deliver after receiving uterine relaxant medications, be prepared with oxytocin for treatment of postpartum hemorrhage
    b. Monitor vital signs and I&O

Table 14-11 **Common Uterine Relaxant Medications**

Generic Name	Category	Route	Notes
Terbutaline sulfate (generic)	Beta-adrenergic agonist	Subcutaneous, IV, PO	Not FDA-approved for preterm labor but most commonly used medication
Nifedipine	Calcium channel blocker	PO	Not FDA-approved for preterm labor but commonly used; may cause oligohydramnios
Indomethacin	NSAID	Rectal, PO	Not FDA-approved for preterm labor but used as third line; increased risk of fetal complications
Magnesium sulfate	mineral	IV infusion	Monitor reflexes and respiratory and cardiovascular status

     c. Nifedipine: avoid grapefruit juice during administration (interferes with effect)

     d. Use indomethacin for a short period of time (2–3 days)

     e. If mother uses terbutaline during pregnancy, monitor the neonate for hypoglycemia

  11. Client education

     a. Possible side effects and coping strategies

     b. Purpose and use of oral medications and importance of taking them on time

     c. Nifedipine: encourage client to change position slowly due to possible orthostatic hypotension

     d. How to self-monitor pulse

     e. Consult prescriber prior to taking over-the-counter (OTC) medications

E. Magnesium sulfate

  1. Action and use

     a. When given parenterally, acts as central nervous system (CNS) depressant and also depresses smooth, skeletal, and cardiac muscle function

     b. Used to arrest preterm labor and to prevent or to treat seizures with preeclampsia and eclampsia

  2. Administration considerations

     a. Used in conjunction with beta adrenergics, which increases risk of pulmonary edema

     b. A 4-gram loading dose is often utilized, which must be given over 20–30 minutes via infusion pump

  3. Contraindications

     a. Preterm labor

     b. Fetal anomaly incompatible with life

     c. Pulmonary edema or heart failure

     d. Anuria, renal failure

     e. Organic central nervous system disease

  4. Significant drug interactions: none reported

  5. Significant food interactions: none reported

  6. Significant laboratory studies: none reported

  7. Side effects

     a. Flushed warm feeling, drowsiness

     b. Decreased deep tendon reflexes

     c. Decreased hand-grasp strength

     d. Fluid and electrolyte imbalance, hyponatremia

     e. Nausea and vomiting

  8. Adverse effects/toxicity

     a. Lack of deep tendon reflexes and/or hand grasp

     b. Respiratory depression leading to respiratory arrest

  9. Client-centered nursing care

     a. Check patellar reflex prior to dose

     b. Monitor hand grasps, deep tendon reflexes, respiratory rate, and serum levels

     c. IV infusion flow rate is generally adjusted to maintain urine flow of at least 30–50 mL/hour, monitor I&O carefully

     d. Monitor IV site closely to avoid extravasation

     e. Monitor vital signs

     f. Take accurate daily weight

  10. Client education

     a. Side effects of medication

     b. Report signs of preeclampsia including headache, epigastric pain, and visual disturbance

     c. Report any signs of confusion

IX. EMERGENCY CONTRACEPTION

A. Plan B

1. The only currently available emergency contraception designed to be taken as soon as possible after unprotected intercourse; less effective if taken more than 72 hours after coitus

2. Contains 750 mcg of levonorgestrel; one pill taken initially, followed by a second pill 12 hours later; prevents ovulation if taken correctly

3. Available over the counter for women 17 years and older; a prescription must be obtained for those younger than 17 years

4. Dispensed by the pharmacist; pharmacies may not have this drug in stock due to insufficient demand or pharmacists may refuse to dispense it based on moral grounds

B. Considerations

1. Side effects include nausea and vomiting, dizziness, abdominal pain, fatigue, and irregular menses

2. Not to be used in place of a primary form of birth control

Case Study

The pregnant client with preeclampsia has been scheduled to have labor induced after cervical ripening. The client is planning to breastfeed her infant.

1. What medications can be used for cervical ripening, and how are they administered?

2. How will the labor be induced physiologically?

3. The client delivered 5 minutes ago and is now experiencing a postpartum hemorrhage. What medication(s) would you anticipate the healthcare provider prescribing at this time?

4. The client has experienced a seizure. What medication should you prepare to administer?

5. A few days postpartum, the client asks what hormonal methods of contraception she can use. How do you answer her question?

For suggested responses, see page 544.

POSTTEST

1 A client beginning oral contraceptive therapy with desogestrel and ethinyl estradiol asks the nurse why two different drugs are needed in the pill. Which explanation by the nurse is best?

1. "This medication is a weak estrogen and progestin combination that requires additional estrogen to work."

2. "Together the hormones prevent the ovum from maturing and the sperm from penetrating through the cervical mucus."

3. "Estrogens alone would prevent pregnancy, but progestins are added so that spotting doesn't occur."

4. "Taking each hormone separately would prevent most pregnancies, but the combination taken together in one pill is more effective."

2 Several clients in an outpatient clinic have requested prescriptions for sildenafil. The nurse anticipates having to inform which client that the request has been denied by the prescriber?

1. Client diagnosed with type 2 diabetes mellitus
2. Client taking medication therapy for angina pectoris
3. Client with benign prostate hypertrophy (BPH) who is being managed medically
4. Client who has chronic sinusitis with flare-ups in the spring

3 The nurse should conclude that a female client has understood medication instruction when she makes which statement about clomiphene?

1. "This medication will help make me ovulate."
2. "I'll take this medicine orally for 1 month."
3. "The medication prepares the wall of the uterus for fertilization."
4. "My husband is going to ask if he can take the medication as well."

4 The nurse should conclude that which client is most likely to have testosterone transdermal prescribed for his condition?

1. A 45-year-old with status-post bilateral vasectomy
2. A 17-year-old with status-post right cryptorchidism repair
3. A 23-year-old with status-post varicocele repair
4. A 32-year-old with status-post bilateral orchidectomy

5 Because the client is being prepared for labor induction with oxytocin, the nurse instructs the licensed practical/vocational nurse (LPN/LVN) to report which client data? Select all that apply.

1. Sudden rise in blood pressure
2. Changes in discomfort level immediately after drug is initiated
3. Gain of more than 2.27 kg (5 lb) during the last month
4. Sensation of nausea without vomiting
5. Changes in level of consciousness

6 The nurse determines teaching regarding the levonorgestrel-releasing intrauterine delivery system has been effective when the client makes which statement?

1. "These devices are 100% effective."
2. "I can keep this device in place for up to 5 years."
3. "I will need to use a barrier method of birth control in addition to this device."
4. "I will have the device removed every 2 years and replaced."

7 After a female client taking an estrogen–progestin combination reports by phone a sudden onset of blurred vision, the nurse at the outpatient clinic should ask what most appropriate question?

1. "Is there someone there with you?"
2. "When was last time you had your eyeglasses prescription changed?"
3. "When is your next appointment with your gynecologist?"
4. "Do you have problems with migraine headaches?"

8 The client in preterm labor who has a history of asthma received 2.5 mg of terbutaline sulfate subcutaneously. After the client expresses concern about the use of this drug, which reply by the nurse would be most appropriate?

1. "The healthcare provider wanted to make sure you did not have asthma problems and early labor."
2. "I am sure the healthcare provider has a very good reason for ordering this medication."
3. "What do you normally take to control your asthmatic attacks?"
4. "Terbutaline sulfate causes the respiratory tract to relax as well as the uterine wall."

POSTTEST

9 The nurse should consult with the healthcare provider after noting that testosterone enanthate has been prescribed for which client?

1. A 16-year-old with moderate acne
2. A 32-year-old client with an increased prostatic antigen level (PSA)
3. A 66-year-old with melanoma
4. A 65-year-old male with a high-density lipoprotein (HDL) level of 88 mg/dL

10 After dinoprostone is administered to a client, a nurse plans to monitor for which of the following?

1. Fetal heart tones on a client who had difficulty conceiving
2. Initiation of contractions for a client desiring an elective abortion
3. Initiation of lactation for a client interested in breastfeeding
4. Early signs and symptoms of pregnancy

➤ *See pages 478–479 for Answers and Rationales.*

ANSWERS & RATIONALES

Pretest

1 **Answer: 1** **Rationale:** Nitroglycerin is commonly used to manage signs and symptoms of coronary artery disease (CAD). A client with CAD who takes sildenafil is at risk for sudden cardiac death because of additive hypotension. Although the drug is contraindicated in clients with severe renal impairment, outcomes of using this drug would not place the client at immediate risk. Blurred vision is a side effect of the drug and could place the client at risk when performing certain activities but is not as life-threatening as cardiac arrest. Although gout is a side effect of the drug, it does not compare to the risk of cardiac arrest. There is no known negative interaction between allopurinol and sildenafil. **Cognitive Level:** Analyzing **Client Need:** Pharmacological and Parenteral Therapies **Integrated Process:** Communication and Documentation **Content Area:** Pharmacology **Strategy:** The critical word in the question is *priority*. This tells you that more than one option may be partially or completely correct but that one is more important than the others. Correlate the drug action that both drugs have in common (vasodilation) to select the correct option. **Reference:** Wilson, B. A., Shannon, M. T., & Shields, K. M. (2017). *Pearson nurse's drug guide 2017.* New York, NY: Pearson, pp. 1439–1440.

2 **Answer: 2, 4, 5** **Rationale:** Synthetic oxytocin enhances endogenous oxytocin. It is administered as a dilute solution of 10 or 20 units in 1 liter IV fluid via infusion pump, with a goal of increasing the frequency, duration, and amplitude of contractions. It also increases the intensity and regularity of uterine contractions. The drug is initiated at a minimal rate to start labor and is administered with increased increments until labor is well established. Hypertension is a side effect of the drug and not a reason to administer it. Contractions that are almost continuous would result in hypoxia, which would damage the fetus and possibly cause uterine rupture. **Cognitive Level:** Analyzing **Client Need:** Pharmacological and Parenteral Therapies **Integrated Process:** Teaching and Learning **Content Area:** Pharmacology **Strategy:** Note the wording of the question indicates that more than one option is likely to be correct. Note the words *further teaching* to identify that the correct options are statements that are factually incorrect. Select the options most indicative of danger to the fetus. **Reference:** Wilson, B. A., Shannon, M. T., & Shields, K. M. (2017). *Pearson nurse's drug guide 2017.* New York, NY: Pearson, pp. 1176–1178.

3 **Answer: 1** **Rationale:** Because IV magnesium sulfate acts as a central nervous system (CNS) depressant, it is prescribed to reduce risk of or to treat seizure activity in an eclamptic or preeclamptic client. The side effects are drowsiness, flushing, heaviness in the limbs, and decreased deep tendon reflexes. Decreased respiratory rate due to depressed neuromuscular function is a sign of magnesium toxicity. Flank and suprapubic assessments are unnecessary. **Cognitive Level:** Applying **Client Need:** Pharmacological and Parenteral Therapies **Integrated Process:** Nursing Process: Assessment **Content Area:** Pharmacology **Strategy:** The critical words in the question are *early side effect.* This tells you the correct answer is an option that represents a mild change rather than an extreme one. Next, associate the function of magnesium with the neurological side effects to choose correctly. **Reference:** Wilson, B. A., Shannon, M. T., & Shields, K. M. (2017). *Pearson nurse's drug guide 2017.* New York, NY: Pearson, pp. 613–614.

4 **Answer: 1 Rationale:** Clomiphene stimulates the production of luteinizing hormone (LH) and follicle-stimulating hormone (FSH), and therefore increases ovulation in women with anovulatory infertility. Clomiphene is used to treat absence of pregnancy. It is unnecessary to monitor temperature. Information about female hormones is appropriate for the client experiencing infertility problems, but does not address the drug specifically. **Cognitive Level:** Applying **Client Need:** Pharmacological and Parenteral Therapies **Integrated Process:** Nursing Process: Planning **Content Area:** Pharmacology **Strategy:** Answer the critical thinking question: What normal reproductive function does clomiphene enhance? **Reference:** Wilson, B. A., Shannon, M. T., & Shields, K. M. (2017). *Pearson nurse's drug guide 2017.* New York, NY: Pearson, pp. 369–371.

5 **Answer: 1 Rationale:** When two pills are missed, the client should "catch up" by taking two pills per day for 2 days and then one pill daily until finishing the pill pack. This will keep her cycle controlled and minimize the chance of midcycle bleeding. The half-life of the drug is 3–27 hours. Since the client could ovulate when missing two or more pills, a backup method such as condoms should be utilized for the rest of the cycle. To prevent midcycle bleeding, the client should take two tablets for 2 days instead of 1 day. **Cognitive Level:** Applying **Client Need:** Pharmacological and Parenteral Therapies **Integrated Process:** Nursing Process: Implementation **Content Area:** Pharmacology **Strategy:** The core issue of the question is how many doses of an oral contraceptive can safely be missed. To determine the correct option, consider the relationship between the half-life of the drug and maintenance of the therapeutic level. **Reference:** Wilson, B. A., Shannon, M. T., & Shields, K. M. (2017). *Pearson nurse's drug guide 2017.* New York, NY: Pearson, pp. 621–624.

6 **Answer: 1 Rationale:** Terbutaline is a beta-adrenergic medication used for tocolysis in the treatment of preterm labor. It stimulates beta$_2$-receptors in uterine smooth muscle, reducing intensity and frequency of uterine contractions and lengthening the gestation period. If a drug is needed to regulate contractions, it is more likely to be oxytocin. Since terbutaline is used to interrupt preterm labor, it could decrease or eliminate the contractions. Oxytocin rather than terbutaline is used for postpartal hemorrhage. An antiepileptic drug such as magnesium sulfate should be administered to a client with signs and symptoms of eclampsia. **Cognitive Level:** Applying **Client Need:** Pharmacological and Parenteral Therapies **Integrated Process:** Nursing Process: Planning **Content Area:** Pharmacology **Strategy:** Specific drug

knowledge is needed to answer the question. Correlate the drug's action with the client's need. **Reference:** Wilson, B. A., Shannon, M. T., & Shields, K. M. (2017). *Pearson nurse's drug guide 2017.* New York, NY: Pearson, pp. 1521–1523.

7 **Answer: 3 Rationale:** Oxytocin is used to control postpartum hemorrhage and promotion of postpartum uterine involution. It causes the least increase in blood pressure of *all* of these oxytocic medications, and considering the history of the client, this drug would be used first in this case. Methylergonovine may result in a severe hypertensive crisis. Ergonovine may raise or lower the blood pressure (BP). If the client is receiving antihypertensives, it could place client at risk for hypotension (consider that this client is already at risk for shock because of postpartal hemorrhage). **Cognitive Level:** Analyzing **Client Need:** Pharmacological and Parenteral Therapies **Integrated Process:** Nursing Process: Planning **Content Area:** Pharmacology **Strategy:** The critical words *most likely* indicate that more than one option may be partially correct but that one is a better choice than the others. The core issue in this question is which drug will stop the bleeding while raising the blood pressure the least. Thus, you need to consider which drug will be effective while minimizing the risk to the client. **Reference:** Wilson, B. A., Shannon, M. T., & Shields, K. M. (2017). *Pearson nurse's drug guide 2017.* New York, NY: Pearson, pp. 1176–1178.

8 **Answer: 1, 3 Rationale:** St. John's wort and many oral antibiotics can decrease the estrogenic effects of oral contraceptives and therefore decrease the efficacy of the pills. Side effects of oral contraceptives include headaches, nausea, cramping, bloating, changes in menstrual flow, and amenorrhea. Oral contraceptives also increase the risk for thromboembolic events, especially in clients with a history of same or who smoke. The use of oral contraceptives is associated with cholelithiasis and gall bladder disease, but since the client has had her gall bladder removed, this is not a concern. Following a vegan diet would not interfere with the action of combined oral contraceptives, but the client taking medroxyprogesterone should increase intake of dairy and calcium-containing foods. **Cognitive Level:** Analyzing **Client Need:** Pharmacological and Parenteral Therapies **Integrated Process:** Nursing Process: Implementation **Content Area:** Pharmacology **Strategy:** Recall specific information about oral contraceptives and their side effects. Correlate the client's risk factors for an increase in these side effects to choose the correct options. **Reference:** Wilson, B. A., Shannon, M. T., & Shields, K. M. (2017). *Pearson nurse's drug guide 2017.* New York, NY: Pearson, pp. 621–624.

9 **Answer: 4 Rationale:** In cases of hypogonadism, too little testosterone is naturally produced. Supplementation may be required to achieve normal hormone levels. Testosterone contributes to muscle development but this is not its only action. It is unnecessary to defer an explanation to the healthcare provider. Stating the drug prevents the client from being feminine-looking is not accurate or therapeutic. **Cognitive Level:** Analyzing **Client Need:** Pharmacological and Parenteral Therapies **Integrated Process:** Teaching and Learning **Content Area:** Pharmacology **Strategy:** Associate the functions of testosterone with the client's need. Use the process of elimination to omit inappropriate responses, and then choose the option that is most complete. **Reference:** Wilson, B. A., Shannon, M. T., & Shields, K. M. (2017). *Pearson nurse's drug guide 2017.* New York, NY: Pearson, pp. 1528–1530.

10 Answer: 1 Rationale: Danazol is an androgen used in the treatment of endometriosis. It suppresses pituitary output of follicle-stimulating hormone (FSH) and luteinizing hormone (LH), which interrupts the progress and pain of endometriosis. The usual period of administration is 3–6 months extending up to 9 months, if needed. Because of potential liver damage, the client would not take it on a lifelong basis. Danazol is only given orally. One of the side effects of danazol is hot flashes. **Cognitive Level:** Applying **Client Need:** Pharmacological and Parenteral Therapies **Integrated Process:** Teaching and Learning **Content Area:** Pharmacology **Strategy:** The critical words in the question are *endometriosis* and *purpose*, which tells you that the correct option is the one that explains the reason for the use of the drug in a client with endometriosis. Eliminate two options first because they are not purposes of the medication. Of the remaining two options, choose the correct option because hot flashes are not associated with endometriosis. **Reference:** Wilson, B. A., Shannon, M. T., & Shields, K. M. (2017). *Pearson nurse's drug guide 2017.* New York, NY: Pearson, pp. 424–425.

Posttest

1 Answer: 2 Rationale: Combining the hormones offers two processes that interrupt conception. Progestins thicken cervical mucous to prevent sperm penetration, follicular maturation, and ovulation. Estrogen prevents the luteinizing hormone (LH) surge that stimulates ova maturation. Additional estrogen is not needed. Progestins are added to reduce sperm penetration, not to prevent spotting. Combining the two ingredients in one pill is more economical rather than effective, but the statement is too vague to have the greatest use to the client. **Cognitive Level:** Analyzing **Client Need:** Pharmacological and Parenteral Therapies **Integrated Process:** Teaching and Learning **Content Area:** Pharmacology **Strategy:** Correlate the drug actions with the therapeutic purposes. Eliminate the false statements first and then choose the most specific option from those remaining. **Reference:** Wilson, B. A.,

Shannon, M. T., & Shields, K. M. (2017). *Pearson nurse's drug guide 2017.* New York, NY: Pearson, pp. 620–624.

2 Answer: 2 Rationale: Nitrates are the most common drugs used in management of angina. Current evidence indicates clients taking nitrates should not ingest sildenafil at the same time because a sudden drop in blood pressure could occur that could lead to sudden death. No endocrine alterations such as diabetes mellitus are associated with the drug, and a diagnosis of diabetes would not be a contraindication for use of sildenafil. Finasteride is used to treat benign prostate hypertrophy (BPH) and may cause impotence and may decrease the effectiveness of sildenafil, but it is not as significant as the risk of cardiac arrest. Sildenafil may worsen chronic sinusitis, but is not as significant as cardiac arrest. **Cognitive Level:** Analyzing **Client Need:** Pharmacological and Parenteral Therapies **Integrated Process:** Nursing Process: Assessment **Content Area:** Pharmacology **Strategy:** The core issue of the question is identification of a client at particular risk if taking sildenafil. Recall that this drug has vasodilating effects and use the process of elimination to select the client in whom vasodilation could pose added risk. **Reference:** Wilson, B. A., Shannon, M. T., & Shields, K. M. (2017). *Pearson nurse's drug guide 2017.* New York, NY: Pearson, pp. 1439–1440.

3 Answer: 1 Rationale: Clomiphene induces ovulation through stimulation of luteinizing hormone (LH) and follicle-stimulating hormone (FSH). It is taken orally in 50-mg dosage for 5 days each month, beginning on day 5 of the menstrual cycle. Clomiphene does not prepare the uterine wall for fertilization. Use of this drug by male clients has occurred but lacks scientific evidence, so therefore this is not the best response. **Cognitive Level:** Applying **Client Need:** Pharmacological and Parenteral Therapies **Integrated Process:** Nursing Process: Evaluation **Content Area:** Pharmacology **Strategy:** Correlate the drug category with the client's statement. The drug is categorized as an ovulation stimulant. **Reference:** Wilson, B. A., Shannon, M. T., & Shields, K. M. (2017). *Pearson nurse's drug guide 2017.* New York, NY: Pearson, pp. 369–371.

4 Answer: 4 Rationale: Orchidectomy is removal of the testicle, which would require hormone replacement. Vasectomy is severing of the vas deferens to prevent the passage of sperm during ejaculation. Cryptorchidism repair is correction of an undescended testicle and would not require hormone replacement. Varicocele repair involves repair of a blood vessel and would require no hormone replacement. **Cognitive Level:** Applying **Client Need:** Pharmacological and Parenteral Therapies **Integrated Process:** Nursing Process: Planning **Content Area:** Pharmacology **Strategy:** Associate the syllable *andro* for *androgen* with the testicles. Recall that it is a male reproductive hormone to help make the correct selection. **Reference:** Wilson, B. A., Shannon, M. T., & Shields, K. M. (2017). *Pearson nurse's drug guide 2017.* New York, NY: Pearson, pp. 1528–1530.

5 **Answer: 1, 5** **Rationale:** One common side effect of oxytocin is hypertensive episodes, so blood pressure should be closely monitored. Subarachnoid hemorrhage is a side effect of the drug and level of consciousness should be monitored. Nausea may occur, as well as an increase in discomfort once the therapy is initiated, but these do not signal the nurse of a serious threat. Weight gain may reflect fluid retention in the later months of pregnancy. **Cognitive Level:** Applying **Client Need:** Pharmacological and Parenteral Therapies **Integrated Process:** Nursing Process: Planning **Content Area:** Pharmacology **Strategy:** Align side effects with management of the client's needs. **Reference:** Wilson, B. A., Shannon, M. T., & Shields, K. M. (2017). *Pearson nurse's drug guide 2017.* New York, NY: Pearson, pp. 1176–1178.

6 **Answer: 2** **Rationale:** Mirena is a levonorgestrel-releasing intrauterine system used for contraception. It releases 20 mcg/day of levonorgestrel over a period of 5 years, at which time it needs to be removed. **Cognitive Level:** Analyzing **Client Need:** Pharmacological and Parenteral Therapies **Integrated Process:** Nursing Process: Planning **Content Area:** Pharmacology **Strategy:** Recall knowledge of intrauterine devices and their duration of action. **Reference:** Adams, M. P., & Urban, C. (2015). *Pharmacology: Connections to nursing practice* (3rd ed.). New York, NY: Pearson, pp. 912–913.

7 **Answer: 1** **Rationale:** Sudden onset of blurred vision may indicate blood clot formation and subsequent pressure on the optic nerves. Hypercoagulation is a common side effect of estrogen derivatives. The client could become suddenly unable to communicate or seek assistance. Sudden onset of blurred vision is not commonly associated with the development of a refractory problem. The client is in need of immediate healthcare unrelated to gynecologic assessment. Clients with migraine headaches often have blurred vision before an attack; however, since the nurse is aware of the risks associated with an estrogen–progestin combination, the high-risk possibilities should be pursued first. **Cognitive Level:** Applying **Client Need:** Pharmacological and Parenteral Therapies **Integrated Process:** Nursing Process: Implementation **Content Area:** Pharmacology **Strategy:** Correlate the client's reported symptom with the drug characteristics and side effects. Select the option that provides the greatest degree of safety. **Reference:** Wilson, B. A., Shannon, M. T., & Shields, K. M. (2017). *Pearson nurse's drug guide 2017.* New York, NY: Pearson, pp. 620–624.

8 **Answer: 4** **Rationale:** Terbutaline sulfate is categorized as a selective beta$_2$-adrenergic stimulant that results in smooth muscle relaxant of the respiratory tract as well as the uterine muscles. Therefore, it is used to treat both bronchospasms as well as premature labor. Asking the client what is used normally to control asthmatic attacks does not address the client's concern and it also provides no actual information. The primary issue is for the nurse to communicate the appropriate information regarding the use of terbutaline sulfate to treat preterm labor. **Cognitive Level:** Analyzing **Client Need:** Pharmacological and Parenteral Therapies **Integrated Process:** Communication and Documentation **Content Area:** Pharmacology **Strategy:** Correlate the differences between common use of the drug and the common physiological processes existing between respiratory function and uterine contraction. **Reference:** Wilson, B. A., Shannon, M. T., & Shields, K. M. (2017). *Pearson nurse's drug guide 2017.* New York, NY: Pearson, pp. 1521–1523.

9 **Answer: 2** **Rationale:** Testosterone is contraindicated in a client suspected of having prostate cancer. Although further assessment is warranted, an increased prostatic antigen level (PSA) may indicate prostate cancer exists. Acne is believed to be stimulated by androgenic hormones and the testosterone could contribute to this, but this is not as much a concern as the client with an elevated PSA level. Etiologic factors associated with melanoma include genetic predisposition, sun exposure, and the presence of moles. Ingestion of testosterone can result in hypercholesterolemia, but this lipoprotein level is within normal limits. **Cognitive Level:** Applying **Client Need:** Pharmacological and Parenteral Therapies **Integrated Process:** Nursing Process: Planning **Content Area:** Pharmacology **Strategy:** Compare and contrast the client characteristics with the characteristics of the drug. Specific drug knowledge is needed to make the correlation. **Reference:** Wilson, B. A., Shannon, M. T., & Shields, K. M. (2017). *Pearson nurse's drug guide 2017.* New York, NY: Pearson, pp. 1528–1530.

10 **Answer: 2** **Rationale:** Dinoprostone is a form of prostaglandin E2 and is used for cervical ripening. It is commonly used as an abortifacient. The client who had difficulty conceiving would be most interested in carrying the fetus to full term so the drug would not be given to this client. Since it is an abortifacient, breastfeeding does not correlate with the drug's actions. **Cognitive Level:** Applying **Client Need:** Pharmacological and Parenteral Therapies **Integrated Process:** Nursing Process: Assessment **Content Area:** Pharmacology **Strategy:** Associate the characteristics of the drug with the needs of the client and use the process of elimination to make a selection. **Reference:** Wilson, B. A., Shannon, M. T., & Shields, K. M. (2017). *Pearson nurse's drug guide 2017.* New York, NY: Pearson, pp. 497–499.

References

Adams, M., Holland, L., & Urban, C. (2017). *Pharmacology for nurses: A pathophysiologic approach* (5th ed.). New York, NY: Pearson.

Adams, M. P., & Urban, C. (2015). *Pharmacology: Connections to nursing practice* (3rd ed.). New York, NY: Pearson.

Burchum, J., & Rosenthal, L. (2016). *Lehne's pharmacology for nursing care* (9th ed.). St. Louis, MO: Mosby.

Drug Facts & Comparisons (2017; updated monthly). St. Louis, MO: Wolters Kluwer.

Karch, A. M. (2016). *Focus on nursing pharmacology* (7th ed.). Philadelphia, PA: Lippincott Williams & Wilkins.

Kee, J. (2017). *Pearson handbook of laboratory and diagnostic tests and nursing implications* (8th ed.). New York, NY: Pearson.

LeMone, P., Burke, K., Bauldoff, G., & Gubrud, P. (2015). *Medical surgical nursing: Clinical reasoning in patient care* (6th ed.). New York, NY: Pearson.

Lilley, L. L., Rainforth Collins, S., & Snyder, K. M. (2017). *Pharmacology and the nursing process* (8th ed.). St. Louis, MO: Mosby.

Vallerand, A. H., Sanoski, C. A., & Deglin, J. H. (2017). *Davis's drug guide for nurses* (8th ed.). Philadelphia, PA: F.A. Davis.

Wilson, B. A., Shannon, M. T., & Shields, K. M. (2017). *Pearson nurse's drug guide 2017.* New York, NY: Pearson.

Integumentary System Medications

Chapter Outline

General Agents
Protective Agents
Antipruritics

Anti-Infectives
Corticosteroids
Keratolytics

Acne Medications
Burn Medications
Debriding Medications

Objectives

➤ Describe the principles related to skin absorption.
➤ Identify the general properties of topical dermatologic medications.
➤ Explain the actions, purposes, and safe use of dermatologic medications.
➤ Describe the nursing considerations when administering medications for the integumentary system.
➤ Describe the general goals of therapy when administering integumentary medications.
➤ List the significant client education points related to integumentary medications.

NCLEX-RN® Test Prep

Access the NEW Web-based app that provides students with additional practice questions in preparation for the NCLEX experience.

Review at a Glance

acne most common chronic skin disease of adolescents and young adults that affects hair follicles and sebaceous glands; characterized by noninflammatory and inflammatory lesions that often involve face, chest, and back

antiseptics chemical agents that inhibit growth of microorganisms but do not necessarily kill them

creams emulsions of oil in water; more complex preparations than ointments

emollients occlusive agents that make skin soft and pliable by increasing hydration of stratum corneum

herpes simplex an acute viral disease marked by groups of vesicles on skin, often on borders of lips or nares or on genitals

lotions liquid suspensions or dispersions intended for external use

ointments water-in-oil emulsions; semisolid preparations of medicinal substances in a base, such as petrolatum or lanolin

papules small, circumscribed, superficial, solid elevations of skin

pediculosis parasitic infestation caused by lice; may involve hair, body, or pubic area

powder finely divided solid drug or mixture of drugs

pruritus intense itching that is relieved fully by controlling the causative primary illness

psoriasis a chronic, genetically influenced skin disorder characterized by periodic exacerbation of erythematous papules and plaques covered by prominent, thick, silvery-white scales

scabies parasitic infestation caused by a mite

tinea pedis a superficial fungal infection of skin of feet; also known as *athlete's foot*

PRETEST

1 A client newly diagnosed with psoriasis has been prescribed betamethasone as treatment for the disorder. What statement made by the client indicates further information is needed about this medication?

1. "This drug will also help cure my acne."
2. "I should report an elevated temperature if it occurs."
3. "After applying the medication, I should either leave the skin exposed or cover it lightly."
4. "It should only be applied to the affected skin area."

2 The nurse teaches the parents of a child with impetigo to apply which topical medication as prescribed to the affected area of the child's skin?

1. Ketoconazole
2. Mupirocin
3. Capsaicin
4. Acyclovir

3 A client is diagnosed with atopic dermatitis. The nurse should expect that which classes of drugs will be prescribed either alone or in combination? Select all that apply.

1. Antihistamines
2. Analgesics
3. Antimicrobials
4. Topical anesthetics
5. Antifungals

4 A participant in a skin care research project asks the nurse educator to justify the recommendation of a sunscreen. Which response by the nurse provides the best rationale?

1. "Sunscreens neutralize the sun's rays."
2. "Sunscreens are waterproof and thus block the sun's rays."
3. "Sunscreens absorb the sun's rays and distribute the heat to other body parts."
4. "Sunscreens prevent sunburn by absorbing and reflecting the sun's rays."

5 An adult client with a pediculosis infestation has a prescription for a drug to treat the condition. The nurse anticipates providing which information as an instruction to the client about application methods?

1. Chlorhexidine: Apply with sterile gloves.
2. Lindane: Leave in place for 12–24 hours.
3. Collagenase: Apply with fingertips.
4. Terbinafine: Apply a thin layer.

6 Permethrin is prescribed for an adult client, and the nurse needs to provide the client with instructions for use. Place the directions in proper sequence that the nurse should provide to the client.

1. Comb hair using a fine-toothed comb.
2. Shampoo hair.
3. Apply permethrin cream to hair and work through to scalp.
4. Let sit for 10 minutes.
5. Wash hair to remove drug.

7 The nurse teaches the client with acne that which preparation is one of the most effective agents for acne treatment?

1. Mafenide
2. Benzoyl peroxide
3. Chlorhexidine
4. Coal tar

8 The school nurse explains to a group of adolescents at a school health fair that which medication is considered to be most effective for the treatment of acne?

1. Tetracycline
2. Penicillin G
3. Clindamycin
4. Isotretinoin

9 After administering silver sulfadiazine to a client with burns, the nurse should perform which assessment to determine the effectiveness of the medication?

1. Measure body temperature
2. Weigh client daily
3. Review serum potassium levels
4. Assess separation of eschar

10 During the first 24 hours, the nurse should manage one of the most common complications associated with burn injury by administering which medications as prescribed for the client?

1. Famotidine 20 mg intravenous every 12 hours
2. Calcium-based antacids by mouth after meals
3. Furosemide 20 mg intravenous twice daily
4. Crotamiton cream, once daily for 2 days

➤ *See pages 502–504 for Answers and Rationales.*

I. GENERAL AGENTS

A. Soaps

1. Action and use
   a. Deodorant soaps are relatively harsh soaps that contain triclosan or triclocarban as topical antibacterial agents and are useful in decreasing body odor, preventing bacterial spread, and assisting in treatment of cutaneous infections
   b. True soaps mechanically remove bacteria and are effective at removing all sebum and environmental dirt
   c. Synthetic detergent bars are generally milder and compose a group of products known as beauty bars
   d. Allergic sensitization can occur to fragrances, dyes, antibacterial agents, or other additives in soaps
   e. Cleansing ingredients in shampoos are detergents that have different abilities to cleanse and lather
   f. Medicated shampoos may be used for dandruff, seborrheic dermatitis, or **psoriasis** (a chronic skin disorder characterized by periodic exacerbations of erythematous papules and plaques covered by prominent, thick, silvery-white scales)
2. Common soap and shampoo preparations: see Box 15-1
3. Client-centered nursing care
   a. Assess any skin symptom, beginning with a history
   b. Monitor for local adverse effects/irritation from use of selected soap(s) and/or shampoo(s)
   c. Read product literature carefully because some shampoos are not recommended for small children
4. Client education
   a. Soaps can be irritating to people with dry skin, especially in winter with low humidity
   b. Apply a moisturizing preparation after bathing if dry skin is a problem
   c. How to use any prescribed shampoo properly

B. Cleansers

1. Action and use
   a. Cleansers are used for preoperative cleansing of skin
   b. Cleansers may be used for treatment of wounds or abrasions
   c. May also be bacteriostatic or bactericidal depending on agent
2. Common cleansing preparations: see Table 15-1
3. Client-centered nursing care
   a. Assess any skin symptom, beginning with a history
   b. Monitor for local irritation and/or drying as an adverse effect of these topical preparations

Box 15-1	**Soaps**
Soaps and Shampoos	**Deodorant Soaps: Harsh**

Soaps

Deodorant Soaps: Harsh

Dial

Lever 2000

Safeguard

True Soaps

Ivory

Synthetic Detergent Soaps: Mild

Dove

Oil of Olay

Neutrogena

Tone

Shampoos
Unmedicated

Too numerous to list

Medicated

Head & Shoulders Intensive Treatment Dandruff Shampoo (selenium sulfide 1%) and other related products

Selsun Blue Dandruff Shampoo and other related products

4. Client education
   a. Proper use of any prescribed cleanser
   b. If wounds or abrasions are present, explain inflammatory process and wound healing process

C. Lotions
   1. Action and use
      a. **Lotions** historically were "shake lotions" or suspensions of a **powder** (finely divided solid drug or mixture of drugs) in water
      b. With a shake lotion, as water in the lotion evaporates, a coating of powder is left on skin, producing a drying effect

Table 15-1 Cleansers

Agent	Use
Povidone-iodine	Bactericidal
Iodine	Cleansing action
Benzalkonium chloride	Bacteriostatic; can support growth of certain *Pseudomonas* species; inactivated by soap; do not cover with an occlusive dressing
Alcohol	Bactericidal; not as effective as povidone-iodine
Hydrogen peroxide	Germicidal; has mechanical effectiveness; do not use after epithelium is formed because it will continue to debride newly growing cells
Chlorhexidine gluconate	Cleansing action
Hexachlorophene	Cleansing action
Oxychlorosene sodium	Cleansing action
Sodium hypochlorite	Cleansing action

      c. Today other types of liquid emulsions of thin, uniform consistency are also referred to as lotions

   2. Common preparation: calamine lotion; a preparation of calamine, zinc oxide, glycerin bentonite magma, calcium hydroxide, and others

   3. Client-centered nursing care

      a. Shake the lotion before application to place powder in suspension

      b. Monitor for local and systemic adverse effects of topical preparation

   4. Client education

      a. Proper use of any prescribed lotion (supervise initial use if appropriate to ensure correct application)

      b. Some preparations of calamine lotion also contain diphenhydramine, which can cause drowsiness; use these products cautiously until effect of these agents is known

D. Emollients

   1. Action and use

      a. **Emollients** are occlusive agents that make skin soft and pliable by increasing hydration of stratum corneum and by filling gaps in stratum corneum created by dry, contracted skin cells

      b. Include silicone oils, propylene glycol, isopropyl palmitate, and octyl stearate

      c. Can also function as skin protectants if they soothe symptoms of **pruritus** (intense itching) due to exposed, traumatized nerve endings

      d. Moisturizers are intended to mimic function of sebum on skin; function is based on mechanisms of occlusion and humectancy

      e. The occlusion function employs petrolatum, lanolin, cocoa butter, or mineral oil to prevent evaporation of water from skin

      f. The humectancy function employs substances that attract moisture to skin (e.g., glycerin, sorbitol, propylene glycol)

   2. Common emollient preparations: common over-the-counter (OTC) products include Aquaphor, Curel, Dermasil, Eucerin, Lubriderm, Neutrogena; there are many others

   3. Client-centered nursing care

      a. Assess any skin symptom, beginning with a history

      b. Unless otherwise directed by product instructions, apply to skin after bathing while skin is slightly moist

   4. Client education

      a. Explain to clients what contents to look for in over-the-counter (OTC) moisturizers that will indicate product is of high quality

      b. Proper use of any prescribed emollient

E. Protectants

   1. Action and use

      a. Several preparations are designed to protect skin from wetness

      b. Help prevent and treat diaper rash, prickly heat, and/or chafing

   2. Common protectant preparations: common OTC ointments contain ingredients such as lanolin, petrolatum, zinc oxide, cod liver oil, balsam Peru, and beeswax; protectant powders may contain cornstarch or calcium undecylenate

   3. Client-centered nursing care

      a. Assess any skin symptom, beginning with a history

      b. Monitor skin for desired effect

   4. Client education

      a. Powders should be kept away from face to avoid inhalation

      b. Some preparations should not be used on broken skin

      c. If diaper rash or skin irritation worsens or does not improve within 7 days of beginning self-care, consult healthcare provider

Practice to Pass

A 6-month-old infant has diaper rash. What would you include in a teaching plan for the mother?

F. Therapeutic baths

1. Action and use
   a. Baths are used for treatment of large affected skin areas; balneotherapy is a type of bath or soak containing minerals
   b. Baths remove crusts, scales, and/or old medications
   c. Assist in the relief of itching and acute dermatoses
   d. Medications can be placed in water
   e. Bath temperature should be 37.7 to 46°C (99.9 to 114.8°F)
   f. Client should be placed in bath for 20–30 minutes
   g. Tub should be filled one-third to one-half full
2. Common therapeutic bath preparations: see Table 15-2
3. Client-centered nursing care
   a. Assess condition of skin including excoriation, drainage, odor, color, and temperature
   b. Assess for pain prior to bathing
   c. Assess range of motion and client safety, particularly in presence of oils
   d. Apply clean gloves to assist client during bath
   e. Fill tub one-third to one-half full
   f. With use of medicated tars, bathroom should be well ventilated due to volatile fumes
   g. Assess skin for achievement of therapeutic effects
   h. Minimize fluctuation in bath and room temperatures during bath
4. Client education
   a. Safety measures when using bath oils and how to prevent falls
   b. Blot skin to dry it after bath
   c. Intended effects of bath
   d. Wear light clothing after bath

G. Soaks and wet dressings

1. Action and use
   a. General rule: acute lesions that are oozing, weeping, and crusting respond best to medication in aqueous, drying preparations
   b. General rule: scaling chronic lesions respond best to medication in moisturizing, lubricating preparations
   c. Open soaks are applied for 20 minutes, three times a day
   d. Closed soaks use a water-impermeable substance (occlusion) over a wet soak; this method causes heat retention, which is excellent for debridement but may lead to maceration; applied for 1–2 hours, 2–3 times a day
   e. Continuous closed soaks are left in place for 24 hours to treat thick crusts; it is important to rewet dressing four to five times a day

Table 15-2 Common Additives to Therapeutic Baths

Therapeutic Bath Solution	Use
Water	Provides wet dressing effect
Saline	Treats wide disseminated lesions
Colloidal	Decreases itching, antipruritic
Sodium bicarbonate	Provides soothing soak, which cools skin, usually a rash
Medicated tars	Psoriasis and eczema
Bath oil	Emollient action and antipruritic for acute generalized eczema
Starch	Soothes skin

Table 15-3	Soaks and Wet Dressings	
Agent	**Use**
Burow's Solution: 5% aluminum acetate solution, 1 Domeboro tablet or packet to 1 pint of tap water	Acts as astringent to decrease exudation by precipitation of protein
Acetic Acid 0.1–1% solution: ½ cup white vinegar to 1 quart water	May be helpful for wounds infected with *Pseudomonas* organisms
Salt solution: 1 tbsp salt to 1 quart of water	Wetting action

    2. Common soaking and wet dressing preparations: see Table 15-3
    3. Client-centered nursing care
        a. Assess any skin symptom, beginning with a history
        b. Monitor for achievement of intended effects
    4. Client education

Practice to Pass

Your cousin, who is fair-skinned, is planning to visit Florida for the first time. She has never seen the ocean and "can't wait to go to the beach." What would you discuss with her before she leaves?

!

        a. In a healthcare institution, carry out prescribed soak procedure
        b. Teach procedure to clients for type of soak recommended or prescribed if scheduled for discharge

H. Rubs and liniments
    1. Action and use: OTC preparations for temporary relief of minor aches and pains of muscles and joints associated with strains, bruises, sprains, sports injuries, simple backache, and arthritis
    2. Common rub and liniment preparations: see Box 15-2
    3. Client-centered nursing care
        a. Assess symptom for which agent is to be used
        b. Monitor for achievement of intended effects
    4. Client education
        a. Clean skin of all other **ointments** (water-in-oil emulsions), **creams** (more complex preparations of oil in water than ointments), sprays, or liniments before applying the product
        b. Apply to affected areas no more than 3–4 times daily
        c. Some products have specific directions (i.e., BenGay should not be used with heating pad or tight bandage)

Box 15-2	
Rubs and Liniments	**Aspercreme External Analgesic Rub with Aloe**
	Available as crème, lotion
	Contains trolamine salicylate, aloe vera gel, many others
	BenGay External Analgesic Products
	Ointment, cream, arthritis formula cream
	Contains menthol in alcohol base gel, methyl salicylate, camphor, others
	Sportscream External Analgesic Rub
	Available as crème, lotion
	Contains trolamine salicylate, acetyl alcohol, others
	Therapeutic Mineral Ice, Pain Relieving Gel, Icy Hot
	Contain menthol, others
	Capsaicin
	Active ingredient from cayenne peppers

I. Powders

   1. Action and use: hygroscopic agents that absorb and retain moisture and assist in reducing friction between bedding and skin

   2. Common preparations: bentonite, cornstarch, talc, and zinc oxide

   3. Client-centered nursing care

     a. Assess skin for breakdown or signs of reduced friction

     b. Keep skin clean and dry

   4. Client education

     a. General skin care and proper application of powder

     b. Importance of changing position to reduce pressure and avoiding friction during repositioning

II. PROTECTIVE AGENTS

  A. Description

   1. This section is limited to discussion of sunscreen preparations and protective dressings

   2. For other preparations that can be defined as offering protection, see previous section on protectants

  B. Sunscreen preparations

   1. Actions and use

     a. Important because they can prevent skin cancer

     b. Chemical sunscreens absorb ultraviolet radiation in the spectrum of ultraviolet light (UVL) most responsible for sunburns

     c. Chemical absorbers formulated against ultraviolet B rays (UVB) include cinnamates, *p*-aminobenzoic acid (PABA) and PABA esters, or salicylates

     d. Chemical absorbers formulated against ultraviolet A rays (UVA) include benzophenones

     e. Physical sunscreens reflect or scatter light to prevent skin penetration

     f. Physical sunscreens contain ingredients such as titanium dioxide, zinc oxide, talc

     g. Effectiveness of a sunscreen is indicated by its sun protection factor (SPF), which is the ratio between exposures to ultraviolet wavelengths and development of skin erythema; an SPF of 6 means product offers six times the protection as the use of no sunscreen

     h. Sunscreens range in SPF

     i. A water-resistant sunscreen should continue to function after 40 minutes in water

     j. A waterproof sunscreen withstands 80 minutes in water

   2. Common sunscreen preparations: see Table 15-4

   3. Nursing considerations: assess skin for degree of burn if not used effectively

Table 15-4   **Common Sunscreen Preparations**

Brand Name	SPF	Active Ingredients
Coppertone Broad Spectrum Lotion	25	Avobenzone, benzophenones, cinnamates
Johnson's Baby Sunblock Lotion	30	Benzophenones, cinnamates, salicylates
Neutrogena Sunblock	30	Cinnamates, menthyl anthranilate, octocrylene
Shade UVA/UVB	15, 25, 30, 45	Avobenzone benzophenones, cinnamates
Sundown Sport	15	Titanium dioxide, zinc oxide
Total Eclipse Lotion	15	Benzophenones, salicylates, PABA
Water Babies UVA/UVB	12, 25, 30, 45	Benzophenones, cinnamates, octocrylene

Table 15-5	Required Skin Protection and SPF
Required Skin Protection	**Recommended SPF**
Minimal	2–11 SPF
Moderate	12–29 SPF
High	30 or above

4. Client education
   a. Follow product directions and avoid contact between product and eyes
   b. Apply sunscreen if outdoors between 10:00 a.m. and 3:00 p.m. daily
   c. Use products with SPF of 15 or greater
   d. Reapply sunscreen every 2 hours or per product directions when swimming or if sweating
   e. Choose sunscreen according to need: see Table 15-5

C. **Protective dressings**
   1. Action and use
      a. Includes occlusive biosynthetic dressings for certain wound therapies
      b. As an example, a hydrocolloid dressing hydrates wound surfaces; wound fluid interacts with wafer of the preparation and melts it, forming a moist, jelly-like substance that keeps wound moist and promotes healing
   2. Common protective wound dressings: see Table 15-6

Practice to Pass

The client has two plantar warts on the ball of his left foot. What would you include in a plan of action for the client?

Table 15-6	Common Types of Dressings
Dressing Type	**Description**
Gauze	Plain or impregnated with an antimicrobial for use on full- and partial-thickness wounds Packs and fills wound; absorbs drainage May be applied dry, wet-to-moist, and wet-to-wet
Transparent film	Adhesive plastic semipermeable dressing that allows oxygen into wound but not liquids and bacteria Protects wound from contamination and friction, prevents fluid evaporation from wound, and aids wound assessment
Impregnated nonadherent	Cotton or synthetic material that is impregnated with saline, zinc-saline, antimicrobials, petrolatum, or others Protects partial- and full-thickness wounds that do not have exudate Requires secondary dressing to keep it in place, hold in moisture, and protect wound
Hydrocolloid	Contains adhesive wafer, paste, or powder; can be worn up to 7 days Inner layer absorbs exudates and forms hydrated gel over wound, while outer film provides occlusive seal Protects wound from contamination and eliminates risk of maceration of surrounding skin
Hydrogel	Water or glycerin is primary component of jelly-like sheet, granules, or gels; maintains moist wound bed and helps liquefy necrotic tissue or slough Permeable to oxygen and can fill dead spaces in a wound Secondary occlusive dressing is required
Alginate (exudate absorbers)	Nonadherent dressings of powder, beads, granules, ropes, sheets, or paste; requires secondary dressing Purpose is to absorb up to 20 times their weight in drainage
Polyurethane foam	Nonadherent hydrocolloid dressing that absorbs large amounts of exudate while keeping wound moist Requires secondary dressing for an occlusive environment, or tape around edges to secure it Skin around area needs protection from maceration
Clear absorbent acrylic	Transparent absorbent wafer with an acrylic layer that absorbs exudates and allows moisture to evaporate Aids in wound assessment while protecting from bacteria and shearing forces; for 5- to 7-day use
Collagen	Derived from animal sources (often pig or cow); comes in a variety of forms Used to halt bleeding and stimulate cell proliferation in wound bed to help healing

3. Client-centered nursing care
   a. Assess any skin wound, beginning with a history
   b. Inspect dressing at least daily for leaks, dislodgment, wrinkling, or odor

   c. Change dressing when it becomes dislodged, leaks, or develops an odor
   d. If wound has substantial drainage, dressing might need to be changed every 24–48 hours, but generally is left in place for 3–7 days
   e. When changing dressing, leave residue that is difficult to remove; it will wear off in time; attempts to remove can irritate surrounding skin
4. Client education: proper use of any prescribed occlusive biosynthetic dressing

III. ANTIPRURITICS

A. Description
1. Antipruritics stop the intense itching known as pruritis
2. Pruritus causes more clients to visit healthcare provider than any other dermatological symptom
3. Pruritus has a multitude of causes and treatment needs to be tailored to specific cause
4. Types of pruritis include winter pruritus, senior pruritus, lichen simplex chronicus, external otitis, pruritus ani (e.g., pinworm infestation in children), and genital pruritus

B. Action and use
1. Antipruritic medication therapy for some types of pruritis might include topical corticosteroids to decrease inflammation and/or methods to promote skin hydration
2. Antipruritic therapy may also necessitate use of a systemic antihistamine
3. Antipruritic lotions contain a powder in water and should be shaken well; powder has active ingredients that treat the affected area; apply to affected area every 3–4 hours or as recommended by healthcare provider

C. Common antipruritic medications: see Box 15-3

Box 15-3

Antipruritic Agents

Lotion or Cream
Aveeno Anti-itch Lotion or Cream
Aveeno Moisturizing Lotion or Cream
Eucerin Crème or Lotion
Sarna Topical Lotion (camphor, menthol, and phenol)
Zonalon Cream
Calamine Lotion

Hydrating Baths
Aveeno (colloidal oatmeal)
Aveeno Oil (e.g., colloidal oatmeal, mineral oil, glyceryl stearate)

Systemic H$_1$ Blockers or Combination
Hydroxyzine hydrochloride
Hydroxyzine pamoate
Chlorpheniramine
Cyproheptadine hydrochloride

Unsafe
Benzocaine and other "-caine" derivatives
Antihistamines such as astemizole

     D. Client-centered nursing care
1. Take a history of this systemic symptom and any associated skin symptoms
2. Monitor for local and systemic adverse effects of any topical preparation
3. Monitor for anticholinergic adverse reactions if systemic antihistamines of the anti-cholinergic type are used

     E. Client education
1. General bathing should be limited to once or twice a week and only mild soaps should be used; any soap chosen should be used sparingly
2. Negative effects of scratching and the need to interrupt any itch-and-scratch cycle
3. Maintain cool environment, especially in the bedroom for sleep

IV. ANTI-INFECTIVES

     A. Antibacterials
1. Action and use
   a. Common causative organisms of skin infections are *Streptococcus pyogenes* and *Staphylococcus aureus*
   b. Certain topical antibiotics are used to inhibit growth of *Propionibacterium acnes* and reduce inflammatory lesions of acne
   c. Topical antibacterial therapy may be useful for prophylaxis of infections in wounds and injuries
2. Common topical antibacterial and antiviral medications: see Table 15-7
3. Client-centered nursing care
   a. Assess any skin symptom, beginning with a history
   b. Assess for hypersensitivity to any ingredient in product to be used; this would constitute a contraindication for use
   c. Monitor for skin irritation and any signs of superinfection
4. Client education
   a. Wash hands before using any topical antibacterial agent and cleanse area to be treated
   b. May wear gloves
   c. Generally topical agents should be applied sparingly and gently to affected area
   d. With some, a dressing should be applied and with some it should not; follow prescriber instructions
   e. Report worsening of condition, lack of healing, or development of a rash around lesion
   f. Protect skin from sunlight if using gentamicin sulfate (risk of photosensitization)

     B. Antivirals
1. Action and use
   a. Used to treat cutaneous **herpes simplex** (an acute viral disease marked by groups of vesicles on skin, often on borders of lips, nares, or on genitals) primarily
   b. May also be used to treat herpes zoster
   c. With some infections an oral agent may be needed instead of a topical agent
2. Common medication: acyclovir 5% ointment; see also Table 15-7
3. Client-centered nursing care
   a. Assess skin symptoms, beginning with a history
   b. Monitor for local adverse effects of topical product, such as mild pain, burning, stinging; report these to prescriber
4. Client education
   a. Wash hands before using topical antiviral drug
   b. Use gloves or finger cot when applying product to avoid autoinnoculation of other body sites
   c. Apply as soon as symptoms of herpes lesions begin

Table 15-7	Topical Antibacterial and Antiviral Agents	
Generic Name	**Action**	**Uses**
Bacitracin	Inhibits cell wall synthesis	Primarily used to treat *Staphylococci* in minor skin abrasions or treat superficial skin infections
Bacitracin, polymixin B, neosporin	Inhibits cell wall synthesis and 30S ribosome	Primarily used to treat *Bacillus subtilis*, *Streptomyces fradiae*, and secondarily infected skin problems
Chloramphenicol	Inhibits cell wall replication; used infrequently due to dose-related bone marrow suppression	*Streptococcus venezuelae*
Clindamycin phosphate	Inhibits protein synthesis, causing cell death	Treat acne vulgaris and bacterial vaginosis
Erythromycin and benzoyl peroxide	Bacteriostatic or bactericidal, binding to cell membrane, changing protein function and causing cell death	Treat acne vulgaris, prophylaxis against infection in minor abrasions, and susceptible skin organisms
Gentamicin sulfate	Inhibits protein synthesis in susceptible Gram-negative bacteria; disrupts cell membrane and causes cell death	Treat minor skin abrasions and superficial infections of skin
Meclocycline sulfosalicylate	Suppresses growth of *Propionibacterium acnes*; synthetic derivative of oxytetracycline	Suppresses growth of *Propionibacterium acnes*
Metronidazole	Inhibits DNA synthesis in anaerobes, causing cell death	Treatment of inflammatory papules, pustules, and erythema of rosacea; treatment of *Gardnerella vaginalis*
Mupirocin	Inhibits bacterial protein synthesis by binding to bacterial transfer-RNA	Treat impetigo due to *S. aureus*, beta-hemolytic *Streptococcus*, and *Streptococcus pyogenes*
Neomycin	Aminoglycoside antibiotic obtained from *Streptomyces fradiae*	Treat short-term eye, ear, and skin infections
Tetracycline	Broad-spectrum antibiotic derived from *Streptomyces aurofaciens*	Treat superficial skin infections
Acyclovir	Inhibits viral DNA replication	Recurrent herpes labialis
Docosanol	Inhibits viral DNA replication	Recurrent herpes labialis
Imiquimod	Inhibits viral DNA replication	Treat external genital and perianal warts; typical nonhyperkeratotic actinic keratoses on face or scalp; basal cell carcinoma in immunocompromised clients
Penciclovir	Inhibits viral DNA replication	Treat cold sores in healthy clients; herpes labialis in lips and face

   d. Apply sparingly and gently to affected area
   e. Wear loose clothing and keep area clean and dry
   f. Avoid sexual intercourse when visible skin lesions are present
C. **Antifungals**
   1. Action and use
      a. Clients with disease and infection limited to glabrous (smooth, hairless) skin can be treated with topical antifungal agents
      b. Clients with extensive disease and infection of hair and nails are best treated with systemic therapy
      c. Advantages of topical use over systemic use: absence of serious adverse reactions, absence of drug interactions, over-the-counter availability of some preparations, ability to localize treatment to affected sites, no need to monitor laboratory tests

d. New drugs have caused decrease in use of keratolytics and **antiseptics** (chemical agents that inhibit growth of microorganisms but do not necessarily kill them) used in the past

2. Common medications
   a. Topical antifungal agents: see Table 15-8
   b. Oral agents include fluconazole, griseofulvin, itraconazole, ketoconazole, and terbinafine
3. Client-centered nursing care
   a. Assess any skin symptom, beginning with a history
   b. Assess for predisposing factors, such as trauma, general health, suppressed immune status, hygiene practices, and exposure to infectious agent

Table 15-8 **Topical Antifungals**

Generic Name	Action	Uses
Amphotericin B	Fungal cell death	Treat mucocutaneous and cutaneous *Candida* infections
Butenafine hydrochloride	Inhibits sterol synthesis	Treat interdigital pedia, tinea corporis, ringworm, tinea cruris
Butoconazole nitrate	Alters fungal cell membrane permeability, preventing cellular replication	Treat vulvovaginal candidiasis
Ciclopirox olamine	Synthetic broad-spectrum antifungal agent; inhibits transport of amino acids within fungal cell; interferes with synthesis of RNA, DNA, and fungal protein	Treat onychomycosis of fingernails and toenails
Clotrimazole	Alters fungal cell membrane permeability, preventing cell replication	Treat tinea pedis, tinea cruris, tinea corporis, tinea versicolor, vulvovaginal and oropharyngeal candidiasis
Econazole nitrate	Fungicidal for certain microorganisms	Active against many dermaphytes. Treatment of tinea pedis, tinea cruris, tinea corporis, cutaneous candidiasis
Gentian violet	Absorbed into skin; should not come in contact with active lesions; alters cellular permeability	Treat topical mycosis
Ketoconazole	Interferes with synthesis of ergosterol, increasing cell membrane permeability and inhibiting fungal growth	Treat tinea corporis, tinea cruris, and tinea versicolor
Naftifine hydrochloride	Interferes with synthesis of ergosterol (principal sterol in fungus cell membrane)	Treat *C. albicans, Epidermophyton floccosum, Microsporum canis, M. audouinii, M. gypseum, Trichophyton rubrum, T. mentagrophytes, T. tonsurans*
Oxiconazole	Alters fungi cell membrane, resulting in increased permeability	Treat tinea pedis, tinea cruris, and tinea corporis
Sertaconazole nitrate	Inhibits CYP-dependent synthesis of ergosterol; alters cell wall permeability and results in cell death	Tinea pedis caused by *Trichophyton mentagrophytes, T. rubrum,* or *Epidermophyton floccosum*
Terbinafine	Inhibits sterol biosynthesis in fungi and results in cell death	Tinea pedis, tinea cruris, and tinea corporis due to *Epidermophyton floccosum, Trichophyton mentagrophyte,* or *T. rubrum*
Tolnaftate	Distorts hyphae and stunts mycelial growth on susceptible fungi	Tinia pedis, tinea corporis, tinea capitis, tinea unguium

        c. Monitor for local adverse effects of topical preparations, which often include irritation, burning, or stinging depending on specific product used

        d. Do not apply gentian violet to active lesions

        e. Monitor for skin sensitization, noted by increased redness, swelling, weeping, or any burning or itching that were not present before treatment began

        f. Systemic effects of topical products are negligible, since absorption rates generally are only 3–6%

        g. Ensure affected area is cultured before starting topical amphoteracin treatment

4. Client education

        a. Use products as directed for full course of therapy (may be prolonged); apply liberally to clean and dry skin

        b. Leave exposed to air; do not apply protective dressing unless specifically prescribed

        c. To prevent such fungal infections as **tinea pedis** (a superficial fungal infection of skin of feet; athlete's foot)

           1) Wear shower shoes or thongs in public or communal showers and locker rooms

           2) Wear footwear of natural fibers (leather shoes, cotton or wool socks)

           3) Avoid going barefoot

           4) Change socks daily

        d. To avoid other fungal infections, practice adequate hygiene

           1) Keep affected areas clean, dry, and well ventilated (loose clothing)

           2) Use powders to keep skin dry and prevent maceration; these may or may not contain antifungal ingredients

D. Antiparasitics

1. Action and use

        a. Used to treat parasitic infestations such as **scabies** (caused by *Sarcoptes scabiei* mite) or **pediculosis** (caused by lice); may involve hair (tinea capitus), body (tinea corporis), or pubic area (tinea pubis)

        b. Recurrence of scabies is generally related to reinfection due to incomplete treatment rather than resistance of mite

        c. Crotamiton can be used in clients with scabies and pediculosis capitis who are ragweed sensitive

2. Common antiparasitic medications: see Table 15-9

3. Client-centered nursing care

        a. Assess any skin symptom, beginning with a history

        b. Although client may bathe, ensure skin is cool and dry before application of scabicide to prevent systemic absorption

        c. Monitor for local adverse effects, including irritation, pruritis, burning, or stinging

        d. Monitor for systemic effect of dizziness with lindane because it affects nervous system; avoid use in infants, children, older adults, and clients with known seizure disorders because of risk of seizures

Table 15-9   **Antiparasitics**

Agent	Uses
Crotamiton	Scabies
Malathion	Pediculosis capitis and their ova
Permethrin	Pediculosis capitis, scabies
Pyrethrin, piperonyl butoxide (liquid, Rid shampoo)	Pediculosis capitis, pediculosis corporis, pediculosis pubis
Lindane	Pediculosis capitis, pediculosis pubis, scabies

4. Client education
    a. After bathing, ensure skin is cool and dry before applying scabicide to reduce risk of seizures from systemic absorption
    b. For scabies
        1) Apply thin layer to dry skin from neck down and rub in thoroughly over entire body
        2) Permethrin and lindane: leave on 8–12 hours, remove thoroughly with washing
        3) Crotamiton: apply again after 24 hours, remove with washing 48 hours after initial application
    c. For pediculosis capitis
        1) Lindane lotion: apply lotion to dry hair, rub in thoroughly, leave on for 12 hours, then remove thoroughly
        2) Lindane shampoo: apply shampoo to dry hair, lather with small amount of water, work into hair for 4 minutes, rinse thoroughly
        3) Second treatment in 7–10 days may be needed with malathion

V. CORTICOSTEROIDS

A. Description
1. Topical corticosteroids are commonly used with skin disorders
2. Systemic corticosteroids may also be used with skin disorders

B. Action and use
1. Corticosteroids enter cell and bind to cytoplasmic receptors to produce an anti-inflammatory, antipruritic, and antiproliferative effect
2. Indicated for relief of inflammatory and pruritic manifestations and for minor skin irritations, rashes, and itching
3. Clinical effectiveness of corticosteroids relates to four properties
    a. Vasoconstriction; decreases erythema
    b. Antiproliferative effects; inhibits DNA synthesis and mitosis
    c. Immunosuppression; mechanism poorly understood
    d. Anti-inflammatory effects; inhibits formation of prostaglandins
4. Responsiveness of diseases to topical corticosteroids varies: highly responsive diseases include psoriasis, atopic dermatitis in children, seborrheic dermatitis, intertrigo
5. Penetration of preparation varies according to skin site
6. Using these products on thin skin, on older adult or pediatric clients, or under occlusion will increase incidence of adverse reactions
7. Adverse effects more common since introduction of higher-potency preparations
8. Local adverse reactions include atrophy, hypopigmentation, striae
9. Topical corticosteroids can cause systemic adverse reactions, including suppression of hypothalamic–pituitary–adrenal axis; occurs most frequently in clients using topical corticosteroids that are covered with an occlusive dressing or in clients with liver failure
10. Low-potency agents are best used for diffuse eruptions, those involving face or occluded areas such as axilla or groin, and chronic dermatoses
11. Medium-potency agents are appropriate for acute flare-ups of chronic dermatoses and acute self-limited eruptions where they can be used for periods of 14–21 days
12. High-potency agents best used for acute localized eruptions for a short time of 7–14 days
13. High-potency agents should be avoided on areas susceptible to increased penetration and adverse reactions, such as face, intertriginous areas, perineum
14. A twice-a-day application is usually sufficient; more frequent application does not appear to improve response
15. Abrupt discontinuation of mid- or high-potency corticosteroids may result in rebound flare-up of disorder

    C. **Common topical corticosteroid medications:** see Table 15-10

    D. **Client-centered nursing care**

       1. Assess any skin symptom, beginning with a history

       2. Apply sparingly and gently in a thin film to affected area, usually two to three times per day

       3. At times, the preparation should be rubbed in thoroughly

       4. Do not use occlusive dressings or tight-fitting diapers, which may increase systemic absorption

       5. Do not apply to open skin lesions

       6. Avoid direct contact to eyes

       7. Monitor for local adverse skin effects, which include acneiform skin lesions, dryness, itching, burning, allergic contact dermatitis, hypopigmentation, overgrowth of bacteria/fungi/viruses (secondary infection), skin atrophy, or striae

       8. Monitor for systemic adverse effects, which are more likely to include hirsutism (usually of face), moon facies, alopecia (scalp), and immunosuppression

       9. These drugs, especially those of higher potency, should be tapered and not discontinued abruptly

Table 15-10   **Topical Corticosteroids**

Potency Class	Generic Name
Lowest potency	Alclometasone 0.05% cream, ointment Desonide 0.05% cream, ointment, lotion Dexamethasone 0.04% aerosol Hydrocortisone 1% cream Hydrocortisone 1% lotion Hydrocortisone 1% ointment, hydrocortisone 2.5% cream, ointment Methylprednisolone acetate 0.25% ointment Methylprednisolone acetate 1% ointment
Low potency	Betamethasone valerate 0.025% cream Clocortolone 0.1% cream Fluocinolone acetonide 0.01% cream, solution Flurandrenolide 0.025% cream, ointment Hydrocortisone valerate 0.2% cream Triamcinolone acetonide 0.025% cream, ointment
Intermediate potency	Betamethasone benzoate 0.025% cream, gel, lotion Betamethasone valerate 0.1% cream, ointment, lotion Desoximetasone 0.05% cream, ointment Fluocinolone acetonide 0.025% cream Halcinonide 0.025% cream, ointment Mometasone furoate 0.1% cream, ointment, lotion Triamcinolone acetonide 0.1% cream, ointment
High potency	Amcinonide 0.1% cream, ointment Betamethasone dipropionate 0.05% cream, ointment, lotion Desoximetasone 0.25% cream, ointment Fluocinolone 0.2% cream Fluocinolone 0.05% cream, ointment Halcinonide 0.1% cream, ointment, solution Triamcinolone acetonide 0.5% cream, ointment
Very high potency	Augmented betamethasone dipropionate 0.05% ointment Clobetasol propionate 0.05% cream, ointment Diflorasone 0.05% gel, ointment Halobetasol propionate 0.05% cream, ointment

E. **Client education**

1. Use exactly as directed; do not overuse
2. Do not apply to open wounds or weeping areas
3. Before using, wash and dry area gently
4. Report worsening of condition, signs of infection, or lack of healing

VI. KERATOLYTICS

A. **Description**
1. Reduce thickness of hyperkeratotic stratum corneum
2. Reduce keratinocyte adhesion (remove or soften horny layer of skin)

B. **Action and use**
1. Used to treat disorders of keratinization (e.g., forms of ichthyosis that generally have genetic component)
2. Some are used to treat certain warts
3. Available in different concentrations
4. Concentration necessary for keratolytic action differs among available agents

C. **Common keratolytic medications:** see Table 15-11

D. **Client-centered nursing care**
1. Assess any skin symptom, beginning with a history
2. Monitor for local adverse effects of topical preparations
3. Warts will become blanched and necrotic in 24–48 hours
4. Assess neurologic function; polyneuropathy may appear in 2 weeks and persist up to 9 months

E. **Client education**
1. Purpose of agent, use, side effects, symptoms of toxicity, and anticipated length of treatment
2. Use as directed; method will vary somewhat depending on condition for which it is used
3. Do not breastfeed while using podofilox
4. Have sex partner examined for warts as applicable

Table 15-11	Keratolytics	
Generic Name	**Action**	**Uses**
Podophyllum resin and podofilox	Cytotoxic and keratolytic agent with caustic action; directly affects epithelial cell metabolism	Benign growths of external genitalia and perianal warts, papillomas, and fibroids
Salicylic acid	Softens scales of outer horny layer of skin	Corns, warts, conditions of scalp, acne, and dermatitis

VII. ACNE MEDICATIONS

A. **Description**
1. Generally a staged approach is used
2. Mild **acne** (noninflammatory and inflammatory lesions that most commonly involve face, chest, back), consisting of some comedones or few inflammatory lesions, is treated by topical therapy with agents such as salicylic acid, azelaic acid, benzoyl peroxide, and topical antibiotics
3. Moderate acne consisting of *comedones* (blackheads) and **papules** (small, circumscribed, superficial, solid elevations of skin) can be managed by gradually increasing strength of topical tretinoin
4. Severe acne consisting of inflammatory papules and nodulocystic disease requires systemic antibiotics and isotretinoin

   B. **Action and use**
1. Choice of vehicle for topical preparation depends on whether client has dry or oily skin
2. Local adverse reactions to some topical preparations include erythema, burning or stinging, excessive dryness, and increased susceptibility to sunburn
3. Most clients will develop tolerance to local side effects within 3–4 weeks

   C. **Common acne medications:** see Tables 15-12 and 15-13

   D. **Client-centered nursing care**
1. Assess skin lesions as baseline and periodically to evaluate effectiveness of therapy
2. Monitor for local adverse effects of topical preparations, such as excessive drying, erythema, and hypersensitivity
3. Monitor for systemic adverse effects as particular to individual product
4. Do not apply adapalene with salicylic acid
5. Do not administer tetracycline to woman who is pregnant or attempting pregnancy

   E. **Client education**
1. Purpose, use, side effects, and anticipated length of treatment
2. Treatment is designed to control, not cure; therefore, periodic breakouts (especially premenstrual flare-ups) may still occur

Table 15-12   **Topical Acne Medications**

Generic/Trade Name	Action	Uses
Adapalene	Retinoidlike compound; modulates cellular differentiation; produces anti-inflammatory action	Acne vulgaris
Azelaic acid	Antibacterial, keratolytic that competitively inhibits tyrosinase; inhibits comedone formation	Acne vulgaris
Benzoyl peroxide	Antibacterial, keratolytic activity	Acne vulgaris
Clindamycin	Antibacterial	Acne vulgaris
Clindamycin and benzoyl peroxide	Antibacterial and keratolytic activity	Acne vulgaris
Sulfacetamide	Antibacterial	Acne vulgaris
Tazarotene	Retinoid	Acne vulgaris
Tetracycline	Suppresses growth of *Propionibacterium acnes* in sebaceous follicles, reducing free fatty acid content in sebum	Acne vulgaris
Tretinoin	Retinoic acid derivative; increases mitotic activity and turnover of follicular epithelial cells; loosens keratin debris; promotes drainage of preexisting comedones; inhibits new comedone formation; maximal result in 6 weeks	Acne vulgaris

Table 15-13   **Oral Medications for Acne Vulgaris**

Generic Name	Action	Uses
Isotretinoin	Regulation of cell differentiation and proliferation of altered lipid composition (highly toxic vitamin A)	Severe recalcitrant cystic acne unresponsive to conventional therapy
Tetracycline, minocycline, doxycycline	Anti-acne action by suppressing growth of *Propionibacterium acnes* in sebaceous follicles, reducing free fatty acid content in sebum	Acne vulgaris

3. With topical preparation, wash and dry skin; massage thin film gently into affected areas twice daily
4. Discontinue use and notify prescriber if severe irritation occurs
5. Avoid getting product into eyes, mouth, and mucous membranes; wash hands after use
6. With certain preparations, minimize exposure to sun and UV light; drying of skin may also lead to photosensitivity
7. Accutane is a teratogen; females of childbearing age must strictly avoid becoming pregnant; they should have negative pregnancy test within 2 weeks before starting therapy and monthly during therapy
8. There is no connection between acne and diet

VIII. BURN MEDICATIONS

A. **Description of burn therapy**
1. Clients who have partial-thickness burns of more than 5–10% of body, full-thickness burns, burns associated with electrical current, or burns of ears, eyes, face, hands, feet, and perineum should be referred to a hospital prepared to handle burn clients
2. Remaining clients who have superficial-thickness burns and partial-thickness burns of less than 5% of body should receive wound care and close follow-up
3. Goals of therapy are to decrease inflammation, prevent infection, relieve pain, and promote healing

B. **Actions and use:** topical agents are used to prevent infection in burn wounds, which could rapidly lead to sepsis

C. **Common burn medications:** see Table 15-14

D. **Adverse effects**
1. Mafenide: pain, burning, or staining at application sites for 20–30 minutes after application; clients with impaired renal function: high blood level of agent may lead to metabolic acidosis; watch for respiratory alkalosis as an indicator
2. Nitrofurazone: must be used with caution in clients with impaired renal function because polyethylene glycol in preparation can be absorbed through denuded skin and may not be excreted normally by compromised kidney; assess for rash, itching, dermatitis, bacterial or fungal superinfection, and allergic reaction at site
3. Silver sulfadiazine: leukopenia, skin necrosis, erythema multiforme, skin discoloration, rashes; up to 10% may be absorbed; hazardous to use in clients with G6PD deficiency

E. **Client-centered nursing care**
1. Agents are applied under sterile conditions once or twice daily to a thickness of approximately 1.5 mm (1/16 in.) to a clean and debrided wound

Table 15-14   **Topical Burn Medications**

Generic Name	Action	Uses
Mafenide	Bacteriostatic against *Pseudomonas aeruginosa* and *Clostridia*	Continue applications after whirlpool baths until healing occurs
Nitrofurazone	Inhibits aerobic and anaerobic cycles in bacterial carbohydrate metabolism	Adjunct treatment of bacterial infection in partial- and full-thickness burns; prevention of infection at skin graft sites
Silver sulfadiazine	Silver released from preparation is toxic to bacteria; silver prevents replication of *S. aureus, E. coli, Klebsiella*, others	Applications of silver sulfiadiazine to burn sites

2. If hospitalized, client may undergo hydrotherapy (bathing in whirlpool) to aid debridement prior to application
3. Client should be premedicated with analgesic, whenever possible, 30 minutes prior to burn wound cleansing; provide emotional support during dressing changes and/or hydrotherapy
4. Wound may be covered or left open
5. Monitor for adverse effects as previously outlined
6. Watch for signs of infection and WBC count in clients receiving silver sulfadiazine because of leukopenic effect

F. **Client education**
1. Purpose, use, side effects, and anticipated length of treatment
2. Use as directed if using preparation as an outpatient

IX. DEBRIDING MEDICATIONS

A. **Description**
1. Debriding agents are used to remove dirt, damaged tissue, and cellular debris from a wound to prevent infection and to promote healing
2. Effectiveness in removing necrotic tissue, clotted blood, purulent exudates, or fibrinous accumulations has been questioned

B. **Action and use**
1. Appear most effective when wound base has collagen that must be removed before epithelialization can proceed
2. Specific indications may vary (e.g., collagenase is indicated for stage 3 and 4 ulcers caused by pressure injury)

C. **Common debriding medications:** see Table 15-15

D. **Client-centered nursing care**
1. Assess skin problem before use
2. Monitor progress in wound healing

E. **Client education**
1. Explain purpose, use, and side effects of medications
2. Assess client's understanding about anticipated length of treatment

Table 15-15 **Debriding Preparations**

Agent	Action	Notes
Collagenase	Digests collagen; active at pH 6–8; takes 10–14 days	Active at pH 6–8, such enzymes tend to be inactivated by extremes of pH; also inactivated by hydrogen peroxide, heavy metals like silver, detergents, and iodine, nitrofurazone, and hexachlorophene
Sutilains	Digests necrotic soft tissues by proteolytic action	See above
Fibrinolysin and deoxyribonuclease	Deoxyribonuclease attacks DNA; fibrinolysin attacks fibrin of blood clots and fibrinous exudates	Hypersensitivity reactions can occur; serious adverse reactions reported when using ointment preparation containing chloramphenicol
Papain and urea	Ointment source is papaya	Chlorophyll derivatives control wound odor
Papain, urea, chlorophyllin copper complex	Source is papaya	See above
Trypsin, balsam Peru, castor oil	Source of trypsin is bovine pancreas	Balsam Peru is capillary bed stimulant used to improve circulation; castor oil used to reduce premature epithelial cornification

Case Study

A 16-year-old male has severe acne vulgaris, which is nonresponsive to conventional treatment with benzoyl peroxide/clindamycin and tetracycline orally. The dermatologist begins isotretinoin 35 mg by mouth twice daily. The client weighs 70 kg (154 lb) and is 1.8 m (6 ft) tall. He is to continue using benzoyl peroxide/clindamycin twice daily.

1. What is the action of benzoyl peroxide/clindamycin?

2. What is the action of isotretinoin?

3. Is this the proper dosage for isotretinoin to be administered to this young man?

4. What client education should be provided to the client and his family?

For suggested responses, see page 544.

POSTTEST

1 A client diagnosed with psoriasis vulgaris is using a prescribed topical corticosteroid. What activity should the nurse perform?

1. Protect the unaffected skin from staining.
2. Heat cream before applying.
3. Provide continuous occlusive therapy.
4. Apply warm, moist dressings over occlusive dressing.

2 After 5-fluorouracil cream is prescribed for a client diagnosed with basal cell carcinoma, what should the nurse teach the client?

1. "The drug will cause increasing tenderness as lesions ooze and erode."
2. "The drug will cause the lesion to become dry, shrink, and fall off."
3. "The drug will decrease the sensitivity of the lesion."
4. "Vigorously massage the lesion after application."

3 The nurse teaches the client how to manage an infestation of scabies with crotamiton by providing which direction?

1. "Rotate the container gently before using. Do not shake."
2. "Vigorously massage the solution into the skin."
3. "Be sure to apply medication also in skin creases and under fingernails."
4. "Apply the product to inflamed areas first."

4 The nurse is most likely to apply a hydrocolloid dressing during wound care for which client?

1. Client who has a necrotic wound with a thick layer of eschar attached
2. Client who has a new, partial-thickness burn
3. Client who has a wound that needs debriding
4. Client who has an uninfected venous stasis ulcer

5 After a healthcare provider prescribed minocycline for a client with acne, the nurse explains to the client which disadvantage of the medication?

1. Suppression of sebum production
2. Lupuslike syndrome and pigmentation changes
3. Open pores promoting excessive production of accumulated sebum
4. Occurrence of spontaneous abortion

POSTTEST

6 A nurse is administering a very high-potency topical corticosteroid clobetasol to certain assigned clients. Which client is most at risk for systemic absorption?

1. 35-year-old with psoriasis
2. 72-year-old with eczema
3. 59-year-old with seborrhea
4. 38-year-old with contact dermatitis

- -

7 A nurse is discussing treatment options for a client with acne vulgaris. The nurse should explain to the client that anti-acne medications work in which ways? Select all that apply.

1. Inhibiting viral replication
2. Inhibiting sebaceous gland overactivity
3. Reducing bacterial colonization
4. Preventing follicles from becoming plugged with keratin
5. Reducing inflammation of lesions

- -

8 After listening to the nurse explain the use of isotretinoin to a 19-year-old female client, the client demonstrates understanding of the most important point by making which statement at the end of the teaching session?

1. "Apply a thick layer of isotretinoin twice a day."
2. "Increase exposure to sun for added benefit."
3. "Have pregnancy test prior to beginning therapy and use contraception."
4. "Keep lips moist and lubricated to prevent inflammation."

- -

9 The client with a burn injury reports a stinging and burning sensation when topical mafenide acetate is applied. Which action should the nurse take?

1. Withhold medication and notify the prescriber.
2. Remove that dose of the medication.
3. Premedicate client with moderate analgesic before applying.
4. Chill preparation before applying.

- -

10 A nurse working in a burn center frequently applies topical burn medications to burn wounds. The nurse should anticipate that which medications may be prescribed topically for a newly admitted client with burns? Select all that apply.

1. Mafenide
2. Sulfisoxazole
3. Silver sulfadiazine
4. Nitrofurazone
5. Trimethoprim

➤ *See pages 504–505 for Answers and Rationales.*

ANSWERS & RATIONALES

Pretest

1 **Answer: 1 Rationale:** Betamethasone is a corticosteroid that is used in the treatment of psoriasis. The client needs to know that acne can occur as a side effect of this medication rather than curing it. The other options indicate correct understanding by the client. The client should report temperature in case symptoms of infection are masked. Only the affected skin area should be treated. The site should be left exposed or covered only lightly with a dressing. **Cognitive Level:** Analyzing **Client Need:** Pharmacological and Parenteral Therapies **Integrated Process:** Teaching and Learning **Content Area:** Pharmacology **Strategy:** The critical words in the question are *further information is needed*. This indicates that the correct option is an incorrect statement on the part of

the client. Recognize this medication as a glucocorticoid and then recall common adverse effects to choose correctly. **Reference:** Adams, M. P., & Urban, C. (2016). *Pharmacology: Connections to nursing practice* (3rd ed.). New York, NY: Pearson, p. 507.

2 **Answer: 2 Rationale:** Mupirocin is a topical antimicrobial agent effective against impetigo caused by *Staphylococcus aureus*, beta-hemolytic streptococci, and *Streptococcus pyogenes*. Ketoconazole is an antifungal agent. Capsaicin is a topical analgesic made from hot peppers. Acyclovir is an antiviral agent. **Cognitive Level:** Applying **Client Need:** Pharmacological and Parenteral Therapies **Integrated Process:** Teaching and Learning **Content Area:** Pharmacology **Strategy:** First recognize that the disease is of bacterial origin. Then associate the drug names with the type of microorganism against which they are effective. Use the process of elimination to choose the antibacterial drug. **Reference:** Adams, M. P., & Urban, C. (2016). *Pharmacology: Connections to nursing practice* (3rd ed.). New York, NY: Pearson, p. 848.

3 **Answer: 1, 2, 4 Rationale:** Pharmacotherapy of dermatitis is symptomatic and involves lotions and ointments to control itching and skin flaking. Antihistamines may be used to control inflammation and reduce itching. Analgesics or topical anesthetics may be prescribed for pain relief. **Cognitive Level:** Applying **Client Need:** Pharmacological and Parenteral Therapies **Integrated Process:** Nursing Process: Planning **Content Area:** Pharmacology **Strategy:** Note that the question is asking for identification of what types of drugs may be used to treat atopic dermatitis. Note that the wording of the question indicates that more than one option will be correct. **Reference:** Adams, M. P., & Urban, C. (2017). *Pharmacology for nurses: A pathophysiologic approach* (5th ed.). New York, NY: Pearson, p. 857.

4 **Answer: 4 Rationale:** The sunscreens frequently recommended are zinc oxide and titanium ointments that include PABA (p-aminobenzoic acid). The sun protective factor (SPF) means that if an individual normally burns in 10 minutes, an SPF 15 would mean sunburn would occur within $10 \times 15 = 150$ minutes. No chemical changes occur between the skin and the sun's rays. The waterproof characteristic limits or prevents washing-away when the skin is exposed to moisture. Heat absorbed by the skin can be distributed to other body parts, but have no relationship to sunscreens. **Cognitive Level:** Applying **Client Need:** Pharmacological and Parenteral Therapies **Integrated Process:** Teaching and Learning **Content Area:** Pharmacology **Strategy:** The core issue of the question is an understanding of the basis of how sunscreens act and the ability to phrase this information in a way that is accurate and understandable to a client. Use basic nursing knowledge and the process of elimination to make a selection. **Reference:** LeMone, P., Burke, K., Bauldoff, G., & Gubrud, P. (2015). *Medical surgical nursing: Clinical reasoning in patient care* (6th ed.). New York, NY: Pearson, p. 452.

5 **Answer: 2 Rationale:** Lindane is the drug of choice because it is well absorbed by the nervous system of the parasite (lice), resulting in death. It should be left in place for at least 12–24 hours. Chlorhexidine is a skin, dental, and wound cleanser. Sterile gloves may be needed for cleansing wounds but not to treat an infestation. Collagenase is an enzyme used in skin debriding and should not be touched with the fingers. Terbinafine is an oral or nasal antifungal agent for tinea infections. **Cognitive Level:** Applying **Client Need:** Pharmacological and Parenteral Therapies **Integrated Process:** Teaching and Learning **Content Area:** Pharmacology **Strategy:** The critical term is *efficient and effective*. Associate the nature of the parasite with the drug and the application method. **Reference:** Adams, M. P., & Urban, C. (2017). *Pharmacology*

for nurses: A pathophysiologic approach (5th ed.). New York, NY: Pearson, p. 850.

6 **Answer: 2, 3, 4, 5, 1 Rationale:** Shampooing the hair prior to application removes oils and cosmetic preparations and leads to increased drug penetration. To be effective the drug needs to be in contact with all infested areas so it is important to saturate the hair and scalp. Once applied, the recommended exposure time is 10 minutes. (Some residue may remain for 8 hours but normal exposure is 10 minutes.) The hair should be washed again to remove the drug after the recommended exposure time is completed. Combing with a fine-toothed comb removes dead lice once the treatment is complete. **Cognitive Level:** Analyzing **Client Need:** Pharmacological and Parenteral Therapies **Integrated Process:** Teaching and Learning **Content Area:** Pharmacology **Strategy:** Note the critical phrase *to sequence the events*, and from there visualize the process of a therapeutic shampoo to place the options in order. **Reference:** Adams, M. P., & Urban, C. (2017). *Pharmacology for nurses: A pathophysiologic approach* (5th ed.). New York, NY: Pearson, p. 850.

7 **Answer: 2 Rationale:** Benzoyl peroxide inhibits growth of *Propionibacterium acnes* (a Gram-positive microorganism). It is effective against inflammatory and noninflammatory acne. The microbe is less likely to develop antibiotic resistance to this agent and it is available in a variety of concentrations. Mafenide is effective against Gram-positive and Gram-negative microorganisms, but the adverse risks are too significant for the treatment of acne. Chlorhexidine is used for the treatment of gingivitis. Coal tar may be prescribed to treat dandruff but is not commonly recommended for acne. The goal is to destroy the skin cells containing the virus. **Cognitive Level:** Applying **Client Need:** Pharmacological and Parenteral Therapies **Integrated Process:** Teaching and Learning **Content Area:** Pharmacology **Strategy:** Specific knowledge of these agents is needed to answer the question. Associate the drug actions with client needs and the offending microbe, and use the process of elimination to make a selection. **Reference:** Adams, M. P., & Urban, C. (2017). *Pharmacology for nurses: A pathophysiologic approach* (5th ed.). New York, NY: Pearson, p. 852.

8 **Answer: 4 Rationale:** Isotretinoin, an oral agent, is effective against acne because it reduces the size of the sebaceous glands and decreases gland cell differentiation and proliferation, as well as lipid composition of sebum on the skin surface. The other products are also used for acne, but are topical preparations and are less effective. Tetracycline suppresses the growth of *P. acne* but lacks the other significant actions. There is no evidence that penicillin or clindamycin act against *P. acne*. **Cognitive Level:** Applying **Client Need:** Pharmacological and Parenteral Therapies **Integrated Process:** Teaching and Learning **Content Area:** Pharmacology **Strategy:** Specific knowledge of the various anti-acne products is needed to answer this question. Review these quickly now if this question was difficult. **Reference:** Adams, M. P., & Urban, C. (2017).

Pharmacology for nurses: A pathophysiologic approach (5th ed.). New York, NY: Pearson, p. 852.

9 **Answer: 1 Rationale:** Infection is one of the primary complications associated with the burned client. Silver sulfadiazine reduces bacterial growth and if treatment is successful, not only will the burned area heal but the client will not experience infection signaled by fever. The drug will not prevent fluid loss through burned tissue. Hypokalemia can occur, but silver sulfadiazine has no direct influence on its prevention or management. Appropriate separation of eschar should be noted as an appropriate assessment if an enzyme such as collagenase was used. **Cognitive Level:** Applying **Client Need:** Pharmacological and Parenteral Therapies **Integrated Process:** Nursing Process: Assessment **Content Area:** Pharmacology **Strategy:** Since burns damage the primary defense or barrier to invasion of microbes, it is logical to address elements associated with infection first. **Reference:** Adams, M. P., & Urban, C. (2017). *Pharmacology for nurses: A pathophysiologic approach* (5th ed.). New York, NY: Pearson, p. 552.

10 **Answer: 1 Rationale:** Curling's ulcer may develop within 24 hours after a severe burn related to decreased blood flow and mucosal damage. For this reason, histamine 2-receptor antagonists such as famotidine are prescribed to reduce secretion of gastric acid. Clients with severe burns are usually NPO. A diuretic such as furosemide increases urinary output at the expense of reducing central circulating volume that results in decreased cardiac output. Crotamiton, an antiparasitic used to treat scabies, is not indicated for use with the burned client. **Cognitive Level:** Applying **Client Need:** Pharmacological and Parenteral Therapies **Integrated Process:** Nursing Process: Implementation **Content Area:** Pharmacology **Strategy:** Consider that burn injury is a major stressor. Next, recall that the body's response to stress includes shunting of blood away from the gastrointestinal (GI) tract, ultimately leading to GI bleeding. Then choose the drug that will reduce secretion of stomach acid. **Reference:** Wilson, B. A., Shannon, M. T., & Shields, K. M. (2017). *Pearson nurse's drug guide 2017.* New York, NY: Pearson, pp. 654–656.

Posttest

1 **Answer: 4 Rationale:** Application of warm, moist dressings enhances the drug's penetration of the skin. Tar preparations are more prone to staining. Subjecting the medication to a change in temperature may reduce its effectiveness. More than 12 hours of occlusive therapy can increase the risk of systemic absorption. **Cognitive Level:** Applying **Client Need:** Physiological Integrity **Nursing/Integrated Concepts:** Nursing Process: Implementation **Content Area:** Pharmacology **Strategy:** Consider that a critical concern with administration of topical medications is their ability to penetrate the skin. With this in mind, determine the best method for maximizing absorption.

Reference: Adams, M. P., & Urban, C. (2016). *Pharmacology: Connections to nursing practice* (3rd ed.). New York, NY: Pearson, p. 1275.

2 **Answer: 1 Rationale:** Clients should be warned about the unsightly appearance of the lesion and that tenderness at the site is to be expected. Sloughing will occur before crusting and dryness occurs. Lesion will be sore and inflamed rather than have decreased sensitivity. Massage may promote systemic absorption and is not recommended. **Cognitive Level:** Applying **Client Need:** Pharmacological and Parenteral Therapies **Integrated Process:** Teaching and Learning **Content Area:** Pharmacology **Strategy:** Because of the depth of the lesion, associate sloughing with the drug. **Reference:** Adams, M. P., & Urban, C. (2016). *Pharmacology: Connections to nursing practice* (3rd ed.). New York, NY: Pearson, p. 971.

3 **Answer: 3 Rationale:** Since some parasites may become resistant to the medications, the hair shaft should be checked regularly for at least a week. The container should be shaken well before use. Vigorous massage will result in systemic absorption. Applying drug to the inflamed areas can result in systemic absorption. **Cognitive Level:** Applying **Client Need:** Pharmacological and Parenteral Therapies **Integrated Process:** Nursing Process: Implementation **Content Area:** Pharmacology **Strategy:** Determine the best method for maximizing the drug's effectiveness. The option that provides for this will be the answer to the question. **Reference:** Adams, M. P., & Urban, C. (2017). *Pharmacology for nurses: A pathophysiologic approach* (5th ed.). New York, NY: Pearson, p. 850.

4 **Answer: 4 Rationale:** A hydrocolloid dressing is a hydrophilic dressing indicated for noninfected ulcers with moderate drainage. The thick eschar at the wound edges should be removed before applying. A hydrocolloid dressing is designed for draining wounds. Fibrinolysin and desoxyribonuclease debride wounds by digesting the fibrin or blood clots inside the wound. **Cognitive Level:** Applying **Client Need:** Pharmacological and Parenteral Therapies **Integrated Process:** Nursing Process: Planning **Content Area:** Pharmacology **Strategy:** Specific knowledge of the purposes of various wound care products is needed to answer the question. Eliminate two options first because they are similar. Next, recall that this is a protective agent that absorbs drainage to help choose the correct option. **Reference:** LeMone, P., & Burke, K. M., Bauldoff, G., & Gubrud, P. (2015). *Medical-surgical nursing: Clinical reasoning in client care* (6th ed.). New York, NY: Pearson, pp. 341, 446.

5 **Answer: 2 Rationale:** Minocycline can lead to development of a lupuslike syndrome and also may cause increased pigmentation changes. It reduces the acne process by reducing the infectious processes. It is an antibiotic and has no effect on the patency of pores. There is no evidence that the drug leads to spontaneous abortions. **Cognitive Level:** Applying **Client Need:** Pharmacological and Parenteral Therapies **Integrated Process:** Teaching and Learning **Content Area:** Pharmacology **Strategy:** Associate the drug with "major" eruptions and increased pigmentation. **Reference:** Wilson, B. A., Shannon, M. T., & Shields, K. M. (2017). *Pearson nurse's drug guide 2017.* New York, NY: Pearson, pp. 1250–1251.

6 **Answer: 2 Rationale:** Excessive absorption is more likely to occur in the older adult because the skin is thinner and more permeable. Excessive absorption is not likely in younger clients, such as those that are 35 years old, 59 years old, and 38 years old. **Cognitive Level:** Applying **Client Need:** Pharmacological and Parenteral Therapies **Integrated Process:** Nursing Process: Planning **Content Area:** Pharmacology **Strategy:** Recall the age-related changes in the skin. Align absorption rates with the client's age. **Reference:** Wilson, B. A., Shannon, M., & Shields, K. (2017). *Pearson nurse's drug guide 2017.* New York NY: Pearson, pp. 360–362.

7 **Answer: 2, 3, 4, 5 Rationale:** Anti-acne medications inhibit sebaceous gland overactivity, reduce bacterial colonization, prevent follicles from becoming plugged with keratin, and reduce inflammation of lesions. They do not inhibit viral replication, as acne is caused by bacteria, not viruses. **Cognitive Level:** Applying **Client Need:** Pharmacological and Parenteral Therapies **Integrated Process:** Nursing Process: Implementation **Content Area:** Pharmacology **Strategy:** Recall the pathophysiology of acne vulgaris and then choose the pharmacological options that address this correctly. **Reference:** Adams, M. P., & Urban, C. (2016). *Pharmacology: Connections to nursing practice* (3rd ed.). New York, NY: Pearson, p. 1268.

8 **Answer: 3 Rationale:** Isotretinoin, an oral preparation, is a known teratogen that may result in spontaneous abortion and/or major fetal abnormalities such as hydrocephalus. Prevention of pregnancy is mandatory during isotretinoin therapy. The drug is not topical. Clients should avoid sun exposure to prevent risk of developing skin cancer. Inflammation of the lips is a side effect of isotretinoin, but this concern does not override the significance of the risk to the fetus. **Cognitive Level:** Applying **Client Need:** Pharmacological and Parenteral Therapies **Integrated Process:** Teaching and Learning **Content Area:** Pharmacology **Strategy:** Associate the drug with

birth defects. Select the option that most represents the knowledge needed to adequately manage isotretinoin therapy. **Reference:** Wilson, B. A., Shannon, M. T., & Shields, K. M. (2017). *Pearson nurse's drug guide 2017.* Upper Saddle River, NJ: Pearson, p. 865.

9 **Answer: 3 Rationale:** Mafenide acetate is a water-soluble cream that is used to treat burns. It may cause a severe stinging or burning sensation for 20 minutes after it is applied. A moderate analgesic may provide some comfort. The prescriber needs to be notified if an analgesic has not been prescribed. Attempting to remove the medication could increase the pain sensation. If the medication is the best application to treat or prevent infection, the focus should be on helping the client manage the discomfort. The temperature of the medication is not the causative factor. Cold application may stimulate a greater sensation of discomfort. **Cognitive Level:** Applying **Client Need:** Pharmacological and Parenteral Therapies **Integrated Process:** Nursing Process: Implementation **Content Area:** Pharmacology **Strategy:** Associate the medication with severe drug-induced pain and use the process of elimination to select the option that matches this concern. **Reference:** Wilson, B. A., Shannon, M. T., & Shields, K. M. (2017). *Pearson nurse's drug guide 2017.* New York, NY: Pearson, p. 839.

10 **Answer: 1, 3, 4 Rationale:** Mafenide, silver sulfadiazine, and nitrofurazone may be prescribed topically for burn treatment. Sulfisoxazole is a short-acting, oral sulfonamide that is taken by mouth for various infections but is not used to treat burns. Trimethoprim is used to treat urinary tract infections and otitis media, not burn wounds. **Cognitive Level:** Applying **Client Need:** Pharmacological and Parenteral Therapies **Integrated Process:** Nursing Process: Implementation **Content Area:** Pharmacology **Strategy:** Note that the question is asking for identification of which topical drugs may be used to treat burn injury. Note that the wording of the question indicates that more than one option will be correct. **Reference:** Adams, M. P., & Urban, C. (2017). *Pharmacology for nurses: A pathophysiologic approach* (5th ed.). New York, NY: Pearson, p. 839.

References

Adams, M., Holland, L., & Urban, C. (2017). *Pharmacology for nurses: A pathophysiologic approach* (5th ed.). New York, NY: Pearson.

Adams, M. P., & Urban, C. (2016). *Pharmacology: Connections to nursing practice* (3rd ed.). New York, NY: Pearson.

Burchum, J., & Rosenthal, L. (2015). *Lehne's pharmacology for nursing care* (9th ed.). St. Louis, MO: Mosby.

Drug Facts & Comparisons (updated monthly). St. Louis, MO: Wolters Kluwer.

Karch, A. M. (2016). *Focus on nursing pharmacology* (7th ed.). Philadelphia, PA: Lippincott Williams & Wilkins.

Kee, J. (2017). *Pearson's handbook of laboratory and diagnostic tests and nursing implications* (8th ed.). New York, NY: Pearson.

LeMone, P., & Burke, K. M., Bauldoff, G., & Gubrud, P. (2015). *Medical-surgical nursing: Clinical reasoning in client care* (6th ed.). New York, NY: Pearson.

Lilley, L. L., Rainforth Collins, S., & Snyder, J. S. (2017). *Pharmacology and the nursing process* (8th ed.). St. Louis, MO: Mosby.

Vallerand, A. H., Sanoski, C. A., & Deglin, J. H. (2017). *Davis's drug guide for nurses* (8th ed.). Philadelphia, PA: F.A. Davis.

Wilson, B. A., Shannon, M. T., & Shields, K. M. (2017). *Pearson nurse's drug guide 2017.* New York, NY: Pearson.

ANSWERS & RATIONALES

16 Visual and Auditory Medications

Chapter Outline

Medications to Treat
    Glaucoma
Mydriatics and Cycloplegics

Anti-Inflammatory and
    Anti-Infective Eye
    Medications

Anesthetic Medications for
    the Eye
Auditory Medications

 NCLEX-RN® Test Prep

Access the NEW Web-based app
that provides students with additional
practice questions in preparation
for the NCLEX experience.

Objectives

➤ Describe general goals of therapy when administering visual or
    auditory medications.
➤ Describe actions and uses of mydriatic, miotic, and cycloplegic
    medications.
➤ Explain the mechanism of action of medications used to treat
    glaucoma.
➤ Describe drug-induced ototoxicity and medications that can lead
    to its development.
➤ Identify correct procedures for administering visual and auditory
    medications.
➤ List significant client education points related to administering
    visual or auditory medications.

Review at a Glance

aqueous humor fluid formed by ciliary body; contained in anterior and posterior chambers of eye; bathes and feeds posterior surface of cornea, lens, and iris

cerumen substance secreted by glands at outer third of ear canal; if accumulated, may cause obstruction of ear canal; also called *earwax*

cornea protective anterior covering of eye; normally transparent and allows light to enter

cycloplegia paralysis of ciliary muscle

external ear outer ear (pinna) and external auditory canal

intraocular pressure pressure within the eye

keratitis inflammation of cornea; usually caused by trauma, microorganisms, or immune-mediated responses

miosis constriction of pupils caused by contraction of sphincter muscle alone or in combination with relaxation of dilator muscle

mydriasis dilation of pupils caused by contraction of dilator muscle and relaxation of sphincter muscle

narrow-angle or closed-angle glaucoma an acute form of glaucoma characterized by increased intraocular pressure caused by impaired rate of outflow of aqueous humor; also called *angle-closure* or *closed-angle glaucoma*

open-angle glaucoma a chronic form of glaucoma that leads to a change in appearance of optic disk and results in visual loss as cup of disk becomes enlarged; increased intraocular pressure may or may not be associated with this

disorder; open-angle glaucoma is most common type

photophobia intolerance to light

systemic absorption entry of drug into body and circulating fluids

tonometry a measurement of tension, such as intraocular tension or pressure; used to detect glaucoma

tympanic membrane thin partition of transparent tissue between external auditory canal and middle ear

uveitis an intraocular inflammatory disorder; may involve iris, ciliary body, choroids, retina, or cornea

vertigo sensation of moving around in space or spinning; also called *dizziness*

PRETEST

1 What should be the priority of the nurse in assessing a client prior to administering the first dose of an ophthalmic medication?

1. Client's understanding of purpose of medication
2. Client's level of consciousness (LOC)
3. Client's history of medication allergies
4. Client's understanding of drug action

2 A nurse should conclude that a client can safely self-administer ophthalmic medications after the client demonstrates which aspects of correct technique? Select all that apply.

1. Pulls lower lid down and instills medication directly onto cornea
2. Pulls lower lid down and instills medication into conjunctival sac
3. Pulls lower lid up and instills medication directly onto the eye
4. Applies gentle pressure to inner canthus for 30 seconds after medication administration
5. Cleanses exudates from eye before instillation of medication

3 The external ear canal of a client with an ear infection is obstructed due to swelling. The nurse should instruct the client to use which techniques during otic medication administration? Select all that apply.

1. Insert gauze ear wick and apply medication to wick.
2. Wait until swelling subsides before instilling medication.
3. Request change in the route of medication.
4. Insert dropper past the edematous canal.
5. Avoid using pressure to insert tip of the fluid container.

4 A client with open-angle glaucoma is being treated with acetazolamide 250 mg tablets by mouth twice daily. Which client statements indicate to the nurse an understanding of therapy with this drug? Select all that apply.

1. "I can take the medication with milk."
2. "I should take the medication in the morning."
3. "I should have a yearly complete blood count."
4. "I can crush the tablet and mix it in juice."
5. "I should avoid foods containing high potassium such as bananas."

5 A client who has a new prescription for dorzolamide asks the nurse how the medication will help treat glaucoma. The nurse's best response should include which item of information?

1. "It decreases production of aqueous humor."
2. "It causes pupil constriction."
3. "It increases the production of aqueous humor."
4. "It increases the outflow of aqueous humor."

6 A client with a history of asthma is describing symptoms that began after starting drug therapy with pilocarpine to treat glaucoma. The nurse should conclude that which symptom indicates a side effect associated with systemic absorption of this drug?

1. Dry mouth
2. Increased blood pressure
3. Wheezing
4. Constipation

7 The nurse should conclude that a 68-year-old client understands proper otic medication administration after observing the client perform which actions during self-administration? Select all that apply.

1. Client pulls pinna down and back before administering medication.
2. Client pulls pinna up and back before administering medication.
3. Client places dropper into the ear canal before administering medication.
4. Client tilts head toward the affected side before administering medication.
5. Client gently massages the anterior ear area after medication administration.

8 The nurse should conclude that a client newly diagnosed with glaucoma understands the purpose for the prescribed timolol when the client makes which statement?

1. "This eyedrop will reduce the intraocular pressure."
2. "I can stop using the eyedrop once my intraocular pressure is normal."
3. "The medicine will help to increase my intraocular pressure."
4. "This eyedrop is the only treatment available for glaucoma."

9 Before administering preoperative medications to a client with a history of glaucoma, the nurse would question which medication prescription?

1. Atropine
2. Diphenhydramine
3. Hydroxyzine
4. Retelase recombinant

10 The nurse should question an order for brinzolamide for a client who has which disorder listed in the health history section of the electronic medical record?

1. Hypertension
2. Chronic renal failure
3. Liver disease
4. Osteoporosis

➤ *See pages 525–527 for Answers and Rationales.*

I. MEDICATIONS TO TREAT GLAUCOMA

A. Prostaglandin analog

1. Action and use
   a. Increases aqueous humor outflow
   b. Used in management of open-angle glaucoma and ocular hypertension
2. Common prostaglandin medications (Table 16-1)
3. Administration considerations

   a. Administer 5 minutes apart from other antiglaucoma ophthalmic medications
   b. If pilocarpine is included in drug regimen, it should be administered 1 hour after administration of prostaglandin analog
   c. May be used in conjunction with other agents to lower intraocular pressure
4. Contraindications: hypersensitivity to latanoprost or benzalkonium, pregnancy, lactation, intraocular infection, conjunctivitis, closed-angle glaucoma
5. Significant drug interactions: if used concurrently with eyedrops that contain thimerosal, precipitation may occur
6. Significant food interactions: none reported
7. Significant laboratory studies: rare adverse effect is abnormal liver function tests
8. Side effects: are usually localized to eye; see Table 16-1 again

9. Adverse effects/toxicity: usually occur with systemic absorption; see Table 16-1 again
10. Client-centered nursing care
    a. Assess for hypersensitivity to latanoprost or benzalkonium chloride
    b. Assess for burning, itching, and stinging after initial administration of medication; preservative-free versions (tafluprost) are available
    c. Monitor visual acuity, vision fields, and intraocular pressure; desired therapeutic effect is intraocular pressure below 21 mmHg and no changes in visual acuity or fields
11. Client education
    a. Drug may cause an increase in iris pigmentation
    b. Do not exceed once-a-day dose
    c. Remove contact lenses before use and for 15 minutes after instillation of medication
    d. Report symptoms of burning, itching, and stinging after administration to prescriber
    e. Report visual disturbances to prescriber
    f. Proper self-administration of ophthalmic medications (see Box 16-1, p. 510)

B. **Beta blockers (beta-adrenergic antagonists)**
    1. Action and use
        a. Decrease production of **aqueous humor** (fluid formed by ciliary body in eye)
        b. Reduce **intraocular pressure** (pressure within eyeball) in **open-angle glaucoma** (a change in appearance of optic disk resulting in visual loss)
        c. Exact mechanism of action is unknown
    2. Common beta-adrenergic blocking medication (Table 16-2)
    3. Administration considerations
        a. Available in ophthalmic solution and ophthalmic suspension
        b. Drugs cross placenta, enter breast milk
        c. Use nasolacrimal occlusion to minimize **systemic absorption** (entry of drug into body and circulating fluids)
        d. Administer with caution to clients receiving cardiovascular agents such as antihypertensives and antidysrhythmics
        e. May mask symptoms of hyperthyroidism

Table 16-1 Prostaglandin Analog Drugs for Glaucoma

Generic Name	Therapeutic Indications	Side/Adverse Effects
Bimatoprost	Glaucoma, open-angle	Local: stinging sensation in eye, sensation of foreign body in eye, darkened iris, longer and thicker lashes. Systemic absorption: flu or respiratory infection, muscle or joint pain, angina
Latanoprost	Glaucoma, open-angle and ocular hypertension	
Tafluprost	Glaucoma, open-angle	
Travaprost	Glaucoma, open-angle	

Table 16-2 Beta-Adrenergic Blocking Agent for Ophthalmic Use

Generic Name	Therapeutic Indications	Side/Adverse Effects
Betaxolol Carteolol Levobunolol Metipranolol Timolol	Ocular hypertension, open-angle glaucoma	Local: stinging or burning sensation, blurred vision, headache. Systemic: angina, exacerbation of heart failure including pulmonary edema, dysrhythmias (sinoatrial or atrioventricular nodal block, tachycardia), hypotension, dizziness or vertigo, bronchoconstriction, constipation, nausea and vomiting

Box 16-1	**Instillation of Eye Drops**
Administration of Ophthalmic Medications	• Wash hands and apply gloves. • Cleanse exudates from eye(s) if necessary. • Tilt client's head toward the side of the affected eye. • Gently pull lower eyelid down, have client look up (this forms a "sac"). • Instill drops in the sac formed by lower lid, *not* onto the eye. • Unless specifically indicated otherwise, apply gentle pressure for 30 seconds to 1 minute over the inner canthus next to the nose. This prevents absorption through the tear duct and drainage of the medication. • Unless specifically indicated otherwise, the client should close the eye(s) gently. Avoid squeezing the eye(s) tightly, as this forms tears, which dilute the medicine and force the medication out.

Instillation of Eye Ointment

• Follow the same procedure for instillation of eye drops, except that the ointment is expressed directly into the conjunctival sac from the inner canthus to the outer canthus.
• Unless specifically indicated otherwise, the client should close the eye(s) and gently massage the eye(s) to distribute the medication.

Note: To avoid contamination and risk of infection, do not touch the dropper or tube to the eye, eyelashes, or any other surface. Remove contact lenses before instilling ophthalmic medications and wait at least 15 minutes before reinserting them.

    f. Drug may be $beta_1$ selective (cardiac), $beta_2$ selective (pulmonary), or both $beta_1$ and $beta_2$ selective

    g. Because it is $beta_1$ selective, betaxolol is usually the drug of choice for clients with pulmonary disease

4. Contraindications

    a. Hypersensitivity

    b. Sinus bradycardia or second- or third-degree heart block

    c. Cardiogenic shock or congestive heart failure (CHF)

    d. Do not administer with other beta blockers (additive effect)

    e. Use cautiously in clients with renal failure, diabetes, asthma, and chronic obstructive pulmonary disease (COPD)

5. Significant drug interactions

    a. Beta-blocking agents may be absorbed systemically, although risk is minimal; review client's current medications to avoid drug–drug interactions; most drug interactions occur because of systemic absorption

    b. Systemic absorption of ophthalmic beta blockers increases effects of insulin, verapamil, prazosin, clonidine, and nonsteroidal anti-inflammatory drugs (NSAIDs)

    c. Adverse cardiovascular effects may occur when beta-adrenergic blockers are used in combination with other cardiovascular agents such as antihypertensives and antidysrhythmics

    d. Use of these agents with ophthalmic epinephrine may decrease effectiveness

6. Significant food interactions: none reported

7. Significant laboratory studies: if systemic absorption occurs, glucose or insulin tolerance tests may be affected

8. Side effects

    a. Primarily local reactions: eye irritation, burning, stinging

    b. Rare occurrences of allergic reaction, eye inflammation, **photophobia** (intolerance to light), burning, stinging, pruritis, blurred vision, and rashes

9. Adverse effects/toxicity
   a. Cardiovascular system: bradycardia or tachycardia, CHF, dysrhythmias, hypotension, and edema of lower extremities
   b. Respiratory system: wheezing, cough, exacerbation of asthma, and bronchospasm
   c. Central nervous system (CNS): weakness, ataxia, confusion, and depression
   d. Gastrointestinal (GI) system: nausea and vomiting
10. Client-centered nursing care
   a. Obtain baseline vital signs and neurologic status
   b. Obtain baseline vision and intraocular pressure data
   c. Assess for cardiovascular disease, renal failure, diabetes mellitus, lactation, or thyrotoxicosis
   d. Assess for signs and symptoms of hypersensitivity such as burning, itching, redness, and swelling occurring after drug administration
   e. Refer to Box 16-1 for procedure for administering ophthalmic medications
11. Client education
   a. Beta-blocking agents may mask symptoms of hypoglycemia in clients with diabetes mellitus
   b. Inform healthcare provider if surgery is being considered; gradual withdrawal of beta-blocking agent 48 hours before surgery may be required (withdrawal is controversial)
   c. Have routine eye examinations and measurement of intraocular pressure (IOP)
   d. Do not stop medication unless instructed to do so by prescriber
   e. Report symptoms of breathing difficulty, swelling of extremities, slow heart rate
   f. Avoid driving if weakness or dizziness occur as drug side effects
   g. Wear dark sunglasses and avoid bright light if photophobia is present
   h. Proper procedure for instillation of ophthalmic medications

C. **Adrenergic medications (alpha-adrenergic agonists), also known as sympathomimetics**
1. Action and use
   a. Decrease production of aqueous humor
   b. Decrease intraocular pressure
   c. Exact mechanism of action is unknown
   d. Used in management of open-angle glaucoma, often in combination with other drugs, and glaucoma secondary to **uveitis** (intraocular inflammatory disorder)
   e. Used to produce **mydriasis** (pupil dilation) for ocular examination
   f. Used to produce local hemostasis during eye surgery to control bleeding
2. Common adrenergic agonist medications (Table 16-3)
3. Administration considerations
   a. Administer with caution to clients with cardiovascular disease, hypertension, asthma, diabetes mellitus, hyperthyroidism, and parkinsonism
   b. Brimonidine crosses the blood–brain barrier; can cause drowsiness, fatigue, and hypotension

Table 16-3 **Adrenergic Agonist Agents for Ophthalmic Use**

Generic Name	Uses	Side/Adverse Effects
Apraclonidine Brimonidine	Increased IOP related to chronic open-angle glaucoma	Local: eye itching and burning, eye tearing, blurred vision, headache, edema of eyelids, allergic conjunctivitis, or hyperemia of conjunctiva, photosensitivity Systemic: unsteady gait, chest pain, dizziness, dysrhythmias, wheezing, dyspnea
Tetrahydrozoline	Redness of eyes, minor irritations	Ocular irritation, photophobia, blurred vision

      c. Assess for sensitivity to sulfites

      d. Avoid concurrent use with MAOIs

      e. Drugs cross placenta, enter breast milk

      f. Do not administer ophthalmic solution that contains precipitates or has turned brown

4. Contraindications: not for treatment of **narrow-angle or closed-angle glaucoma** or abraded **cornea** (protective anterior covering of eye) because pupil dilation will further restrict ocular fluid outflow, precipitating an acute attack of glaucoma

5. Significant drug interactions

      a. Significant drug interactions are related to systemic absorption of adrenergic agonists and may result in adverse cardiovascular reactions and adverse CNS reactions, especially in clients with cardiovascular disease

      b. Systemic absorption of adrenergic agonists interferes with actions of beta-blocking agents and some antihypertensive agents

6. Significant food interactions: none reported

7. Significant laboratory studies: none reported

8. Side effects

      a. Local reactions include eye pain and stinging on initial instillation; a frequent cause for discontinuation is allergic-type reaction that causes a sensation of a foreign body, itching, and hyperemia

      b. CNS side effects include headache, blurred vision, brow ache, photophobia, and difficulty with night vision

9. Adverse effects/toxicity: systemic adverse effects are unusual, but may occur especially in clients with cardiovascular disease; symptoms include confusion, tachycardia, hypertension, diaphoresis, and tremors

10. Client-centered nursing care

      a. Obtain history of allergies or hypersensitivity to specific agents

      b. Be alert for vasovagal episode with bradycardia, pallor, nausea, and pain

      c. Obtain baseline vital signs

      d. Obtain baseline vision and intraocular pressure data

      e. Assess cardiac, respiratory, and renal function routinely

11. Client education

      a. Drugs may discolor contact lenses

      b. Do not blink for at least 30 seconds after instilling medication

      c. Report a decrease in visual acuity, floating spots, sensitivity to light, eye redness, acute eye pain, or headache to healthcare provider

      d. Proper self-administration of ophthalmic medications

D. Cholinergic agents (miotics, cholinesterase inhibitors)

1. Action and use

      a. Increase outflow of aqueous humor, decrease resistance to aqueous flow

      b. Produce **miosis** (pupil constriction) and contraction of ciliary muscles

      c. Used in treatment of open-angle and angle-closure glaucoma

      d. Used to facilitate miosis before ophthalmic examination or after ophthalmic surgery

      e. Generally used for clients who fail to respond to first-line agents (such as prostaglandin analogs or beta blockers)

2. Common cholinergic medications (Table 16-4)

3. Administration considerations

      a. Drug crosses placenta, enters breast milk

      b. Do not administer ophthalmic solution that contains precipitates or has turned brown

      c. Pilocarpine can be stored at room temperature

Table 16-4 **Cholinergic Agents for Ophthalmic Use**

Generic Name	Uses	Side/Adverse Effects
Carbachol	Glaucoma, miosis during surgery	Ataxia, confusion, seizures, coma, respiratory failure, hypotension, death
Echothiophate iodide	Open-angle glaucoma, accommodative esotropia	Conjunctival thickening, chest pain, dysrhythmia, ocular irritation
Pilocarpine	Acute or chronic glaucoma	Burning of eye, tearing, ciliary spasm, hypertension, nausea and vomiting, pulmonary edema, salivation, sweating, bronchial spasm, respiratory failure

4. Contraindications
   a. Acute iritis
   b. Conditions in which pupillary constriction is not desirable
5. Significant drug interactions: concurrent use with beta-adrenergic blocking agents may increase risk of cardiovascular reactions
6. Significant food interactions: none reported
7. Significant laboratory studies: none reported
8. Side effects: local effects include visual blurring, myopia, irritation, brow pain, and headache
9. Adverse effects/toxicity
   a. Systemic reactions include abdominal pain, bronchoconstriction, diarrhea, hypotension, nausea and vomiting, diuresis, diaphoresis, exacerbation of asthma
   b. Toxic effects produce ataxia, confusion, seizures, coma, respiratory failure, hypotension, and death
   c. Prolonged use of cholinergics may lead to retinal detachments, obstruction of tear drainage, and cataracts

   d. Acute toxicity is reversible by intravenous (IV) administration of atropine (anticholinergic agent) as an antidote
10. Client-centered nursing care
    a. Obtain baseline vital signs and neurologic status
    b. Obtain baseline vision and intraocular pressure data
    c. Assess for cardiovascular disease, renal failure, diabetes, lactation, or thyrotoxicosis
    d. Assess for signs and symptoms of hypersensitivity such as burning, itching, redness, and swelling occurring after medication administration
11. Client education
    a. Difficulty adjusting quickly to changes in illumination and decreased vision in low light may occur as a result of miosis
    b. Proper self-administration of ophthalmic medications
E. **Carbonic anhydrase inhibitors**
   1. Action and use
      a. Interfere with synthesis of carbonic acid, lowering intraocular pressure by decreasing aqueous production
      b. Oral carbonic anhydrase inhibitors are used to treat open-angle, secondary, and angle-closure glaucoma when other agents have not been effective
      c. Ophthalmic carbonic anhydrase inhibitors are used to treat open-angle glaucoma and ocular hypertension
      d. Commonly used preoperatively in intraocular surgery
      e. Tablet, capsule, or injection; other therapeutic uses include as diuretic and antiepileptic

Table 16-5	Carbonic Anhydrase Inhibitors			
Generic Name	**Route**	**Uses**		**Side/Adverse Effects**
Acetazolamide	PO	Increased IOP related to open-angle glaucoma		Drowsiness, Stevens–Johnson syndrome, transient myopia, nausea and vomiting, hyperchloremic acidosis, hypokalemia, aplastic anemia, renal calculi, bone marrow depression
Brinzolamide	Ophthalmic			Headache, dry eyes, altered taste
Dorzolamide hydrochloride	Ophthalmic			Altered taste, fatigue, dizziness, ocular burning, keratitis, conjunctivitis, photophobia, bronchospasm, dyspnea, angioedema
Methazolamide	PO			Photophobia, photosensitivity, urticaria, anorexia, vomiting, constipation, bone marrow depression, hepatic insufficiency

2. Common carbonic anhydrase inhibitor medications (Table 16-5)
3. Administration considerations
   a. Oral acetazolamide is administered for maintenance
   b. Observe for signs of hypokalemia and hyperglycemia
   c. To minimize nocturia, schedule doses early in day
   d. Administer with caution to clients with adrenocortical insufficiency
4. Contraindications
   a. Hypersensitivity to antibacterial sulfonamides
   b. Chronic noncongestive angle-closure glaucoma
   c. Hyponatremia, hypokalemia, or other electrolyte imbalances
   d. Hepatic or renal dysfunction
5. Significant drug interactions
   a. Interference with renal excretion of quinidine, salicylates, lithium
   b. Carbonic anhydrase inhibitors decrease excretion of amphetamines, mecamylamine, and quinidine, which could result in prolonged duration of drug actions
6. Significant food interactions: none reported

Practice to Pass

A client with open-angle glaucoma is having the medication regimen changed to acetazolamide. What important teaching and information do you provide to the client?

7. Significant laboratory studies
   a. False-positive results in tests for urinary protein and falsely high values for urine urobilinogen
   b. Monitor sodium, potassium, bicarbonate levels for imbalances
   c. May increase uric acid level
   d. May decrease thyroid iodine uptake, WBC count
8. Side effects
   a. Oral agents: anorexia, diarrhea, diuresis, nausea and vomiting, lethargy, weakness, weight loss, metallic bitter taste, and paresthesia of fingers, hands, and toes
   b. Ophthalmic agents: topical allergic reaction, photosensitivity, superficial **keratitis** (inflammation of cornea)
9. Adverse effects/toxicity
   a. Stevens–Johnson syndrome with acetazolamide
   b. Bone marrow depression with acetazolamide
   c. Acidosis
   d. Blood dyscrasias
   e. Hypokalemia
10. Client-centered nursing care
    a. Potential exacerbation of renal stones; monitor renal function
    b. Monitor for fluid volume depletion related to diuresis

      c. Monitor intake and output (I&O), skin turgor, mucous membranes, and weight

      d. Monitor urinalysis, complete blood cell count (CBC), electrolytes

  11. Client education

      a. Unless contraindicated, eat a diet high in potassium and low in sodium

      b. Unless contraindicated, increase fluid intake to at least 2 liters per day to decrease risk of renal stones

      c. Report changes in urine color, rashes, fever

      d. Proper self-administration of ophthalmic medications

      e. Monitor weight for weight loss and report to prescriber

      f. Report symptoms of bone marrow toxicity such as weakness, unusual bleeding, numbness, or tingling of extremities

F. Immunomodulators

  1. Action and use

      a. Used to increase tear production if the cause of dry eye is inflammation

      b. Immunosuppressant

  2. Common medication: cyclosporine

  3. Administration considerations: with concurrent use of ophthalmic NSAIDs, tear production is *not* increased

  4. Contraindications: administer cautiously in clients with decreased immune function

  5. Significant drug interactions: none noted

  6. Significant food interactions: none noted

  7. Significant laboratory studies: renal studies in case of systemic absorption

  8. Side effects: immunosuppression and nephrotoxicity (if systemically absorbed)

  9. Adverse effects/toxicity: irritation, blurred vision

  10. Client-centered nursing care: gently mix the emulsion prior to use

  11. Client teaching: adverse effects/toxicity

Practice to Pass

A client receiving pilocarpine ophthalmic solution for glaucoma is prescribed latanoprost for concurrent therapy with the pilocarpine. What teaching and information do you provide to this client?

II. MYDRIATICS AND CYCLOPLEGICS

A. Anticholinergics

  1. Action and use

      a. Produce mydriasis (pupil dilation), thus allowing for better visualization of retinal structures

      b. Produce **cycloplegia** (paralysis of ciliary muscle) to prevent the lens from moving during assessment

      c. Used in treatment of ocular pain secondary to inflammatory disorders such as uveitis and keratitis

      d. Used to relax ciliary muscle to improve measurement of refractive errors

      e. Used preoperatively and postoperatively for intraocular surgery

  2. Common mydriatic and cycloplegic medications (Table 16-6)

  3. Administration considerations

      a. Apply ointment several hours before vision examination

      b. Compress lacrimal duct during administration and for 2–3 minutes after administration

  4. Contraindications

      a. Severe systemic reactions to atropine

      b. Hypersensitivity to anticholinergic drugs

      c. Use with caution in clients with primary glaucoma as mydriatics can impair aqueous humor outflow

      d. Use with caution in clients with predisposition to angle-closure glaucoma

  5. Significant drug interactions: results from systemic absorption; decreases effectiveness of phenothiazines and haloperidol

Table 16-6	Mydriatic and Cycloplegic Agents for Ophthalmic Use	
Generic Name	**Uses**	**Side/Adverse Effects**
Atropine	Mydriasis, inflammation of iris and uveal tract, cycloplegia	Transient stinging, dry mouth, nausea and vomiting, bradycardia, palpitations, tachycardia, increased IOP, photophobia, urinary hesitancy, heat prostration, decreased sweating
Cyclopentolate	Mydriasis, cycloplegia	Allergic reaction, conjunctivitis
Homatropine Scopolamine	Mydriasis, inflammation of iris and uveal tract	Transient stinging, dry mouth, nausea and vomiting, bradycardia, palpitations, tachycardia, increased IOP, photophobia, urinary hesitancy, heat prostration, decreased sweating
Tropicamide	Mydriasis, cycloplegia	Allergic reaction, conjunctivitis
Hydroxyamphetamine/ Tropicamide	Mydriasis, cycloplegia	Blurred vision, headache, dizziness, enlarged pupils, tachycardia, nervousness, stomach pain, photosensitivity, nausea and vomiting, flatulence, dyspepsia

6. Significant food interactions: none reported
7. Significant laboratory studies: none reported
8. Side effects
    a. Local: blurred vision, photophobia, allergic lid reactions
    b. Systemic: confusion, delirium, drowsiness, dry mouth, flushing, and tachycardia
9. Adverse effects/toxicity

    a. Hallucinations, tachycardia, slurred speech, psychiatric and behavioral problems, fever, respiratory depression, coma
    b. Acute glaucoma can be precipitated by pupillary dilation; if not recognized and treated, acute glaucoma can result in blindness
    c. Dry mouth and tachycardia may be symptoms of scopolamine toxicity
10. Client-centered nursing care
    a. Obtain baseline intraocular pressure and vision status data
    b. Combination drugs produce greater mydriasis
    c. Systemic side effects are more pronounced in infants and children with blond hair and blue eyes
    d. Monitor for tachycardia, confusion, slurred speech, dry mouth, dry skin, weakness, drowsiness
11. Client education
    a. Mydriasis may last from 3 days (scopolamine) to 12 days (atropine)
    b. Blurred vision may occur
    c. Wear dark sunglasses and avoid bright light as counteractive measures for photophobia
    d. Intraocular pressure and vision should be monitored over course of therapy
    e. Withhold medication if experiencing tachycardia or dry mouth (symptoms of toxicity) and report these symptoms to prescriber
    f. Use sugarless hard candy to combat dry mouth
    g. Proper self-administration of ophthalmic medications
B. **Lubricants and vasoconstrictors**
    1. Phenylephrine is a sympathomimetic that is used during eye exam; it has general properties similar to other adrenergic drugs (Section I, Medications to Treat Glaucoma)
    2. Lubricants are useful in treating minor eye irritation due to dryness, while vasoconstrictors are useful in treating minor eye irritations (see Box 16-2)
    3. These are generally well tolerated with no serious adverse effects
    4. Local side effects may include temporary burning or stinging and headache

Box 16-2	Lanolin alcohol (ointment)
Lubricants and Vasoconstrictors for Minor Eye Conditions	Naphazoline (eyedrops)
	Oxymetazoline (eyedrops)
	Polyvinyl alcohol (eyedrops)
	Tetrahydrozoline (eyedrops)

III. ANTI-INFLAMMATORY AND ANTI-INFECTIVE EYE MEDICATIONS

A. **Nonsteroidal anti-inflammatory drugs (NSAIDs)**
1. Action and use
   a. In general, used for pain and inflammation following surgery
   b. Flurbiprofen and suprofen are used to inhibit intraoperative miosis
   c. Diclofenac is used to treat postoperative inflammation after cataract extractions
   d. Ketorolac is used to treat conjunctivitis and seasonal allergic ophthalmic pruritis
2. Common NSAID medications (Table 16-7)
3. Administration considerations
   a. Systemic effect may be produced if absorbed
   b. NSAIDs have potential to cause increased bleeding; therefore, clients with increased bleeding tendencies should be monitored closely
4. Contraindications: sensitivity to aspirin, phenylacetic acid derivatives, or systemic NSAIDs
5. Significant drug interactions: none reported
6. Significant food interactions: St. John's wort (herb) and ciprofloxacin lead to increased photosensitivity
7. Significant laboratory studies: potential for bleeding; monitor CBC and coagulation studies
8. Side effects: local—transient burning or stinging on application, itching, allergic reaction, pain, and redness
9. Adverse effects/toxicity: bleeding
10. Client-centered nursing care: assess for hypersensitivity symptoms such as burning, itching, redness, and swelling occurring after administration of dose
11. Client education
    a. NSAIDs may potentiate bleeding in clients with known bleeding tendencies
    b. Proper self-administration of ophthalmic medications

B. **Antibacterial, antifungal, and antiviral agents**
1. Action and use
   a. Antibacterial agents are used to treat bacterial infections such as conjunctivitis, blepharitis, keratitis, uveitis, and hordeolum (sty)
   b. Antifungal agents are used to treat fungal blepharitis, conjunctivitis, and keratitis

Table 16-7	**Nonsteroidal Anti-Inflammatory Agents for Ophthalmic Use**	
Generic Name	**Uses**	**Side/Adverse Effects**
Diclofenac	Postoperative inflammation after cataract surgery	Headache, dizziness, dyspepsia, ophthalmic effects, renal impairment, anaphylactic shock, constipation
Flurbiprofen	Constriction of pupil prior to surgery	Eye irritation
Ketorolac	Relief of ocular itching, postoperative inflammation after cataract surgery	Eye irritation
Suprofen	Inhibit intraoperative miosis	Eye irritation

Table 16-8	Antibacterial, Antifungal, and Antiviral Agents for Ophthalmic Use	
Generic Name	**Uses**	**Side/Adverse Effects**
Bacitracin	Eye infection caused by *Staphylococcus*	Blurring of vision
Chloramphenicol	Eye infection for susceptible organisms when less dangerous anti-infectives are ineffective	Bone marrow hypoplasia, irritation, burning, itching, angioneurotic edema, superinfection, aplastic anemia
Ciprofloxacin	Eye infection for susceptible organisms when less dangerous anti-infectives are ineffective, otitis externa	Dry eye, eye pain, keratopathy
Erythromycin	Superficial ocular infections, ophthalmia neonatorum caused by *Neisseria gonorrhoeae* or *Chlamydia trachomatis*	Edema, urticaria, dermatitis, angioneurotic edema, irritation, burning, itching at application site
Gentamicin	Superficial ocular infections	Transient irritation, burning, stinging, itching, angioneurotic edema, urticaria, maculopapular dermatitis, photosensitivity, superinfection
Ofloxacin	Bacterial conjunctivitis, otitis externa from *E. coli, P. aeruginosa, S. aureus*	Visual disturbances
Polymyxin B	Bacterial infection caused by *Proteus aeruginosa*	Eye irritation, blurred vision, itching, stinging, burning
Sulfisoxazole	Conjunctivitis, corneal ulcer, superficial ocular infection	Stevens–Johnson syndrome, nausea and vomiting, abdominal pain, headache, hematuria, crystalluria, agranulocytosis, photosensitivity, alopecia
Tobramycin	Superficial ocular infection	Pain, irritation, superinfection, ocular toxicity, hypersensitivity, erythema, punctuate keratitis
Trifluridine	Keratoconjunctivitis, epithelial keratitis, viral infections of the eye	Burning, stinging, palpebral edema, epithelial keratopathy, keratitis sicca, hyperemia, increased IOP
Vidarabine	Varicella zoster virus, cytomegalovirus, vaccinia, and HBV	Increased IOP glaucoma, cataracts

c. Antiviral agents are used to treat herpes simplex virus keratitis and herpes simplex virus keratoconjunctivitis

2. Common antibacterial, antifungal, and antiviral medications (Table 16-8)

3. Administration considerations

   a. If indicated, obtain culture specimen from eye(s) before administering first dose of medication

   b. Remove exudates from eyes before administering dose

   c. Continue medications for full course of prescribed treatment, which allows full healing to occur (antibacterials and antivirals) and help prevent development of antibiotic-resistant strains (antibacterials)

4. Contraindications: hypersensitivity

5. Significant drug interactions

   a. Para-aminobenzoic acid (PABA) reduces the action of sulfonamides

   b. Ophthalmic anesthetics should not be administered within 30 minutes of sulfonamides

   c. Sulfonamides are incompatible with thimerosol and silver preparations

6. Significant food interactions: none reported

7. Significant laboratory studies: monitor CBC and coagulation studies in clients with potential for bleeding

8. Side effects: local dermatitis, itching, stinging, swelling

9. Adverse effects/toxicity: blood dyscrasias with chloramphenicol

Practice to Pass

A client with an eye infection has crusty drainage in and around the eye. Before administering the prescribed ophthalmic solution, what nursing measures do you implement?

Table 16-9	Common Corticosteroid Agents for Ophthalmic Use	
Generic Name	**Uses**	**Side Effects**
Dexamethasone	Conjunctivitis	Cataracts, glaucoma
Prednisone	Ophthalmic disorders	Cushing syndrome, hyperglycemia, muscle weakness, nausea and vomiting, dyspepsia, increased appetite, delayed wound healing, superinfection, cataracts, glaucoma, thrombus formation

10. Client-centered nursing care
    a. Monitor infected eye(s) for pain, drainage, redness, and swelling
    b. Monitor for unusual bleeding or bruising with chloramphenicol
11. Client education
    a. Inform prescriber of photosensitivity, redness, or swelling
    b. Inform prescriber of increased drainage, pain, or if no improvement is seen within a few days
    c. Proper self-administration of ophthalmic medications

C. **Corticosteroids**
1. Action and use: management of allergic and inflammatory ophthalmic disorders of conjunctiva, cornea, and anterior segment of eye
2. Common corticosteroid medications (Table 16-9)
3. Administration considerations
    a. Corticosteroids should be used for short-term treatment only
    b. Use with caution in clients with cataracts and chronic open-angle glaucoma
4. Contraindications: hypersensitivity and corneal abrasion
5. Significant drug interactions: corticosteroids may mask hypersensitivity reactions to other drugs
6. Significant food interactions: none reported
7. Significant laboratory studies: none reported
8. Side effects: local—stinging after application
9. Adverse effects/toxicity: visual disturbances, headache, and eye pain
10. Client-centered nursing care
    a. Corticosteroids may mask symptoms of infection and hypersensitivity reactions
    b. Corticosteroids may increase susceptibility to infection
11. Client education
    a. Avoid use of contact lenses during and for the prescribed time after use of corticosteroid therapy
    b. Do not discontinue medication without instructions from prescriber
    c. Have eye(s) examined periodically for progress
    d. Proper self-administration of ophthalmic medications

IV. ANESTHETIC MEDICATIONS FOR THE EYE

A. **Action and use**
1. Prevent initiation and transmission of nerve impulses
2. Used to prevent pain during procedures such as **tonometry** (measurement of intraocular tension, used to detect glaucoma), subconjunctival injections, removal of foreign bodies, and removal of sutures

B. **Common medications**
1. Proparacaine hydrochloride: one to two drops of 0.5% solution (single dose) to affected eye(s)
2. Tetracaine hydrochloride: one to two drops of 0.5–1% solution (single dose) to affected eye(s)

C. Administration considerations
1. Rapid onset within 20 seconds and duration is 15–20 minutes
2. Tetracaine hydrochloride can cause systemic toxicity

D. Contraindications: hypersensitivity

E. Significant drug interactions: may interact with ophthalmic cholinesterase inhibitors, increasing risk of toxicity

F. Significant food interactions: none reported

G. Significant laboratory studies: none reported

H. Side effects: proparacaine causes allergic contact dermatitis, cycloplegia, conjunctival congestion, delayed corneal healing

I. Adverse effects/toxicity
1. CNS excitation symptoms: blurred vision, dizziness, nervousness, restlessness, trembling
2. CNS depression (follows CNS excitation): dyspnea, drowsiness, dysrhythmias

J. Client-centered nursing care
1. To protect cornea, apply eye patch until blink reflex has returned
2. Assess for hypersensitivity symptoms such as burning, itching, stinging

K. Client education: do not touch or rub the eye until anesthesia has worn off

V. AUDITORY MEDICATIONS

A. Antibiotics for the ear
1. Action and use
   a. Used to manage infections of **external ear** (external auditory canal surface); note that infections of middle ear (otitis media) are treated with oral (systemic) antibiotics
   b. Chloramphenicol is used to treat infections caused by such organisms as *Enterobacter aerogenes, Escherichia coli, Haemophilus influenzae, Pseudomonas aeruginosa,* and others
2. Common medications
   a. Chloramphenicol: two to three drops instilled in ear canal every 6–8 hours
   b. Gentamicin sulfate otic solution: three to four drops instilled in ear canal three times daily
   c. *Note:* Otic preparation of gentamicin sulfate has not been approved by Food and Drug Administration (FDA); prescribers in United States use the *ophthalmic* preparation for otic infections
3. Administration considerations
   a. Unless contraindicated, warm ear drops by running medication bottle under warm water, immersing bottle in a cup of warm water, or holding bottle in the hand or pocket for 30 minutes prior to administration
   b. Assess client's baseline hearing status
   c. Assess client for ear drainage, earache, erythema, pain, and **vertigo** (dizziness)
   d. Assess that ear canal is clear and not impacted with **cerumen** (earwax) before medication administration
   e. Assess for intact **tympanic membrane** (thin membrane between external auditory canal and middle ear)
4. Contraindications: hypersensitivity; perforation of tympanic membrane
5. Significant drug interactions: none reported
6. Significant food interactions: none reported
7. Significant laboratory studies: assess CBC for blood dyscrasias with chloramphenicol
8. Side effects
   a. Local: burning, rash, redness, swelling, blurred vision
   b. Systemic: hypersensitivity reaction

Box 16-3	**For instillation of eardrops in older children and adults:**
Administration of Otic Medications	• Assess the ear canal for cerumen or edema
	• Tilt client's head toward the unaffected side
	• Gently pull the pinna of the ear up and back
	• Instill the eardrops—*do not* insert dropper into the ear canal
	• Gently massage the area anterior to the ear to facilitate entry of the drops into the ear canal
	For instillation of eardrops in children 3 years and younger:
	• Assess the ear canal for cerumen or edema
	• Tilt client's head toward the unaffected side
	• Gently pull the pinna of the ear slightly down and back
	• Instill the eardrops—*do not* insert dropper into the ear canal
	• Gently massage the area anterior to the ear to facilitate entry of the drops into the ear canal

9. Adverse effects/toxicity
   a. Hypersensitivity reaction
   b. Rare occurrence of systemic hematologic toxicity
10. Client-centered nursing care
    a. Assess for signs of hypersensitivity such as burning, rash, redness, and swelling after administration of dose
    b. Discontinue use if hypersensitivity reaction occurs
    c. Monitor auditory canal for drainage and pain
    d. Monitor for hearing disturbances
11. Client education
    a. Inform healthcare provider of increased pain, drainage, or no improvement in symptoms within a few days of treatment
    b. Refer to Box 16-3 for instillation of otic medications

B. Corticosteroids
   1. Action and use
      a. Used for anti-inflammatory effects
      b. Used for antipruritic and anti-allergic effects
   2. Common otic corticosteroid medications (Table 16-10)
   3. Administration considerations
      a. Assess client's hearing status
      b. Assess client for ear drainage, earache, erythema, pain, and vertigo
      c. Assess that ear canal is clear and not impacted with cerumen before medication administration

Table 16-10   Corticosteroid Agents for Otic Use

Generic Name	Uses	Side/Adverse Effects
Betamethasone Hydrocortisone Dexamethasone Hydrocortisone with acetic acid Hydrocortisone with alcohol Hydrocortisone with acetic acid and benzethonium	Inflammatory conditions of ear	Cushing syndrome, hyperglycemia, muscle weakness, nausea and vomiting, dyspepsia, increased appetite, delayed wound healing, superinfection, cataracts, glaucoma, thrombus formation

        d. Assess for intact tympanic membrane

        e. May be given in combination with antibiotics to treat infections of external ear canal or mastoid cavity

   4. Contraindications

        a. Hypersensitivity to sulfites

        b. Perforation of tympanic membrane

   5. Significant drug interactions: none reported

   6. Significant food interactions: none reported

   7. Significant laboratory studies: none reported

   8. Side effects: corticosteroids may mask infection or exacerbate an existing infection

   9. Adverse effects/toxicity: corticosteroids may mask infection or exacerbate an existing infection

   10. Client-centered nursing care: assess for hypersensitivity after administration of dose

   11. Client education

        a. Have hearing monitored for duration of treatment

        b. Inform healthcare provider of new onset of ear drainage, heat, fever, odor, or pain

        c. Inform healthcare provider if no improvement is seen within a few days of treatment

        d. Refer to Box 16-3 for administration of otic medications

C. Other medications (over-the-counter medications)

   1. Action and use

        a. Acetic acid (alcohol, glycerin, or propylene glycol) is used after swimming or bathing to restore normal acid pH to the ear canal

        b. Glycerin, mineral oil, and olive oil are used as emollients to relieve itching and burning in ear

        c. Propylene glycol enhances antibacterial effects and acidity of acetic acid

        d. Carbamide peroxide is an antibacterial agent used to help remove accumulated cerumen

   2. Common OTC medications for otic use (refer to Box 16-4)

   3. Administration considerations

        a. Follow manufacturer's directions for number and timing of drops

        b. If cotton wick is used because of swelling in outer ear canal, saturate wick before insertion, moisten it as directed, and remove wick after 24 hours

   4. Contraindications: hypersensitivity; otherwise generally considered safe

   5. Significant drug interactions: none reported

   6. Significant food interactions: none reported

   7. Significant laboratory studies: none reported

   8. Side effects: generally considered safe without side effects

   9. Adverse effects/toxicity: generally considered safe without side effects

   10. Client-centered nursing care: assess for hypersensitivity

---

Practice to Pass

A client returns to the clinic reporting that the medication prescribed for an ear infection "runs right back out of my ear." What assessment and instructions do you provide for this client?

Box 16-4	Hydrocortisone, propylene glycol, alcohol, benzyl benzoate
Common Over-the-Counter (OTC) Agents for Otic Use	Boric acid and isopropyl alcohol
	Carbamide peroxide
	Carbamide peroxide and glycerin
	Isopropyl alcohol
	Isopropyl alcohol in glycerin

11. Client education

    a. Seek evaluation by healthcare provider if symptoms do not improve within several days

    b. Inform healthcare provider if adverse reactions occur or if symptoms worsen

    c. Refer to Box 16-3 for administration of otic medications

! **D. Medications that cause ototoxicity**

    1. Analgesics: aspirin and other salicylates, NSAIDs

    2. Antibiotics: aminoglycosides, clarithromycin, erythromycin, vancomycin

    3. Antineoplastic agents: cisplatin, mechlorethamine

    4. Loop diuretics: bumetanide, furosemide, torsemide

Case Study

A client with newly diagnosed open-angle glaucoma is prescribed betaxolol. The client also has a history of chronic obstructive pulmonary disease.

1. How does the nurse explain glaucoma and the purpose of the medication to this client?

2. The client expresses concern about the new medication and the possible interference with the treatment and course of the preexisting pulmonary disease. What information should be provided to the client?

3. What information does the client need regarding the side effects and signs and symptoms of hypersensitivity to betaxolol?

4. What instructions does the nurse provide specifically related to the potential side effect of photophobia?

5. What instructions does the client need regarding proper administration of ophthalmic medications?

For suggested responses, see page 544.

POSTTEST

1 A client with diabetes and glaucoma has NPH insulin and carteolol listed on the medication administration record. The nurse should consider which assessment to be of priority when seeing the client?

    1. Blood pressure
    2. Blood glucose
    3. Headache
    4. Diarrhea

2 The nurse should conclude that a client understands instructions about how to self-administer a prescribed otic solution when the client makes which statement?

    1. "I place the bottle of medication under cool running water before using."
    2. "I place the bottle of medication under warm running water before using."
    3. "I warm the bottle of medication in the microwave before using."
    4. "I warm the bottle of medication in my hand for 5 minutes before using."

POSTTEST

POSTTEST

3 After a nurse provides instructions about betaxolol to a client with chronic obstructive pulmonary disease (COPD), the client asks, "How can eyedrops affect my lungs?" The nurse's best response includes which information?

1. The medication does not have any effects on the pulmonary system.
2. Client is only at risk if prescribed ophthalmic medication is cardioselective.
3. Client is at risk if betaxolol is taken at same time as oral medications for pulmonary disease.
4. If betaxolol is systemically absorbed, it can exert the same systemic effects as other beta-blockers.

4 A client telephones the outpatient clinic and reports severe ear pain that ceased suddenly when copious drainage came from the ear. The client wants to instill remnants of a 2-month-old otic antibiotic prescription left over from a previous ear infection. What is the best response by the nurse?

1. "See a healthcare provider. Do not treat the ear with the antibiotic."
2. "If the medication has been stored properly, it should be okay to instill."
3. "Begin treatment and seek help if no improvement is seen within 2 days."
4. "The shelf-life of otic medications is 3 months; therefore, the medication would be safe to use."

5 The nurse should conclude that a client is demonstrating appropriate technique for instilling ophthalmic medication when the client performs which action?

1. Cleanses crust from eye by applying petroleum jelly and wiping with a washcloth
2. Cleanses crust from eye by wiping from the inner canthus outward with a cotton ball
3. Cleanses crust with mild soapy water using 4 × 4 gauze
4. Cleanses crust with a cotton-tipped swab

6 Because a prescription of gentamicin sulfate for an ear infection reads "for ophthalmic use," the client refuses to instill the medication. After verifying the prescription with the client's chart, what is the most appropriate conclusion by the nurse?

1. An error is likely in the dispensing of the medication since the clinician is treating an otic infection.
2. It is an accepted and safe practice in the United States for clinicians to prescribe ophthalmic gentamicin for otic use.
3. An error was likely committed by the clinician in prescribing the medication.
4. The client requires further teaching on proper medication administration.

7 Because a client with glaucoma is scheduled for removal of a cataract from the left eye, the nurse should anticipate a prescription from the surgeon to administer which drug?

1. Atropine sulfate
2. Glycopyrrolate
3. Acetazolamide
4. Pralidoxime

8 A client is receiving an ophthalmic anesthetic agent prior to removal of sutures. The nurse should consider implementing which priority nursing measures?

1. Measures to protect the airway
2. Measures to reduce hypersensitivity
3. Measures to control body temperature
4. Measures to protect the eye

9 A client is prescribed the ophthalmic medication latanoprost. The nurse should teach the client about what common effects of this drug? Select all that apply.

1. Maintenance of visual fields
2. Thickening of eyelashes
3. Changes in liver function tests
4. Bronchoconstriction
5. Blue pigmentation of the iris

10 A client is scheduled for an annual eye exam. What instructions should the nurse provide? Select all that apply.

1. "Wear sunglasses after the exam because atropine will cause photophobia."
2. "Tropicamide may be administered to dilate the pupil."
3. "Proparacaine drops are used to paralyze the ciliary muscle."
4. "Because you have dry eyes the doctor may prescribe cyclosporine drops."
5. "Phenylephrine may be prescribed to decrease your ocular pressures."

➤ *See pages 527–528 for Answers and Rationales.*

ANSWERS & RATIONALES

Pretest

1 **Answer: 3** **Rationale:** Assessment of allergies and reactions to medications is essential when administering a new medication. Hypersensitivity responses can occur with ophthalmic medications, and severe adverse reactions may occur with hypersensitivity to the medication because it may be systemically absorbed. Knowledge of the purpose of a drug is not unique to ophthalmic drugs. Assessment of level of consciousness (LOC) would not override the risks of a topical allergic reaction or the risks of systemic responses to the medications. Teaching about the drug's action is very important but should follow assessment. **Cognitive Level:** Analyzing **Client Need:** Pharmacological and Parenteral Therapies **Integrated Process:** Nursing Process: Assessment **Content Area:** Pharmacology **Strategy:** The critical words in the question are *first dose*. Use principles of safety in medication administration to consider that a risk for allergy is present whenever a client receives a new medication. Correlate this risk with the likely reaction to choose the option that indicates the critical assessment. **Reference:** Adams, M. P., Holland, N., & Urban, C. (2017). *Pharmacology for nurses: A pathophysiologic approach* (5th ed.). New York, NY: Pearson, p. 870.

2 **Answers: 2, 4, 5** **Rationale:** The correct technique for administration of ophthalmic medications includes pulling the lower eyelid down and instilling medication into the conjunctival sac, which ensures retention of the medication as well as exposure to a highly vascular area. Applying gentle pressure to inner canthus for 30 seconds to 1 minute after medication administration prevents absorption through the tear duct and subsequent drainage of medications. Cleaning exudates from the eye before instillation of medication promotes the absorption of medication. Placing medications directly on the cornea can be extremely painful and can cause tissue injury. The lower eyelid is pulled down, not up. **Cognitive Level:** Applying **Client Need:** Pharmacological and Parenteral Therapies **Integrated Process:** Nursing Process: Evaluation **Content Area:** Pharmacology **Strategy:** Select the options most likely to result in retaining the medication within the eye for the longest period of time and that also promotes absorption of medication. **Reference:** Adams, M. P., Holland, N., & Urban, C. (2017). *Pharmacology for nurses: A pathophysiologic approach* (5th ed.). New York, NY: Pearson, p. 29.

3 **Answers: 1, 5** **Rationale:** When an external ear canal is obstructed by edematous tissue, a gauze wick is inserted past the edematous segment. The medication is then applied to the outside wick, allowing the medication to be absorbed along the path of the wick. Forcing the tip of the container or forcing the stream of liquid could result in damage to the ear canal or ear drum. The occluded canal is related to the infection and probably will not subside without intervention. Topical medications are prescribed because it provides direct contact with the microorganism. Since an alternative to expensive systemic medications exists, it is the best method. Inserting an object (such as a dropper) into a canal without visualization is an unsafe technique. Since an infected ear is usually very painful, forcing an object into the canal would be painful. **Cognitive Level:** Applying **Client Need:** Pharmacological and Parenteral Therapies **Integrated Process:** Nursing Process: Implementation **Content Area:** Pharmacology **Strategy:** Evaluate each option considering its effect on tissue that is edematous and most likely uncomfortable. Select the options that are most likely to achieve the goal while protecting the safety of the client. **Reference:** Adams, M. P., Holland, N., & Urban, C. (2017). *Pharmacology for nurses: A pathophysiologic approach* (5th ed.). New York, NY: Pearson, pp. 29–30.

4 **Answers: 1, 2, 4** **Rationale:** To minimize gastrointestinal distress, the client may take the medication with milk. Acetazolamide is taken in the morning to avoid nocturnal diuresis. It reduces intraocular pressure, which is related to increased aqueous humor formation. The client may crush the tablet and mix it with juice. A side effect of acetazolamide is suppression of bone marrow, which may result in decreased platelets, RBCs, and WBCs. Since the signs and symptoms of bone marrow suppression can be vague, the client should have regular blood counts performed several times during the year. A high-potassium diet should be encouraged (unless there is a specific contraindication) because acetazolamide can cause hypokalemia. **Cognitive Level:** Applying **Client Need:** Pharmacological and Parenteral Therapies **Integrated Process:** Teaching and Learning **Content Area:** Pharmacology **Strategy:** Specific knowledge of adverse effects of acetazolamide is needed to answer the question. Associate the drug with the side effect of hematologic alterations and hypokalemia to help make the correct selection. **Reference:** Wilson, B. A., Shannon, M. T., & Shields, K. M. (2017). *Pearson nurse's drug guide 2017.* New York, NY: Pearson, pp. 13–15.

5 **Answer: 1 Rationale:** Carbonic anhydrase inhibitors such as dorzolamide decrease aqueous humor production by approximately one-half of baseline, thereby lowering intraocular pressure (IOP). Cholinergic agonists such as carbachol cause pupil constriction, which does not affect aqueous humor production but increases its drainage. The glaucoma results from an increased production of aqueous humor, so increasing the production of aqueous humor would not resolve the problem. Increased outflow of aqueous humor is accomplished by a cholinergic agonist and nonselective sympathomimetics. **Cognitive Level:** Analyzing **Client Need:** Pharmacological and Parenteral Therapies **Integrated Process:** Teaching and Learning **Content Area:** Pharmacology **Strategy:** Recall that glaucoma is characterized by increased intraocular pressure (IOP). Associate the drug with the reversal of the disease process to make the correct selection. **Reference:** Wilson, B. A., Shannon, M. T., & Shields, K. M. (2017). *Pearson nurse's drug guide 2017.* New York, NY: Pearson, pp. 525–526.

6 **Answer: 3 Rationale:** Because the drug is a cholinergic agent, it will reverse the effects of sympathomimetic drugs, often used to treat asthma. Precipitation of an asthma attack is a systemic side effect of pilocarpine. Other side effects include salivation, hypotension, diarrhea, and nausea and vomiting. Since the drug is a cholinergic agent, the client is more likely to have excessive salivation than dry mouth. This drug is more likely to cause hypotension rather than hypertension and diarrhea rather than constipation. **Cognitive Level:** Applying **Client Need:** Pharmacological and Parenteral Therapies **Integrated Process:** Nursing Process: Assessment **Content Area:** Pharmacology **Strategy:** Associate the word *asthma* in the stem of the question with the word *wheezing* in the correct option. **Reference:** Wilson, B. A., Shannon, M. T., & Shields, K. M. (2017). *Pearson nurse's drug guide 2017.* New York, NY: Pearson, pp. 1259–1260.

7 **Answers: 2, 5 Rationale:** In the adult client, the medication is most likely to flow into the canal if the pinna is pulled up and back before instilling otic solutions. The client can massage the anterior ear after medication administration. The pinna is pulled down in a child under age 3, not in an adult. Droppers should never be inserted into the ear canal. The head should be tilted toward the unaffected side rather than the affected side. **Cognitive Level:** Applying **Client Need:** Pharmacological and Parenteral Therapies **Integrated Process:** Nursing Process: Evaluation **Content Area:** Pharmacology **Strategy:** Select the option that is most likely to promote appropriate flow of the medication into the ear canal. **Reference:** Adams, M. P., Holland, N., & Urban, C. (2017). *Pharmacology for nurses: A pathophysiologic approach* (5th ed.). New York, NY: Pearson, p. 29.

8 **Answer: 1 Rationale:** Ophthalmic beta blockers such as timolol reduce intraocular pressure (IOP) by decreasing production of aqueous humor. The medication must be continued as lifelong therapy to maintain a stable IOP. Glaucoma already involves increased IOP so the medication is not given to raise it. Other drug groups may be utilized for the treatment of glaucoma as well as surgical intervention. **Cognitive Level:** Applying **Client Need:** Pharmacological and Parenteral Therapies **Integrated Process:** Nursing Process: Evaluation **Content Area:** Pharmacology **Strategy:** Recall first that timolol is a beta-blocking agent since it ends in the suffix *-olol*. Next, recall the pathophysiology of glaucoma and select the option that correlates closest to the reversal of the disease process. **Reference:** Adams, M. P., Holland, N., & Urban, C. (2017). *Pharmacology for nurses: A pathophysiologic approach* (5th ed.). New York, NY: Pearson, pp. 870–871.

9 **Answer: 1 Rationale:** Because pupillary dilation pushes the iris over the area where aqueous humor normally drains, atropine (an anticholinergic agent) can precipitate an acute glaucoma crisis. Blurred vision, diplopia, photosensitivity, and dry eyes are the visual alterations associated with diphenhydramine. No visual alterations are associated with hydroxyzine. Contraindications associated with retelase recombinant include bleeding disorders, stroke, and severe uncontrolled hypertension. **Cognitive Level:** Applying **Client Need:** Pharmacological and Parenteral Therapies **Integrated Process:** Nursing Process: Implementation **Content Area:** Pharmacology **Strategy:** First recall the pathophysiology of glaucoma. Select the drug that represents a drug category that is most likely to cause structural changes that could increase intraocular pressure. Alternatively, recall that atropine dilates the pupil and associate this with blockage of the outflow of aqueous humor to make the correct selection. **Reference:** Adams, M. P., Holland, N., & Urban, C. (2017). *Pharmacology for nurses: A pathophysiologic approach* (5th ed.). New York, NY: Pearson, p. 698.

10 **Answer: 2 Rationale:** If systemically absorbed, brinzolamide (a carbonic acid inhibitor) is eliminated via the kidneys. In chronic renal failure with a urine output less than 30 mL/hr, the drug is retained. The drug is a systemic diuretic that could result in electrolyte imbalances, but not hypertension. The drug has no known contraindications or side effects associated with the liver. The drug does not affect the skeletal system. **Cognitive Level:** Applying **Client Need:** Pharmacological and Parenteral Therapies **Integrated Process:** Nursing Process: Implementation **Content Area:** Pharmacology **Strategy:** Correlate the drug category (carbonic anhydrase inhibitor) with the potential outcome of drug accumulation. **Reference:** Adams, M. P., Holland, N., & Urban, C. (2017). *Pharmacology for nurses: A pathophysiologic approach* (5th ed.). New York, NY: Pearson, p. 1687.

Posttest

1 **Answer: 2** **Rationale:** Carteolol is a beta-adrenergic blocker useful for treatment of glaucoma. If systemically absorbed, the medication could mask symptoms of hypoglycemia. A serum glucose level significantly lower than normal can place the client at great risk more rapidly than an elevated blood pressure. Many clients live for long periods with hypertension without immediate risks to their health. Headache is not a common effect and if present would not be the first priority. Diarrhea needs to be controlled because of the potential fluid and electrolyte loss, but this is not the *first priority*. **Cognitive Level:** Applying **Client Need:** Pharmacological and Parenteral Therapies **Integrated Process:** Nursing Process: Evaluation **Content Area:** Pharmacology **Strategy:** Note that insulin is given for diabetes mellitus and that carteolol is a beta-adrenergic blocker. Determine the relationship between these drugs to conclude that the carteolol could mask some signs of hypoglycemia. **Reference:** Wilson, B. A., Shannon, M. T., & Shields, K. M. (2017). *Pearson nurse's drug guide 2017.* New York, NY: Pearson, pp. 271–273.

2 **Answer: 2** **Rationale:** Warming eardrops under running water (if not contraindicated) makes administration of the medication more comfortable than it would be as a cold solution. Eardrops that are cooled under running water could lead to dizziness upon instillation. Microwaving the solution could result in hot spots that burn the tissue or could change the composition of the medication. The client is least likely to spend 5 minutes holding a bottle in the hands to warm it before each use. **Cognitive Level:** Analyzing **Client Need:** Pharmacological and Parenteral Therapies **Integrated Process:** Nursing Process: Evaluation **Content Area:** Pharmacology **Strategy:** Correlate the temperature of solution with common otic responses and use the process of elimination to make a selection. **Reference:** Adams, M. P., Holland, N., & Urban, C. (2017). *Pharmacology for nurses: A pathophysiologic approach* (5th ed.). New York, NY: Pearson, pp. 29–30.

3 **Answer: 4** **Rationale:** If systemic absorption occurs after the administration of betaxolol, adverse effects such as increased airway resistance may override the effect of medications given to decrease airway resistance, leading to possible dyspnea. **Cognitive Level:** Analyzing **Client Need:** Pharmacological and Parenteral Therapies **Integrated Process:** Teaching and Learning **Content Area:** Pharmacology **Strategy:** The core issue of the question is an understanding of the characteristics of the drug with the primary alterations associated with chronic obstructive pulmonary disease (COPD). **Reference:** Wilson, B. A., Shannon, M. T., & Shields, K. M. (2017). *Pearson nurse's drug guide 2017.* New York, NY: Pearson, pp. 180–181.

4 **Answer: 1** **Rationale:** Because the tympanic membrane may be ruptured, the ear should be assessed before instilling medication. Because of the risk of a ruptured tympanic membrane, the client should not instill an old prescription (drug deterioration and storage are other lower priority but appropriate concerns). It is inappropriate for the nurse to have the client use the old medication and seek help if not better in two days. The shelf-life of the medication is not the concern; the client must be assessed by a healthcare provider before starting a medication. **Cognitive Level:** Applying **Client Need:** Pharmacological and Parenteral Therapies **Integrated Process:** Communication and Documentation **Content Area:** Pharmacology **Strategy:** Associate the sudden change with increased pressure often occurring with an infection. With this in mind, conclude that this is a situation that warrants direct assessment and treatment by a healthcare provider. **Reference:** Adams, M. P., & Urban, C. (2015). *Pharmacology: Connections to nursing practice* (3rd ed.). New York, NY: Pearson, p. 1298.

5 **Answer: 2** **Rationale:** Wiping from the inner canthus out prevents movement of microorganism-laden crusts from reaching the lacrimal duct. The client should avoid applying oil-based products on the eye and a washcloth is too coarse. To prevent irritation, the client should avoid using soap. If a cotton swab is used, sudden movement by the client could result in injury. **Cognitive Level:** Applying **Client Need:** Pharmacological and Parenteral Therapies **Integrated Process:** Nursing Process: Evaluation **Content Area:** Pharmacology **Strategy:** Utilize knowledge of the sterility of the mucous membranes of the eye in choosing the correct option. **Reference:** Berman, A., Snyder, S., & Frandsen, G. (2016). *Kozier & Erb's fundamentals of nursing: Concepts, process, and practice* (10th ed.). New York, NY: Pearson, p. 703.

6 **Answer: 2** **Rationale:** Because otic gentamicin is not approved for use in the United States, it is a safe and accepted practice for clinicians to prescribe ophthalmic gentamicin for otic use. The client should be informed of this practice. The pharmacist did not make an error in dispensing the medication. The clinician did not make an error in prescribing the medication. The client has not provided evidence of lack of ability to correctly self-administer the medication; the client's question was about the actual medication itself. **Cognitive Level:** Analyzing **Client Need:** Pharmacological and Parenteral Therapies **Integrated Process:** Teaching and Learning **Content Area:** Pharmacology **Strategy:** Compare and contrast ophthalmic medications with otic medications. Specific medication knowledge is needed to answer this question. **Reference:** Wilson, B. A., Shannon, M. T., & Shields, K. M. (2017). *Pearson nurse's drug guide 2017.* New York, NY: Pearson, pp. 733–736.

7 **Answer: 3 Rationale:** Acetazolamide inhibits carbonic anhydrase, which reduces the formation of aqueous humor, preventing an increase in intraocular pressure. Because of the anticholinergic effects, atropine sulfate, glycopyrrolate, and pralidoxime are contraindicated in clients with glaucoma. **Cognitive Level:** Analyzing **Client Need:** Pharmacological and Parenteral Therapies **Integrated Process:** Nursing Process: Implementation **Content Area:** Pharmacology **Strategy:** Correlate the drug's action with the primary problem associated with glaucoma. **Reference:** Wilson, B. A., Shannon, M. T., & Shields, K. M. (2017). *Pearson nurse's drug guide 2017.* New York, NY: Pearson, pp. 13–15, 136–139, 744–746, 1290–1292.

8 **Answer: 4 Rationale:** Ophthalmic anesthetic agents block the blink reflex. Because the eye is at risk for injury, an eye patch is applied for protection. Priority is given to protecting the cornea from irritants, debris, and rubbing. Since the medication is local, the airway is not compromised. Hypersensitivity reactions are not related directly to administration of ophthalmic anesthesia. The anesthesia would not change body temperature. **Cognitive Level:** Analyzing **Client Need:** Pharmacological and Parenteral Therapies **Integrated Process:** Nursing Process: Planning **Content Area:** Pharmacology **Strategy:** The primary concept is safety. Correlate the function of the eyelid movement with risks to the client. **Reference:** Adams, M. P., & Urban, C. (2016). *Pharmacology: Connections to nursing practice* (3rd ed.). New York, NY: Pearson, p. 1294.

9 **Answers: 1, 2 Rationale:** Latanoprost is a prostaglandin analog prescribed to treat open-angle glaucoma. The therapeutic effect is maintenance of visual fields, vision, and intraocular pressures below 21 mmHg. A common side effect is lengthening and thickening of eyelashes. Rare side effects include alterations in liver function tests. Bronchoconstriction is a side effect of beta-adrenergic blockers such as timolol. The pigmentation of the iris could change to brown, not blue. **Cognitive Level:** Applying **Client Need:** Pharmacological and Parenteral Therapies **Integrated Process:** Nursing Process: Implementation **Content Area:** Pharmacology **Strategy:** Determine the intended outcomes of the medication and the most common side effects. **Reference:** Adams, M. P., & Urban, C. (2016). *Pharmacology: Connections to nursing practice* (3rd ed.). New York, NY: Pearson, pp. 1287–1288.

10 **Answers: 1, 2, 4 Rationale:** Medications commonly used in eye examinations include tropicamide or atropine to dilate the pupil and paralyze the ciliary muscle. The client should wear sunglasses after the exam because the client will experience temporary photophobia secondary to pupil dilation. Proparacaine drops are used to anesthetize the eye, not paralyze ciliary muscle. Cyclosporine drops can be prescribed to decrease dry eyes. Phenylephrine eye drops cause vasoconstriction, thus dilating the eyes and reducing redness. **Cognitive Level:** Analyzing **Client Need:** Pharmacological and Parenteral Therapies **Integrated Process:** Nursing Process: Implementation **Content Area:** Pharmacology **Strategy:** Connect the drugs to their uses. **Reference:** Adams, M. P., & Urban, C. (2016). *Pharmacology: Connections to nursing practice* (3rd ed.). New York, NY: Pearson, pp. 1293–1294.

References

Adams, M. P., & Urban, C. (2016). *Pharmacology: Connections to nursing practice* (3rd ed.). New York, NY: Pearson

Adams, M. P., Holland, N., & Urban, C. (2017). *Pharmacology for nurses: A pathophysiologic approach* (5th ed.). New York, NY: Pearson.

Berman, A., Snyder, S., & Frandsen, G. (2016). *Kozier & Erb's fundamentals of nursing: Concepts, process, and practice* (10th ed.). New York, NY: Pearson.

Burchum, J., & Rosenthal, L. (2016). *Lehne's Pharmacology for nursing care* (9th ed.). St. Louis, MO: Mosby.

Drug Facts & Comparisons (Updated monthly). St. Louis, MO: A. Wolters Kluwer.

Karch, A. M. (2016). *Focus on nursing pharmacology* (7th ed.). Philadelphia, PA: Lippincott Williams & Wilkins.

Kee, J. L. (2017). *Pearson handbook of laboratory and diagnostic tests with nursing implications* (8th ed.). New York, NY: Pearson.

LeMone, P., Burke, K., Bauldoff, G., & Gubrud, P. (2015). *Medical surgical nursing: Clinical reasoning in patient care* (6th ed.). New York, NY: Pearson.

Skidmore-Roth, L. (2016). *Mosby's 2017 nursing drug reference* (30th ed.). St. Louis, MO: Mosby.

Wilson, B. A., Shannon, M. T., & Shields, K. M. (2017). *Pearson nurse's drug guide 2017.* New York, NY: Pearson.

Appendix A Practice to Pass and Case Study Suggested Answers

➤ Practice to Pass Suggested Answers

Chapter 1

Page 6: *Suggested Answer*—The pregnant client should be advised to avoid all medications during the pregnancy. Since she reports these discomforts occasional in frequency, the nurse may recommend some nonpharmacologic remedies for the headaches and backaches, such as taking a rest period or lying down during the day or application of ice to the forehead or back.

Page 11: *Suggested Answer*—Most medications depend on a functioning renal system for excretion from the body. For a client with chronic renal failure, the priority considerations are related to appropriate dosing with the drug and to careful assessment of the client for toxic effects of the drug. The drug regimen for clients with chronic renal failure is often complex; the nurse should review with the client the prescribed drugs and the schedule for administration. If the client is being treated with hemodialysis for chronic renal failure, the nurse should review with the client which drugs are taken before and after the dialysis treatment.

Page 12: *Suggested Answer*—The correct volume to administer morphine sulfate 15 mg in this example is 0.6 mL. The problem can be set up this way: 25 mg: 1 mL = 15 mg: x mL.

$$25x = 15, x = 15 \div 25, x = 0.6 \text{ mL}$$

The nurse should review the answer and note that, if 25 mg is contained in 1 mL, then 15 mg must be contained in a volume less than 1 mL—in this case 0.6 mL. The nurse enhances client safety through accurate dosing by performing a "common-sense" check at the end of each drug calculation.

Page 12: *Suggested Answer*—A topical dose of nitroglycerin is commonly applied in the morning and removed at hour of sleep. This allows for continual absorption and effect during the day when the client is active. Removing it at bedtime helps prevent medication tolerance (decreased physiological response to the medication).

Page 15: *Suggested Answer*—There are several strategies the nurse can use in this situation:

- When teaching the client, use short, simple sentences and provide a demonstration where possible.
- Use an interpreter or, if unavailable, ask a member of client's family to interpret.
- Search online or use other resources to find drug information materials in the client's language.
- Develop a diagram of the drug schedule that uses pictures and numbers.
- Observe the client for cues that signal lack of effective communication during the teaching session.

Chapter 2

Page 32: *Suggested Answer*—Three types of phytomedicines that are contraindicated in the client with a history of hemorrhagic stroke are bilberry, feverfew, and garlic (also ginkgo and ginger). Since a hemorrhagic stroke is caused by a bleed, any medication or herb (such as these) that prolongs coagulation time should be avoided.

Page 33: *Suggested Answer*—Ginkgo is recommended for age-related mental decline. By increasing cerebral circulation, it is believed to improve short-term memory and concentration. New evidence suggests effective use in the treatment of Alzheimer's disease and dementia. The appropriate phytotherapy for this client would be American ginseng, which will help the client (student) improve concentration and stamina and increase the body's ability to resist stress.

Page 38: *Suggested Answer*—Milk thistle is known as the liver herb. It has been shown to protect hepatocytes from toxins and enhance regeneration of the liver cells. It has also been shown to be effective in reducing hepatotoxicity with concomitant use of psychoactive drugs such as phenothiazines and in treating overdose of the death cap mushroom.

Page 39: *Suggested Answer*—Some other names used to identify St. John's wort are amber goatweed, Johnswort, klamanthweed, God's wonder plant, touch-and-heal, witch's herb, chassediable, and devil's scourge. Since many of the herbs are identified by several names, including the English common, brand name, or foreign translation, it is important to be familiar with these names to help the client identify them appropriately.

Page 41: *Suggested Answer*—The nurse should tell the client to read the label for the specific, intended use of phytomedicines. Also, the client should read the label for dosage, placing more trust in phytomedicines that contain a standardized form of the herb. The dosage should be clear and include length of therapy required for expected results. The client should also read the label to determine where the herb was manufactured. Although some European herbs are highly regulated and standardized, caution should be taken with those herbs manufactured or purchased outside of the United States because the herbs may be contaminated. The letters *USP* demonstrate standards were followed in the herb's manufacture and that the herb has an approved use by the FDA. If use of the herb has not been approved by the FDA, the label should read "NF," meaning that the manufacturer has at least followed the same standards of quality and purity.

Chapter 3

Page 52: *Suggested Answer*—Discontinue the patient-controlled analgesia (PCA), contact the healthcare provider stat, and be prepared to give an antihistamine or epinephrine for an allergic reaction.

Page 55: *Suggested Answer*—The client is probably experiencing acetaminophen toxicity because of taking acetaminophen as well as cold medication with acetaminophen in it. Acetaminophen is toxic to the liver and should not be taken in doses exceeding 4 grams per 24 hours.

Page 63: *Suggested Answer*—The tube feeding usually needs to be turned off for 30 minutes to 1 hour prior to the medication administration and for 1–2 hours afterward. A nurse who has questions about the effects of a change in rate can also consult the agency pharmacist.

Page 69: *Suggested Answer*—Because of the multiple medication profile, medications such as antihypertensives and antidiabetic medications, including insulin, may need adjustment.

Page 73: *Suggested Answer*—The opioid medication meperidine should not be administered because it increases the risk of respiratory depression, hypotension, and serotonin syndrome. Severe interactions can lead to coma or possibly death.

Chapter 4

Page 91: *Suggested Answer*—Neuroleptic malignant syndrome (NMS) is a potentially fatal reaction to antipsychotic drugs. At one time it was thought to occur in about 1% of the clients taking antipsychotics with an accompanying mortality rate of up to 30%. Increased awareness and vigilance by nurses and others has significantly reduced both morbidity and mortality rates. It occurs most often when high-potency antipsychotic drugs are prescribed. Haloperidol is frequently cited as the causative neuroleptic. Onset is from 3 to 9 days after initiation of an antipsychotic. It is manifested by muscular rigidity, tremors, impaired ventilation, muteness, altered consciousness, and autonomic hyperactivity. The cardinal symptom is high body temperature. Temperatures as high as 108°F (42.2°C) have been reported. More likely, temperatures are 101–103°F. Dantrolene and bromocriptine are the drugs of choice for treating NMS and should be continued for 8–12 days after improvement. Antipsychotics should not be reinstituted for at least 2 weeks after complete resolution of NMS symptoms.

Page 103: *Suggested Answer*—A common adverse effect of fluoxetine includes sexual dysfunction (e.g., anorgasmia, delayed ejaculation, decreased libido), occurring in about 70% of men and women. Other common adverse effects include nausea, headache, and manifestations of CNS stimulation, including nervousness, insomnia, and anxiety. Dizziness, fatigue, and anorexia associated with weight loss are also seen in clients taking fluoxetine.

Page 109: *Suggested Answer*—The teaching plan for the medication regimen should include that lithium should be taken exactly as prescribed even if feeling "well." Other important points are:

- If a dose is missed, take as soon as remembered unless within 2 hours of next dose (6 hours if extended release).
- Medication may cause dizziness or drowsiness—do not drive or perform activities that require alertness or precision until response to medication is known.
- Low sodium levels may predispose client to toxicity; need to drink 2,000–3,000 mL of fluid each day and eat a diet with consistent and moderate sodium intake.
- Avoid excessive amounts of coffee, tea, and cola because of diuretic effect.
- Avoid activities that cause excess sodium loss—especially being exposed to summer sun, hot weather, saunas, and exertion.
- Notify healthcare professional of fever, vomiting, and diarrhea.
- Advise client that weight gain may occur—review principles of low-calorie diet.
- Instruct client to discuss any OTC medication with healthcare professional before taking.
- Advise client to use contraception—notify healthcare professional if pregnancy suspected.
- Review side effects and symptoms of toxicity with client.
- Instruct client to stop medications and report signs of toxicity to healthcare professionals promptly.
- Explain to clients with cardiovascular disease or who are over 40 years of age about the need for electrocardiogram (ECG) evaluation before and periodically during therapy. Always report fainting, irregular pulse, or difficulty breathing immediately.

Page 116: *Suggested Answer*—Common side effects of lorazepam that should be included in client teaching are daytime sedation, ataxia, dizziness, headache, blurred vision, hypotension, tremors, and slurred speech.

Page 117: *Suggested Answer*—The primary nursing priority for this client is maintaining physiological stability during the withdrawal phase. Other important priorities include to promote client safety, provide appropriate referral and follow-up, and encourage client to participate in the intervention process and become familiar with self-help, rehabilitation, and aftercare.

Chapter 5

Page 138: *Suggested Answer*—This client appears to be experiencing bronchoconstriction as evidenced by wheezing and the dusky color. The pulse oximeter reading of 88% is too low. The client's color also indicates a low oxygen level. Appropriate actions by the nurse include administration of oxygen with continuous pulse oximetry to evaluate the effects of the oxygen. Since we do not know this client's history, starting oxygen at 2 L/min via nasal cannula is appropriate in case there is a history of chronic obstructive pulmonary disease. Further actions include obtaining an order for a bronchodilator and administration of the medication. Obtaining a nursing history and keeping the client on bedrest to conserve energy are also appropriate nursing interventions.

Page 139: *Suggested Answer*—The client's theophylline level of 25 mg/dL is too high. More data are needed to determine the reason for the increased level. Dosage should be checked to be sure that the client is taking the medication as prescribed. Theophylline doses should be based on lean body weight as theophylline does not enter the adipose tissue; therefore, the proper dose should be calculated and adjusted accordingly. The reason for the elevated BUN and creatinine should be explored. Some theophylline is excreted via the kidneys; if there is renal disease, it could partially account for the increased theophylline level. A liver profile will likely be prescribed as theophylline is metabolized via the liver. The age of this client is not mentioned, but the nurse should consider the client's age (there is potential for increased sensitivity to theophylline in older adults and dosages may need to be decreased). The nurse should monitor the client for toxic effects of theophylline due to the elevated level. These include seizures, tachycardia, tremors, dizziness, hallucinations, restlessness, agitation, headaches, insomnia, nausea and vomiting, tachydysrhythmias, and chest pain. Adverse cardiac effects are not usually seen until the theophylline level exceeds 30 mg/dL. Seizure activity is not usually seen until levels exceed 40 mg/dL.

Page 142: *Suggested Answer*—The client needs to know the therapeutic action of these medications. Albuterol is given to dilate the constricted airways and can be used to prevent or treat acute bronchoconstrictive attacks. Of the two medications listed, albuterol is the one that can be taken in the event of an acute attack, as beclomethasone is preventative. The difficulty with ventilation should improve with the administration of these agents; if it does not, the client should seek medical attention. Beclomethasone is an inhaled corticosteroid and is administered to decrease inflammation in the airways. Reassure the client that inhaled corticosteroids are not as likely to cause systemic side effects as corticosteroids that are administered orally. In addition to drug actions

and intended effects, the nurse should provide information about potential side effects. Side effects of albuterol include hypotension, headaches, tremors, decreased potassium levels, increased blood glucose, nausea and vomiting, chest pain, irregular heart rhythm, restlessness, agitation, and insomnia. Side effects of beclomethasone include pharyngeal irritation, coughing, dry mouth, oral fungal infections, sore throat, and sinusitis. The client may also experience diarrhea and nausea and vomiting. The nurse should use wording that the client understands and not give too much information in the first session depending on the client's response (a client with anxiety about a new diagnosis might not hear all that is said). The basic information that is needed in this case is the way the medications work, how to take them, signs that the medications are working properly or not working properly, and potential side effects of the medications. Additional information can be given at a later date or as indicated by the individualized needs of the client.

Page 149: *Suggested Answer*—Fexofenadine is an antihistamine. It blocks the action of histamine by competing with it for receptor sites and therefore interrupts the allergic response. This medication should ease breathing and decrease allergic secretions. It is used prophylactically to decrease allergic reactions and should be taken regularly, not during an acute allergic attack. Fexofenadine is a nonsedating antihistamine that has a rapid onset after oral administration. Although it treats the symptoms, the cause of the allergic reaction should be avoided when possible. Fexofenadine may be tolerated better if taken with meals. Some side effects can include drowsiness, dry mouth, visual changes, constipation, and difficulty with urination. The client may also experience nausea and vomiting, diarrhea, dizziness, syncope, muscular weakness, unsteady gait, restlessness, and nervousness. Fluid intake should be increased to decrease the potential dry mouth effect and also to thin respiratory secretions and therefore ease expectoration. The medication should be taken exactly as prescribed. The prescriber should be contacted prior to taking any over-the-counter (OTC) medications. Alcohol and other central nervous system depressants should be avoided while on this medication. Hard, sugarless candy may help if the client has a problem with dry mouth. Prolonged exposure to the sun can cause sunburn.

Page 154: *Suggested Answer*—Dimetane-DC is an opioid antitussive medication containing brompheniramine, phenylpropanolamine, and codeine. There is a risk for respiratory depression with these medications. The client is 80 years old, which makes her more at risk for side effects, which are intensified in older adults. She may have decreased renal function and not be able to excrete the medication as readily. The client is definitely in respiratory difficulty as evidenced by a respiratory rate of 8 per minute and cyanosis. The client is also lethargic, which may be because of the narcotic but also could be related to decreased oxygenation and increased CO_2 levels. The client should be started on oxygen, and oxygen saturation should be measured continuously. Respiratory effort should be monitored. Arterial blood gases should be drawn, and a workup should be done to determine the cause of the cough. No more antitussive agents should be administered. The client will likely have a chest x-ray and be admitted to the hospital for possible intubation and mechanical ventilation. The daughter and the client (when she is more responsive) should be taught about the adverse effects of opioid antitussive medications and the time limits on their use (2 weeks is too long). The underlying reason for the cough (such as respiratory disease) should be determined. The client should be assessed for liver, renal, thyroid, and adrenal diseases as any of these can intensify the effects of opioid antitussive medications. The nurse should also obtain a history as to the concurrent use of central nervous system depressants such as alcohol and antianxiety agents, as these can intensify the effects of opioid antitussive medications.

Chapter 6

Page 169: *Suggested Answer*—OTC diet pills contain many unknown chemicals that might interact with transdermal nitroglycerin, an anti-anginal medication. This could put the client at risk for additional cardiac problems. The client should be praised for wanting to lose the weight, but advise her to contact the prescriber prior to taking OTC medications.

Page 173: *Suggested Answer*—Your client may be experiencing an adverse reaction to the beta-adrenergic blocking medication. The beta$_2$ receptors in the lungs are probably being affected. Evaluate the vital signs, check the pulse oximetry, and notify the prescriber. Be prepared to take further actions as prescribed to relieve the client's symptoms and increase gas exchange.

Page 175: *Suggested Answer*—Assess the vital signs, including heart rate, BP, respiratory rate, and mental status. Assess whether the client is experiencing any chest pain. The diltiazem drip is a calcium channel blocker and may be causing a second-degree, Mobitz I heart block. Reduce the rate of the diltiazem drip by half if allowed by a standard protocol order set and agency policy and notify the prescriber. Do not leave the client alone.

Page 184: *Suggested Answer*—Turn off the infusion pump; remove the tubing but maintain a patent IV site with a saline lock or an NS infusion directly into the site. *Do not use the tubing containing the sodium nitroprusside.* The client is experiencing profound hypotension with compensatory tachycardia from the nitroprusside drip. Notify the prescriber urgently. Assess the client's vital signs, including mental status, HR, and BP. Maintain an airway and the IV site, and monitor the client continuously.

Page 185: *Suggested Answer*—The client may be experiencing digitalis toxicity. Assess vital signs including mental status, heart rate, and blood pressure. Discuss the need to obtain a digoxin level and potassium with the prescriber. If necessary, draw the venous blood sample and send to the laboratory. Ask the client if he or she is taking other medications that might have interacted with digoxin.

Chapter 7

Page 214: *Suggested Answer*—The nurse must teach a client who has been placed on anticoagulation therapy that this treatment regimen will require close follow-up and long-term monitoring. Explain that the anticoagulant medication will make the client more susceptible to bleeding. Provide safety instructions about how to prevent bleeding episodes, such as using soft toothbrushes, electric razors, and avoiding trauma. Explain potential drug and food interactions. Discuss with the client that compliance with the treatment regimen is important to help the client achieve health goals. Provide verbal and written instruction to the client to enhance understanding and provide a reference postdischarge.

Page 217: *Suggested Answer*—Low-dose aspirin (ASA) therapy is used as a "blood thinner" for its antiplatelet effect. The dosage used is normally one baby ASA or 81 mg per day. The normal adult dose of 650 mg q 4–6 hours is used to treat fever, aches, and pains. Since the client will be taking ASA, the nurse should have the client consult with the healthcare provider about whether acetaminophen or an NSAID should be used for aches and pains. Taking too much ASA can lead to potential health consequences such as ASA toxicity. Gastrointestinal hemorrhage can occur with the prolonged use of ASA at high doses. The client can always be referred back to the prescriber to clarify the intended dose in writing.

Page 219: *Suggested Answer*—Nursing interventions aimed at preventing or reducing the likelihood of increased bleeding would include (1) minimizing the number of injections, (2) coordinating lab draws to avoid increased risk, (3) applying pressure after venipuncture and lab draws, (4) maintaining aseptic technique and limiting (if possible) the number of invasive procedures, (5) taking vital signs (using automatic blood pressure cuffs), and (6) continued assessment for possible bleeding sources (internal, retroperitoneal, intracranial, and gastrointestinal). The nurse must monitor the client closely and keep in close communication with the healthcare provider.

Page 223: *Suggested Answer*—It is important to know how long the topical agent has been in contact with the client's skin because there can be potential for skin damage upon removal of the agent. If the area is dry, then the nurse should irrigate the area gently with normal saline to minimize tissue irritation. Consult the healthcare provider or the pharmacist regarding removal and application procedures if needed.

Page 232: *Suggested Answer*—Since anemia is a broad category and is sometimes a symptom of an illness as well as a disease entity, medication alone may not restore adequate blood cell levels to correct anemia. Medication in conjunction with adequate dietary sources is a very effective treatment plan. However, it would be important to verify the type of anemia that the client has in order to fully explore the answer. Clients who have vitamin B_{12}, folic acid, and iron-deficiency anemias can be treated successfully with combination diet and medication therapy in order to restore adequate blood cell levels.

Page 238: *Suggested Answer*—Cholesterol-lowering medications should be taken at bedtime because the body normally performs the function of cholesterol synthesis at night. If the body were normally undergoing that function, using the medication at that time would increase its biologic effect and efficiency.

Chapter 8

Page 249: *Suggested Answer*—The nurse should teach the client to report tinnitus, hearing impairment, deafness, vertigo, or sense of fullness in the ears as signs of drug-induced ototoxicity.

Page 253: *Suggested Answer*—Because spironolactone is a potassium-sparing diuretic that is often used to manage hypertension and induce diuresis in other fluid-retaining disorders, the nurse should assess the client's blood pressure, fluid balance, and weight (weight loss may occur from loss of excess fluid volume). The nurse should also question the client about possible signs of hyperkalemia.

Page 257: *Suggested Answer*—Client teaching about potassium supplements should include sitting upright when taking dose, take dose with meals to decrease GI irritation, take dose exactly as prescribed, avoid salt substitutes (high in potassium) while taking a potassium supplement, and notify prescriber of adverse effects such as confusion, irregular heartbeat, shortness of breath, anxiety, excessive fatigue, weakness of legs, or numbness of feet, fingers, or lips.

Page 261: *Suggested Answer*—Although the antibiotic must be taken for the full course of therapy, phenazopyridine can be stopped once symptoms of UTI resolve (usually 24–48 hours) because it is a urinary analgesic. It discolors the urine because it is reddish-orange and may stain undergarments. The main side effects are headache, nausea, GI distress and sometimes vertigo.

Page 262: *Suggested Answer*—Finasteride works by blocking alpha-1 receptors in the prostate gland. This leads to relaxation of prostate smooth muscle, which in turn improves the ability to urinate and reduces symptoms of hesitancy, weak urine stream, and incomplete bladder emptying.

Chapter 9

Page 277: *Suggested Answer*—The client should contact a healthcare provider if diarrhea lasts longer than 2 days, which will allow the healthcare provider to rule out any infectious or colonic disorder.

Page 287: *Suggested Answer*—Misoprostol can cause miscarriage. This information is vital for the pregnant client to be aware of so that she can make informed decisions about whether or not to take this medication.

Page 289: *Suggested Answer*—The nurse should assess swallowing ability, which can be impaired in some clients after stroke. Certain proton pump inhibitors must be swallowed whole whereas others may be opened and sprinkled on applesauce.

Chapter 10

Page 305: *Suggested Answer*—The nurse should assess the client for signs of hypersensitivity, which include any of the following: rash, urticaria, angioedema, and difficulty breathing. Hypersensitivity reaction is a medical emergency and must be assessed for and treated promptly.

Page 305: *Suggested Answer*—The nurse should ensure that the client has prescriptions to obtain a complete blood count (CBC) with differential and platelet count prior to therapy with colony-stimulating factors. They should also be measured following the administration of medication. The nurse should report a neutrophil count of 20,000/mm^3 to healthcare provider. If the CBC, particularly hematocrit, is rising rapidly (greater than 4% in 2 weeks), assess carefully for hypertension and seizure activity.

Page 310: *Suggested Answer*—The following items should be considered when determining learning objectives for a client who will be receiving immunosuppressant agents:

1. Educate regarding the prevention of infection (e.g., avoid overcrowded areas or people with known infections, take in adequate nutrition, maintain good hygiene practices).
2. Educate regarding all laboratory studies that should be conducted, such as CBC, platelet count, and renal and liver function.
3. Educate regarding supportive care for flulike symptoms.
4. Educate regarding action, side effects, and nursing implications of medications being administered.

Page 315: *Suggested Answer*—The following items should be incorporated into client teaching during an outbreak of hepatitis A:

1. Hepatitis A is transmitted by fecal–oral route.
2. Instruct on proper hygiene and sanitation.
3. Instruct on proper food preparation.
4. Hepatitis A transmission occurs from person-to-person contact and has been noted in areas with overcrowding, such as schools or daycare centers.

Page 319: *Suggested Answer*—The following nursing interventions should be implemented to relieve flulike symptoms caused by medications used to treat multiple sclerosis:

1. Administer acetaminophen for relief of pain or fever.
2. Provide adequate fluid intake to prevent dehydration.

3. Assess intake and output every 8 hours.
4. Provide adequate rest to promote healing.
5. Assess vital signs every 4 hours and administer anti-pyretic agents for temperatures over 101°F.

Chapter 11

Page 339: *Suggested Answer*—Assess number and characteristics of stools, abdominal cramping, if there is newly developed fever, and length of time on antibiotic therapy. If pseudomembranous colitis is suspected, arrange for a stool specimen for culture and sensitivity for *Clostridium difficile*. If specimen is positive for *C. difficile*, collaborate with the prescriber about discontinuing the antibiotic, initiating therapy with vancomycin PO or IV or with metronidazole to treat the pseudomonas colitis, and maintaining fluid and electrolyte balance. If the diarrhea is mild and no *C. difficile* is present, the antibiotic may be continued, and an absorbent antidiarrheal such as kaolin and pectin may be prescribed. Monitoring hydration status and potassium level will be important. Provide for good hygiene.

Page 354: *Suggested Answer*—Take tetracycline on an empty stomach with a full glass of water. Take 1 hour before and 2 hours after meals, and avoid ingestion of milk or milk products or antacids, which would interfere with drug efficacy. If the client is taking oral contraceptives, advise use of an alternative contraceptive method during therapy and for 1 month after discontinuation of tetracycline (which interferes with effectiveness of oral contraceptives). Breakthrough bleeding may occur as well. Report severe side effects and clinical manifestations of Candida infection. Avoid direct sunlight and ultraviolet lights including tanning beds because of risk for photosensitivity. If in the sun, advise client to wear long sleeves, long-legged pants, hat, and sunglasses. Sunscreen and sunblocks may be used but may not prevent a photosensitivity reaction. Teach the client to store tetracycline in a tightly covered container protected from moisture and light. Keep health care appointments for follow-up exams and tests.

Page 356: *Suggested Answer*—Peak and trough laboratory findings guide dosage and dosing schedule for certain drugs such as vancomycin. Changes will be prescribed based on these findings and the client's clinical manifestations. Apparently, the trough level was low and so the dosing frequency was increased from every 8 hours to every 6 hours. The dosage may also have been increased. If the trough is low, the therapeutic drug level is not being maintained, which could limit therapeutic effectiveness and allow microorganisms to replicate, causing continuation or exacerbation of the infection. Explain the rationale for the change to the client. Ask for clarification of what the client means by "tied down," and facilitate the client's exploration of possible options to not being "tied down." Client adherence is necessary for effective outcomes.

Page 369: *Suggested Answer*—Explain to the client that taking the acyclovir before symptoms occur better enables the antiviral drug to be effective in reducing the viral load and preventing complications. The drug's efficacy is best when the virus is residing in the body's cells and before the virus is released from the cell. The drug's effectiveness will diminish over time, but its effectiveness is optimized with early introduction, as evidenced by persons with HIV not becoming symptomatic for longer periods. There are other antiviral agents available that are used in combination for future needs and to retard development of drug resistance. Offer to arrange for the client to discuss the treatment strategy with the prescriber if concerns persist.

Page 372: *Suggested Answer*—Xerostomia is dryness of the mouth. Amantadine, an antiviral, is also an anticholinergic agent that can cause dry mucous membranes, such as in the mouth. Oral care is important for comfort and also to protect the integrity of the oral cavity that harbors pathogenic microorganisms. Frequent mouth rinses with water or warm saline solution can be refreshing and cleansing. Avoid hydrogen peroxide and commercial mouthwashes that contain alcohol because both can contribute further to mouth dryness. Sucking on hard candy may stimulate secretion of saliva, and there are artificial saliva products available. Keep the client hydrated.

Page 376: *Suggested Answer*—Determine first what the client means by "stuff" (the drug, the central line, or some other concern) and what the client's understanding is of the "bad things that can happen." Based on the client's response, reaffirm the purpose of the therapy and explain how risks or possible deleterious effects are minimized. For example, explain that premedication is provided to mitigate adverse reactions of amphotericin B, including antiemetic, antihistamine, and antipyretic agents. Analgesics are available if needed to maintain comfort as well. The client will also be hydrated before, during, and after the antifungal administration that will facilitate removal of toxins. Allow the client to verbalize concerns. Offer to arrange for the client to discuss concerns further with the prescriber if necessary. The client may prefer not to be alone, so arrange for someone (family, friend, pastoral care, volunteer) to be with the client during the drug administration, if possible. Prudent nursing interventions can help this acutely ill client through a difficult time of treatment.

Chapter 12

Page 395: *Suggested Answer*—Three measures to prevent renal toxicity secondary to cisplatin administration include the following:

1. Assess BUN and creatinine before administration and periodically during treatment.
2. Provide adequate intravenous or oral hydration (1,000–1,500 mL in 6–8 hours) before administration.
3. Administer mannitol or furosemide to promote diuresis as prescribed.

Page 397: *Suggested Answer*—To prevent or decrease the severity of stomatitis:

1. Promote oral hygiene before meals and at bedtime with fluorinated toothpaste, a soft-bristled toothbrush, and diluted baking soda rinse.
2. Assess oral cavity daily and report any redness, irritation, or white patches observed (monilia).
3. Teach the client to report soreness at the first sign of irritation.

Page 401: *Suggested Answer*—Before administering a chemotherapeutic drug that is a vesicant:

1. Ensure that IV site was not started more than 48 hours before administration.
2. Assess IV site for any redness or irritation, and restart if present.
3. Assess blood return and ensure that the vein is easily accessible and full.
4. Remove opaque or gauze dressing from the site to provide clear visualization during administration.
5. Ensure IV site is not positioned in the area of a joint (with underlying tendons and nerves nearby) or on the dorsal side of the hand.

Page 404: *Suggested Answer*—To prevent constipation related to chemotherapy with vinca or plant alkaloid medications:

1. Assess client's usual bowel history prior to administration.
2. Provide a high-fiber diet.
3. Obtain a prescription for stool softeners at least twice daily.
4. Auscultate bowel sounds and assess for bowel movement Q shift.
5. Obtain a prescription for laxatives if the client has no bowel movement by 48 hours after administration.

Page 409: *Suggested Answer*—Measures to reduce the potential for infection after chemotherapy administration include:

1. Take oral temperature at the same time every day and report to healthcare provider if greater than or equal to 101°F.
2. Maintain oral hygiene before meals and at bedtime.
3. Avoid eating raw fruits and vegetables.
4. Avoid proximity to fresh flowers or plants.
5. Refrain from emptying boxes filled with kitty litter or fish tanks or aquariums.
6. Avoid large crowds and young children and those with known infections.

Chapter 13

Page 428: *Suggested Answer*—A cold (rhinitis) or upper respiratory infection may decrease the effectiveness of this therapy. The nurse should advise the client to notify the prescribing healthcare provider. The client should also be advised to contact the nurse again if there is any increase in urine output.

Page 430: *Suggested Answer*—Clients taking mineralocorticoid therapy are instructed to weigh themselves and notify the nurse if there is a weekly gain of more than 5 lbs (mineralocorticoids can alter fluid and electrolyte balance). Since this client has gained 5½ lbs in 2 days, the nurse should assess vital signs, edema, lung sounds, and skin to gather additional data related to fluid overload. Once the nurse has a comprehensive picture, the information should be reported to the prescriber.

Page 432: *Suggested Answer*—The nurse should encourage the client to carry or wear some type of medic alert identification. If the client should become ill or injured, the health information contained in this identification will have an impact on treatment. The most common side effects of glucocorticoid therapy are mental status changes, including affect, mood, behavior, aggression, and depression. Clients taking glucocorticoids should have medic alert identification in the event that they become mentally incapacitated and cannot care for themselves temporarily.

Page 434: *Suggested Answer*—Increased effects of anticoagulant therapy can result when taken with thyroid medications. The nurse should monitor the client's prothrombin time (PT) or International Normalized Ratio (INR) to determine whether the warfarin is being maintained in an appropriate dosage range.

Page 437: *Suggested Answer*—Digoxin toxicity and increased risk of dysrhythmias may result when digoxin and calcium supplements are taken together. Thus, the nurse should monitor serum digoxin levels and look for early signs of digoxin toxicity, such as anorexia and nausea. The nurse should also observe the cardiac monitor (if in use) for dysrhythmias or look for an irregular pulse or change in pulse rate of a client who does not have a cardiac monitor in place.

Page 439: *Suggested Answer*—A musculoskeletal assessment needs to be performed, including inspection and gentle palpation of the vertebral column, particularly the lower thoracic and lumbar vertebrae. Back pain along with restriction of spinal movement and tenderness could be related to one or more compression fractures. Fractures in the distal end of the radius and the upper third of the femur may also occur.

Page 441: *Suggested Answer*—Insulin not in use should be refrigerated. Temperatures less than 36°F or greater than 86°F need to be avoided and all insulin should be kept away from direct heat and light. A slight loss of potency may occur if the bottle has been in use for more than 30 days, even when the expiration date has not been passed. Therefore, a spare bottle of insulin should always be available.

Page 443: *Suggested Answer*—The client's healthcare provider needs to be notified. Also, the client needs to monitor blood glucose level at least every 4 hours and test urine for ketones if the blood glucose level is greater than 240 mg/dL. Also, the client should continue to take regularly prescribed insulin or oral antidiabetic agents and sip sugar-free liquids to total 8–12 ounces every hour if possible.

Page 446: *Suggested Answer*—The nurse needs to assess the client's financial status and initiate an immediate social service referral to determine what resources may be available. The American Diabetes Association (ADA) has a toll-free phone number (800-232-2383) in the United States) and will refer a diabetic client to the appropriate agencies or resources. The American Association of Diabetes Educators (800-338-3633) can also refer a diabetic client to a certified diabetes educator in the client's own area.

Chapter 14

Page 457: *Suggested Answer*—Instructions on use of estradiol depend on the route. Oral doses should be taken at the same time each day; doses should not be skipped or missed since this therapy is hormone replacement. A transdermal patch should be changed as prescribed and applied to intact skin on a clean, dry area on the trunk of the body (including buttocks and abdomen), not over a skin area that has any type of impairment. For intravaginal use, the client should squeeze the prescribed amount of cream into the applicator and insert the cream deep into the vagina one to three times per week as directed. The client should remain recumbent for at least 30 minutes and preferably use at bedtime to retain medication for a longer time. The client should not douche.

Page 459: *Suggested Answer*—Include these points when providing information about testosterone enanthate:

1. Secondary sex characteristics such as pubic, axillary, chest, and facial hair; deepening voice; and enlargement of the testes and penis will begin to develop.
2. Testosterone can cause premature closure of the epiphyseal plates with subsequent loss of potential adult height; therefore, the healthcare provider may prescribe wrist x-rays every 6 months to monitor for this condition.
3. Acne may develop.
4. Libido may increase.

Page 460: *Suggested Answer*—Laboratory studies that will be prescribed include liver function tests to detect hepatotoxicity and HIV and hepatitis B and C panels because of possible needle sharing.

Page 463: *Suggested Answer*—Other medications can be used, such tadalafil and vardenafil. In addition, alprostadil is available IV and in transurethral pellets.

Page 466: *Suggested Answer*—Questions to ask a client considering combination oral contraceptive therapy may include:

1. Has she ever had a deep vein thrombus (DVT), embolus, myocardial infarction (MI), or cerebrovascular accident (CVA)?
2. Is she taking any other medications, especially antibiotics and antiepileptics?
3. When was her last monthly period? Could she be pregnant at this time?

Chapter 15

Page 485: *Suggested Answer*—Assess the "diaper rash" before presenting a teaching plan. Take a history of the rash, the infant's usual foods, and the usual skin care the infant is now receiving. There can be several reasons for diaper rash (e.g., remaining in diaper too long, overingestion of a food to which the child is sensitive, or some topical agent the mother is using). It also might be caused by a substance being used elsewhere, such as at a childcare center. Sensitizers could be in soap, "baby wipes," topical powders, ointments, and even diapers. Thus, the first step is to eliminate any food and any topical substance being used that seem likely to be sensitizers. The interventions aimed at restoring intact skin should be as simple as possible. There are skin protectants that might be helpful, such as vitamins A and D–medicated diaper rash ointment or zinc ointment. However, these are unlikely to be helpful if the culprit is a food. Directions for any topical preparation should be followed closely (e.g., "thicker is not better"). Exposure of the skin to air for 15 minutes four times a day can be helpful in drying out a rash. If the steps are followed and there is no improvement after 7 days, a healthcare provider should be seen, since it could be a different problem, such as a fungal infection.

Page 487: *Suggested Answer*—The cousin needs advice on a photoprotection program. Sunscreens are a key ingredient in such a program and should be applied 30 minutes before exposure. Probably a strong sunscreen with a SPF of 15 or above would be prudent in this situation. Reapplication may be advisable after swimming or sweating. A broad-brimmed hat shields the face, neck, and ears. Planning to do outdoor activities early in the morning (before 10:00 A.M.) or late in the afternoon (after 3:00 P.M.) is a simple form of photoprotection.

Page 488: *Suggested Answer*—A typical client with head lice (pediculosis capitis) has few, if any, easily observable signs of infestation. The child may complain of itching around the ears and over the sides of the neck, but these changes occur so gradually that clients frequently give them little attention.

Nits represent eggs cemented to the side of hairs, and they cannot be removed easily. Lice are spread from human to human by direct physical contact and through fomites.

A shampoo with permethrin, lindane 1%, or pyrethrin and piperonyl butoxide combination would be used to treat pediculosis capitis. Lindane is the least desirable product for children because of risk of seizures. A nit comb is usually packaged with the shampoo and is used to contribute to the removal of nits from the hair. Even if no nits are visible, the shampoo can be used in case they are present. All potentially contaminated articles of clothing, bedding, and personal hygiene products need to be disinfected. For head lice, the focus would be brushes, combs, hats, scarves, and coats. Items can be treated with rubbing alcohol or placed in home dishwasher. Towels, sheets, pillowcases, and bedding should be laundered in hot water. Items that are difficult to clean can be placed in a sealed plastic bag for at least 48 hours (lice need blood to survive and cannot live long away from host). It is not necessary to fumigate the house to rid the client of head lice.

Page 489: *Suggested Answer*—The client should use a topical product that contains salicylic acid to treat the wart. The product should be used as per its directions. General foot hygiene measures should be followed, including proper washing and drying of feet, wearing clean socks that are changed daily, and making sure to wear shoes (rather than go barefoot). If the wart does not heal within the time specified on the product directions, further treatment should be sought.

Chapter 16

Page 514: *Suggested Answer*—Oral acetazolamide may cause gastrointestinal (GI) side effects such as anorexia, nausea and vomiting, and weight loss. To reduce risk of GI side effects, teach the client to take the medication with food or milk. Because acetazolamide also causes diuresis, instruct the client to take medication early in the day to avoid nocturia. Acetazolamide may also exacerbate renal stones. Unless contraindicated, the client should consume at least 2,000 mL of fluid per day and a diet high in potassium and low in sodium. The client should also maintain follow-up visits to monitor for fluid and electrolyte imbalances.

Page 515: *Suggested Answer*—Instruct the client to administer pilocarpine 1 hour after the administration of latanoprost. Inform client of side effects such as blurred vision, photophobia, burning, stinging, and itching. Latanoprost may also cause an increase in iris pigmentation. The client should remove contact lenses before use and leave them out for 15 minutes after medication instillation.

Page 518: *Suggested Answer*—The eye needs to be cleansed of crust and drainage before administering the ophthalmic solution. To properly clean the eye, use a cotton ball moistened with sterile normal saline or other prescribed solution. Wipe the eye from the inner canthus toward the outer canthus. To avoid contamination of the other eye, use a separate cotton ball for each eye. Clean both the eyelid and eyelashes.

Page 520: *Suggested Answer*—Proparacaine hydrochloride temporarily causes a loss of the blink reflex due to the effects of anesthesia. To protect the cornea, an eye patch is applied until the blink reflex returns. Instruct the client to avoid touching or rubbing the eye until the anesthesia has worn off. Because the client had a foreign body removed, instructions also include reporting drainage, severe irritation, delayed healing, or any other symptoms that may indicate an infection.

Page 522: *Suggested Answer*—Initially, the client's ear canal should be examined to determine the presence of cerumen or edema, which would prevent the flow of medication into the canal. If cerumen is present, it is removed by the clinician. If edema is present, a wick may be inserted to allow absorption of the medication. If the ear canal is clear, evaluate the client's administration technique. Instruct the client to pull the pinna up and back, tilt head toward the unaffected side, or lie on the side with the affected ear up. After the medication is instilled, allow time for the medication to flow into the ear canal by remaining in the position for 2–3 minutes.

➤ *Case Study Suggested Answers*

Chapter 1

1. The nurse should always be concerned when a new drug is added to a client's regimen. There are no significant interactions between metoprolol and furosemide, but if the client is taking ibuprofen with regularity or frequency, it many decrease the effect of metoprolol. Phenytoin many increase the effects of warfarin and furosemide. It is important to review drug literature for any drug–drug interactions when a new medication is prescribed for a client.

2. Protein-binding plays a very significant role in the above interactions. The portion of a drug bound to protein is not biologically active in the body. Warfarin is a highly protein-bound drug (99%), meaning 99% of the drug is bound to albumin and only 1% of the drug is free and biologically active. Phenytoin is 95% protein bound, furosemide 95%, and metoprolol 12%. So when phenytoin is added to the medication regimen, there will be competition for the protein sites and some of the other drugs may be displaced from albumin binding sites, which results in greater percentage of free drug. Since furosemide and warfarin are also highly protein bound, this may lead to more biological action of these medications and could contribute to toxicity.

3. Metoprolol: monitor for bradycardia, hypotension, signs of heart failure, fatigue, and dizziness. Furosemide: monitor for increased diuresis, dehydration, hyponatremia, hypokalemia, weakness, and fatigue. Warfarin: monitor for signs of increased bleeding such as nosebleeds, petechiae, and increased ecchymosis and bleeding from venipuncture sites. Phenytoin: monitor for rash, bradycardia, and confusion.

4. It is important to monitor CBC, platelets, prothrombin time, electrolyte levels (in particular sodium and potassium), and liver and renal function tests. It would also be important to check the albumin level; if this is decreased, there will be fewer protein-binding sites, and a greater risk for higher levels of free drug and toxicity. Because the client is an older adult, it would be important to check the albumin level and liver and renal function tests, as they may be decreased.

5. There are important nursing considerations related to phenytoin administration. Phenytoin should not be administered with high-protein meals, as this may interfere with drug absorption. Phenytoin levels should be monitored with initial therapy and periodically for toxicity. Assess client for rash and signs of gingival hyperplasia (a common adverse effect with long-term therapy). Monitor labs for thrombocytopenia and agranulocytosis).

Chapter 2

1. Possible unintended effects of St. John's wort are GI distress, fatigue, pruritus, weight gain, headache, dizziness, restlessness, and photosensitivity. Possible unintended effects of garlic are contact dermatitis, vertigo, garlic breath, hypothyroidism, GI irritation, and nausea and vomiting (with large doses). Possible unintended effects of gingko biloba are, in large doses, restlessness, headache, nausea and vomiting, and diarrhea.

2. Concerns related to this combination of herbs include increased risk for GI distress or nausea and vomiting (all three herbs) and headache (St John's wort and gingko biloba). Gingko biloba and garlic should not be used together because both play a role in blood clotting and could increase the risk for bleeding. Specifically, the terpene lactones in ginkgo biloba inhibit the platelet-activating factor, which can increase bleeding time. Garlic also inhibits platelet aggregation and could prolong bleeding.

3. The client will need to inform the surgeon of his use of these herbal products. He will need to stop use of the ginkgo for 2 weeks prior to surgery to reduce his risk for bleeding postoperatively. Garlic has a very transient effect (only a few hours) on blood clotting; he should stop use of the garlic a few days prior to surgery.

4. The client should be taught to refrain from resuming herbal therapy until completely recovered from surgery and advised by the healthcare provider, since many medications can interact with herbal agents. In particular, herbs that may play a role in blood clotting should be avoided, including bilberry, garlic, ginger, and gingko. If he will be on any anticoagulant or platelet aggregate inhibitor medication, he will need to remain off these supplements while taking these medications because this would increase the risk for bleeding. The client should be taught to report any unusual bleeding or bruising. St. John's wort should not be used concomitantly with opioids or other CNS depressants because it could contribute to serotonin syndrome. Since he may be given these types of medications postoperatively, there would be an increased risk. He should also avoid use of alcohol, OTC cold and flu preparations, and foods containing tyramine, as they could cause a hypertensive crisis. St. John's wort can also cause photosensitivity and precautions should be taken when exposed to direct sunlight.

Chapter 3

1. Questions to ask the family upon arrival should include:
   - When did the client have his last seizure?
   - When did the client last take his seizure medication?
   - What other medications is the client taking, both prescription and nonprescription?
   - Is the client currently experiencing an unusual amount of stress?

2. Initial assessments should include level of consciousness (LOC), mental status, and vital signs. These provide a baseline measurement of the client's neurologic, cardiac, and respiratory status.

3. The priorities of care for the client while he is in the emergency department include to keep him seizure-free and explore why the client experienced the seizure.

4. The client education points that are of highest priority prior to discharge home include:
   - Medication regimen including dose, schedule, side effects, and adverse effects
   - When to call healthcare provider
   - The importance of always taking prescribed medication
   - Healthcare follow-up needed to ensure therapeutic dosage levels

5. Medications or foods that could interfere with the client's antiepileptic medication include:
   - Phenytoin: alcohol, antacids, antineoplastics, and antihistamines (*Note:* The only foods that interfere with phenytoin are tube feedings, which do not apply to this client.)
   - Phenobarbital: theophylline, corticosteroids, and doxycycline

Chapter 4

1. Some significant concerns are the client's lack of access to medical care and the need to maintain a consistent diet and water intake. Sudden changes in sodium intake may alter lithium resorption, which would change the amount of drug that is available in the bloodstream. Since lithium has such a narrow therapeutic blood level, this places her at a greater risk to develop lithium toxicity. A decrease in water intake could also alter the lithium balance. Since she will be camping in the Southwest, a concern for potential for dehydration is significant. The increased heat and physical exertion can predispose her to increased loss of body fluids and sodium through sweating. A constant level of sodium and fluid intake is important to avoid any fluctuation in lithium level. She will most likely need to increase fluid and sodium intake if she does a lot of hiking and is sweating.

2. The client needs to be aware of the potential for increased fluid and sodium loss while engaging in camping activities. The healthcare provider should explore with her how she plans to have sufficient water available each day and discuss what kinds of foods she will be eating. The sodium content of the food should be similar to what she consumes currently, since she has been well controlled for the past 6 months, but she may need to increase intake to compensate for increased losses with sweating. It is important for her to remain hydrated (2–3 liters/day or more if sweating) and maintain sufficient salt intake to keep lithium level stable and prevent lithium toxicity.

3. The client should be alert to these common adverse effects of lithium: increased thirst, frequent urination, nausea, fine hand tremors, and muscle weakness.
4. The client should be alert for these signs of lithium toxicity:slurred speech, unsteady gait, weakness, drowsiness, diarrhea, vomiting, confusion, hyperirritability of muscles, and irregular heartbeat.
5. Other client teaching points include:
   - Avoid alcohol and caffeine-containing food and beverages such as coffee, tea, and chocolate, as these can increase lithium excretion.
   - Avoid over-the-counter products containing NSAIDs, except aspirin, as they can decrease renal clearance of lithium.
   - Maintain an intake of 2,000–3,000mL/day of fluid.
   - If signs of toxicity develop, an increase of sodium and/or fluid intake may be needed.
   - If diarrhea should occur, take measures to correct this and increase fluid intake.

Chapter 5

1. Albuterol is a beta-adrenergic agent that is given orally or by inhalation and is used to treat and prevent bronchoconstriction. Albuterol dilates constricted airways to ease breathing and should be taken exactly as prescribed. Beta$_2$-specific actions may be diminished at larger-than-prescribed doses. Therefore, the client may experience cardiac symptoms such as increased heart rate and, at larger doses, she may also experience nausea, anxiety, and tremors. Albuterol effects can be intensified by decongestants and some antihistamines. The prescriber should be notified prior to taking any OTC medications. Some clients experience hypotension and vascular headaches with albuterol. The client should have blood pressure and heart rate monitored regularly to ensure there are no cardiac side effects. She should be taught the proper use of an inhaler. The client should note the color, amount, and character of sputum. Oral doses of this medication should be taken with meals to decrease gastric upset. She should keep a record of when medications are taken and whether or not symptoms subside to determine the medication effectiveness. Inhalations of different medications should be taken at least 1 minute apart or longer depending on product literature. The client should avoid eye contact with the spray of an inhaled medication. Wheezing and dyspnea should decrease with the administration of this medication; if not, the prescriber should be notified. She should take the inhaler to school with her so that it can be used as needed in the event of an acute asthmatic attack. She should begin to note which allergens cause her difficulty and attempt to avoid them. Also, increased fluid intake will help liquefy any secretions and ease expectoration.
2. Beclomethasone is an inhaled corticosteroid that is thought to decrease the release of bronchoconstricting substances. Swelling in the airways is thought to diminish. This medication is to be used preventatively and not for an acute attack. She should take the medication whether or not symptoms are present. Inhaled corticosteroids are not as likely to cause the typical systemic effects of oral corticosteroids. Symptoms of a cold or the flu should be reported to the provider immediately due to the potential for suppression of the immune system. Again, this is less likely with inhaled corticosteroids than with oral corticosteroids. Allergens should be identified and avoided. She should be aware of symptoms and notice any increase or decrease. Difficulty should be reported to the healthcare provider. She should be taught to note the amount, color, and character of sputum. Increased fluid intake helps thin secretions and ease removal. Hard candy decreases difficulty with mouth dryness. She should wear a bracelet that identifies her medication. The medication should be taken exactly as prescribed and not overused. The medication should not be stopped abruptly. The correct use of the inhaler should be taught as well as the need to rinse the mouth after inhalation of medication.
3. It is important for the nurse to understand the needs of an adolescent client. Acceptance by and being similar to the peer group is very important to the 14-year-old. Exploring how the client can self-administer medications without making her appear different from her peers would be beneficial. Another aspect to consider is that adolescents are normally healthy. Sickness in an adolescent makes the young person different from the norm. Attempting to help the client incorporate the illness into her self-concept will aid in acceptance as well as compliance. The nurse should respond with compassionate understanding of the real issues faced by the client. Assisting her to determine ways that she can participate in the normal activities of a 14-year-old in spite of her illness will help with acceptance and compliance.
4. The anticipated effect of albuterol is to dilate the airway and ease breathing. With proper medication use, she should experience less wheezing and dyspnea. Some of the side effects of albuterol are listed in the answer to question 1. Additional side effects include tremors, hypokalemia, hyperglycemia, nausea and vomiting, chest pain, dysrhythmias, paradoxical bronchospasms, and urinary retention. The anticipated effect of beclomethasone is to decrease inflammation of the airway and therefore ease breathing. She should notice a decrease in the symptoms of dyspnea and wheezing. Potential side effects include pharyngeal irritation, coughing, dry mouth, oral fungal infections, sore throat, and sinusitis. Some clients experience diarrhea, nausea and vomiting, and stomach upset. Menstrual disturbances are possible and should be reported to the prescriber.
5. The nurse should assess respiratory function, talk to the client about the disease, and assess her acceptance of the disease and treatment. The nurse should determine whether or not medications are taken regularly and

properly. It would be helpful to observe the client self-administer inhaled medication to be sure her technique is appropriate. Determine whether or not the client is experiencing any side effects. Explore her thoughts and feelings about the disease and its treatment and about whether or not medications are controlling the symptoms. Determine whether or not she can participate in activities that are important to her. Talk to her about whether or not she feels accepted by her friends and if she has any feelings about being different from her friends. This will provide information about her acceptance of the disease and her tolerance not only of the disease, but of the treatment as well. Acceptance of the disease and its treatment will aid in adherence.

Chapter 6

1. The nurse should assess the client's cardiac rhythm (amiodarone) and blood pressure (atenolol and morphine) and should be aware of the client's baseline coagulation studies, such as PTT (heparin and aspirin). Although not directly related to administration of the prescribed medications, the nurse would also want to assess whether the client is having chest pain or whether it was relieved by the morphine administered in the ED.

2. Amiodarone is a Class III antidysrhythmic that exerts its effects by blocking potassium channels in myocardial cells. It is commonly used to treat ventricular dysrhythmias that can occur during and after myocardial infarction. Aspirin is an antipyretic and analgesic drug and has antiplatelet properties. It is used in this client for its antiplatelet effect to help prevent the propagation of the thrombus that has formed in the affected coronary artery. Heparin is an anticoagulant drug that interferes with the clotting cascade and is also used to prevent further thrombus formation. Morphine is an opioid analgesic that acts on the central nervous system to provide pain relief. It also causes arterial and venous vasodilation, so it may help reduce cardiac preload and afterload.

3. Nursing implications of amiodarone are to monitor the cardiac rhythm and BP during infusion and to titrate the dose using prescribed protocols to prevent hypotension and bradycardia. Nursing implications of aspirin and heparin are to assess the client for bleeding and to monitor results of CBC and coagulation studies such as PTT. Nursing implications of atenolol are to monitor BP, check pulse before each dose, and withhold dose and consult with prescriber if pulse is less than 60/minute.

4. Because the client is in a highly stressful situation (life-threatening health event and admission to ICU), the nurse should provide medication explanations in simple terms and expect that the client will need to have explanations repeated because of situational anxiety. The nurse should explain that morphine was given to relieve chest pain and to let the nurse know immediately if pain recurs; amiodarone will help regulate the heart rhythm by treating dysrhythmias that often accompany MI; aspirin and heparin will help prevent excess clotting of blood so that the MI cannot extend or get worse. Atenolol will reduce blood pressure, which indirectly reduces the workload of the heart because it has to pump against less pressure in the arterial circulation.

5. The nurse should assess for these adverse effects of medication:
   - Amiodarone: bradycardia or other dysrhythmias, hypotension, cardiac arrest, heart failure or cardiogenic shock, fever, elevated liver function tests
   - Heparin: easy bruising, bleeding from gums and IV or other injection sites, occult bleeding in urine or stool, and heparin-induced thrombocytopenia (HIT)
   - Aspirin: bleeding and ototoxicity, hearing loss from cochlear branch of cranial nerve (CN) VIII; vertigo, dizziness, and ringing in ears from vestibular branch of CN VIII
   - Atenolol: dizziness, orthostatic hypotension, bradycardia, depression, decreased libido or impotence, nausea or diarrhea, and bronchospasm (difficulty breathing, wheezing)
   - Morphine: sedation, respiratory depression, hypotension, constipation, nausea and vomiting, or allergic reaction

Chapter 7

1. A weight-based heparin therapy protocol is being used as it is the most effective method for achieving a therapeutic anticoagulation level in a short amount of time. Weight-based therapy helps individualize the dosage, client response, and therapeutic level. Many times, in adult clients, the dosage will be the same for all clients regardless of size and weight (e.g., antibiotic therapy). However, in most acute-care settings, it is important to go back to weight-based dosing to achieve a safe and therapeutic effect.

2. Activated partial thromboplastin time (APTT) would help to establish therapeutic blood levels of heparin administration. It would be important to obtain baseline complete blood count (CBC) with differential, serum chemistry, and coagulation studies. In addition, labs should be done per protocol and the results trended to establish therapeutic levels. A Doppler/vascular study may be necessary to evaluate the client's deep vein thrombosis (DVT).

3. The nurse can help to decrease the client's anxiety by explaining why lab tests are necessary. It is important to offer the client information and emotional support to make the client feel a part of the healthcare team. It is important to spend time with the client and determine whether or not this anxiety is related to "frequent blood tests" or if there are any other underlying reasons that could be causing the client to be anxious.

4. It is important to give both verbal and written instructions regarding warfarin therapy to the client before discharge. Referral to a dietitian and continued follow-up

will help the client feel that the healthcare team is available to supply necessary information and support. It would be important to include family members in the client teaching so that the client can meet therapeutic goals in a safe environment. It may be helpful to share with the client that many people are on this medication on a long-term basis and live well within the guidelines without adverse effects.

Chapter 8

1. Lisinopril is an ACE inhibitor, which will block peripheral vasoconstriction and will help to control his hypertension. Because he also has a history of heart failure (HF), it will help to prevent ventricular remodeling and enlargement of his heart, which would worsen the HF. Furosemide is a loop diuretic and will promote fluid loss and aid in controlling blood pressure as well as heart failure. Spironolactone is a potassium-sparing diuretic and is often used to help balance the loss of potassium that frequently occurs with loop diuretics; notice that the client is not on a potassium supplement. A daily baby aspirin is used in the presence of cardiac disease to prevent cardiovascular events.

2. His potassium is elevated as well as the BUN and creatinine, and GFR is slightly low. The potassium level could be related to the potassium-sparing diuretic as well as impaired renal function. The elevated BUN and creatinine along with a decrease in GFR raise a concern of impaired renal function. This could be secondary to impaired cardiac output due to his history of HF as well as an age-related decline in renal function.

3. Even though he is taking a loop diuretic, the dose is fairly low; the potassium-sparing diuretic he is receiving may balance the potassium losses. He is also 78 years old and renal function decreases with age, so this may contribute to inability to excrete potassium sufficiently. The ACE inhibitor blocks aldosterone, which promotes sodium loss, but can contribute to potassium retention, so this may also be a factor. His diet should also be explored to determine if he eats many foods high in potassium.

4. The nurse should notify the primary care provider and surgeon of the abnormal labs. The client should be monitored for signs of hyperkalemia, balanced intake and output, signs of dehydration (possible cause of elevated BUN) and/or fluid overload (since renal function is impaired), confusion, dysrhythmias, hypertension, and signs of HF.

5. The client should be taught the following information about potassium-sparing diuretics:
   - Signs and symptoms of hyperkalemia to be alert to
   - Avoid use of salt substitutes that contain potassium (since he has history of HF, he may be on a sodium restricted diet)
   - Foods high in potassium to restrict or avoid
   - Take dose with food to increase absorption and reduce GI upset
   - Report any decrease in urine output to healthcare provider.

Chapter 9

1. During an episode of gastroesophageal reflux, gastric acid (which has a low pH) from the stomach backs up through the lower esophageal sphincter into the esophagus and irritates esophageal tissue. This explains why the client is experiencing heartburn and cough, particularly at night when the client is lying down and the force of gravity is removed.

2. The client should eat several small meals per day rather than three larger ones. The client should also limit or eliminate alcohol because it increases gastric acid leading to reflux. It is important that he understands that lying recumbent after a meal will increase the chance of gastric acid reflux. The client should not consume food or fluids prior to bedtime. Foods that tend to contribute to acid reflux include coffee, mints, and dairy products as examples.

3. In the event of *H. pylori*, omeprazole (or another proton pump inhibitor) can be combined with clarithromycin or other approved antibiotic to eradicate the infection. Sometimes medications can be packaged together for convenience of medication therapy.

4. Antacids and proton pump inhibitors reduce gastric secretions and promote healing of erosive esophagitis. These medications will also relieve symptoms of heartburn. The client should maintain his medication schedule to prevent complications, such as Barrett's esophagus, from occurring. Barrett's esophagus is caused by a change in cells lining the esophagus and increases the risk of esophageal cancer.

Chapter 10

1. The priority nursing concerns preoperatively include a risk for bleeding because of impaired clotting, a reduced ability to engage in activity because of illness state and fatigue, risks to tissue integrity because of edema, pain because of liver enlargement, insufficient knowledge about the surgical experience, and possible reduced family coping ability because of a fear of the unknown. Postoperatively, the priority nursing concerns would include pain, possible reduced ability to cough and clear airway because of pain and location of incision near diaphragm, possible disturbed body image (incisions), and insufficient knowledge about postoperative care, medication administration, and infection-related side effects of immunosuppressant medications.

2. It is important for the following laboratory studies to be assessed prior to and during medication therapy:
   - Aspartate aminotransferase (AST)/alanine aminotransferase (ALT)
   - Blood glucose
   - Blood urea nitrogen (BUN) and creatinine
   - Electrolytes: sodium, potassium, calcium, magnesium, and phosphorus
   - Complete blood count (CBC) and platelet count
   - Uric acid

3. The teaching plan for the client and family should include the following elements:
   - Discuss medications that have been prescribed by the healthcare provider.
   - Discuss potential side effects of medications.
   - Instruct the client and family on prevention of infection, since the goal of immunosuppressant therapy is to decrease the immune response and prevent rejection of the transplanted liver.
   - Instruct about pain relief measures.
   - Instruct on coping mechanisms to assist in preventing anxiety and depression.
4. Nursing interventions that should be implemented prior to discharge after portal vein repair include:
   - Instruct on signs and symptoms of bleeding, and report any sign of bleeding to the healthcare provider.
   - Instruct on care of the incision site.
   - Instruct on prevention of infections.
   - Instruct on proper nutrition.
   - Assess for signs and symptoms of liver failure.
   - Assess AST/ALT periodically as available.
   - Assess vital signs frequently.
   - Instruct the client on turning, coughing, and deep breathing to prevent atelectasis.
   - Provide pain relief measures.
5. Methylprednisolone is administered following the portal vein repair to decrease the inflammation within the liver and diminish the likelihood of organ rejection.

Chapter 11

1. Assess allergies to previous penicillin therapy and to cephalosporins because there is cross-sensitivity between the two classes of antibiotics; occurrence of mild erythematous, maculopapular rash is not a hypersensitivity reaction but needs to be reported to the healthcare provider. Gastrointestinal side effects do not preclude the client from taking amoxicillin.

   Assess vital signs, especially temperature, to establish baseline febrile status, to assess the immunologic response, to determine if interventions are indicated for client's comfort, and to determine baseline for future evaluation of drug therapy effectiveness.

   Determine if the client is pregnant. Safe use during pregnancy has not been established, although antibiotic therapy will probably be implemented. The risks for rheumatic heart disease and acute glomerulonephritis as sequelae to a "strep throat" infection are significant.

   Assess renal function since the drug is usually excreted through the kidneys; periodic assessment of BUN and creatinine would be indicated for prolonged therapy.

   If complete blood count (CBC) results are available, leukocytosis with elevated neutrophils, bands, and stabs would be expected with this diagnosis of an acute bacterial infection.

   Assess concurrent medications that may interact, such as tetracycline, which may interfere with the anti-infective property of the amoxicillin, and probenecid, which delays excretion of the antibiotic and prolongs its effect.

2. Assess for improvement of clinical manifestations such as resolution of fever, dysphagia, malaise, and inflamed, erythematous posterior oropharynx and tongue with white pustules. Improvement of signs and symptoms should be observed within 48–72 hours of antibiotic therapy. Identify negative results on reculture of oropharynx and resolution of leukocytosis if respective laboratory findings are available. No or minimal side effects occur.

3. Assess number and characteristics of stools. Pseudomembranous colitis is characterized by at least four to six watery stools a day with blood and/or mucus, a newly developed fever, and abdominal cramping. If pseudomembranous colitis is suspected, arrange for culture and sensitivity on a stool specimen. If positive, collaborate with the prescriber regarding discontinuation of the antibiotic and initiation of vancomycin or metronidazole to treat the colitis.

   If the diarrhea is mild, yogurt or buttermilk can be added to the diet to counter eradication of the normal intestinal flora. An absorbent antidiarrheal agent as kaolin and pectin may be prescribed. In either case, ensure hydration and assess for hypokalemia, which often demonstrates nonspecific symptoms such as muscle weakness, fatigue, anorexia, nausea, irritability, and depressed T wave.

4. The full course of antibiotic therapy must be completed in order to better ensure eradication of the pathogenic organisms, to prevent regrowth of organisms that can occur with premature discontinuation of the antibiotic, and to decrease the risk for drug resistance to develop.

   The antibiotic should be continued for at least 48–72 hours after clinical manifestations of the infection are resolved. Furthermore, this client with a hemolytic streptococcal infection needs at least 10 days of antibiotic therapy to prevent complications such as acute glomerulonephritis and acute rheumatic fever.

   The two infectious sequelae that could occur are acute rheumatic fever and acute glomerulonephritis.

5. If the client is taking oral contraceptives, advise client that the antibiotic may interfere with the effectiveness of the oral contraceptive and an alternate method of contraception will need to be used during therapy with amoxicillin and for 1 month after treatment has been discontinued. Breakthrough bleeding may occur.

   Take medication around the clock at evenly spaced intervals without interrupting sleep, as possible. This schedule better ensures sustaining a therapeutic drug level.

   If a dose is missed, take as soon as remembered, but do not double-dose at the next administration time. Report side effects such as rash, urticaria, wheezing, and GI adverse effects that are severe such as nausea and vomiting and diarrhea. May take dose with food to minimize gastrointestinal distress. Practice good hygiene including washing hands frequently, disposing of tissues properly, and not sharing eating utensils. Encourage fluid intake of at least eight glasses a day. Explain rationale for completing full course of treatment and for follow-up.

Chapter 12

1. The most important prioritized nursing concerns include risk for infection because of myelosuppression caused by chemotherapy, possible reduced cardiac output because doxorubicin is cardiotoxic, risk for bleeding because of possible effects on platelets during myelosuppression, possible insufficient nutrient intake because of chemotherapy-induced nausea and vomiting, insufficient knowledge of side effects of chemotherapy, possible stomatitis related to chemotherapy, and risk for damage to local tissue if IV vesicant infiltrates. The nursing concerns are listed in priority from the most life-threatening to the least. Since the development of infection is the most life-threatening, it is listed first. Doxorubicin can cause cardiomyopathy and is therefore listed second. All of the agents can cause myelosuppression; therefore, the risk for development of thrombocytopenia needs to be assessed. Excessive nausea and vomiting can cause nutritional alteration. Although insufficient knowledge is an actual problem, the potential problems that precede it are more life-threatening, should they occur. Methotrexate and 5-FU commonly cause stomatitis, which can also promote nutritional alterations. While extravasation of a vesicant is a potential problem, it is listed last since it is rare.

2. The following are important diagnostic or assessment values that need to be obtained before initiating the chemotherapy:
   - Ejection fraction from the multigated acquisition (MUGA) scan. If less than 50%, the prescriber should be notified before administration of doxorubicin.
   - Liver function studies (LFS) and complete blood count (CBC). If LFS are elevated, the prescriber should be notified for potential dosage reduction. The WBC and differential should be assessed to ensure the absolute granulocyte count (AGC) is greater than or equal to $1,500/mm^3$.
   - Obtain ultrasound of the liver and ensure no abnormality is found.
   - Client's vital signs, including weight, height, temperature, blood pressure, and pulse.

3. A pretreatment teaching plan for this client could include the following outlined elements:
   - Discuss chemotherapy agents prescribed.
   - Discuss potential side effects and mechanisms of preventing them, including nausea and vomiting, stomatitis, extravasation, hemorrhagic cystitis, and sterility.
   - Teach client to report burning or stinging of chemotherapy upon administration.
   - Teach client mechanisms to prevent infection.
   - Teach oral care and demonstrate mixing of solutions.
   - Discuss contraceptive methods if appropriate.

4. The prescriptions that need further clarification with the prescriber are:
   - Loading dosage of ondansetron exceeds the recommended dose of 20 mg.
   - The dose of 5-FU seems to be too low. Is it a transcription error?
   - Since this is the client's first dose of chemotherapy and he does not have a central venous line (CVC), does the healthcare provider intend on placing a temporary CVC such as a peripherally inserted central catheter (PICC) or triple-lumen catheter (TLC)?

5. The following should be done to prepare the client for discharge from the hospital:
   - Reinforce continuation of oral hygiene after discharge.
   - Reinforce mechanisms to prevent infection.
   - Identify primary caregiver and/or financial resources to obtain one temporarily.
   - Teach anticipated nadir period and signs and symptoms to report to the healthcare provider.

Chapter 13

1. It is important to inform the client that type 1 diabetes mellitus (DM) can occur at any age but is most likely to occur in childhood and adolescence. Type 1 DM is an autoimmune disease in which the immune system destroys the insulin-producing beta cells of the pancreas, creating a need for insulin injections. It is important to inform the client of the genetic predisposition to diabetes mellitus. Approximately 1 in 20 children of a parent with diabetes will become diabetic.

2. The clinical manifestations of DM are caused by glucose molecules, which accumulate in the blood causing hyperglycemia. This leads to increased blood volume because of increased osmolality and increased renal flow with osmotic diuresis (polyuria). Glucose is then excreted in the urine, which is known as glucosuria. Since these factors cause dehydration, the client experiences polydipsia (increased thirst). The client will then become lethargic and experience excessive hunger. The excessive hunger is called polyphagia. Thus, polyuria, polydipsia, and polyphagia are the cardinal signs of diabetes mellitus.

3. Hyperglycemia is a blood glucose (BG) level above 110 mg/dL (normal 70–110 mg/dL). The client should understand that a sudden BG decrease to 45–60 mg/dL is considered hypoglycemia and should be treated with a quick-acting sugar. Severe hypoglycemia can cause coma and ultimately death. An increase in blood glucose can result from overconsumption of food, lack of exercise, decrease in insulin administration, or onset of illness or infection. Manifestations of diabetic ketoacidosis are a blood glucose level of 250 mg/dL or higher and a plasma pH less than 7.3. The client's bicarbonate level will be less than 15 mEq/L. The client will present with glycosuria and ketonuria, which could also lead to coma or death if untreated.

4. It is important that the client understand that she should know the times of onset, peak, and duration of prescribed insulin therapy. Medications are timed so that their peak effect occurs at a mealtime. If the client is taking a long-acting insulin, it should be taken at the same time each day as prescribed. Meals should be eaten at regular times to work in conjunction with the timing of insulin therapy to avoid hyper- or hypoglycemia.

5. Diet, exercise, and insulin therapy all work together to maintain normal blood glucose levels. Diet is important for adequate nutrients and the prescribed diet should be adhered to in order to help maintain glycemic control. The diet should be nutrient dense and maintained at the prescribed number of calories. Exercise helps prevent weight gain and it requires adequate glucose and insulin to prevent episodes of hypoglycemia during exercise. Insulin therapy is customized to the client's needs, according to dietary requirements and exercise level. The three must be in balance to prevent hyper- or hypoglycemia from occurring.

Chapter 14

1. Dinoprostone is FDA-approved for cervical ripening prior to the induction of labor. Prepidil intracervical gel contains 0.5 mg of dinoprostone and is inserted into the cervix after direct visualization via speculum. Cervidil vaginal insert contains 10 mg dinoprostone, and one insert is placed into the posterior cul-de-sac, with the string protruding out of the vagina. The client should remain recumbent after administration.

2. Labor induction is accomplished by starting a peripheral IV, using either Y-tubing or piggy-backing into the main line, and infusing oxytocin via infusion pump. The oxytocin solution is most commonly diluted as 10 units in 1 liter of IV fluid (although some practitioners will prescribe 20 units in 1 liter). Oxytocin is begun at 1 or 2 milliunits, and increased every 20–30 minutes until adequate contractions occur.

3. Because of the hypertension of preeclampsia, the oxytocin solution infusion rate would be increased. If this did not control the hemorrhage, carboprost tromethamine would be utilized, as it produces less increase in blood pressure than do either methylergonovine or ergonovine.

4. Magnesium sulfate is most commonly used for the seizures of eclampsia. A 4- to 6-gram loading dose is given over 20 minutes, and then 1–2 grams per hour is usually given via IV infusion.

5. Breastfeeding women can use progestin-only preparations for contraception. This includes medroxyprogesterone acetate IM, levonorgestrel intradermal implants, or oral norethindrone.

Chapter 15

1. Benzoyl peroxide has keratolytic activity and clindamycin is an antibacterial agent. This product is applied directly to the skin twice daily after cleansing of the affected areas.

2. Isotretinoin is a retinoic acid derivative used for severe recalcitrant nodular acne that is unresponsive to conventional therapy. It should only be administered for 15–20 weeks. The action of the medication is that it normalizes keratinization and decreases the size of the sebaceous glands, reducing the amount of oil released by the glands. It is important that the young client be assessed for any psychiatric disorders, asthma, liver disease, anorexia, and diabetes.

3. This is the proper dose for this client (0.5–1 mg/kg/day) but it could be raised to 2–4 mg/kg/day in divided doses.

4. The client should protect his skin from the sun and use sunscreen during exposure because of the photosensitive nature of both medications. He should avoid using vitamin A products. He should not use tetracycline due to increased potential for the development of pseudotumor cerebri. He should be aware that food taken with medication increases absorption, thus it should be taken with food. Instruct him that alcohol use may increase hypertriglyceridemia. The client should report any visual disturbances, joint pain, or muscle pain. Although this is not particular to this case, any sexually active woman of childbearing age should be taking oral or topical contraceptives.

Chapter 16

1. Glaucoma is a disease of the eye characterized by elevated intraocular pressure. The increase in intraocular pressure results from excessive production of aqueous humor or a decrease in the outflow of aqueous humor. Persistent high intraocular pressure may lead to blindness. The medication prescribed, betaxolol, is a beta-adrenergic blocking agent that decreases the production of aqueous humor, thereby reducing intraocular pressure.

2. Because of its β_1 cardioselectivity, betaxolol is the drug of choice for clients with pulmonary disease. However, beta-blocking agents are used cautiously in clients with pulmonary disease (risk of bronchospasm). The client should be monitored for cardiopulmonary complications.

3. Local side effects include burning, stinging, and eye irritation. Systemic absorption may lead to bradycardia, heart failure, cardiac dysrhythmias, bronchospasm, insomnia, dizziness, vertigo, and gastrointestinal disturbances. The client should report these symptoms to the healthcare provider.

4. Photophobia may result from use of betaxolol. The client should wear dark sunglasses and avoid bright lights.

5. Instruct the client to wash hands, look up toward the ceiling, pull down the lower eyelid to form a sac, and then instill the medication into the sac. Instruct the client to avoid touching the eye and to avoid touching the eyedropper to the eye or any other object. Instruct the client to use nasolacrimal occlusion (press on the tear duct) to minimize systemic absorption.

Appendix B
Reference Tables

Appendix B-1	Common Abbreviations in Pharmacology		
ac	before meals	mg	milligram
ACE	angiotensin converting enzyme	ml, mL	milliliter
ARB	angiotensin II receptor blocker	NSAID	nonsteroidal anti-inflammatory drug
ASA	acetylsalicylic acid (aspirin)	OTC	over-the-counter
bid	2 times a day	OU	both eyes
cc	cubic centimeter	pc	after meals
COX	cyclo-oxygenase	PO	oral, by mouth
DMARD	disease modifying antirheumatic drug	PPD	purified protein derivative
DPI	dry powder inhaler	PR	per rectum
h, hr	hour	PRN	as needed
HRT	hormone replacement therapy	q	every
IM	intramuscular(ly)	qid	4 times a day
IV	intravenous(ly)	qod	every other day
kg	kilogram	Subcut/SubQ	subcutaneous(ly)
KVO	keep vein open	sl	sublingual
LKVO	liter	stat	immediately
MAOI	monoamine oxidase inhibitor	tid	3 times a day
MDI	metered dose inhaler		

Appendix B-2	Common Equivalent General Weights and Measures

1 gram = 1000 milligrams (mg) = 1,000,000 micrograms (mcg)

1 mg = 1,000 mcg

1 mcg = 0.001 mg

1 pound = 16 ounces (oz) = 454 grams = 0.454 kilograms (kg)

1 kg = 2.2 pounds (lb)

1 cubic centimeter (cc) = 1 milliliter (mL)

Temperature in degrees Fahrenheit (F)— = (Celsius degrees $\times$ 9/5) + 32

Temperature in degrees Celsius (C) = (Fahrenheit degrees −32) $\times$ 5/9

Appendix B-3 Clinically Useful Approximate Liquid Measure Equivalents

Milliliter (mL)	Liter (L)	Teaspoon (tsp)	Tablespoon (Tbsp)	Ounces (oz)	Cups (c)	Pint (Pt)	Quart (Qt)	Gallon (Gal)
5	-	1	0.33	-	-	-	-	-
15	-	3	1	0.5	-	-	-	-
29.6 (~30)	-	6	2	1	-	-	-	-
237	-	-	-	8	1	0.5	0.25	-
473	-	-	-	16	2	1	0.5	-
946	0.946	-	-	32	4	2	1	0.5
1000	1	-	-	33.8	-	2.11	1.06	-
3785	3.785	-	-	128	-	-	~4	~1

—, not clinically useful; ~, approximate

Appendix B-4 Therapeutic Drug Levels

Generic (Trade) Names	Level in Conventional Units	Level in SI Units
acetaminophen	0.2–0.6 mg/dL; toxic: greater than 5 mg/dL	13–40 micromoles/L
carbamazepine	4–12 mcg/mL	375–900 nmol/L
digoxin	0.5–2 ng/mL	1–2.6 nmol/L
lidocaine	1.5–6 mcg/mL	6–21 micromoles/L
lithium	0.5–1.5 mEq/L	0.5–1.5 mmol/L
phenytoin	10–20 mcg/mL	40–80 mcg/mL
procainamide	4–8 mcg/mL	17–40 micromoles/L
quinidine	2–6 mcg/mL	4.6–9.2 micromoles/L
salicylate (acetylsalicylic acid; aspirin)	100–200 mg/L; toxic: greater than 200mg/L	724–1448 micromoles/L; toxic: greater than 1450 micromoles/L
theophylline	10–20 mcg/mL	55–110 micromoles/L
valproic acid	50–100 mcg/mL	350–700 micromoles/L
vancomycin	30–40 mg/mL (peak); 5–10 mg/mL (trough)	20–40 mg/dL (peak); 5–10 (trough)

dL, deciliter; L, liter; mcg, microgram; mEq, milliequivalent; mg, milligram; mL, milliliter; ng, nanogram; nmol, nanomole

| Appendix B-5 | Selected Medication/Poison Toxicities and Antidotes |

Substance at Toxic/Poisonous Level	Antidote
Acetaminophen	acetylcysteine
Anticholinergics	physostigmine
Benzodiazepines	flumazenil
Calcium channel blockers	calcium chloride, calcium gluconate
Copper	penicillamine
Cyanide or nitrate	methylene blue
Digoxin	digoxin immune fab
Doxorubicin	dexrazoxane
Heparin	protamine sulfate
Insulin	glucagon
Iron	deferoxamine
Isoniazid	pyridoxine
Lead	succimer
Methotrexate	leucovorin calcium
Nondepolarizing neuromuscular blockers	neostigmine
Opioids	naloxone; nalfemene
Warfarin	vitamin K

Preparing for the NCLEX-RN® Exam

SAFE AND EFFECTIVE CARE ENVIRONMENT: MANAGEMENT OF CARE

Management of Care makes up 17–23% of the questions on the NCLEX-RN® exam.

Key Testing Strategies:

- Recognize questions that require priority setting through words in the question such as first, initial, best, most important, essential, and most therapeutic.

- When answering questions related to delegation to caregivers, such as float registered nurses from other clinical specialties, LPNs/LVNs, and unlicensed assistive personnel (UAPs), recall that the task being delegated needs to be part of that caregiver's skill set and that the other rights of delegation must be upheld.

- Immediately eliminate distracters that violate client rights or ethical principles.

Areas of Focus for Management of Care Questions	Ethical and legal concepts for nursing practice	Performance or quality improvement
	Maintaining client rights, including confidentiality and informed consent	Communication with interdisciplinary team (collaboration, client advocacy, case management, making referrals, and maintaining continuity of care)
	Assisting client with self-determination (such as with life planning, advance directives, and organ donation)	
	Nursing management concepts	Skills involving clinical reasoning, such as priority setting, assignment-making, delegation, and supervision
	Using information technology in clinical care	

Essential Rights of Delegation

1. **Right Task:** Nurses determine those activities team members may perform. For each situation, the nurse must consider the client's condition, the complexity of the activity, the UAP's capabilities, and the amount of supervision the nurse will be able to provide.

2. **Right Circumstances:** The nurse evaluates the individual clients and the individual UAPs and matches the two. The nurse assesses the client's needs, looks at the care plan, and considers the setting, ensuring that UAPs have the proper resources, equipment, and supervision to work safely.

3. **Right Person:** The nurse follows organizational policies, which are congruent with state law, in determining the appropriate staff to which to delegate a nursing activity.

4. **Right Direction and Communication:** The nurse needs to communicate the acceptable tasks and activities. The nurse needs to clearly understand the organization's policies and procedures to carry out effective delegation. In turn, staff nurses need to direct UAPs' actions and communicate clearly about each delegated task. Nurses must be specific about how and when UAPs should report back to them. Nurses should feel comfortable asking, Do you know how to do this? Where did you learn? How many times have you done it in the past? Where is your experience documented?

5. **Right Supervision and Evaluation:** Nurse managers must ensure that each unit has adequate staffing and time, identify the task inherent to each staff role, and evaluate the impact of the organization's nursing service on the community. The delegating nurse then must supervise, guide, and evaluate the UAPs' task implementation. The nurse must ensure that UAPs meet expectations and must intervene if they aren't performing well.

Based on the April 2016 Test Plan

	Guiding Principles Physiology	First Priority Airway, breathing, and circulation	Second Priority
Strategies for Setting Priorities in Clinical Practice	Maslow's Hierarchy of Needs theory	Physiological (primary) needs: air, breathing, circulation, water, food (oxygen therapy, circulatory support, IV hydration, nutrition, critical lab values, treatment of pain)	Safety and security (primary) needs: prevention of falls, reorientation to surroundings, abnormally high or low values that are not critical, may include some client teaching (e.g. insulin administration)
	Policies and Procedures	Activities governed by agency policy or procedure that involves strict timelines (e.g., restraints, falls, stat medications)	Activities governed by policy or procedure that directly affect client care (e.g., non-stat, regularly scheduled medications, dressings)
	Care activities related to clinical condition of client	Life-threatening or potentially life-threatening occurrences (adverse changes in VS, change in LOC, potential for respiratory or circulatory collapse); often unanticipated	Activities essential to safety: life-saving medications and equipment that protect clients from infections or falls
	Medication or IV therapy priorities	Medications that prevent or treat physiological distress (e.g., analgesics, updrafts or inhalers); medications ordered more frequently (e.g., every 4 hours) because late medication delivery could affect next dose; IV therapy for hydration in clients who are NPO because of nonfunctional GI tract	Medications that prevent reoccurrences of symptoms of disease processes (such as digoxin or antibiotics); medications ordered once per shift, routine maintenance of IV therapy or heparin/saline lock care

Ethical Principles and Decision-making	Autonomy	Beneficence
	Accountability	Justice
	Fidelity	Veracity
	Confidentiality	Nonmaleficence

Informed Consent

- Requirements of client: has mental capacity to consent; it is voluntarily done; and client understands treatment and information presented
- Requirements of healthcare provider (performing treatment, procedure, or surgery): shares information about planned treatment, procedure or surgery, its associated risks and benefits, and alternatives to treatment; gives client opportunity to ask questions and have them answered
- If a client waives right to informed consent, document this in the medical record
- If client is deemed incompetent to make informed decisions about healthcare in court of law, a court-appointed guardian makes these decisions
- Informed consent for minors is obtained from parent or legal guardian, except in emergency situations, when minor is married or emancipated from parents, or has special care needs, such as with sexually transmitted infection or pregnancy

Upholding HIPAA (Health Information Portability and Accountability Act)

- Protect personal identifying information (such as name, social security number, date of birth) and information about diagnosis or treatment
- Share information only with individuals involved directly in client's care, payment for care, and/or management of client's care
- Verify identify of persons asking for client information
- Dispose of confidential documents in accord with agency policy (such as shredder, locked recycle bin)

- Keep contents of medical record out of public view by placing in a secure area and turning computer screens displaying client data away from general view
- Discuss client's care only in areas where cannot be overheard

SAFE AND EFFECTIVE CARE ENVIRONMENT: SAFETY AND INFECTION CONTROL

Safety and Infection Control makes up 9–15% of the questions on the NCLEX-RN® exam.

Key Testing Strategies

- Questions that focus on assessing the home environment of a client may be seeking to determine knowledge of risks to safety in the home, such as risk of falls (e.g., throw rugs, no night lights, handrails, or bathroom safety bars) or risk of fire (e.g., oxygen in the home, frayed electrical cords, lack of smoke detectors).
- When answering a question that addresses an infectious disease, consider that the question may be determining knowledge of precautions to prevent disease transmission, and discriminate the need to use contact, airborne, or droplet precautions.
- When answering a question that addresses a client with a compromised immune system or who is receiving chemotherapy, consider that the question may be determining whether the client has a need for neutropenic precautions (for low white blood cell count) or thrombocytopenic precautions (for low platelet count).

Areas of Focus for Safety and Infection Control Questions	Using ergonomic principles	Preventing accidents, errors, and injuries
	Using equipment safely	Implementing infection control practices such as standard precautions, transmission-based precautions, and surgical asepsis
	Using equipment for client safety (such as restraints or safety devices) correctly	
	Workplace safety measures such as security plan/emergency response plan and reporting adverse events using incident/irregular occurrence/variance reports	Safe handling of hazardous materials or infectious materials
		Assessing and assisting with home safety

4 Steps to Maintain Client Safety During a Fire	Remove clients from danger	Contain the fire
	Activate the fire alarm	Evacuate the area (do horizontal evacuation if possible before vertical evacuation)

Fall Risk Factors in Older Adults	**Intrinsic Age-Related Changes**	**Intrinsic Disease Related Changes**	**Extrinsic Risk Factors**
	Gait (step length and height)	Orthostatic hypotension	Floor surface; waxed, scatter rugs, tears in carpeting
	Gait (symmetry and path)	Dehydration	Steps uneven, without hand rails
	Balance when sitting	Cardiac arrhythmias and anemias	Edges and curbing without contrasting colors
	Balance when standing	Urinary tract and other infections	Dim lighting, bright lights that cause glare
	Balance when turning	Osteoporosis and fractures	Bathrooms without grab bars and tub or shower seats
	Stability	Hypoglycemia	High-heeled shoes
	Cognition	Seizures, TIA, CVA, adverse effects of medication, delirium	Clutter

Principles of Surgical Asepsis

- All objects used in a sterile field must be sterile.
- Sterile objects that touch unsterile objects become unsterile.
- Sterile items that are out of vision or below waist level are considered unsterile.
- Sterile objects can become unsterile by prolonged exposure to airborne microorganisms.
- Fluids flow in the direction of gravity.
- Moisture that passes through a sterile object exerts capillary action to draw microorganisms from unsterile surfaces above or below to the sterile surface.
- The edges of a sterile field are considered unsterile.
- The skin is unsterile and cannot be sterilized.
- Conscientiousness, alertness, and honesty are essential qualities in maintaining surgical asepsis.

Centers for Disease Control and Prevention (CDC) Precautions	**Tier 1: Standard Precautions** Hand hygiene Gloves Face protection (mask, goggles, face shield) Gowns and other protective apparel Others **Tier 2: Transmission Based Precautions** **Airborne Precautions:** Use when small ($<5\ \mu$m) pathogen-infected droplet nuclei may remain suspended in air over time and travel distances greater than 3 feet. *Examples: varicella, measles, tuberculosis* **Droplet Precautions:** Use with large ($>5\ \mu$m) pathogen-infected droplets that travel 3 feet or less via coughing, sneezing, etc. or during procedures (suctioning). *Examples: Haemophilus influenzae, Neisseria meningitides, others* **Contact Precautions:** Use with known or suspected microorganisms transmitted by direct hand-to-skin client contact or indirect contact with surfaces or care items in the environment. *Examples: Clostridium difficile, diphtheria (cutaneous), herpes simplex (mucocutaneous or neonatal), impetigo, pediculosis, scabies, zoster (disseminated, immunocompromised host), viral/hemorrhagic infections (Ebola, Lassa, Marburg), others*

HEALTH PROMOTION AND MAINTENANCE

Health Promotion and Maintenance makes up 6–12% of the questions on the NCLEX-RN® exam.

Key Testing Strategies

- Make note of whether the client's age is identified in the question. If so, the question may be determining ability to apply concepts of normal growth and development.
- Because health promotion often involves client education, be prepared to apply principles of teaching and learning to questions in this area.
- When determining interventions to enhance a client's wellness, consider options that promote healthy nutrition, regular exercise, proper weight maintenance, proper rest, and avoidance of harmful chemicals, such as nicotine, and risk-taking behaviors, such as not wearing a seat belt.

Areas of Focus for Health Promotion and Maintenance Questions	Growth and development concepts, including the aging process, developmental stages, and assisting clients with transitions Assisting clients with self-care Activities to promote health and prevent disease, including health screenings	Client lifestyle choices and high-risk behaviors Maternal-newborn concepts such as antepartum, intrapartum, postpartum, and newborn care Physical assessment techniques

Health Screening for Cancer	*Use common sense when monitoring for signs of cancer in clients or yourself:*
	Pay attention to body changes: • Unexplained weight loss • Changes in the characteristics or timing of bowel movements • Alterations in tissue (moles, thicknesses, lumps)	• Hoarseness, cough, difficulty swallowing Follow recommended guidelines (USPSTF, ACS, other) for screening recommendations at different ages Ensure family history of cancer is reviewed as part of record

ABCDE Rule for Evaluating a Suspicious Skin Lesion	A = Asymmetry (one half of lesion does not match the other half) B = Border irregularity (edges are blurred, jagged, or have a notched appearance) C = Color variation is present or has a dark black color change D = Diameter is greater than 6 millimeters in size E = Evolving (color, size, or shape is changing)

Techniques of Physical Assessment

- Inspection: utilizes observation to obtain important information about a client's state of health; have adequate lighting to visually inspect the body without distortions or shadows; lighting can be sunlight or artificial
- Palpation: uses the sensation of touch and pressure of the hands and fingers to determine masses, elevations, temperature, organ position, and any abnormal findings; can be light or deep depending on the area of the body being examined
  - Light palpation is 1 cm in depth
  - Deep palpation is about 4 cm in depth
  - Deep palpation should occur after light palpation
- Percussion: a skill in which the finger of one hand touches or taps a finger of the other hand to generate vibration, which in turn produces a specific, diagnostic sound; the sound changes as the practitioner moves from one area to the next
- Auscultation: uses the sense of hearing to identify sounds produced by the body; some sounds can be heard and identified without a stethoscope; others can only be identified in a quiet environment with a stethoscope

Basic Teaching Principles

- Set priorities for client's learning needs.
- Use appropriate timing.
- Organize materials so that learning proceeds from simple to complex.
- Promote and maintain learner attention and participation.
- Build on the client's existing knowledge.
- Select appropriate teaching methods, including discussion, question and answer, role-play, or discovery, or computerized instruction.
- Use appropriate teaching aids: visual aids (drawings, charts, models, printed materials), audiotapes, films or videotapes, programmed instruction, games, and others.
- Provide teaching related to developmental level.

Age-Related Changes

Skin: Subcutaneous tissue loss and dermal thinning, leading to wrinkling; increase in lentigines (brown age spots); hair thins and loses pigment; nail growth slows and nails may become thicker; skin tissue is more fragile

Sensory/perceptual: Visual acuity changes; ocular changes lead to near vision problems (presbyopia), increased sensitivity to glare, decreased ability to adjust to darkness; cataracts may develop; eyelids lose elasticity; ear canal narrows with calcification of ossicles and increased cerumen, resulting in progressive hearing loss (presbycusis); reduced ability to smell and discriminate odors; sense of taste decreases (especially to sense sweet taste); touch sensation changes with reduced ability to sense heat and cold

Neurologic: Conduction speeds of neuron firing and transmission decrease; memory retrieval is slower; sleep stages 2–4 shorten, leading to a decrease in deep sleep; proprioception decreases

Musculoskeletal: Muscles atrophy; joint cartilage deteriorates; intervertebral disks atrophy, resulting in a loss of height of 1–3 inches

Pulmonary: Chest wall becomes rigid; thoracic muscles weaken; ciliary activity decreases; delivery and diffusion of O_2 to tissues decreases

Cardiovascular: Cardiac output and stroke volume decrease; valves stiffen; conductivity is altered; blood vessels are less elastic, leading to increasing blood pressure

Renal: Decreased glomerular filtration rate and creatinine clearance; possible residual urine or nocturia

Gastrointestinal: Thirst decreases; swallowing time is delayed; possible loss of teeth; decreased saliva; decreased gastric enzymes; weaker intestinal walls

Endocrine: Slowed basal metabolism; insulin levels increase but insulin sensitivity decreases

Genital: Males: prostate enlarges (often benign); decreased sperm protection. Females: vaginal dryness and atrophy

Immune: First sign of infection in an older adult may be a fall; temperature pattern may be lower than younger adult with the same infection

PSYCHOSOCIAL INTEGRITY

Psychosocial Integrity makes up 6–12% of the questions on the NCLEX-RN® exam.

Key Testing Strategies

- For communication questions, select answers that use therapeutic communication techniques and eliminate options that represent communication blocks.
- If a question suggests that a client is at risk for abuse, assess the client without caregivers present and be aware of mandatory reporting laws.
- When responding to a client's communication, look for options that address the client's concern or issue.
- When answering questions of a psychosocial nature when all options seem of equal importance, follow the SEAs: **s**afety, **e**xpressing feelings, and **a**ssisting with problem solving.

Areas of Focus for Psychosocial Integrity Questions	Cultural and spiritual/religious influences on health
	Therapeutic communication and environment
	Coping mechanisms, stress management, support systems, and crisis intervention
	Mental health concepts
	Supporting client who has sensory-perceptual alterations
	Assisting clients with grief and loss; end-of-life care
	Family dynamics
	Recognizing and intervening with client abuse or neglect
	Working with clients who have chemical or other dependencies or substance use disorders
	Using behavioral interventions

Components of a Mental Status Exam

General Appearance	Appears stated age? Hygiene? Body odors? Dressed to season? Layered? Cleanliness?
Orientation	Person, place, time, and situation?
Thought Process	Clear, coherent, appropriate to topic? Concentration? Hallucinations or delusions?
Memory	Short-term (What did you have for breakfast?), long-term (Who is the president, and the president before that?)
Judgment	Appropriate? Safe? Impaired? Poor?

Communication Techniques to Avoid	Self-disclosure	Giving personal opinions or advice
	Inattentive listening	Prying to satisfy personal curiosity
	Overuse of medical jargon	Changing the subject

Suicide Precautions

When a client is acutely or actively suicidal, the following precautions should be taken:

- If not already hospitalized, someone should stay with the client until he or she can be admitted to prevent self-harm and maintain the safety of the client.
- Remove all sharp or dangerous objects from the client and the immediate vicinity, including knives or forks, scissors, mirrors, glass, and other objects that could be used for self-harm.
- Remove clothing that could be used as a tourniquet to cause self-harm, including belts of all kinds, neckties, stockings, handbags with long straps, etc.
- Remove all substances that could be ingested to toxic levels, including alcohol, recreational drugs, and medications. Keep client's medications locked.
- Ensure that the client swallows all pills, tablets, or other oral forms of medication, so that they are not kept in the cheek and then stored for later overdose.
- Keep the client in seclusion under one-to-one supervision while actively suicidal; explain in a gentle manner that this is for the client's safety until he or she is able to resist suicidal urges.
- Monitor a client who is not under one-to-one supervision with a nursing unit staff member every 10 to 15 minutes on an irregular schedule of observation.

Ensuring Your Safety on the Psychiatric Unit

1. Never be with a client by yourself. Alert staff to your whereabouts at all times.
2. Always have the ability to exit; do not put yourself in a position where your back is toward a closed-in area without an escape route.
3. Dress in casual clothes. Avoid sexually provocative clothing. Avoid having too much skin exposed.
4. Psychotic clients generally experience three delusional themes: 1) sexual, 2) political, and 3) religious. Avoid these topics unless you are experienced in managing them.
5. Remember that staff members are trained in managing client behavioral problems. Obtain the assistance of more experienced staff members when encountering unsafe situations early in practice.
6. Avoid wearing necklaces or other items that can be used as a weapon to strangle. Wear closed-toe shoes. Do not wear loop earrings (or rings).
7. Remember safety first. Always listen to your primary or gut instinct. Enlist the aid of other staff to help in maintaining control.

Therapeutic Communication Techniques	Acknowledging:	Gives nonjudgmental recognition to a client for a certain behavior or contribution, or indicates attention to and care of the client
	Clarifying:	Asks for additional information to ensure understanding of the message sent; a statement like "Would you tell me more about what you have just said?" indicates that understanding the client's message is important to the nurse
	Focusing:	Focuses the client on information that is pertinent and helps the client expand on that information; this technique directs the client towards information that is important
	Giving information:	Provides specific information to a client either with or without the client's request
	Offering self:	Offers the nurse's presence without attaching any expectations or conditions about the client's behavior during that time
	Restating or paraphrasing:	Ensures the nurse understands the message sent; utilizing this technique the nurse repeats the main thought of the message sent
	Reflecting:	Redirects the content of a client's message back to the client for further thought or consideration
	Summarizing:	May be used at the end of an interaction to identify material discussed; it helps to sort out relevant information from irrelevant
	Using silence:	Allows for quiet time without conversation for several seconds or minutes to allow for reflection about the discussion that just occurred, to reduce tension, or to gather thoughts about how to proceed

PHYSIOLOGICAL INTEGRITY: BASIC CARE AND COMFORT

Basic Care and Comfort makes up 6–12% of the questions on the NCLEX-RN® exam.

Key Testing Strategies

- Use principles of administering basic physiological care to clients when answering questions in this part of the test plan.
- When questions address a client's mobility, select answers that will preserve muscle tone and joint function and prevent contractures or skin breakdown.
- Keep principles of safety in mind when answering questions about the use of assistive devices, such as canes, walkers, and crutches.
- Promote good nutrition by selecting meal choices that are balanced and that address any diet restrictions, such as low sodium or reduced fat.
- Use principles of gravity when considering how to position the clients or when working with clients who have drainage or wound tubes.

Areas of focus for Basic Care and Comfort Questions	Assisting with or supporting client self-care needs for hygiene, elimination, rest and sleep, and nutrition and oral hydration
	Assisting client with mobility, including use of assistive devices, and caring for clients who are immobile
	Maintaining client comfort using nonpharmacological interventions

Safety Precautions During Oxygen Therapy

- Instruct the client and visitors about the danger of smoking when oxygen is in use. If necessary, remove matches, lighters, and ashtrays.
- If oxygen therapy is used at home, instruct family members or caregivers to smoke only outside. If smoking is permitted, teach visitors to use smoking room.

- Avoid materials that generate static electricity such as woolen blankets and synthetic fabrics; instead use cotton fabrics.
- Avoid use of volatile, flammable substances such as acetone in nail polish removers, alcohol, ether, and oils near clients using oxygen.
- Remove any friction type or battery operated gadgets, devices, or toys.
- Make sure electric devices such as radios, razors, and televisions are in good working order to prevent short-circuit sparks.
- Ensure that electric monitoring equipment and suction machines are properly grounded. Disconnect any ungrounded equipment.
- Personnel need to be aware of the location of fire extinguishers and be able to use them properly.
- Know location of oxygen meter turn-off value.

Therapeutic Diets		
Regular diet	High-residue/high-fiber diet
Clear liquids	Low-residue/low-fiber
Full liquids	Carbohydrate controlled
Pureed diet	Fat controlled
Dysphagia diet	Protein controlled
Soft diet	Gastric bypass diet
Mechanical soft diet	Restricted diets (gluten, tyramine, others)
Bland diet	

Types of Dressings

Dressing Type	Description
Gauze	Plain or impregnated with an antimicrobial • Packs and fills wound • Absorbs drainage • Used for full- and partial-thickness wounds with drainage • May be apply dry, wet-to-moist, and wet-to-wet
Transparent film	Adhesive plastic semipermeable membrane that allows oxygen into wound but is occlusive to liquids and bacteria • Protects wound from contamination and friction
Impregnated nonadherent	Cotton or synthetic material impregnated with saline, zinc-saline, antimicrobials, petrolatum or others • Protects nonexudative partial- and full-thickness wounds • Requires secondary dressing to keep in place, hold in moisture, and protect wound
Hydrocolloid	Adhesive made of gelatin • Is occlusive to microorganisms and liquids and promotes absorption of wound exudates • Enhances autolysis of necrotic tissue within wound bed • Duo-Derm and Tegasorb are examples
Hydrogel	Water or glycerin is primary component of jelly-like sheet, granules, or gels • Maintains moist wound bed and helps liquefy necrotic tissue or slough • Permeable to oxygen and can fill dead spaces in a wound • Secondary nonadhesive dressing is required
Alginate (exudate absorbers)	Nonadherent dressings with granules, ropes, paste or other materials; requires secondary dressing • Purpose is to absorb up to 20 times their weight in drainage
Polyurethane foam	Nonadherent dressings that absorb large amounts of exudates while keeping wound moist • Use secondary dressing or tape around edges to secure it
Clear absorbent acrylic	Absorbs exudate and allows moisture to evaporate • Aids in wound assessment and protects from bacteria and shearing forces

PHYSIOLOGICAL INTEGRITY: PHARMACOLOGIC AND PARENTERAL THERAPIES

Pharmacologic and Parenteral Therapies makes up 12–18% of the questions on the NCLEX-RN® exam.

Key Testing Strategies

- Use knowledge of drug action, intended effects and key side and adverse effects to answer a question about a specific medication.
- For questions addressing medication history, do not forget to ask about over-the-counter and herbal supplements as well as prescription medications.
- Double-check drug dosages and make sure the answer passes the common sense test (e.g., answer for a subcutaneous dose should not be more than 1 milliliter for an adult).
- Look for certain prefixes and suffixes in drug names to help identify the drug if the name is unfamiliar.

Areas of Focus for Pharmacologic and Parenteral Therapies Questions	Expected medication actions and client outcomes	Calculating drug dosages
	Unintended medication effects such as side and adverse effects, drug interactions; contraindications to specific medications	Pharmacological pain management
		Maintaining central venous access devices
		Administering blood and blood products
	Administering medications and parenteral/intravenous therapies	Administering total parenteral nutrition

Calculating Medication Dosages

Formula 1

$$\frac{\text{dose ordered (desired)}}{\text{dose on hand (have)}} \times \text{amount available (quantity)} = \text{amount to give}$$

Formula 2 (ratio and proportion)

$$\frac{\text{dose ordered}}{\text{dose on hand}} = \frac{\times}{\text{quantity available}}$$

Formula 3 (dimensional analysis)

Rule 1: Multiplying one side of an equation by a conversion factor will not change the value of the equation.

Rule 2: Set up the problem so that all labels cancel from the numerator and denominator except the label desired in the answer.

Calculating IV Drip Rates

$$\frac{\text{volume (of fluid)}}{\text{time (in minutes)}} \times \text{drop factor} = \text{flow rate}$$

Steps for Calculating Pediatric Medication Dosages

1. Convert the child's weight from pounds (lb) to kilograms (kg); 1kg = 2.2 lb.
2. Calculate the safe total daily dose in mg/kg or in mcg/kg for a child of this weight as recommended in a standard drug reference book (mg/kg recommended × weight in kg). Then calculate the amount of one dose (total daily dose divided by the number of doses/day).
3. Compare the ordered dose to the recommended dose and determine if the dose is safe.
4. If the dose is safe, calculate the amount of one dose using one of the medication dosage formulas shown. If unsafe, consult prescriber before administering.

Reducing the Risk of Medication Errors

- Question any medication order that is not written clearly, has an unusual dose, or is not in keeping with treatment for client's known health problems.
- Prepare medications in a quiet area away from noise and distractions.
- Check client drug allergies before giving medications; if there is no notation in the allergy section(s) of the medical record, STOP and be sure to obtain allergy history prior to administration. Verify order for a medication that is questionable based on allergy history before administration.
- Be knowledgeable about medications: various names, correct dosage ranges, method of administration, and side/adverse effects.
- Have another nurse check dosage of parenteral medications (such as heparin, digoxin, and insulin) that could pose immediate harm to client if given incorrectly.
- Be aware of drug-food and drug-drug interactions to reduce risk of either ineffective treatment or toxic effects. Sometimes interactions reduce drug's effectiveness and sometimes they heighten its effect.
- Identify client correctly by asking client to state his or her name; checking identification bracelet is the next best method if client is nonverbal. Be especially careful when there are two clients or more in room. Use two unique identifiers per agency policy. If medication bar coding technology is in use, scan medication per agency policy.
- If client questions a medication or states it is different than one taken at home, STOP and recheck medication order and client history. Verify order as necessary before proceeding to administer.
- Carefully and promptly document medication administration.
- Check results of ordered therapeutic drug levels as soon as they are expected to be available and report results promptly.
- Teach clients and significant others/family members about medications well in advance of discharge so they are prepared for safe self-administration following discharge.

Memory Aid for Drugs by Generic Name Prefix, Root, or Suffix*	Syllable in Generic Name	Interpretation	Examples by Generic Name
	-ase, -plase	Thrombolytic agent (-ase usually indicates enzyme)	alteplase, anistreplase, reteplase, streptokinase, tenecteplase
	-azole	Antifungal antimicrobial	itraconazole, fluconazole, clotrimazole, miconazole
	cef-, ceph-	Cephalosporin, antibiotic; check allergy to this class and penicillins	cefazolin, cephalexin, cefotetan, ceftazidime, ceftriazone
	-cillin	Penicillin, antibiotic; check allergy	amoxicillin, penicillin, piperacillin, ticarcillin, nafcillin, oxacillin
	-cycline	Tetracycline, antibiotic	doxycycline, minocycline, tetracycline
	-dipine	Calcium channel blocker, antianginal, antihypertensive	amlodipine, nicardipine, nifedipine, felodipine
	-dronate	Bisphosphonate, bone resorption inhibitor	alendronate, etidronate, pamidronate, risedronate
	-floxacin	Fluoroquinolone, antibiotic	ciprofloxacin, levofloxacin, norfloxacin, sparfloxacin
	-micin, -mycin	Aminoglycoside, antibiotic**	gentamicin, kanamycin, netilmicin, tobramycin
	nitr-, -nitr-	Nitrate, vasodilator, antianginal	nitroglycerin, isosorbide dinitrate
	-olol, -lol	Beta adrenergic blocker, antihypertensive and/or antianginal	propranolol, atenolol, metoprolol, nadolol, labetalol, timolol

Syllable in Generic Name	Interpretation	Examples by Generic Name
-parin	Anticoagulant, heparin or heparinoid	heparin, dalteparin, enoxaparin
-phylline	Xanthine type of bronchodilator	aminophylline, theophylline
-prazole	GI proton pump inhibitor, antiulcer	omeprazole, lansoprazole
-pril	Angiotensin converting enzyme (ACE) inhibitor, antihypertensive	captopril, enalapril, fosinopril, lisinopril, quinapril
sal-, -sal-	Contains salicylate; check allergy to salicylates or aspirin	salsalate (nonopioid analgesic), sulfasalazine (GI anti-inflammatory)
-sartan	Angiotensin II receptor antagonist, antihypertensive	candesartan, eprosartan, losartan, valsartan
-sone, -lone, pred-	Corticosteroid	prednisone, betamethasone, dexamethasone, cortisone, triamcinolone, prednisolone
-statin	HMG-Coenzyme A reductase inhibitor, lipid lowering agent	atorvastatin, fluvastatin, lovastatin, pravastatin, simvastatin
sulfa-	Sulfonamide, antibiotic; check allergy to sulfa	sulfacetamide, sulfamethoxazole
-terol	Adrenergic type of bronchodilator	albuterol, formoterol, levabuterol, pirbuterol, salmeterol
-tidine	Histamine H2 antagonist (GI), antiulcer	cimetidine, ranitidine, famotidine, nizatidine
-triptan	Vascular headache suppressant, serotonin (5-HT1) agonist	almotriptan, naratriptan, sumatriptan, zolmitriptan
-vir	Antiviral antiinfective	acyclovir, cidofovir, famciclovir, gangciclovir, valacyclovir
-zepam, -zolam	Benzodiazepine, antianxiety, sedative/hypnotic	diazepam, lorazepam, oxazepam, alprazolam, midazolam
-zosin	Peripherally acting anti-adrenergic, antihypertensive	doxazocin, prazosin, terazosin

* This is not an exhaustive list and may not be inclusive of every drug in each category.
** This category does not include erythromycin, azithromycin, or clarithromycin, all of which are a macrolide type of antibiotic.

PHYSIOLOGICAL INTEGRITY: REDUCTION OF RISK POTENTIAL

Reduction of Risk Potential makes up 9–15% of the questions on the NCLEX-RN® exam.

Key Testing Strategies

- Memorize common laboratory values and use them to answer questions about specific laboratory test results.
- Always ask if a female client of childbearing age is pregnant before she has x-rays taken.
- Remove all metal objects before a client has an x-ray.
- Ask routinely about allergies to contrast dyes or media before a client undergoes a diagnostic test using injectable contrast material.
- Recall that clients cannot wear or have imbedded metal (prostheses, for example) to be eligible for magnetic resonance imaging (MRI).

Key Assessments in the Immediate Post-surgical Period

- Adequacy of airway
- Adequacy of ventilation
- Cardiovascular status
- Level of consciousness
- Presence of protective reflexes (e.g., gag, cough)
- Activity, ability to move extremities
- Skin color (pink, pale, dusky, blotchy, cyanotic, jaundiced)
- Fluid status: intake and output, status of IV infusions (type of fluid, rate, amount in container, patency of tubing), signs of dehydration or fluid overload
- Condition of operative site, dressing and presence of drainage
- Patency of and character and amount of drainage from catheters, tubes, and drains
- Discomfort (i.e., pain) (type, location, and severity), nausea, vomiting
- Safety (e.g., necessity for side rails, call bell within reach)

Areas of Focus for Reduction of Risk Potential Questions		
Recognizing changes and abnormal trends in vital signs	Potential for complications of diagnostic tests, client treatments or procedures, client health alterations, or surgery	
Laboratory and diagnostic tests		
Potential for body system alterations	Assessments specific to one or more body systems	
Implementing therapeutic procedures		

Vital Signs by Age

Age	Heart Rate Range & (Avg) in bpm*		Respiratory Rate Range in rpm**		Median Blood Pressure (mm Hg)***	
Newborn (NB)–1 mo	NB	110–170 (120)		30–60	NB	73/55
	1 mo	90–130 (110)			1 mo	86/52
6 months–1 year		80–130 (110)	6 mo	24–36	6 mo	90/53
			1 yr	20–40	1 yr	90/56
2 years		70–120 (100)		20–40		90/56
3–5 years		70–120 (100)		20–30		92/55
6–9 years		70–110 (90)		16–22	6 yrs	96/57
					9 yrs	100/61
10–15 years		60–100 (85)		16–20	10 yrs	100/61
					12 yrs	107/64
					15 yrs	114/65
18 years		60–100 (85)		12–20		121/70

* Beats per minute.
** Respirations per minute; higher when awake; slower during sleep.
*** Blood pressure varies by gender as well as age.

Normal Arterial Blood Gas Values

Arterial Blood Gas Parameter	Normal Value
pH	7.35–7.45
PCO_2	35–45 mm Hg
HCO_3^-	22–26 mEq/L
PO_2	80–100 mm Hg

Adult Reference Range for Common Laboratory Tests	Coagulation Studies	Prothrombin time (PT): 10–13 seconds; 1.5–2.0 times the control in seconds for anticoagulant therapy; Activated partial thromboplastin time (APTT): 20–35 seconds (1.5–2.5 times the control in anticoagulant therapy); Partial thromboplastin time (PTT): 60–70 seconds; 1.5–2.5 times the control in anticoagulant therapy; International normalized ratio (INR): 2.0–3.0 for most anticoagulation needs
	Electrolytes	Sodium (Na^+): 135–145 mEq/L; Potassium (K^+): 3.5–5.1 mEq/L Chloride (Cl^-): 95–105 mEq/L CO_2 combining power: 22–30 mEq/L; 22–30 mmol/L Calcium, total (Ca^{++}): 4.5–5.5 mEq/L, 9–11 mg/dL, 2.3–2.8 mmol/L Calcium (ionized): 4.25–5.25 mg/dL, 2.2–2.5 mEq/L, 1.1–1.24 mmol/L Magnesium (Mg^{++}): 1.5–2.5 mEq/L, 1.8–3.0 mg/dL
	Glucose	Fasting (FBS): 70–110 mg/dL (serum, plasma); 60–100 mg/dL (whole blood); 70–120 mg/dL (elderly); panic values: < 40 or > 700 mg/dL Fingerstick glucose (self-monitoring device): 60–100 mg/dL
	Hematology	White blood cells (WBC): 5000–10,000 microliter or 4500–11,500/mm^3 Neutrophils: 1935–7942 (absolute count) or 45–75% Red blood cells (RBC): 4.5–5.3 million or (10^6)/mm^3 (men), 4.1–5.1 million or (10^6)/mm^3 (women) Hemoglobin (Hgb): 13.0–18.0 grams/100 mL (men), 12–16 grams/100 mL (women) Hematocrit (Hct): 37–49 % (men), 36–46 % (women) Platelet count: 150,000–400,000/mm^3 (or microliter)
	Renal Function Studies	Blood urea nitrogen (BUN): 5–25 mg/dL Serum creatinine: 0.5–1.5 mg/dL
	Therapeutic Drug Levels	Digoxin: 0.5–2.0 ng/mL; Phenytoin: 10–20 mcg/mL Theophylline derivatives: 10–20 mcg/mL or 10–20 mg/mL

PHYSIOLOGICAL INTEGRITY: PHYSIOLOGICAL ADAPTATION

Physiological Adaptation makes up 11–17% of the questions on the NCLEX-RN® exam.

Key Testing Strategies

- Think about the underlying pathophysiology when selecting interventions to assist a client with a health problem affecting a particular body system.
- Remember when a client's status is deteriorating rapidly, follow the ABCs—airway, breathing, and circulation.
- When evaluating the condition of a client with a particular health problem, use knowledge of normal findings or the client's usual baselines as a gauge as to the effectiveness of care.

Areas of Focus for Physiological Adaptation Questions	Body system alterations and pathophysiology	Responding to medical emergencies
	Management of illness	Assessment and treatment of fluid and electrolyte imbalances
	Recognizing and providing care during unexpected response to therapies	Client hemodynamics

Symptom Analysis	**O** When was the onset of symptom and what was the client doing? **P** What was the provoking incident (aggravating factor[s]) that caused the symptom, if any? Any palliating factors? **Q** What is the quality of the symptom? Is it burning, throbbing, aching, stabbing, other? **R** Where is the region of symptom? Does it radiate? Does anything relieve the symptom? **S** How severe is the symptom? (intensity, quantity) **T** What is the timing of the symptom? When does it occur; how long does it last? (pattern, duration)

Glasgow Coma Scoring System

Type of Response Tested	Score	Indicator
Physical (Motor) Response	6	Acts out a simple command
	5	Reacts to a localized discomfort and offensive stimulus
	4	Moves purposelessly or flexes in response to pain
	3	Exhibits abnormal flexion (decorticate posture)
	2	Exhibits abnormal extension (decerebrate posture)
	1	Has no motor response
Verbal Response	5	Has full orientation (time, place, person)
	4	Shows confusion and disorientation
	3	Uses disorganized or inappropriate words; cannot sustain a conversation
	2	Uses sounds instead of words
	1	Makes no verbal response
Eye Response	4	Open when a person approaches (spontaneous response)
	3	Open when a person speaks
	2	Open only when in pain
	1	Open never, even in presence of painful stimuli

Note: Add numbers to find score from 3 (profound coma) to 15 (normal conscious state).

Neurovascular Status: Checking the "6 Ps"	**Pain:** is there pain or discomfort in the extremity? **Pallor:** is the skin color paler than normal or baseline? **Polar:** is the skin cooler to the touch than normal or baseline in the area? **Paresthesia:** are there any unusual sensations, such as numbness or tingling? **Paralysis:** is the extremity without movement or weaker than normal or baseline? **Pulse:** is the affected pulse (or pulses) diminished or absent?

Nursing Care of the Client in a Cast

- Casts made from plaster of Paris should not get wet and cast padding should not be removed; if cast becomes soiled, clean with a damp cloth. Casts made of synthetic material dry more quickly and allow mobility in less than an hour.
- Smooth rough edges to prevent skin injury; explain that no foreign objects should be inserted into the cast (sticks, food crumbs, etc.) to prevent skin breakdown.
- Avoid covering a new plaster cast with blanket or plastic for extended periods (air cannot circulate, and heat builds up in cast).
- Turn client from side to side (using palms, not fingertips) every 2 hours to facilitate drying for the first 24 to 72 hours.
- Apply ice (crushed or small cubes to avoid denting cast) for the first 24 hours over fracture site to control edema, ensuring that ice is securely contained to avoid wetting cast.
- Elevate extremity above the level of the heart to promote venous return for the first 24 hours after application.
- Encourage active range of motion (AROM) to joints above and below immobilized extremity.
- Report to healthcare provider: increasing pain in immobilized extremity, excessive swelling and discoloration of exposed limb, burning or tingling under cast, sores, or foul odor under cast.

Rule of Nines for Calculating Burn Injury

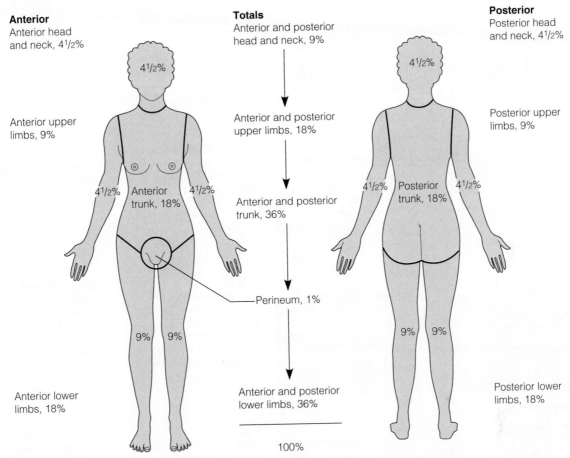

Anterior
Anterior head and neck, 4 1/2%

Anterior upper limbs, 9%

Anterior trunk, 18%

Anterior lower limbs, 18%

Totals
Anterior and posterior head and neck, 9%

Anterior and posterior upper limbs, 18%

Anterior and posterior trunk, 36%

Perineum, 1%

Anterior and posterior lower limbs, 36%

100%

Posterior
Posterior head and neck, 4 1/2%

Posterior upper limbs, 9%

Posterior trunk, 18%

Posterior lower limbs, 18%

Clinical Manifestations of Chronic Renal Failure

Body System	Clinical Manifestations	Cause of Manifestations
Cardiovascular	Hypervolemia, hypertension, tachycardia, arrhythmias, congestive heart failure, pericarditis	Increased fluid volume, build-up of metabolic wastes, chronic hypertension, change in renin-angiotension mechanism
Hematologic	Anemia, leukocytosis, decreased platelet function, thrombocytopenia	Decreased production of erythropoietin and RBCs, decreased survival of RBCs, decreased platelet activity; blood loss through dialysis and bleeding
Gastrointestinal	Anorexia, nausea, vomiting, abdominal distention, diarrhea, constipation, bleeding	Build-up of uremic toxins, electrolyte imbalances, changes in platelet activity, conversion of urea to ammonia by saliva
Neurologic	Lethargy, confusion, convulsions, stupor, coma, sleep disturbances, behavioral changes, muscle irritability	Uremic toxins, electrolyte imbalances, cerebral swelling caused by fluid shifts
Dermatologic	Pallor, pigmentation, pruritus, ecchymosis, excoriation, uremic frost	Anemia, decreased activity of sweat glands, dry skin, phosphate deposits on skin
Urinary	Decreased urine output, decreased specific gravity, proteinuria, casts and cells in the urine	Damage to the nephron
Skeletal	Osteoporosis, renal rickets, joint pain	Decreased calcium absorption, decreased phosphate excretion

Priority Cardiac Dysrhythmias

Rhythm/ECG Appearance
Supraventricular Rhythms

	ECG Characteristics	Management

Sinus tachycardia

ECG Characteristics
Rate: 101 to 150 bpm
Rhythm: regular
P:QRS ratio is 1:1 (with very fast rates, P wave may be hidden in preceding T wave)
PR interval: 0.12–0.20 sec
QRS complex: 0.06–0.10 sec

Management
Treat only if client is experiencing symptoms or is at risk for myocardial damage; treat underlying cause (e.g., hypovolemia, fever, pain); beta blockers or verapamil may be used

Sinus bradycardia

ECG Characteristics
Rate: less than 60 bpm
Rhythm: regular
P:QRS ratio is 1:1
PR interval: 0.12–0.20 sec
QRS complex: 0.06–0.10 sec

Management
Treat only if client is experiencing symptoms; intravenous atropine and/or pacemaker therapy may be used

Atrial fibrillation

ECG Characteristics
Rate: atrial 300–600 bpm (too rapid to count); ventricular 100–180 bpm in untreated clients
Rhythm: irregularly irregular
P:QRS ratio is variable
PR interval: not measured
QRS complex: 0.06–0.10 sec

Management
Synchronized cardioversion; medications to reduce ventricular response rate: verapamil, propranolol, digoxin, anticoagulant therapy to reduce risk of clot formation and stroke

Ventricular Rhythms

Premature ventricular contractions (PVC)

ECG Characteristics
Rate: variable
Rhythm: irregular, with PVC interrupting underlying rhythm and followed by a compensatory pause
P:QRS ratio: no P wave noted before PVC
PR interval: absent with PVC
QRS complex: wide (greater 0.12 sec), bizarre in appearance; differs from normal QRS complex

Management
Treat if client is experiencing symptoms; advise against stimulant use (caffeine, nicotine); drug therapy includes intravenous lidocaine, procainamide, quinidine, propranolol, phenytoin, amiodarone

Ventricular tachycardia (VT or V tach)

ECG Characteristics
Rate: 100–250 bpm
Rhythm: regular
P:QRS ratio: P waves usually not identifiable
PR interval: not measured
QRS complex: 0.12 sec or greater; bizarre shape

Management
Treat if VT is sustained or if client is experiencing symptoms; treatment includes intravenous procainamide or lidocaine and/or immediate defibrillation if the client is unconscious or unstable

Ventricular fibrillation (VF or V fib)

ECG Characteristics
Rate: too rapid to count
Rhythm: grossly irregular
P:QRS ratio: no identifiable P waves
PR interval: none
QRS: bizarre, varying in shape and direction

Management
Immediate defibrillation

Index